Kinesiology: The Mechanics of Body Movement

Kinesiology: The Mechanics of Body Movement

Edited by Randall Calloway

hayle medical

New York

Hayle Medical,
750 Third Avenue, 9th Floor,
New York, NY 10017, USA

Visit us on the World Wide Web at:
www.haylemedical.com

ISBN: 978-1-63241-449-6

The publisher's policy is to use permanent paper from mills that operate a sustainable forestry policy. Furthermore, the publisher ensures that the text paper and cover boards used have met acceptable environmental accreditation standards.

Printed in China.

Cataloging-in-Publication Data

Kinesiology : the mechanics of body movement / edited by Randall Calloway.
p. cm.
Includes bibliographical references and index.
ISBN 978-1-63241-449-6
1. Kinesiology. 2. Human mechanics. 3. Human locomotion. 4. Movement education.
I. Calloway, Randall.

QP303 .K56 2017
612.76--dc23

Table of Contents

Preface

Kinesiology is an upcoming field of science associated with the study of body movement. It has undergone rapid development over the past few decades. This book on kinesiology deals with the application of kinesiology in physical therapy and physical movement. The study of human kinetics can help design and execute improved exercise and physiotherapy routines. Health education, athletic training and disability management are some of the fields that are aided by this field. The topics covered in this book offer the readers new insights in the field of kinesiology. This book, with its detailed analyses and data, will prove immensely beneficial to professionals and students involved in this area at various levels.

This book unites the global concepts and researches in an organized manner for a comprehensive understanding of the subject. It is a ripe text for all researchers, students, scientists or anyone else who is interested in acquiring a better knowledge of this dynamic field.

I extend my sincere thanks to the contributors for such eloquent research chapters. Finally, I thank my family for being a source of support and help.

Editor

SMAD3 Is Associated with the Total Burden of Radiographic Osteoarthritis

Erfan Aref-Eshghi[1], Yuhua Zhang[1], Deborah Hart[2], Ana M. Valdes[2], Andrew Furey[1], Glynn Martin[1], Guang Sun[1], Proton Rahman[1], Nigel Arden[3], Tim D. Spector[2], Guangju Zhai[1,2]*

1 Faculty of Medicine, Memorial University of Newfoundland, St. John's, Newfoundland, Canada, **2** Department of Twin Research & Genetic Epidemiology, King's College London, London, United Kingdom, **3** Musculoskeletal Epidemiology and Biobank, University of Oxford, Oxford, United Kingdom

Abstract

Background: A newly-described syndrome called Aneurysm-Osteoarthritis Syndrome (AOS) was recently reported. AOS presents with early onset osteoarthritis (OA) in multiple joints, together with aneurysms in major arteries, and is caused by rare mutations in *SMAD3*. Because of the similarity of AOS to idiopathic generalized OA (GOA), we hypothesized that *SMAD3* is also associated with GOA and tested the hypothesis in a population-based cohort.

Methods: Study participants were derived from the Chingford study. Kellgren-Lawrence (KL) grades and the individual features of osteophytes and joint space narrowing (JSN) were scored from radiographs of hands, knees, hips, and lumbar spines. The total KL score, osteophyte score, and JSN score were calculated and used as indicators of the total burden of radiographic OA. Forty-one common SNPs within *SMAD3* were genotyped using the Illumina HumanHap610Q array. Linear regression modelling was used to test the association between the total KL score, osteophyte score, and JSN score and each of the 41 SNPs, with adjustment for patient age and BMI. Permutation testing was used to control the false positive rate.

Results: A total of 609 individuals were included in the analysis. All were Caucasian females with a mean age of 60.9±5.8. We found that rs3825977, with a minor allele (T) frequency of 20%, in the last intron of *SMAD3*, was significantly associated with total KL score ($\beta = 0.14$, $P_{permutation} = 0.002$). This association was stronger for the total JSN score ($\beta = 0.19$, $P_{permutation} = 0.002$) than for total osteophyte score ($\beta = 0.11$, $P_{permutation} = 0.02$). The T allele is associated with a 1.47-fold increased odds for people with 5 or more joints to be affected by radiographic OA ($P_{permutation} = 0.046$).

Conclusion: We found that *SMAD3* is significantly associated with the total burden of radiographic OA. Further studies are required to reveal the mechanism of the association.

Editor: Masaru Katoh, National Cancer Center, Japan

Funding: The study was supported financially by Newfoundland and Labrador RDC Ignite program, and Memorial University of Newfoundland. EAE was supported by The Dean's Fellowship of Faculty of Medicine, Memorial University of Newfoundland. The Chingford Study was supported by Welcome Trust and Arthritis Research UK. The funders had no role in study design, data collection and analysis, decision to publish, or preparation of the manuscript.

Competing Interests: The authors have declared that no competing interests exist.

* E-mail: guangju.zhai@med.mun.ca

Introduction

Osteoarthritis (OA) is the most common form of arthritis in the elderly, characterized pathologically by focal areas of damage to the articular cartilage centered on load-bearing areas. It is associated with new bone formation at the joint margins (osteophytosis), changes in the subchondral bone, variable degrees of mild synovitis, and thickening of the joint capsule [1] which lead to the presentation of pain, stiffness and disability. Its prevalence—already high—is increasing due to population aging and the increase in obesity. Eighty percent of individuals over 75 years of age have radiographic OA changes in at least one of their joints [2]. According to a report from the Arthritis Community Research & Evaluation Unit in April 2010, the prevalence of self-reported and physician-diagnosed OA in individuals over age 45 ranged from 2.3%–11% in the third world to 8%–16% in the USA [3]. In the same year it affected 27 million people in the USA, imposing a burden of over 11 million dollars on outpatient visits and over 13 billion dollars on OA-related job absence [4]. Half of all adults will develop symptomatic OA of the knee at some points in their lives [5].

OA is a multifactorial disease whose etiology is incompletely understood. It is believed that a number of different environmental and genetic factors interact in its initiation and progression [6]. Evidence suggests that genetic factors play a major role in OA, although they may be site- and sex-specific. From twin studies, this genetic influence has been estimated to be between 40% and 65% on hand and knee OA [7]. First-degree relatives of individuals with spine, hand, hip, or polyarticular OA have a two- to three-fold increased risk of the disease [8,9]. The nature of the genetic influence in OA is still unclear but it is likely to involve a combination of effects on structure (i.e. collagen), alterations in cartilage, bone metabolism and inflammation [10]. Although the genetic influence on OA was recognized more than 130 years ago [11], genetic variants identified so far account only for a small fraction of its heritability [12]. This may reflect several factors including the heterogeneous nature of the disease, the tendency to use less severe phenotypes in genetic searches and the reliance on underpowered studies [13]. Generalized OA—a subtype of primary OA—is characterized by the involvement of multiple joints, and is believed to have a stronger genetic component than individual joint OA [14]. However, genetic data on generalized OA are limited.

Recently, a new syndrome called Aneurysm-Osteoarthritis Syndrome (AOS) was reported [15]. Patients with AOS present with early-onset OA affecting multiple joints including feet/ankle, hand/wrist, knee, hip, facet joints, uncovertebral joints and also exhibit degeneration of the intervertebral discs [15,16]. Eight rare mutations in the *SMAD3* gene (Similar to Mothers Against Decapentaplegic type 3) were identified as responsible for AOS in eight unrelated families.[15, 16] Subsequent studies reported additional *SMAD3* mutations [17,18] and also a CNV (copy number variant) [19] linked to AOS. The *SMAD3* gene encodes a protein that belongs to the SMAD protein family, that are downstream mediators of the transforming growth factor beta (*TGF-β*) signaling pathway [20], which inhibits terminal hypertrophic differentiation of chondrocytes and is essential for maintaining the integrity of articular cartilage [20,21]. This regulatory pathway also stimulates osteogenesis and bone formation [22]. *SMAD3* knock-out mice develop degenerative joint disease similar to human OA [23]. Although a few studies on *SMAD3* and single-joint OA have been reported, no data are available regarding the role *SMAD3* plays in generalized OA. Because of the similarity with AOS, in which multiple joints are also affected, we hypothesized that the *SMAD3* gene plays a role in idiopathic generalized OA. We tested our hypothesis in a large population-based cohort of individuals who had radiographic assessment of multiple joints.

Methods and Subjects

Subjects

The study subjects were women aged 43-67 years at baseline (1988–1989) who were participating in the Chingford Study, a prospective population-based study of OA and osteoporosis. The Chingford Study cohort comprises 1003 women derived from the register of a large general practice in North London, who are similar to the UK population for most demographic variables [24].

Height, weight and details of concomitant diseases, operations and medications were recorded for all subjects. DNA was extracted from blood by standard phenol or salting-out methods. At both baseline and 10 years later, all subjects completed a standardized medical history questionnaire.

Ethics

The Guys & St Thomas' Trust and the Waltham Forest Trust ethics committees approved the study protocol. Written consent was obtained from all participants.

Radiography

Plain films of all joints were obtained from a standard postero-anterior view at baseline and again 9–11 years later. The distal interphalangeal (DIP), proximal interphalangeal (PIP) and first carpometacarpal (CMC) joints of the thumbs, the knee- and hip-joints, as well as four lumbar spinal joints (L1–L5) were assessed for radiographic OA according to the Kellgren & Lawrence (KL) score using a 0–4 scale [25]. Joint Space Narrowing (JSN) and osteophyte characteristics were each scored on a 0–3 scale using a standard atlas [26]. All radiographs were independently assessed by two trained observers (DJ Hunter and DJ Hart). In cases of disagreement, a third adjudicator was used. The intra- and inter-observer reproducibility of the scoring measured on a subgroup of 50 hands had a Kappa statistic of approximately 0.68 for all sites and features.

For the current study, the most recent radiographic and demographic data were used, including cross sectional radiographic data for hip, spine, knee and hand from years 8, 9, 10, and 11 and the age and body mass index (BMI) from the 8th year of the study. All patients were visited at year 8, when the demographic information was collected. Due to the schedule of the radiology department, different joints were assessed in different years (between year 8 and year 11). Total KL score, osteophyte and JSN scores were used as indicators of the total burden of radiographic OA, which was calculated by summing up the individual scores of each joint. Total radiographic scores have been used by researchers in clinical, biomedical, and genetic studies of OA [14,27–29] as an indicator for total burden of OA. In addition, individuals were evaluated for the criteria required for a diagnosis of generalized OA. To this end, joints were defined as being affected by OA if the KL score was ≥2. OA of either the DIP or PIP joint groups was defined as the presence of OA in at least two of the relevant joints. A diagnosis of GOA was based on the definition used by Cooper et al [30]. Fourteen joints or joint groups were considered: the four lumbar joints together with the left and right knee, hip, DIP group, PIP group and thumb CMCs. GOA was defined as the presence of OA in at least five of these 14 joints. Those with fewer than five joints affected were designated as controls.

Genotyping

The samples were genotyped using the Illumina HumanHap610Q array. The normalized intensity data was used by the Illluminus calling algorithm [31] to assign genotypes. No calls were assigned if an individual's most likely genotype was called with a posterior probability threshold of less than 0.95. Sample exclusion criteria were: (i) sample call rate <98%, (ii) heterozygosity across all SNPs ≥2 s.d. from the sample mean; (iii) evidence of non-European ancestry as assessed by PCA comparison with HapMap3 populations; (iv) observed pair-wise IBD probabilities suggestive of sample identity errors; (v). SNP exclusion criteria included (i) Hardy-Weinberg p-value$<10^{-6}$, assessed in a set of unrelated samples; (ii) MAF<1%, assessed in a set of unrelated samples; (iii) SNP call rate <97% (SNPs with MAF≥5%) or < 99% (for 1%≤MAF<5%). For the current study, we retrieved genotype data for all 41 SNPs within the *SMAD3* gene which were available on the array.

Statistics

Since the distribution of the total KL, JSN, and osteophyte scores was skewed, a logarithmic transformation was performed to approximate a normal distribution. Subsequent analyses were performed on the log-transformed values. A linear regression model, testing for an additive genetic model, was used to test the association between each of the 41 candidate SNPs and the total KL, JSN, and osteophyte scores individually. A logistic regression model was used to test the association between each of the 41 SNPs and GOA. Potential confounders such as age and BMI were considered in both models. All SNP associations with $p<0.05$ in the initial analyses were subject to permutation testing in order to control the false positive rate. The permutation method is well established as a robust approach for obtaining empirical significance levels while minimizing Type I errors [32,33], and has been used to correct for multiple testing in genetic association studies [34]. Because of the infinite permutation with our sample size, we used a Monte Carlo permutation procedure and the phenotype labels were reshuffled 10,000 times. The permutation-based p-value was calculated as the proportion of the statistic on all the reshuffled data sets greater than the observed statistic [34]. The significance level was defined as a permutation-based p-value of less than 0.05. All analyses were conducted using STATA/SE 11.2 (Stata Corp, College Station, Texas, USA).

Results

All study subjects were Caucasian females. Radiographic data for spine, hips, knees and hand joints were available for 796, 794, 614, and 687 individuals, respectively. The age and BMI data were available for 843 participants with a mean age of 61.2±5.8 and a mean BMI of 26.7±4.7. Total KL, osteophyte and JSN scores were available for 609, 603, and 607 individuals respectively. As expected, patients with GOA—defined as having 5 or more joints affected—were, on average, older than those with fewer than 5 affected joints, and also had a higher BMI (Table 1). The frequency of subjects with different number of affected joints is presented in Table 2.

Forty-one common SNPs within the *SMAD3* gene were genotyped and passed quality control. They were scattered randomly throughout the *SMAD3* gene, but none were located in exons (Figure 1). The average pairwise R^2 between SNPs was 0.07.

We found that SNP rs3825977 was significantly associated with all phenotypes analyzed, *viz.* total KL, osteophyte and JSN scores. The differences in these traits among individuals with different genotypes are presented in Figures 2, 3, 4. After adjustment for age and BMI, the minor (T) allele of rs3825977—with 20% allele frequency—was associated with a 0.14% increase in log total KL score (95% CI 0.04–0.20, $P_{permutation} = 0.002$). The association is stronger for log total JSN score with $\beta = 0.19$ (95%CI 0.07–0.31, $P_{permutation} = 0.002$) than for log total osteophyte score with $\beta = 0.11$ (95%CI 0.01–0.20, $P_{permutation} = 0.02$). Two other SNPs—rs6494629 and rs2118612—were significant for only total osteophyte score in the univariate analysis but not in a multivariate analysis. All the results of univariate and multivariate linear regression analyses for total KL, osteophyte and JSN scores for all 41 SNPs are presented in Tables S1–S3 in File S1, respectively.

Furthermore, we categorized the study participants into two groups: one with ≥5 joints affected (GOA) and one with <5 joints affected and examined the association of each group with each of the 41 SNPs. We found that the T allele of rs3825977 was significantly associated with a 1.47-fold increased risk of GOA (95% CI 1.02–2.1, $P_{permutation} = 0.046$) after adjustment for age and BMI (Table 3). All results of the associations with each of the 41 SNPs are presented in Table S4 in File S1.

Table 2. Frequency of patients with different number of joints affected.

Number of Joints affected	Frequency (%)
0	43 (7.06%)
1	62 (10.18%)
2	83 (13.63%)
3	93 (15.27%)
4	80 (13.14%)
5	51 (8.37%)
6	64 (10.51%)
7	38 (6.24%)
8	36 (5.91%)
9	22 (3.61%)
10	15 (2.46%)
11	12 (1.97%)
12	9 (1.48%)
13	1 (0.16%)
Total	609 (100%)

Discussion

In the present study we demonstrate a significant association of SNP rs3825977—located in the last intron of *SMAD3*—with the total burden of radiographic OA. This SNP is more strongly associated with total JSN score than with total KL score or osteophyte score, suggesting that the potential mechanism for the association is more likely through cartilage loss rather than osteophyte formation. The same SNP has previously been reported as associated with increased breast cancer risk for *BRCA2* mutation carriers [35]. Although the possible effect of the SNP on *SMAD3* function is still unclear, it is believed that the effects on both breast cancer and generalized OA susceptibility are mediated through the *TGF-β* signaling pathway.

Data on the associations between the *SMAD3* gene and GOA are limited and, to our knowledge, no genetic or genome-wide association study has been performed on GOA. A study by Yao JY, *et al.* [36] was the first to report a connection between *SMAD3* and OA. This paper described a missense mutation located in the linker region of the SMAD3 protein which resulted in an increased expression of matrix metalloproteinase (MMP) 2 and 9 in the serum of one OA mutation carrier compared to MMP expression in other OA patients and in controls. Another study by A. Valdes and colleagues [37] reported the association of a variant in the *SMAD3* gene with hip and knee OA. In that study the frequency of the major (G) allele of rs12901499—located in the first intron of *SMAD3*—was increased in patients undergoing hip or knee

Table 1. Descriptive statistics of the study population.

	GOA (n = 247)	Controls (n = 360)	P-Value
Age	64.21±0.34	58.71±0.3	P<0.0001
BMI	27.50±0.26	26.02±0.2	P<0.0001

Figures are mean ± SD, and Student's T-test was used for the comparison.

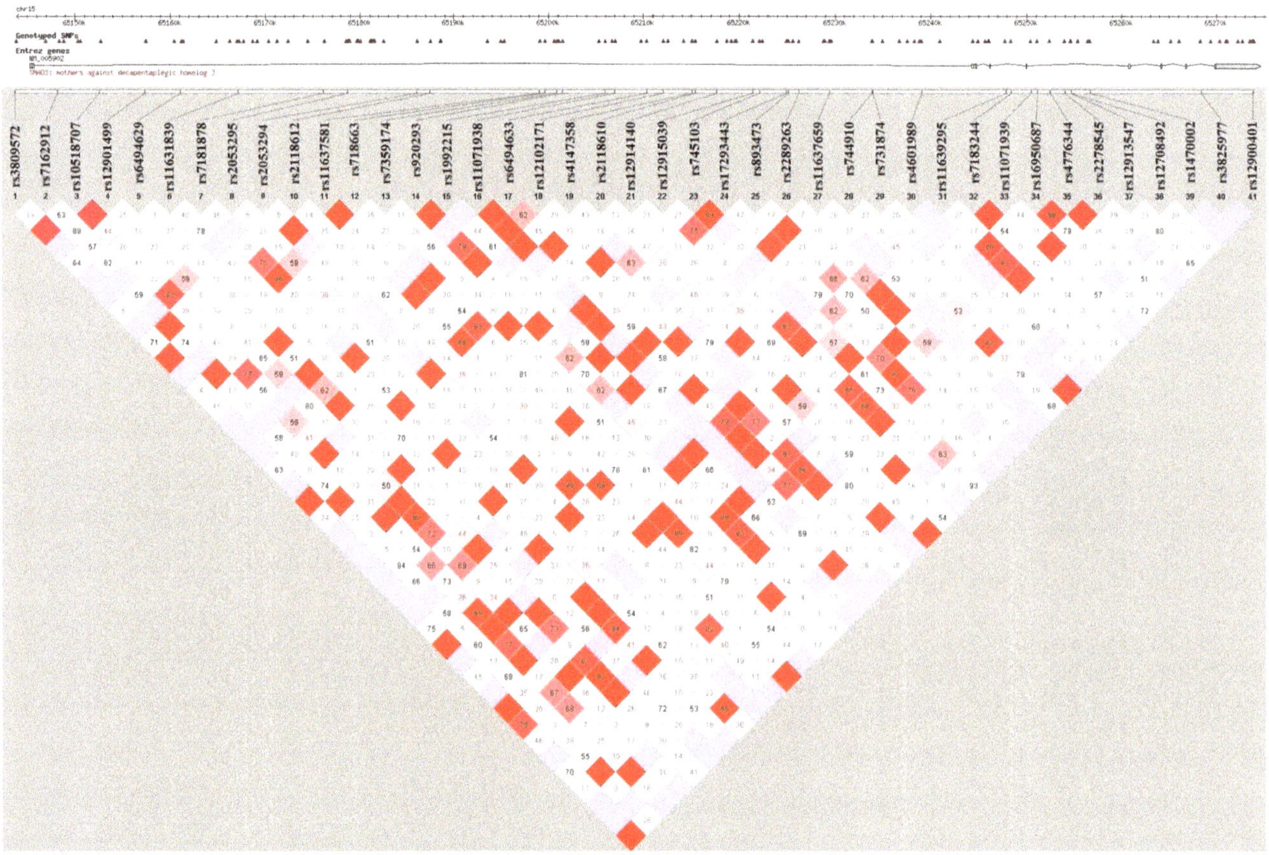

Figure 1. Distribution and LD pattern of 41 genotyped SNPs in SMAD3 gene.

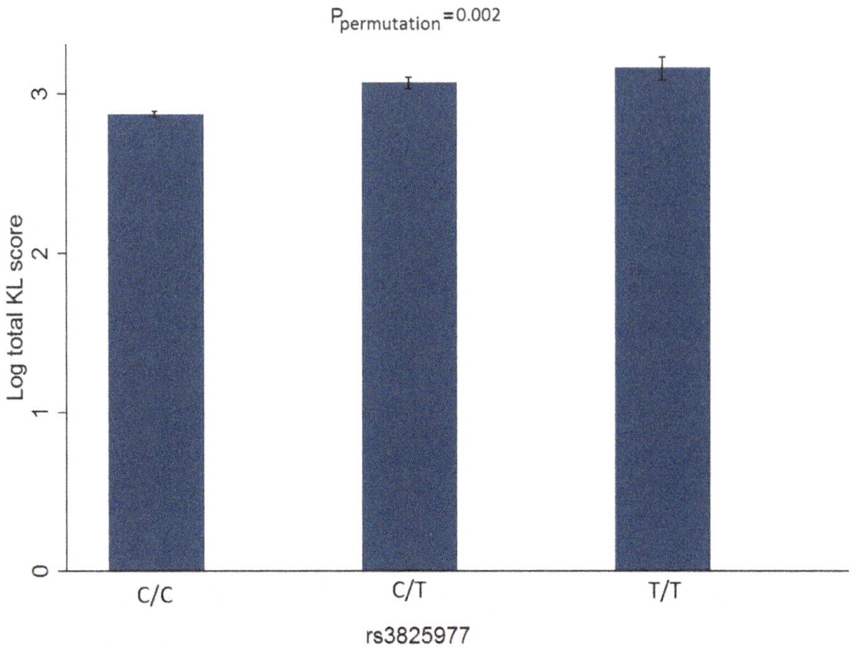

Figure 2. Total KL and each genotype of rs3825977. Error bars indicate Standard Error of the mean.

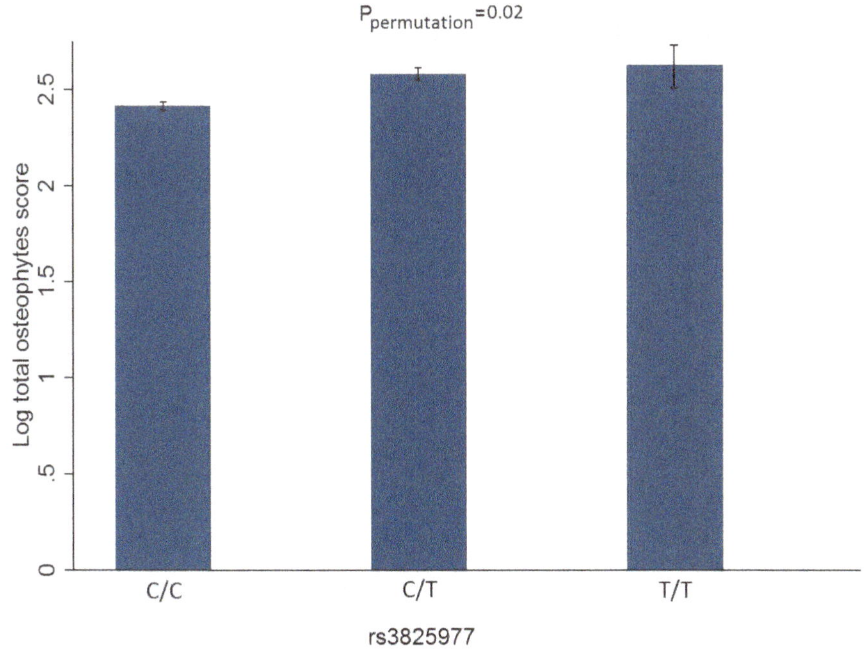

Figure 3. Total osteophyte and each genotype of rs3825977. Error bars indicate Standard Error of the mean.

replacement as compared to controls. A recent study by Jiang Liying *et al.* [38] found this SNP was also associated with hand and knee OA in a northeast Chinese population. However, we did not observe a significant association with rs12901499, which is not in LD with rs3825977 ($R^2 = 0.01$). This may have resulted from the different methods used for the definition and classification of OA in our study and the previous studies which used either end-stage OA (requiring total joint replacement) or symptomatic OA, neither of which is necessarily concordant with radiographic OA [39]. Alternatively, one or both of these SNPs may be non-functional but rather in LD with causal variants in the gene that were not typed in these studies.

Cartilage homeostasis depends on a balance between the catabolic and anabolic activities of chondrocytes being controlled

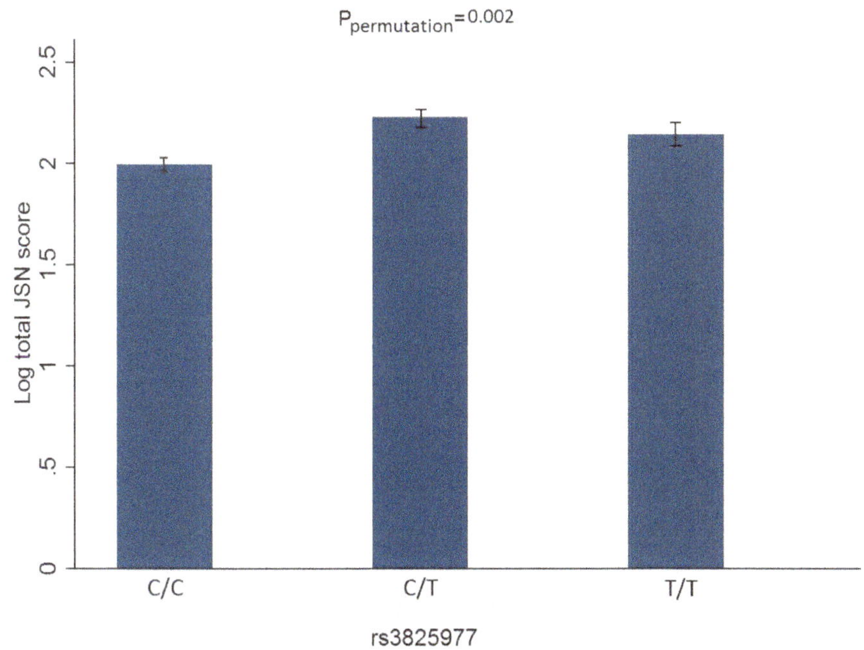

Figure 4. Total JSN and each genotype of rs3825977. Error bars indicate Standard Error of the mean.

Table 3. Association between GOA and rs3825977*.

Variables	Multivariable Analysis OR (95% CI)	P-value	$P_{permutation}$	MAF Cases	MAF Controls
rs3825977 (T vs. C allele)	1.47 (1.02–2.1)	0.037	0.046	0.23	0.17
Age (per year)	1.2 (1.16–1.25)	<0.0001	-	-	-
BMI (per kg/m²)	1.09 (1.04–1.15)	<0.0001	-	-	-

*Logistic regression was used. MAF: Minor allele frequency, OR: Odds Ratio, CI: Confidence interval.

by numerous cytokines and growth factors. *TGF-β* is an important molecule that plays a critical role in the development, growth, maintenance and repair of articular cartilage by modifying the metabolism of the chondrocyte. Deregulation of *TGF-β* signaling and responses have been shown to be involved in OA [20]. The SMAD family proteins, including SMAD3, are important intracellular signals in the *TGF-β* pathway [21]. Another possible mechanism by which SMAD3 acts to maintain cartilage homeostasis is by inducing the expression of type II collagen and repressing *MMP-13*. A recent study by Chen and colleagues [40] showed that *SMAD3* $^{(fl/fl)}$ mice were severely deficient in both type II collagen and aggrecan due to the proteolytic activity of *MMP-13*, which is normally down-regulated by *TGF-β* signals mediated through *SMAD3*.

There are some limitations in the study. All the participants were female, which limits the generalizability. Given its unknown function, it is not clear whether the associated SNP is causal.

Conclusions

We demonstrated that the *SMAD3* gene is associated with the total burden of radiographic OA. As a marker, it has a potential in identifying those with increased risk of OA, thus permitting earlier joint-preserving intervention. It also has potential as a molecular target for developing new OA drugs.

Supporting Information

File S1 Contains the files: Table S1 Univariate and multivariate linear regression for total KL score and each SNP. **Table S2** Univariate and multivariate linear regression for total osteophytes score and each SNP. **Table S3** Univariate and multivariate linear regression for total JSN score and each SNP. **Table S4** Univariate and multivariate logistic regression for GOA and each SNP.

Acknowledgments

We thank all the study participants who made this study possible. Thanks also go to all the staff in the Chingford Study who helped data collection and managing the database. We thank Dr. Roger Green for proofreading the manuscript.

Author Contributions

Conceived and designed the experiments: GZ EAE. Performed the experiments: DH AMV NA TDS. Analyzed the data: EAE GZ YZ. Contributed reagents/materials/analysis tools: GZ EAE AF GM GS PR. Wrote the paper: EAE GZ. Revision: YZ DH AMV AF GM GS PR NA TDS GZ.

References

1. Paitzker K (2003) Pathology of osteoarthritis. In: Osteoarthritis. Edited by K Brandt, M Doherty, L.S. Lohmander, 2nd edn. Oxford: Oxford University Press 49–58.
2. Arden N, Nevitt MC (2006) Osteoarthritis: Epidemiology. Best Practice & Research Clinical Rheumatology Vol. 20, No. 1, pp. 3–25.
3. Arthritis community research & evaluation unit, Toronto Western Research Institute (2010) Prevalence of Arthritis and Rheumatic Diseases around the World, A Growing Burden and Implications for Health Care Needs. Available from: http://www.modelsofcare.ca/pdf/10-02.pdf (last accessed 27 April 2014)
4. Center for disease control and prevention (2010) National Public Health Agenda for Osteoarthritis. Available from: http://www.cdc.gov/arthritis/docs/OAagenda.pdf (last accessed 27 April 2014)
5. Murphy L, Schwartz TA, Helmick CG, Renner JB, Tudor G, et al (2008) Lifetime risk of symptomatic knee osteoarthritis. Arthritis & Rheumatism 59(9):1207–1213
6. Felson DT (2004) An update on the pathogenesis and epidemiology of osteoarthritis. Radiol Clin North Am 42(1):1–9.
7. Tim D Spector, Cicuttini F, Baker J, Loughlin J, Hart D (1996) Genetic influences on osteoarthritis in women: a twin study. BMJ 312: 940–4.
8. Hirsch R, Lethbridge-Cejku M, Hanson R, Scott WW, Reichle R, et al (1998) Familial aggregation of osteoarthritis: data from the Baltimore Longitudinal Study on Aging. Arthritis Rheum 41(7):1227–1232.
9. Riyazi N, Meulenbelt I, Kroon HM, Ronday KH, Le Graverand MH, et al (2005) Evidence for familial aggregation of hand, hip, and spine but not knee osteoarthritis in siblings with multiple joint involvement: the GARP study. Ann Rheum Dis 64(3):438–443.
10. Valdes AM, Spector TD (2011) Genetic epidemiology of hip and knee osteoarthritis. Nat Rev Rheumatol 7(1):23–32.
11. Charcot J (1881) The New Sydenham Society; Clinical lectures on senile and chronic diseases. London 1881.
12. Meulenbelt I (2012) Osteoarthritis year 2011 in review: genetics. Osteoarthritis and Cartilage 20: 218–222.
13. Loughlin J (2011) Genetics of osteoarthritis. Current Opinion in Rheumatology 23(4):479–483.
14. Bijkerk C, Houwing-Duistermaat JJ, Valkenburg HA, Meulenbelt I, Hofman A, et al (1999) Heritabilities of radiologic osteoarthritis in peripheral joints and of disc degeneration of the spine. Arthritis Rheum. 1999 Aug;42(8):1729–35.
15. Van de Laar IM, Oldenburg RA, Pals G, Roos-Hesselink JW, De Graaf BM, et al (2011) Mutations in SMAD3 cause a syndromic form of aortic aneurysms and dissections with early-onset osteoarthritis. Nature Genetics 43: 121e6.
16. Van de Laar IM, Van der Linde D, Oei EH, Bos PK, Bessems JH et al. (2012) Phenotypic spectrum of the SMAD3-related aneurysmseosteoarthritis syndrome. J Med Genet 49: 47–57.
17. Wischmeijer A, Van Laer L, Tortora G, Bolar NA, Van Camp G, et al (2013) Thoracic aortic aneurysm in infancy in aneurysms-osteoarthritis syndrome due to a novel SMAD3 mutation: further delineation of the phenotype. Am J Med Genet A. 161A(5):1028–35.
18. Regalado ES, Guo DC, Villamizar C, Avidan N, Gilchrist D, et al (2011) Exome sequencing identifies SMAD3 mutations as a cause of familial thoracic aortic aneurysm and dissection with intracranial and other arterial aneurysms. Circ Res 109(6):680–6.
19. Hilhorst-Hofstee Y, Scholte AJ, Rijlaarsdam ME, van Haeringen A, Kroft LJ, et al (2013) An unanticipated copy number variant of chromosome 15 disrupting SMAD3 reveals a three-generation family at serious risk for aortic dissection. Clin Genet 83(4):337–44.
20. Finnson KW, Chi Y, Bou-Gharios G, Leask A, Philip A (2012) TGF-b signaling in cartilage homeostasis and osteoarthritis. Front Biosci (Schol Ed) 4: 251–68.
21. Alvarez J, Serra R (2004) Unique and redundant roles of Smad3 in TGF-beta-mediated regulation of long bone development in organ culture. Dev Dyn 230(4):685–99.

22. Chen G, Deng C, Li YP (2012) TGF-β and BMP signaling in osteoblast differentiation and bone formation. Int J Biol Sci 8(2):272–88
23. Yang X, Chen L, Xu X, Li C, Huang C, Deng CX (2001) TGF-beta/Smad3 signals repress chondrocyte hypertrophic differentiation and are required for maintaining articular cartilage. J Cell Biol 2;153(1):35–46.
24. Hart DJ, Spector TD (1993) The relationship of obesity, fat distribution and osteoarthritis in the general population: the Chingford Study. J Rheumatol 20: 331–5.
25. Kellgren JH, Lawrence JS (1963) Atlas of standard radiographs of arthritis; The epidemiology of chronic rheumatism. Oxford: Blackwell Scientific Publications.
26. Burnett S, Hart DJ, Cooper C, Spector TD (1994) A radiographic atlas of osteoarthritis. London: Springer Verlag; 1994.
27. Livshits G, Kato BS, Zhai G, Hart DJ, Hunter D, et al (2007) Genomewide linkage scan of hand osteoarthritis in female twin pairs showing replication of quantitative trait loci on chromosomes 2 and 19. Ann Rheum Dis. 66(5):623–7.
28. Bucsi L, Poór G (1998) Efficacy and tolerability of oral chondroitin sulfate as a symptomatic slow-acting drug for osteoarthritis (SYSADOA) in the treatment of knee osteoarthritis. Osteoarthritis Cartilage. 6 Suppl A:31–6
29. Jordan KM, Syddall HE, Garnero P, Gineyts E, Dennison EM, et al (2006) Urinary CTX-II and glucosyl-galactosyl-pyridinoline are associated with the presence and severity of radiographic knee osteoarthritis in men. Ann Rheum Dis. 65(7):871–7
30. Cooper C, Egger P, Coggon D, Hart DJ, Masud T, et al (1996) Generalized osteoarthritis in women: pattern of joint involvement and approaches to definition for epidemiological studies. J Rheumatol. 23(11):1938–42
31. Teo YY, Inouye M, Small KS, Gwilliam R, Deloukas P, et al (2007) A genotype calling algorithm for the Illumina BeadArray platform. Bioinformatics 15;23(20):2741–6
32. Good P (1994) A practical guide to resampling methods for testing hypotheses. New York: Springer-Verlag
33. Doerge RW, Churchill GA (1996) Permutation tests for multiple loci affecting a quantitative character. Genetics 142: 285–94.
34. Knüppel S, Rohde K, Meidtner K, Drogan D, Holzhütter HG, et al (2013) Evaluation of 41 candidate gene variants for obesity in the EPIC-Potsdam cohort by multi-locus stepwise regression. PLoS ONE 8(7): e68941.
35. Walker LC, Fredericksen ZS, Wang X, Tarrell R, Pankratz VS, et al (2010) Evidence for SMAD3 as a modifier of breast cancer risk in BRCA2 mutation carriers. Breast Cancer Res. 12(6):R102.
36. Yao JY, Wang Y, An J, Mao C, M Hou, et al (2003) Mutations analysis of the SMAD3 gene in human osteoarthritis. European journal of Human Genetics. 11(9):714–7.
37. Valdes AM, Spector TD, Tamm A, Kisand K, Doherty SA, et al (2010) Genetic variation in the SMAD3 gene is associated with hip and knee osteoarthritis. Arthritis and rheumatism 62(8):2347–52.
38. Liying J, Yuchun T, Youcheng W, Yingchen W, Chunyu J, et al (2013) A SMAD3 gene polymorphism is related with osteoarthritis in a Northeast Chinese population. Rheumatology international 33(7), 1763–1768.
39. Hannan MT, Felson DT, Pincus T (2000) Analysis of the discordance between radiographic changes and knee pain in osteoarthritis of the knee. J Rheumatol 27(6):1513–7
40. Chen CG, Thuillier D, Chin EN, Alliston T (2012) Chondrocyte-intrinsic Smad3 represses Runx2-inducible matrix metalloproteinase 13 expression to maintain articular cartilage and prevent osteoarthritis. Arthritis Rheum 64(10):3278–89.

2

Exercise-Induced Bone Formation Is Poorly Linked to Local Strain Magnitude in the Sheep Tibia

Ian J. Wallace[1]*, Brigitte Demes[2], Carrie Mongle[1], Osbjorn M. Pearson[3], John D. Polk[4], Daniel E. Lieberman[5]

1 Department of Anthropology, Stony Brook University, Stony Brook, New York, United States of America, **2** Department of Anatomical Sciences, Stony Brook University, Stony Brook, New York, United States of America, **3** Department of Anthropology, University of New Mexico, Albuquerque, New Mexico, United States of America, **4** Department of Anthropology, University of Illinois at Urbana-Champaign, Urbana, Illinois, United States of America, **5** Department of Human Evolutionary Biology, Harvard University, Cambridge, Massachusetts, United States of America

Abstract

Functional interpretations of limb bone structure frequently assume that diaphyses adjust their shape by adding bone primarily across the plane in which they are habitually loaded in order to minimize loading-induced strains. Here, to test this hypothesis, we characterize the *in vivo* strain environment of the sheep tibial midshaft during treadmill exercise and examine whether this activity promotes bone formation disproportionately in the direction of loading in diaphyseal regions that experience the highest strains. It is shown that during treadmill exercise, sheep tibiae were bent in an anteroposterior direction, generating maximal tensile and compressive strains on the anterior and posterior shaft surfaces, respectively. Exercise led to significantly increased periosteal bone formation; however, rather than being biased toward areas of maximal strains across the anteroposterior axis, exercise-related osteogenesis occurred primarily around the medial half of the shaft circumference, in both high and low strain regions. Overall, the results of this study demonstrate that loading-induced bone growth is not closely linked to local strain magnitude in every instance. Therefore, caution is necessary when bone shaft shape is used to infer functional loading history in the absence of *in vivo* data on how bones are loaded and how they actually respond to loading.

Editor: David Carrier, University of Utah, United States of America

Funding: This research was supported by NSF (www.nsf.gov) grant no. IBN 96-03833 to DEL. The funder had no role in study design, data collection and analysis, decision to publish, or preparation of the manuscript.

Competing Interests: The authors have declared that no competing interests exist.

* E-mail: ian.wallace@stonybrook.edu

Introduction

Functional analyses of limb bone structure, without prior knowledge of loading history, commonly assume that the distribution of bony material within diaphyseal cross sections is affected by the magnitude of local mechanical strains (deformations) generated by habitual physical activities such as locomotion [1]. In this strategy, bone tissue's formative and resorptive activity is considered an optimization process that acts primarily to maximize resistance to loading-induced strains with a minimum of material. Functional loading is expected to have a predictable effect on diaphyseal shape by promoting bone formation disproportionately in areas of the shaft surface that are routinely subject to the highest levels of strain. Thus, bone shaft cross-sectional shapes that display structural reinforcement in a particular plane (e.g., elliptically shaped cross sections) are hypothesized to have experienced more frequent bending loads and higher strains across the axis about which the bulk of bone tissue is distributed [2–4].

However, studies documenting *in vivo* diaphyseal strains in a variety of animals have shown that limb bone shaft cross sections are not always reinforced in the planes in which they are habitually loaded [5–8]. For example, during quadrupedal walking, the ulna of a macaque monkey primarily experiences coronal bending, with the highest strains produced on the medial and lateral shaft surfaces; however, macaque ulnar diaphyses are shaped to better resist sagittal bending [7]. Some functional morphologists have downplayed the relevance of these results by pointing to other strain studies that found the correspondence between maximum strain distribution and maximum bending rigidity in diaphyses to improve during more vigorous activities [1]. For example, when macaques transition from walking to galloping, the greatest strains engendered in tibial shafts begin to approximate the direction of maximal diaphyseal bending rigidity [9]. This suggests to some that diaphyseal shape indeed reflects patterns of functional loading, particularly activities involving vigorous loading [1].

In order to rigorously evaluate the relationship between limb bone loading history and diaphyseal shape, experiments are required that directly relate *in vivo* functional strains to patterns of bone growth. To date, however, few studies of this kind have been conducted. In the present study, we characterize the *in vivo* strain environment of the tibial midshaft in sheep during treadmill exercise and test whether bone formation induced by this activity occurs primarily in diaphyseal regions that experience the highest strains. Such a growth response would structurally reinforce the shaft across its bending axis and, likewise, would influence diaphyseal shape in a manner consistent with the model within

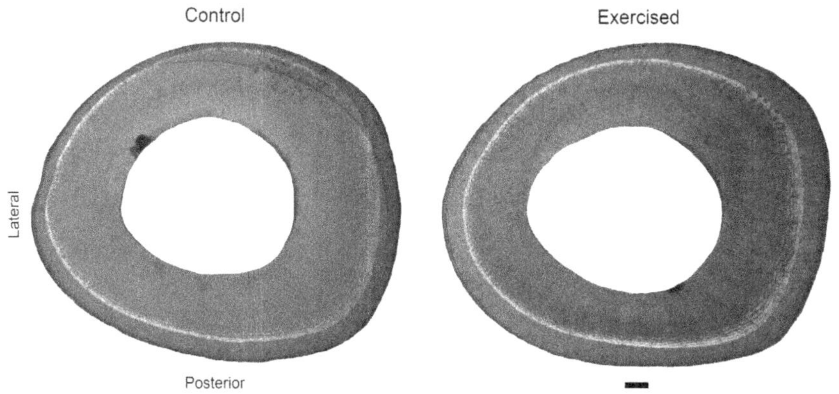

Figure 1. Tibial midshaft cross sections. The sedentary control sheep (subject 4) and the exercised sheep (subject 3) had similar body masses throughout the experiment. The calcein labels injected after the first week of the exercise treatment are visible as the light grey rings within the sections. Scale equals 1 mm.

which functional morphologists often interpret shaft structure in the absence of information on loading history.

Materials and Methods

Ethics Statement

All experimental procedures were reviewed and approved by the Institutional Animal Care and Use Committee of Harvard University.

Experimental Procedures

Juvenile animals were employed because the osteogenic response to exercise is typically greatest during the growth period [10–12]. At 40 days of age, rams (*Ovis aries*; Dorset) were divided into three groups. In the first group (N = 5), strain gauges were attached to the tibial midshaft, and strain data were recorded during treadmill trotting at a Froude speed of 0.5 (approximately 4 km h^{-1}). A second group (N = 5) was exercised on a treadmill at the same Froude speed for 30 min day^{-1} (approximately 6,000 loading cycles day^{-1}) for 90 days. Subjects were injected (i.p.) with calcein (20 mg kg^{-1}) after the first week of the exercise treatment to record bone growth on the periosteal surface of the tibia. The third group (N = 5) served as sedentary controls and received a calcein injection but no exercise treatment. All subjects were individually housed and were given the same *ad libitum* diet of food and water. After the 90-day treatment period, subjects were euthanized and tibiae were extracted.

Strain Gauge Recordings

Following induction and maintenance of isoflurane general anaesthesia, triple-rosette strain gauges (Sokki Kenkyujo, Tokyo, Japan) were affixed to the anterior, medial, and posterior diaphyseal surfaces of the left tibia through small skin incisions using aseptic technique. At each gauge site, 5 mm^2 of periosteum was removed, the bone surface was degreased with 100% chloroform, and a gauge was glued to the prepared surface with methyl-2-cyano-acrylate. Care was taken to align one gauge element with the long axis of the bone. Gauge leads were passed extracutaneously beneath flexible bandages to the hip, where they were sutured to a belt worn around the subject's abdomen. Strain relief was provided by attaching the leads to dressing wrapped around the leg near the incision sites.

Strain data were recorded 4 and 24 h after surgery, when subjects were moving with normal gaits and showed no signs of lameness or discomfort. During each recording session, gauges were connected with insulated wire to Vishay 2120A amplifiers (MicroMeasurements Inc., Raleigh, NC) to form one arm of a Wheatstone quarter-bridge circuit. Bridge excitation was 1 V. Voltage outputs were recorded on a Teac RD-145T DAT tape recorder (Teac Corp., Tokyo, Japan). Gauges were calibrated when subjects were stationary with their instrumented limb off the ground, and were periodically balanced during experiments to adjust for zero offsets.

Strain Gauge Analyses

Strain data sequences were sampled from tape recordings using an Ionet A-D board (GW Instruments, Somerville, MA) at 250 Hz. A custom-written Superscope 3.0 (GW Instruments, Somerville, MA) virtual instrument was used to determine the zero offset, calculate strains of principal tension and compression from raw voltage data using shunt calibration signals recorded during experiments, and calculate the orientation of principal tensile strain relative to the bone's long axis using standard engineering equations [13]. Igor Pro 4.0 (Wavemetrics Inc., Lake Oswego, OR) was used to calculate these strains at temporal midstance—when peak strains occur [8]—for at least 10 gait cycles per subject. To characterize the average tibial midshaft strain environment among all subjects, a custom-written macro [8] for ImageJ (NIH, Bethesda, MD) was used to compute the mean location and orientation of the neutral axis, as well as mean gradients of cross-sectional normal strain, using linear beam theory [13].

Histological Analyses

In the exercised and control subjects, bone formation on the tibial periosteal surface during the treatment period was quantified on midshaft transverse cross sections (100-µm thickness) using an Olympus SZH-10 microscope (Olympus America, Melville, NY) with epifluorescence (Fig. 1). Using ImageJ, digitized cross sections were divided into 16 equal-angle sectors positioned about the experimentally determined neutral axis, with the axis orthogonal to the neutral axis projected through the area centroid [8]. Bone area added in each sector during the treatment period was measured from the calcein line to the periosteal surface. Bone areas were standardized by body $mass^{0.67}$, calculated as mean mass during the final 3 weeks of the experiment. Two-sample Wilcoxon tests were performed to evaluate differences in bone formation between exercised and control animals.

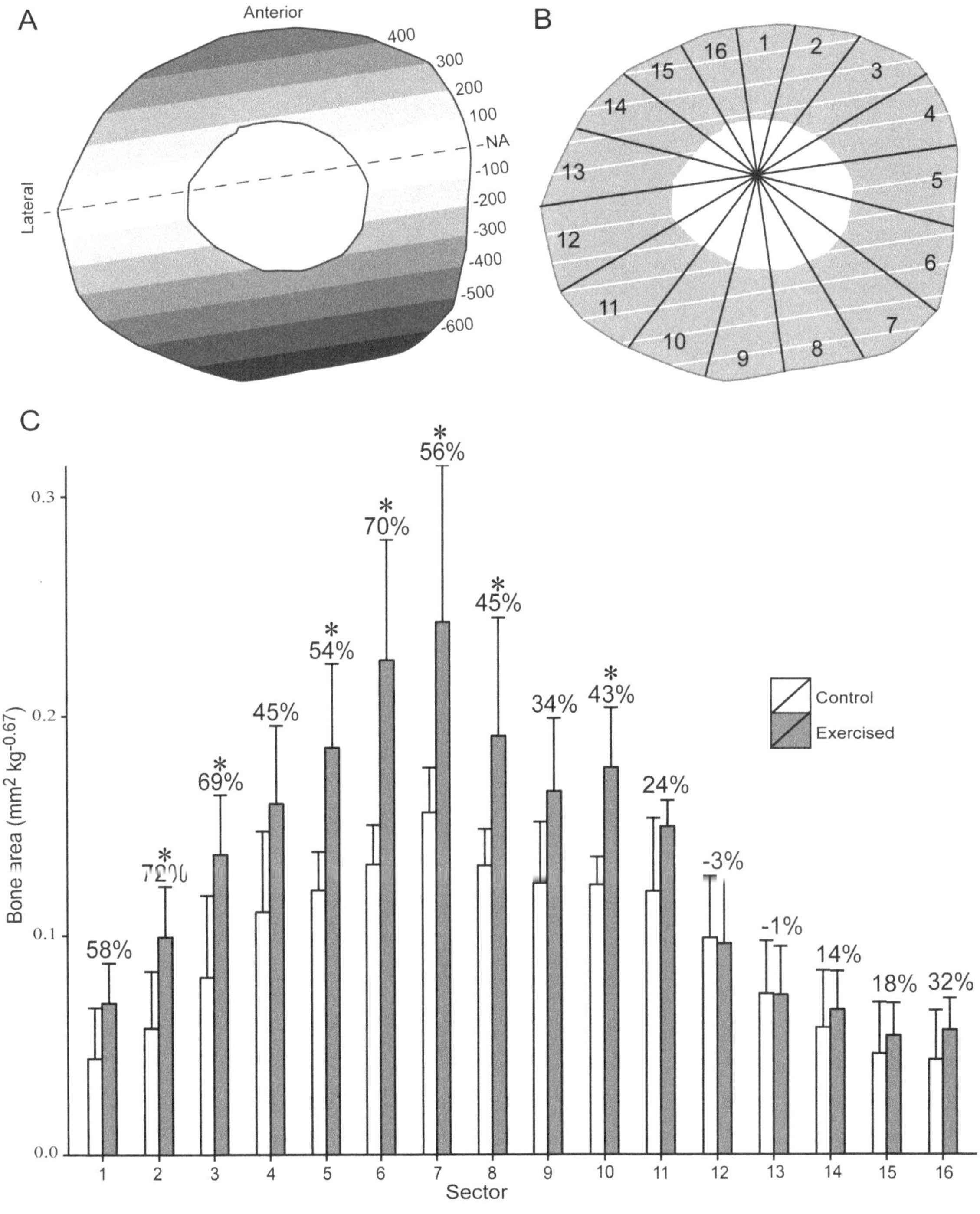

Figure 2. Bone strain and bone formation. (A) Mean distribution of peak longitudinal normal strain (με) across the tibial mid-diaphysis during treadmill exercise. The neutral axis (NA) is dashed with compressive and tensile strain isopleths plotted parallel to it. Maximal compressive strains (negative sign) were produced on the posterior shaft surface, and maximal tensile strains were produced on the anterior shaft surface. (B) Tibial midshaft cross section subdivided into 16 equal-angle sectors positioned about the neutral axis, with the axis orthogonal to the neutral axis projected through the area centroid. (C) Distribution of periosteal bone added in exercised animals and sedentary controls during the experimental period (means + SD). Asterisks indicate statistically significant ($P<0.05$) differences between exercised animals and controls as determined by two-sample Wilcoxon tests. Numbers indicate percent difference between the mean of the exercised animals relative to the control mean.

Additional details of the experimental and analytical methods are provided elsewhere [8,11]. Raw bone strain and histological data are available in [8] and Dataset S1, respectively.

Results and Discussion

Treadmill exercise caused a highly non-uniform strain environment in the sheep tibial midshaft (Fig. 2A). During peak loading, maximal compressive strains were generated on the posterior shaft surface, and maximal tensile strains were produced on the anterior surface. The neutral axis was oriented within 10° of a mediolateral axis and shifted toward the anterior diaphyseal surface, indicating that bones were bent in an anteroposterior direction. Maximal compressive strains were approximately 40% higher than tensile strains, as expected in a loading regime that includes both bending and axial compression. Based on these data, if functional loading stimulates bone formation disproportionately in diaphyseal regions that experience the highest strains, as is often assumed in functional interpretations of bone shaft structure, then one would expect treadmill exercise to promote osteogenesis primarily on the anterior and posterior tibial shaft surfaces.

However, in the sheep in this study, locations of exercise-induced bone formation were poorly linked to local strain magnitude during peak loading (Fig. 2B,C). Instead of being biased toward areas of maximal strains across the anteroposterior shaft axis, significant exercise-induced bone formation occurred primarily around the medial half of the diaphyseal circumference, in both high strain regions and directly adjacent to the neutral axis where strains were lowest. In nearly all areas of the lateral shaft surface, exercise failed to stimulate significant bone formation, including in multiple sectors that experienced maximal strains. Relative differences in bone added between exercised sheep and sedentary controls were greatest in an area of high tensile strains (sector 2) and smallest in the two lateral sectors adjacent to the neutral axis (sectors 12 and 13), yet relative group differences were very similar between other regions of maximal and minimal strains (e.g., sector 4 vs. 8). In sum, these results demonstrate that, although it might be assumed that the primary purpose of bone response to loading is to adjust its morphology to best resist maximal strains, this is not necessarily what is achieved in every instance.

These findings accord well with those of previous experiments with bird models involving both exogenous limb loading [14] and weight-bearing exercise [6] that failed to find any significant correlation between bone formation stimulated by loading and local strain magnitude. In contrast, however, peak magnitude strains have been associated with sites of increased bone formation in experiments involving external loading of rodent limbs [15,16] and natural physiological limb loading in goats [17]. A notable difference between these previous studies is that in the bird experiments, subjects were skeletally mature and the surfaces of their bones were primarily quiescent, whereas subjects in the mammal experiments were growing and had bones with active surfaces. Bone's response to loading is known to be affected by age [10–12], and has been hypothesized to differ between distantly related taxa [1,18]. Therefore, the agreement between the results of bird studies and the present experiment involving growing mammals is important because it implies that the bone functional response observed in sheep was not due to their specific age, nor is it unusual for vertebrates in general. Also important is the disparity between our results and those of other mammal studies because it suggests that a universal relationship between bone growth and local strain magnitude probably does not exist.

Previous *in vivo* strain studies demonstrating that, in many animals, limb bone shafts are structurally reinforced about the bending axis rather than in the direction of bending have led to the suggestion that bone turnover may not be optimized to minimize strains, but instead to confine strains to a relatively narrow range of orientations [5,6]. According to this view, loading-induced bone formation should occur primarily in low strain areas across the neutral axis, rather than in high strain regions, as a way of ensuring that bones are loaded in a predictable fashion. In the present study, however, although significant bone formation was stimulated by exercise near the neutral axis (at least on the medial shaft surface), it was also induced in areas distant from the neutral axis in the plane of maximum strain distribution. Thus, our results are inconsistent with hypotheses that limb bone shaft shape results from an adaptive process that either minimizes strains or makes them more predictable. Nevertheless, it possible that the patterns of exercise-induced bone formation observed in this study reflect some sort of compromise between maintaining equilibrium strain levels while still ensuring that bones maintain a sufficient safety factor to withstand atypical loading [17].

The lack of a predictable relationship between bone formation and strain magnitude highlights the inherent problem with inferring loading history from bone shaft shape in the absence of *in vivo* data on how bones are loaded and how they actually respond to loading. Without a doubt, functional loading has a critical influence on limb bone shaft morphology, and strains either directly or indirectly (e.g., through cortical interstitial fluid flow) play an important role in regulating bone mechanorespon-siveness. However, strain parameters such as frequency [19], rate [20], orientation [21], and gradients [6,14], may be as influential as magnitude in the control of bone turnover. Biophysical signals independent of strain, such as cellular oscillations, might also have an effect on bone growth [22]. Ultimately, the mechanical environment of limb bone shafts produced by functional loading is complex, and it is unlikely that any single dimension of loading history is solely responsible for causing changes in bone cell activity [23]. More likely, the distribution of bone tissue within diaphyses is affected by numerous aspects of the constant barrage of biophysical signals, spanning a wide range of magnitudes, to which bone cells are exposed throughout the daily course of functional activities. However, in terms of the precise local mechanical conditions under which bone turnover results in net formation (or resorption), gaps exist in our understanding. Until those gaps are filled, there is risk in assuming any simple relationship between limb bone diaphyseal shape and functional loading history [10].

Author Contributions

Conceived and designed the experiments: IJW DEL. Performed the experiments: BD OMP JDP DEL. Analyzed the data: IJW BD CM OMP JDP DEL. Contributed reagents/materials/analysis tools: DEL. Wrote the paper: IJW.

References

1. Ruff CB, Holt B, Trinkaus E (2006) Who's afraid of the big bad Wolff? "Wolff's Law" and bone functional adaptation. Am J Phys Anthropol 129: 484–498.
2. Larsen CS (1997) Bioarchaeology: Interpreting behavior from the human skeleton. Cambridge: Cambridge University Press. 473 p.
3. Ruff CB (2008) Biomechanical analyses of archaeological human skeletons. In: Katzenberg MA, Saunders SR, editors. Biological anthropology of the human skeleton.New York: Alan R. Liss. pp. 183–206.
4. Moore MK (2013) Functional morphology and medical imaging. In: DiGangi EA, Moore MK, editors. Research methods in human skeletal biology.Waltham, MA: Academic Press. pp. 397–424.
5. Lanyon LE, Rubin CT (1985) Functional adaptation in skeletal structures. In: Hildebrand M, Bramble DM, Liem KF, Wake BD, editors. Functional vertebrate morphology.Cambridge, MA: Belknap Press. pp. 1–25.

6. Judex S, Gross TS, Zernicke RF (1997) Strain gradients correlate with sites of exercise-induced bone-forming surfaces in the adult skeleton. J Bone Miner Res 12: 1737–1745.
7. Demes B, Stern JT Jr, Hausman MR, Larson SG, McLeod KJ, et al. (1998) Patterns of strain in the macaque ulna during functional activity. Am J Phys Anthropol 106: 87–100.
8. Lieberman DE, Polk JD, Demes B (2004) Predicting long bone loading from cross-sectional geometry. Am J Phys Anthropol 123: 156–171.
9. Demes B, Qin Y-X, Stern JT Jr, Larson SG, Rubin CT (2001) Patterns of strain in the macaque tibia during functional activity. Am J Phys Anthropol 116: 257–265.
10. Bertram JEA, Swartz SM (1991) The "law of bone transformation": a case of crying Wolff? Biol Rev 66: 245–273.
11. Lieberman DE, Pearson OM, Polk JD, Demes B, Crompton AW (2003) Optimization of bone growth and remodeling in response to loading in tapered mammalian limbs. J Exp Biol 206: 3125–3138.
12. Pearson OM, Lieberman DE (2004) The aging of Wolff's "Law": ontogeny and responses to mechanical loading in cortical bone. Yrbk Phys Anthropol 47: 63–99.
13. Biewener AA (1992) *In vivo* measurement of bone strain and tendon force. In: Biewener AA, editor. Biomechanics—structures and systems: a practical approach,Oxford: Oxford University Press. pp. 123–147.
14. Gross TS, Edwards JL, McLeod KJ, Rubin CT (1997) Strain gradients correlate with sites of periosteal bone formation. J Bone Miner Res 12: 982–988.
15. Mosley JR, March BM, Lynch J, Lanyon LE (1997) Strain magnitude related changes in whole bone architecture in growing rats. Bone 20: 191–198.
16. Warden SJ, Fuchs RK, Turner CH (2004) Steps for targeting exercise towards the skeleton to increase bone strength. Eur Med Phys 40: 223–232.
17. Main RP (2007) Ontogenetic relationships between *in vivo* strain environment, bone histomorphometry and growth in the goat radius. J Anat 210: 272–293.
18. Carter DR, Beaupré GS (2001) Skeletal function and form: Mechanobiology of skeletal development, aging, and regeneration. Cambridge: Cambridge University Press. 332 p.
19. Rubin C, Turner AS, Bain S, Mallinckrodt C, McLeod K (2001) Anabolism: low mechanical signals strengthen long bones. Nature 412: 603–604.
20. O'Connor JA, Lanyon LE, MacFie H (1982) The influence of strain rate on adaptive bone remodelling. J Biomech 15: 767–781.
21. Wallace IJ, Kwaczala AT, Judex S, Demes B, Carlson KJ (2013) Physical activity engendering loads from diverse directions augments the growing skeleton. J Musculoskelet Neuronal Interact 13: 283–238.
22. Garman R, Rubin C, Judex S (2007) Small oscillatory accelerations, independent of matrix deformations, increase osteoblast activity and enhance bone morphology. PLoS ONE 2: e653.
23. Thompson WR, Rubin CT, Rubin J (2012) Mechanical regulation of signaling pathways in bone. Gene 503: 179–193.

3

Mechanosensing by the Primary Cilium: Deletion of Kif3A Reduces Bone Formation Due to Loading

Sara Temiyasathit[1,2], W. Joyce Tang[1], Philipp Leucht[7], Charles T. Anderson[9], Stefanie D. Monica[8], Alesha B. Castillo[1,6], Jill A. Helms[8], Tim Stearns[3,5], Christopher R. Jacobs[1,2,4,6]*

1 Bone and Joint Rehabilitation R&D Center, Department of Veterans Affairs, Palo Alto, California, United States of America, **2** Department of Bioengineering, Stanford University, Stanford, California, United States of America, **3** Department of Biological Sciences, Stanford University, Stanford, California, United States of America, **4** Department of Biomedical Engineering, Columbia University, New York, New York, United States of America, **5** Department of Genetics, Stanford University, Stanford, California, United States of America, **6** Department of Mechanical Engineering, Stanford University, Stanford, California, United States of America, **7** Department of Orthopaedic Surgery, Stanford University, Stanford, California, United States of America, **8** Department of Surgery-Plastic and Reconstructive Surgery, Stanford University, Stanford, California, United States of America, **9** Energy Biosciences Institute, University of California, Berkeley, California, United States of America

Abstract

Primary cilia, solitary microtubule-based structures that grow from the centriole and extend into the extracellular space, have increasingly been implicated as sensors of a variety of biochemical and biophysical signals. Mutations in primary cilium-related genes have been linked to a number of rare developmental disorders as well as dysregulation of cell proliferation. We propose that primary cilia are also important in mechanically regulated bone formation in adults and that their malfunction could play a role in complex multi-factorial bone diseases, such as osteoporosis. In this study, we generated mice with an osteoblast- and osteocyte-specific knockout of Kif3a, a subunit of the kinesin II intraflagellar transport (IFT) protein; IFT is required for primary cilia formation, maintenance, and function. These *Col*α*1(I) 2.3-Cre;Kif3a*$^{fl/fl}$ mice exhibited no obvious morphological skeletal abnormalities. Skeletally mature *Col*α*1(I) 2.3-Cre;Kif3a*$^{fl/fl}$ and control mice were exposed to 3 consecutive days of cyclic axial ulna loading, which resulted in a significant increase in bone formation in both the conditional knockouts and controls. However, *Col*α*1(I) 2.3-Cre;Kif3a*$^{fl/fl}$ mice did exhibit decreased formation of new bone in response to mechanical ulnar loading compared to control mice. These results suggest that primary cilia act as cellular mechanosensors in bone and that their function may be critical for the regulation of bone physiology due to mechanical loading in adults.

Editor: Nic D. Leipzig, The University of Akron, United States of America

Funding: This work was supported by a National Institutes of Health grant R21AR054156 (CRJ), and ST was granted a fellowship by the Department of Veterans Affairs. The funders had no role in study design, data collection and analysis, decision to publish, or preparation of the manuscript.

Competing Interests: The authors have declared that no competing interests exist.

* E-mail: crj2111@columbia.edu

Introduction

Primary cilia are nearly ubiquitous microtubule-based cellular structures that, although discovered almost a century ago, have received less attention than the motile cilia found in the respiratory and reproductive tracts. However, a recent flurry of research into the function of the non-motile primary cilium has implicated it in the Sonic hedgehog (Shh) [1,2,3,4], Wnt [5,6], and platelet derived growth factor (PDGF) [7] signaling pathways, as well as mechanosensing in the kidney [8,9,10] and embryonic node [11]. The emerging picture is that the primary cilium acts as a versatile nexus where extracellular signals are sensed and integrated to initiate a coordinated cellular response. In terms of human disease, mutations in primary cilium proteins have been linked to a number of rare developmental disorders as well as the dysregulation of cell proliferation [12]. However, the role of primary cilia in complex multi-factorial bone diseases, such as osteoporosis, is unknown.

A number of important tissues and organs are regulated not only by biochemical but also by mechanical factors. Abnormal response to mechanical loading leads to the development of diseases such as osteoporosis and atherosclerosis [13]. Understanding the mechanism by which the cells within these tissues sense mechanical loads is critical in understanding the etiology of such diseases. Primary cilia have been shown to act as mechanosensors in the kidney and liver [8,9,14], regulating cell proliferation in these tissue types. There is *in vitro* evidence that they act as mechanosensors in bone as well, with cultured osteoblasts and osteocytes responding to mechanical stimulation with primary cilium-dependent osteogenic gene expression [15]. Germ line deletion of the primary cilium-associated gene Pkd1 in mice results in polycystic kidney disease and reduced bone mass [16], however this finding is difficult to interpret due to potential cross-talk between bone and impaired kidney function. Conditional deletion of Pkd1 in bone tissue results in skeletal developmental abnormalities [17], with reduced bone formation in development of the cranium that has been ascribed to abnormal sensing of mechanical loads during cranial expansion [18]. It is unclear how these findings relate to adult human bone pathologies such as osteoporosis because the cranial stresses and strains that occur during development are difficult to relate to the skeletal loading in adults that is due to habitual activities such as ambulation.

In this study, we investigate the role of primary cilia in regulating skeletal mechanosensing *in vivo*. Since genetic ablation of the primary cilium is embryonic lethal, we used mice with a conditional deletion of Kif3a, an essential subunit of the kinesin II intraflagellar transport (IFT) motor protein, in osteoblasts and osteocytes. Intraflagellar transport along the microtubule core of the primary cilium is required for its formation, maintenance, and function [19,20]. Deletion of Kif3a has been linked to cell signaling dysfunction through disruption of IFT [4,21]. Using this method of primary cilium disruption, we found no substantial difference in skeletal morphology in embryonic and skeletally mature mice without loading, suggesting that primary cilia in osteoblasts and osteocytes do not play a role in skeletal development. We show, however, that a tissue-specific conditional knockout of Kif3a in mice leads to attenuated sensitivity of bone to mechanical loading. This suggests that primary cilia are important for the regulation of bone formation in adults and may be involved in a larger number of complex human diseases than previously appreciated.

Results

We first generated mice with a bone-specific knockout of *Kif3a*, a subunit of kinesin II which is required for functional primary cilia, by crossing mice possessing a floxed *Kif3a* allele with mice expressing *Cre* recombinase specifically in bone driven by the 2.3 kb fragment of the α1(I)-collagen promoter [22,23]. Resulting *Colα1(I) 2.3-Cre;Kif3a*$^{fl/+}$ and *Kif3a*$^{fl/+}$ offspring were selected for subsequent breeding to generate *Colα1(I) 2.3-Cre;Kif3a*$^{fl/fl}$ (experimental) mice and control mice, which were identified by PCR-based genotyping of genomic DNA (Fig. 1A). The growth and survival of *Colα1(I) 2.3-Cre; Kif3a*$^{fl/fl}$ mice were similar to that of wild-type controls. To assess the specificity of *Cre* expression, *Colα1(I) 2.3-Cre* mice were crossed with *Rosa26R* reporter mice, and effective Cre recombination was detected by LacZ staining in osteoblasts and osteocytes of *Colα1(I) 2.3-Cre;R26R* mice but not in littermates lacking *Cre* (Fig. 1B). Cre recombination did not occur in non-bone tissue of *Colα1(I) 2.3-Cre* mice.

To determine whether *Colα1(I) 2.3-Cre;Kif3a*$^{fl/fl}$ mice exhibit abnormalities in skeletal morphology, we compared embryos at different developmental stages using histological and whole mount techniques. Embryo size and limb patterning were indistinguishable between E18.5 *Colα1(I) 2.3-Cre;Kif3a*$^{fl/fl}$ and control mice (Fig. 2A,B). There were also no differences between E16.5 *Colα1(I) 2.3-Cre;Kif3a*$^{fl/fl}$ and control mice with regards to osteogenic (Fig. 2C–H) and chondrogenic (Fig. 2C,D,I,J) differentiation. These data indicate that primary cilia in osteoblasts and osteocytes are not critical for embryonic viability, unlike the systemic knockout of *Kif3a*, which is embryonic lethal [24]. Also, disruption of *Kif3a* in osteoblasts and osteocytes does not affect skeletal size and patterning, unlike *Kif3a* deletion in messenchyme tissue [25,26].

We then assessed whether mature *Colα1(I) 2.3-Cre;Kif3a*$^{fl/fl}$ mice exhibit altered skeletal morphology. *Colα1(I) 2.3-Cre;Kif3a*$^{fl/fl}$ and control mice were compared using whole mount staining and micro-computed tomography. There were no significant differences in the size of adult skeletons between *Colα1(I) 2.3-Cre;Kif3a*$^{fl/fl}$ and control mice (Fig. 3). There were also no significant effects of *Kif3a* deletion on ulna length or cortical bone architecture at the ulnar midshaft (Table 1). Although most of the static histomorphometric measurements of trabecular bone did not show a difference between control and cKO animals (Table 2), there were some minor differences. For example, there was a 4% higher bone volume fraction in the distal femur that was also reflected in altered trabecular number and spacing. In all cases the differences were statistically significant, but small in magnitude and often inconsistent. Thus, they appear to be statistical anomalies rather than evidence of altered bone architecture. Taken together, these data suggest that disruption of intraflagellar transport in osteoblasts and osteocytes did not affect bone formation during development, and resulted in no difference in skeletal morphology between adult *Colα1(I) 2.3-Cre;Kif3a*$^{fl/fl}$ mice and controls.

Since the *Colα1(I) 2.3-Cre;Kif3a*$^{fl/fl}$ mice were devoid of developmental abnormalities observed with other *Kif3a* knockouts [24,25,26], we could determine whether primary cilia play a role in regulating mechanosensing in bone in the absence of complicating developmental effects. To ensure that we were introducing the same strain in both *Colα1(I) 2.3-Cre;Kif3a*$^{fl/fl}$ and control mice, we performed a strain calibration test prior to *in vivo* ulna loading studies (Fig. 4A). We determined that strain in cortical bone at a given load level was the same between *Colα1(I) 2.3-Cre;Kif3a*$^{fl/fl}$ and control mice (Fig. 4B).

Mutants and littermate controls were then exposed to a cyclic ulnar loading regimen of one minute per day for three consecutive

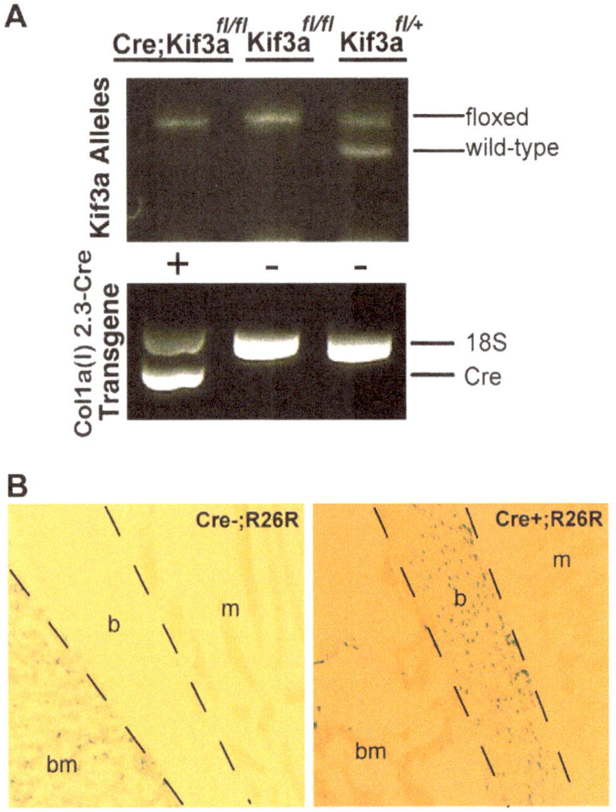

Figure 1. Generation and confirmation of bone-specific Kif3a conditional knockout mice. (**A**) A typical agarose gel resulting from PCR genotyping of genomic DNA from tail biopsies of transgenic mice. Bands indicate floxed (490 bp) and wild-type (360 bp) *Kif3a* and *Cre* recombinase (650 bp). 18S (870 bp) used as a positive control in the *Cre* PCR reactions. Floxed and recombined *Kif3a* allele present in *Colα1(I) 2.3-Cre;Kif3a*$^{fl/fl}$ mice due to heterogeneous tissue in tail biopsies. (**B**) To assess *Cre* specificity, *Colα1(I) 2.3-Cre* mice were crossed with *Rosa26R* reporter mice. Effective *Cre* recombination was detected by LacZ staining in osteoblasts and osteocytes of *Colα1(I) 2.3-Cre;R26R* mice (right) but not in littermates lacking *Cre* (left). LacZ staining was not visible in muscle tissue of *Colα1(I) 2.3-Cre;R26R* mice. (b- bone, bm- bone marrow, m- muscle).

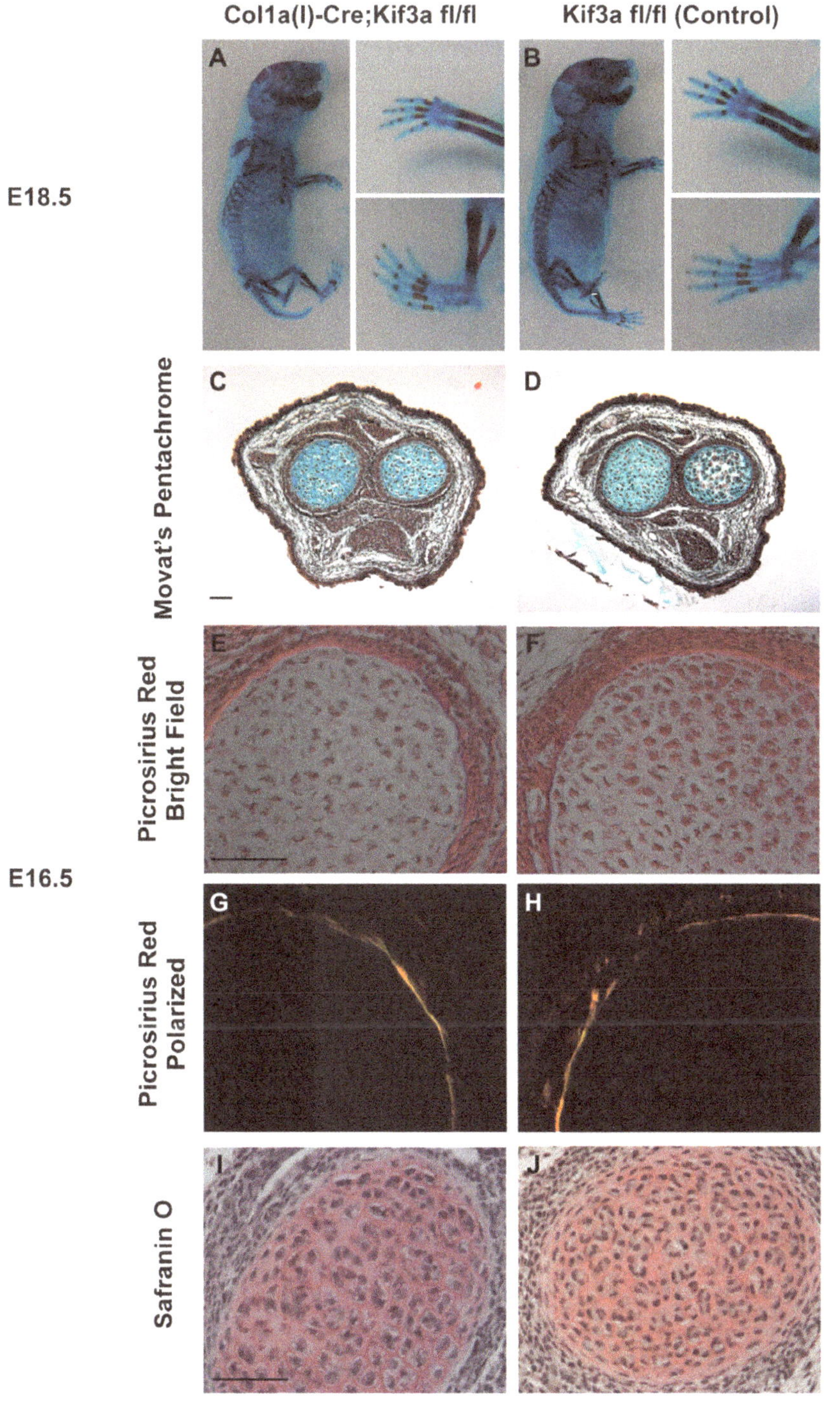

Figure 2. Kif3a expression in osteoblasts and osteocytes is not critical for embryonic skeletal development. (**A,B**) Whole mount Alizarin Red (bone) and Alcian Blue (cartilage) staining of E18.5 *Colα1(I) 2.3-Cre;Kif3a*$^{fl/fl}$ (A) and control (B) embryos. The size and limb patterning of *Colα1(I) 2.3-Cre;Kif3a*$^{fl/fl}$ mice was similar to that of the control mice. (**C,D**) Movat's pentachrome staining of cross-sections of the radial/ulnar growth plates (cartilage-blue) in E16.5 *Colα1(I) 2.3-Cre;Kif3a*$^{fl/fl}$ (C) and control (D) mice. (**E–J**) Cross-sections of E16.5 long bones stained with Picrosirius red (E,F-bright field; G,H-polarized light) to illuminate collagen and Safranin O (I,J) to demarcate cartilage. Both control and *Colα1(I) 2.3-Cre;Kif3a*$^{fl/fl}$ mice have similar patterns of osteogenic and chondrogenic differentiation. Scale bar: 100 μm.

days (Fig. 4A) and bone formation was assayed with injected fluorescent tracers and dynamic histomorphometry (Fig. 5A) [27]. After 3 consecutive days of loading, there was a significant increase in rMS/BS (Fig. 5B), rMAR (Fig. 5C), and rBFR/BS (Fig. 5D) in both *Colα1(I) 2.3-Cre;Kif3a* mutant and control mice (Table 3). However, the increase was significantly less in *Colα1(I) 2.3-Cre;Kif3a*$^{fl/fl}$ mice, by approximately 32% in rMAR and 33% in rBFR/BS, as compared to control mice (Fig. 5C,D). Collectively, our data show that an osteoblast- and osteocyte- specific knockout of Kif3a avoids the developmental abnormalities of other primary

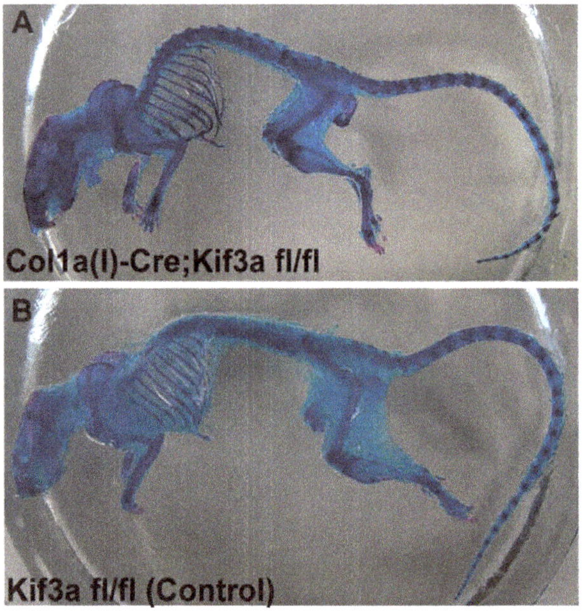

Figure 3. Skeletal morphology of adult *Colα1(I) 2.3-Cre;Kif3a$^{fl/fl}$* mice is similar to control mice. (**A,B**) Comparison of 16 week old *Colα1(I) 2.3-Cre;Kif3a$^{fl/fl}$* (A) and control (B) mice stained with Alizarin Red (bone) and Alcian Blue (cartilage) revealed no differences in size or morphology of the axial or appendicular skeleton.

cilium knockouts, but that primary cilia play a critical role in the response of adult bone to mechanical loading *in vivo*.

Discussion

The current primary cilium-related diseases are relatively rare, genetic disorders (e.g. Bardet-Biedl syndrome, Meckel-Gruber syndrome, and polycystic kidney disease); however, it is possible that primary cilia play a role in complex, multi-factorial diseases as well. For example, osteoporosis, a common and costly disease that fundamentally results from an imbalance of bone formation and bone resorption, can result from low levels of sex hormones, vitamin and mineral deficiencies, and lack of physical loading [28,29]. In this study, we found that loading of *Colα1(I) 2.3-Cre;Kif3a$^{fl/fl}$* mutant ulnae resulted in reduced loading-induced bone formation when compared to controls. We have previously shown that cultured osteoblasts and osteocytes respond to mechanical stimulation with primary cilia-dependent osteogenic gene expression [15]. Taken together these data support the idea that primary cilia may be more important in formation of bone in adults and in complex multi-factorial bone diseases, such as osteoporosis, than was previously appreciated.

In addition to their established role in development, our study provides further evidence that primary cilia play a role in maintaining adult tissue, specifically adult bone, due to mechanical loading. Recently, mice bearing global mutations in Pkd1 have been shown to form less cortical and trabecular bone with lower bone density and reduced osteogenic gene expression during skeletal development [16]. Further evidence suggests that Pkd1 might mediate sensing of mechanical stresses that occur with skeletal development [18]. In our study, there was no skeletal defect resulting from disrupting IFT in osteocytes and osteoblasts, suggesting that bone primary cilia do not participate in skeletogenesis. However, our loading results demonstrate that these primary cilia play an important role in mechanosensing in adult bone. There is precedence for the mechanisms of skeletal development and skeletal remodeling being distinct in the osteopontin-dependent response to mechanical loading [30] and integrin-dependent responses to mechanical loading and unloading [31,32]. Thus, although the mechanisms of ciliary mechanotransduction in adult bone are not fully understood, our findings suggest that the primary cilium plays a significant role in the connection between extracellular sensing and bone formation in adult bone.

While numerous *in vivo* studies have shown that primary cilia act as chemosensors in several important chemical signaling pathways, there has been less *in vivo* evidence that primary cilia are involved in mechanosensing. Studies of primary cilia and mechanosensing have shown that there is a primary cilium-dependent Ca^{2+} response when cultured kidney cells are mechanically stimulated [8,33]. More recently, *ex vivo* studies of primary cilia in the embryonic node and liver ducts implicated primary cilia as sensors of fluid flow [11,14,34]. In addition, Xiao et al. examined bone morphology of mice heterozygous for mutation of *pkd1*, a gene that encodes polycystin 1 [35]; polycystin 1 is a transmembrane protein that is found at the cilium, and the polycystin 1/2 complex is thought to have mechanosensing capabilities [36]. They found that these mice are osteopenic; however, mechanical loads were not applied directly [35]. Our results provide the first direct *in vivo*

Table 1. *Kif3a* deletion in osteoblasts and osteocytes has no effect on tibial midshaft geometry.

	Control (n = 25)	Col2.3-Cre;Kif3a fl/fl (n = 22)	p-value
Ulna			
Bone Length (mm)	14.4 ± 0.2	13.99 ± 0.2	N.S.
Imin (mm^4)	0.0046 ± 0.0002	0.0048 ± 0.0002	N.S.
Imax (mm^4)	0.0160 ± 0.0009	0.0147 ± 0.0006	N.S.
Tibia Midshaft			
Cortical Thickness (mm)	0.238 ± 0.003	0.239 ± 0.008	N.S.
Imin (mm^4)	0.077 ± 0.005	0.066 ± 0.006	N.S.
Imax (mm^4)	0.128 ± 0.006	0.109 ± 0.010	N.S.
pMOI (mm^4)	0.205 ± 0.011	0.175 ± 0.016	N.S.

Imin and Imax are maximum and minimum second moment of inertia, respectively. pMOI is polar moment of inertia. Cortical bone geometry in 16 week old skeletally mature *Colα1(I) 2.3-Cre;Kif3a$^{fl/fl}$* and control mice was assessed using as microCT. Data presented as mean±SEM. N.S. is not significant ($p > 0.15$).

Table 2. *Kif3a* deletion in osteoblasts and osteocytes has minimal effect on trabecular bone architecture.

	Control (n = 25)	Col2.3-Cre;Kif3a fl/fl (n = 22)	p-value
Proximal Tibia			
BV/TV (%)	12.6 ± 0.9	14.6 ± 1.3	N.S.
Tb.N (1/mm)	3.75 ± 0.21	4.41 ± 0.26	N.S.
Tb.Th (mm)	0.058 ± 0.002	0.055 ± 0.002	N.S.
Tb.Sp (mm)	0.289 ± 0.019	0.246 ± 0.02	N.S.
Conn.D (1/mm^3)	60.4 ± 10.3	97.0 ± 16.5	N.S.
Distal Femur			
BV/TV (%)	15.1 ± 1.0	19.0 ± 1.5	0.036
Tb.N (1/mm)	4.31 ± 0.17	4.94 ± 0.18	0.019
Tb.Th (mm)	0.057 ± 0.002	0.055 ± 0.001	N.S.
Tb.Sp (mm)	0.238 ± 0.011	0.200 ± 0.009	0.014
Conn.D (1/mm^3)	104.4 ± 12.7	141.1 ± 13.4	N.S.
L5			
BV/TV (%)	26.0 ± 0.9	24.1 ± 1.0	N.S.
Tb.N (1/mm)	4.35 ± 0.16	4.34 ± 0.16	N.S.
Tb.Th (mm)	0.64 ± 0.002	0.059 ± 0.002	0.043
Tb.Sp (mm)	0.236 ± 0.009	0.233 ± 0.009	N.S.
Conn.D (1/mm^3)	119.7 ± 10.5	125.2 ± 8.5	N.S.

Trabecular bone volume fraction (BV/TV, %), trabecular number (Tb.N, μm^{-1}), trabecular thickness (Tb.Th, μm), trabecular spacing (Tb.Sp, μm), and connectivity density (Conn.D, μm^{-3}) of the proximal tibia, distal femur, and L5 vertebra were measured using microCT. Data presented as mean±SEM. N.S. is not significant (p>0.15).

evidence that primary cilia in bone sense physical extracellular signals. They extend prior studies by demonstrating that primary cilia in bone sense physical extracellular signals and are important in cellular mechanosensing in bone in adults via a mechanism that might be distinct from the role of Pkd1 in skeletal development.

Because disrupting intraflagellar transport via the deletion of *Kif3a* may or may not result in missing or stunted primary cilia, demonstration of ciliary dysfunction is challenging. In vivo imaging of primary cilia would be inconclusive, and the associated technical difficulties have greatly limited the assessment of primary cilia in bone. Culturing primary osteocytes is another strategy, but the isolation of these cells and their return to a proliferative state would again make presence or absence of primary cilia, per se, inconclusive. Thus, verification of the Kif3a-deleted genotype, as shown in this study, may be the more effective approach.

This work raises a number of intriguing points for future research. There are a number of studies showing that disruption of IFT has led to a clear breakdown in signaling pathways, such as the hedgehog signaling [4,21,37] and Wnt signaling [5,38]. In this study, we showed that response to loading was decreased in *Colα1(I) 2.3-Cre; Kif3a$^{fl/fl}$* mice, and indeed, a number of studies have explored primary cilium-dependent mechanotransduction pathways in musculoskeletal systems [15,39,40]. However, we did not link disruption of any specific pathway to the deletion of Kif3a or primary cilia disruption in this study. In addition, while Kif3a is widely accepted to be essential to IFT in the primary cilium [19,20] and Kif3a deletion to be a method of disrupting cilia formation and function [22,41,42], there are studies that show that Kif3a is associated with non-ciliary microtubules in some cell types [43,44,45]. Finally, there are a number of potential mechanosensors in bone, including integrins [31,32,46] and mechanically-activated membrane channels [47,48,49]. The existence of other mechanosensors is suggested by our studies since deletion of the Kif3a resulted in a decrease in loading-induced response when compared to wild-type mice, rather than a failure to respond to loading.

In summary, these findings represent an *in vivo* demonstration of a link between the disruption of primary cilia function and decreased bone mechano-responsiveness, suggesting that the primary cilium acts as cellular mechanosensors. Our results also suggest that primary cilia may play a broader role in regulating

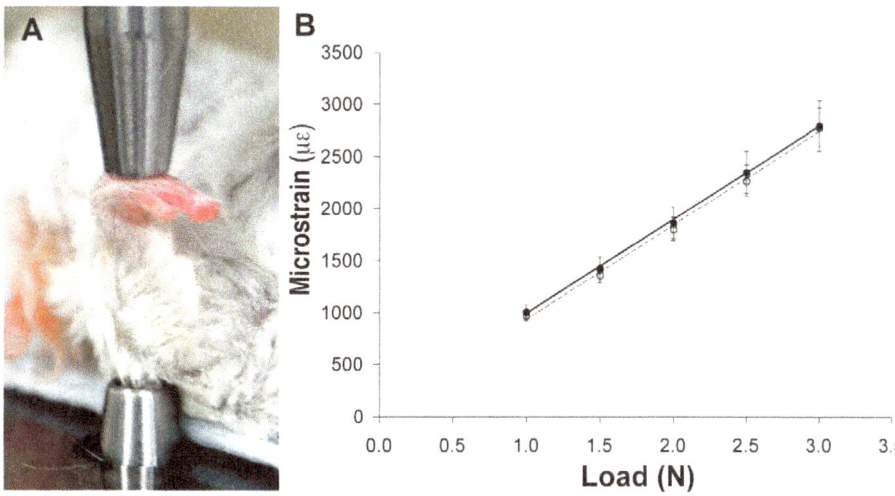

Figure 4. Axial ulnar loading leads to similar strain at the ulnar midshaft of *Colα1(I) 2.3-Cre;Kif3a$^{fl/fl}$* and control mice. (**A**) Image of strain gaging and axial ulnar loading experimental set-up. The right forearms of 16 week old skeletal mature mice were axially loaded for 120 cycles per day for 3 consecutive days with a 2 Hz sine wave using an electromagnetic loading system with feedback control. The left forearms were not loaded and used as non-loaded internal controls. (**B**) Strain in cortical bone at given mechanical loading levels. Open and closed circles indicate *Colα1(I) 2.3-Cre;Kif3a$^{fl/fl}$* (n = 35) and control (n = 27) mice, respectively. Data presented as mean ± SEM. * p<0.05.

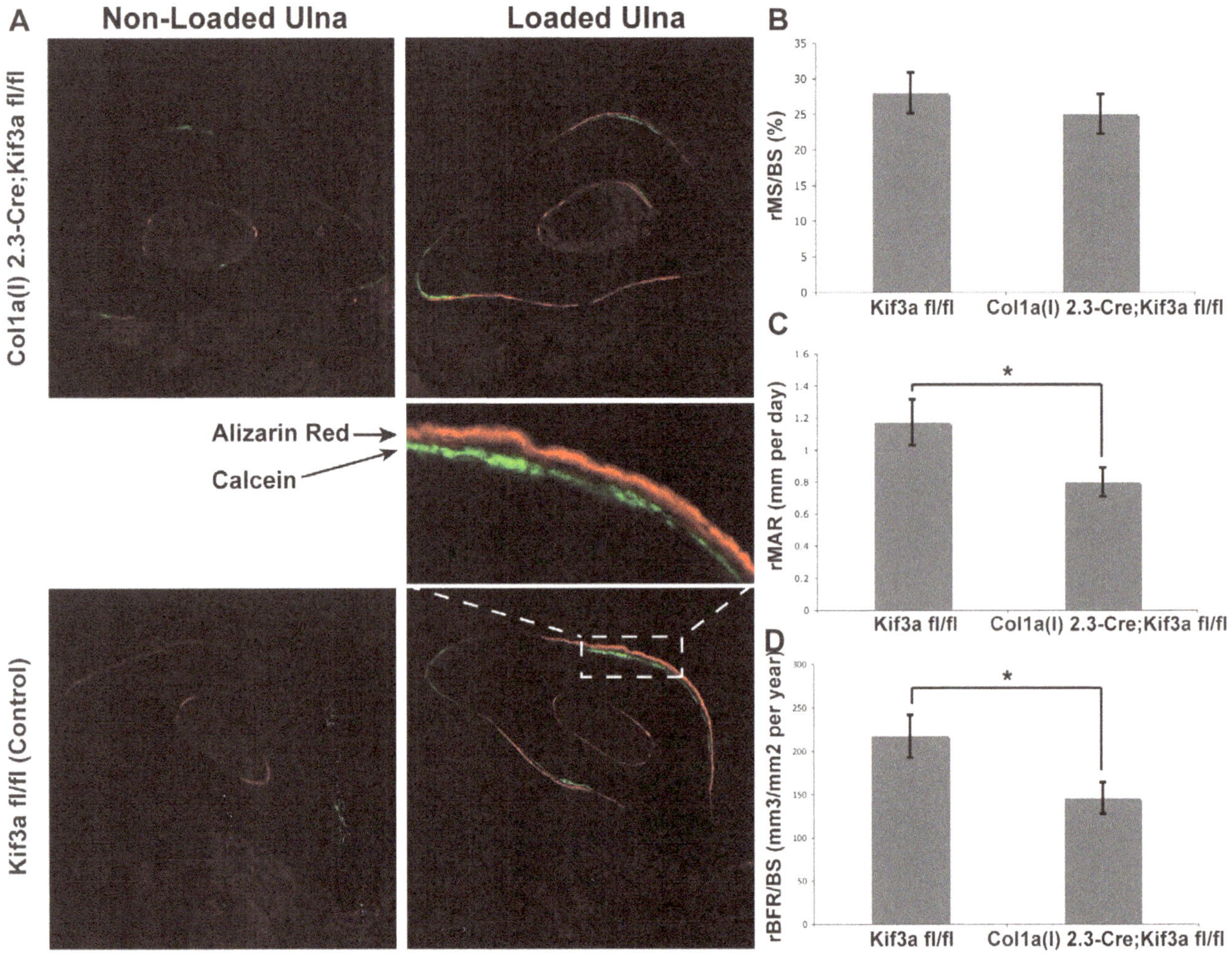

Figure 5. Skeletally mature *Colα1(I) 2.3-Cre;Kif3a$^{fl/fl}$* mice exhibit less responsiveness to mechanical loading compared to control mice. (**A**) Representative images of non-loaded (left) and loaded (right) ulnae of *Colα1(I) 2.3-Cre;Kif3a$^{fl/fl}$* (top) and control (bottom) mice. Fluorochrome labels (Calcein-green and Alizarin Red-red) given on Days 5 and 12 after the onset of mechanical loading. (**B to D**) Relative mineralizing surface (rMS/BS, %, B), mineral apposition rate (rMAR, μm per day, C), and bone formation rate (rBFR/BS, $\mu m^3/\mu m^2$ per year, D) of mechanically loaded mice. *Colα1(I) 2.3-Cre;Kif3a$^{fl/fl}$* mice exhibited a decrease of 32% in rMAR and 33% in rBFR/BS when compared to control mice. Data presented as mean ± SEM. * $p<0.05$.

Table 3. *Colα1(I) 2.3-Cre;Kif3a$^{fl/fl}$* were significantly less responsive to mechanical loading than control mice.

	MS/BS (%)		MAR (um per day)		BFR/BS (um3/um2 per year)	
***Col2.3-Cre;Kif3a fl/fl* (n = 35)**						
left (non-loaded)	12.30+/−2.05		0.316+/−0.046		21.62+/−5.41	
right (loaded)	36.82+/−2.58	+++	1.089+/−0.086	+++	166.78+/−18.55	+++
relative (loaded - non-loaded)	25.01+/−2.79		0.798+/−0.090	*	145.52+/−18.23	*
***Control* (n = 27)**						
left (non-loaded)	12.96+/−2.49		0.481+/−0.074		31.64+/−7.78	
right (loaded)	40.59+/−2.51	+++	1.644+/−0.120	+++	248.71+/−24.92	+++
relative (loaded - non-loaded)	27.98+/−2.88		1.171+/−0.143		217.07+/−24.62	

Colα1(I) 2.3-Cre;Kif3a$^{fl/fl}$ and control mice responded to mechanical loading with increased mineralizing surface (MS/BS), mineral apposition rate (MAR), and bone formation rate (BFR/BS), however, *Colα1(I) 2.3-Cre;Kif3a$^{fl/fl}$* were significantly less responsive to mechanical loading than control mice. Data presented as mean±SEM.
$^{+++}p<0.001$ for loaded vs. non-loaded values.
*$p<0.05$ for *Colα1(I) 2.3-Cre;Kif3a$^{fl/fl}$* vs. control mice.

bone formation in adults and in complex multi-factorial bone diseases than was previously appreciated.

Materials and Methods

Animals

Kif3a$^{fl/fl}$ and *Colα1(I) 2.3-Cre* mice were created as described previously [22,23]. Male *Colα1(I) 2.3-Cre* and female *Kif3a*$^{fl/fl}$ mice founder mice were used to generate *Colα1(I) 2.3-Cre;Kif3a*$^{fl/fl}$ (experimental) and *Kif3a*$^{fl/fl}$ (control) for experimentation. The *Cre* transgene was transmitted through the male to avoid undesirable Cre activity in the female germline. To assess Cre expression, *Colα1(I) 2.3-Cre* mice were mated with *Rosa26R* reporter mice [50]. For staged embryos, *Colα1(I) 2.3-Cre;Kif3a*$^{fl/fl}$ and *Kif3a*$^{fl/fl}$ mating pairs were set up in the afternoon and checked for vaginal plugs the next morning. Noon of the day of the vaginal plug was designated as embryonic day E0.5. Genotypes of transgenic mice were determined by PCR analysis of genomic DNA from tail biopsies. The heterogeneous mix of tail tissue, some of which did express *Cre* recombinase (e.g. bone) and some of which did not (e.g. skin, muscle, etc.), often resulted in a combination of floxed and recombined alleles in PCR results, depending on the portion of the tail biopsy that was digested. In these samples, a band representing the recombined allele was present at 200 bp. *Cre* and *Kif3a* floxed and wildtype primers were previously described [22,23]. 18S was used as a positive control for the *Cre* PCR reaction with P1: 5′ CAA GGA AGG CAG CAG GCG CGC AAA T 3′; P2: 5′TGC ACC ACC ACC CAC GGA ATC GAG AA 3′. Mice were housed up to 5 per cage and provided with standard mouse chow and water ad libitum throughout the study. All procedures performed in this study were approved by the Palo Alto IACUC with ACORP protocol approval number JAC050806MOU.

LacZ Staining, Histology and Whole Mount Skeletal Staining

Tissues were harvested at specified time points, fixed in 4% paraformaldehyde for 24 h at 4°C, decalcified for 10–14 days in 19% EDTA at 4°C, and embedded in paraffin or OCT. Sections were cut at 8–12 µm thickness. For histology, sections were stained with Movat's pentachrome [51]. Adjacent sections were stained with Picrosirius red and Safranin O. For LacZ staining, tissue sections were fixed, permeabilized, and stained for 4–5 days in a 1 mg/mL X-gal (5-bromo-4-chloro-3-indolyl-D-β-galactosidase) solution, adapted from Colnot et al. [52]. Whole mount skeletal staining with Alizarin Red and Alcian Blue was performed as previously described [53,54].

Micro-Computed Tomography

Bone samples from sixteen week old *Colα1(I) 2.3-Cre;Kif3a*$^{fl/fl}$ and control mice were dissected, fixed in 70% ethanol, and scanned using micro-computed tomography (Scanco vivaCT 40, Bassersdorf, Switzerland) at 10 µm isotropic resolution. Cortical bone analysis on the mid-diaphysis included cortical thickness and maximum and minimum second moment of inertia (Imax and Imin). Trabecular bone analysis was completed at the proximal tibia, distal femur and L5 lumbar vertebra. Trabecular bone was designated using contours inside the cortical shell on two-dimensional slices. Histomorphometric analysis included bone volume fraction (BV/TV, %), trabecular number (Tb.N, μm^{-1}), trabecular thickness (Tb.Th, µm), trabecular spacing (Tb.Sp, µm), and connectivity density (Conn.D, μm^{-3}).

Strain Measurement During Axial Ulnar Loading

Strain calibration test were performed prior to the *in vivo* ulna loading study to ensure that the same strain was introduced in both *Colα1(I) 2.3-Cre;Kif3a*$^{fl/fl}$ and control mice. Peak mechanical strain at the medial aspect of the ulnar midshaft was measured based on a previously described protocol [55]. The forearm of 16 week old *Colα1(I) 2.3-Cre;Kif3a*$^{fl/fl}$ and control mice were loaded in axial compression, using the same device and frequency used for *in vivo* loading (Fig. 3A). Forearms were loaded at magnitudes of 1.0, 1.5, 2.0, 2.5, and 3.0 N, during which peak-to-peak voltage was measured using a digital oscilloscope. Voltage was converted to strain as previously described [55]. We determined that strain in cortical bone at a given load level was the same between *Colα1(I) 2.3-Cre;Kif3a*$^{fl/fl}$ and control mice (Fig. 3B).

In Vivo Axial Ulnar Loading

The *in vivo* axial ulnar loading protocol was modified from Robling and Turner [55]. Because the experimental animals were of mixed genetic background resulting from the cross of C57Bl/6 and FVB mice, we did not know a priori what load level would produce a robust bone formation. Thus, we conducted an initial dose-response experiment with 2.8N, 3.0N, and 3.4N applied load. A consistent formative response was found in the 3.4N group only, thus we chose this load level for the in vivo axial ulnar loading experiments. While under isofluorane anesthesia (2.5%) the right forearm from each mouse was axially loaded for 120 cycles per day for 3 consecutive days with a 2 Hz sine wave using an electromagnetic loading system with feedback control (Fig. 3A; EnduraTEC, Bose, Eden Prairie, MN). The left forearms were not loaded and used as non-loaded internal controls. All mice were allowed normal cage activity in between loading sessions. All mice received subcutaneous injections of Calcein (30 mg/kg body weight; Sigma Chemical Co., St. Louis, MO) 5 days after the first day of loading and Alizarin Red (50 mg/kg body weight; Sigma Chemical Co., St. Louis, Mo, USA) 12 days after the first day of loading. All animals were euthanized 19 days after the first day of loading and processed for dynamic histomorphometric analysis

Dynamic Histomorphometry

The right and left ulnae were isolated, cleaned of soft tissue, measured for total length and stored in 70% ethanol for histomorphometry. The ulnae were then dehydrated in graded alcohol (70–100%), infiltrated with three changes of methyl methacrylate (Aldrich Chemical Co., Milwaukee, WI), and embedded in methyl methacrylate in the presence of benzoyl peroxide. Transverse sections of the ulnar midshaft were collected using a diamond saw (Isomet, Buehler, Lake Bluff, IL) and imaged on a laser scanning confocal microscope (Nikon C-1) using a 0.45 NA 10× objective.

Using Image J, the following data were collected from the periosteal surface: bone perimeter (B.Pm), single label perimeter (sL.Pm), double label perimeter (dL.Pm), and double label area (dL.Ar). From these primary data, the following were calculated for each bone: mineralizing surface (MS/BS = [1/2 sL.Pm+dL.Pm]/B.Pm×100; %), mineral apposition rate (MAR = dL.Ar/dL.Pm/7days; µm per day) and bone formation rate (BFR/BS = MAR×MS/BS×3.65; $\mu m^3/\mu m^2$ per year). Relative (r) measurements of rMS/BS, rMAR, rBFR/BS, were calculated by subtracting the non-loaded from loaded values to show increases due to mechanical loading.

Statistical Analysis

Data were expressed as mean ± SEM. Differences in slope and intercept for the linear regressions between *Colα1(I) 2.3-Cre;Kif3a*$^{fl/fl}$ and control mice were analyzed by analysis of covariance. Differences between right (loaded) and left (non-loaded) ulnae were analyzed using paired t-tests (two-tailed). All other comparisons between *Colα1(I) 2.3-Cre;Kif3a*$^{fl/fl}$ and control mice were analyzed using unpaired t-tests (two-tailed). For all tests, $\alpha = 0.05$.

Acknowledgments

We thank Jeremiah M. Jones for technical assistance, Ronald Y. Kwon for assistance in taking the axial ulna loading image, and Ronald Y. Kwon and Julie B. Litzenberger for discussion.

Author Contributions

Conceived and designed the experiments: ST JAH TS CRJ. Performed the experiments: ST WJT PL CTA SDM. Analyzed the data: ST WJT ABC JAH TS CRJ. Wrote the paper: ST CRJ.

References

1. Corbit KC, Aanstad P, Singla V, Norman AR, Stainier DY, et al. (2005) Vertebrate Smoothened functions at the primary cilium. Nature 437: 1018–1021.
2. Rohatgi R, Milenkovic L, Scott MP (2007) Patched1 regulates hedgehog signaling at the primary cilium. Science 317: 372–376.
3. Kovacs JJ, Whalen EJ, Liu R, Xiao K, Kim J, et al. (2008) Beta-arrestin-mediated localization of smoothened to the primary cilium. Science 320: 1777–1781.
4. Huangfu D, Liu A, Rakeman AS, Murcia NS, Niswander L, et al. (2003) Hedgehog signalling in the mouse requires intraflagellar transport proteins. Nature 426: 83–87.
5. Corbit KC, Shyer AE, Dowdle WE, Gaulden J, Singla V, et al. (2008) Kif3a constrains beta-catenin-dependent Wnt signalling through dual ciliary and non-ciliary mechanisms. Nat Cell Biol 10: 70–76.
6. Gerdes JM, Liu Y, Zaghloul NA, Leitch CC, Lawson SS, et al. (2007) Disruption of the basal body compromises proteasomal function and perturbs intracellular Wnt response. Nat Genet 39: 1350–1360.
7. Schneider L, Clement CA, Teilmann SC, Pazour GJ, Hoffmann EK, et al. (2005) PDGFRalphaalpha signaling is regulated through the primary cilium in fibroblasts. Curr Biol 15: 1861–1866.
8. Praetorius HA, Spring KR (2001) Bending the MDCK cell primary cilium increases intracellular calcium. J Membr Biol 184: 71–79.
9. Praetorius HA, Frokiaer J, Nielsen S, Spring KR (2003) Bending the primary cilium opens Ca2+-sensitive intermediate-conductance K+ channels in MDCK cells. J Membr Biol 191: 193–200.
10. Nauli SM, Alenghat FJ, Luo Y, Williams E, Vassilev P, et al. (2003) Polycystins 1 and 2 mediate mechanosensation in the primary cilium of kidney cells. Nature Genetics 33: 129–137.
11. McGrath J, Somlo S, Makova S, Tian X, Brueckner M (2003) Two populations of node monocilia initiate left-right asymmetry in the mouse. Cell 114: 61–73.
12. Berbari NF, O'Connor AK, Haycraft CJ, Yoder BK (2009) The primary cilium as a complex signaling center. Curr Biol 19: R526–535.
13. Ingber DE (2003) Mechanobiology and diseases of mechanotransduction. Annals of Medicine 35: 1–14.
14. Masyuk AI, Masyuk TV, Splinter PL, Huang BQ, Stroope AJ, et al. (2006) Cholangiocyte cilia detect changes in luminal fluid flow and trasmit them into intracellular Ca2+ and cAMP signaling. Gastroenterology 131: 911–920.
15. Malone AM, Anderson CT, Tummala P, Kwon RY, Johnston TR, et al. (2007) Primary cilia mediate mechanosensing in bone cells by a calcium-independent pathway. Proceedings of the National Academy of Sciences of the United States of America 104: 13325–13330.
16. Xiao Z, Zhang S, Magenheimer BS, Luo J, Quarles D (2008) Polycystin-1 regulates skeletogenesis through stimulation of the osteoblast-specific transcription factor runx2-II. Journal of Biological Chemistry 283: 12624–12634.
17. Xiao Z, Zhang S, Cao L, Qiu N, David V, et al. (2010) Conditional disruption of Pkd1 in osteoblasts results in osteopenia due to direct impairment of bone formation. J Biol Chem 285: 1177–1187.
18. Hou B, Kolpakova-Hart E, Fukai N, Wu K, Olsen BR (2009) The polycystic kidney disease 1 (Pkd1) gene is required for the responses of osteochondroprogenitor cells to midpalatal suture expansion in mice. Bone 44: 1121–1133.
19. Rosenbaum JL, Witman GB (2002) Intraflagellar transport. Nat Rev Mol Cell Biol 3: 813–825.
20. Scholey JM (2003) Intraflagellar transport. Annu Rev Cell Dev Biol 19: 423–443.
21. Huangfu D, Anderson KV (2005) Cilia and Hedgehog responsiveness in the mouse. Proc Natl Acad Sci U S A 102: 11325–11330.
22. Lin F, Hiesberger T, Cordes K, Sinclair AM, Goldstein LS, et al. (2003) Kidney-specific inactivation of the KIF3A subunit of kinesin-II inhibits renal ciliogenesis and produces polycystic kidney disease. Proc Natl Acad Sci U S A 100: 5286–5291.
23. Dacquin R, Starbuck M, Schinke T, Karsenty G (2002) Mouse alpha1(I)-collagen promoter is the best known promoter to drive efficient Cre recombinase expression in osteoblast. Dev Dyn 224: 245–251.
24. Marszalek JR, Ruiz-Lozano P, Roberts E, Chien KR, Goldstein LS (1999) Situs inversus and embryonic ciliary morphogenesis defects in mouse mutants lacking the KIF3A subunit of kinesin-II. Proc Natl Acad Sci U S A 96: 5043–5048.
25. Haycraft CJ, Zhang Q, Song B, Jackson WS, Detloff PJ, et al. (2007) Intraflagellar transport is essential for endochondral bone formation. Development 134: 307–316.
26. Kolpakova-Hart E, Jinnin M, Hou B, Fukai N, Olsen BR (2007) Kinesin-2 controls development and patterning of the vertebrate skeleton by Hedgehog- and Gli3-dependent mechanisms. Dev Biol 309: 273–284.
27. Parfitt AM, Drezner MK, Glorieux FH, Kanis JA, Malluche H, et al. (1987) Bone histomorphometry: standardization of nomenclature, symbols, and units. Report of the ASBMR Histomorphometry Nomenclature Committee. J Bone Miner Res 2: 595–610.
28. Burge R, Dawson-Hughes B, Solomon DH, Wong JB, King A, et al. (2007) Incidence and economic burden of osteoporosis-related fractures in the United States, 2005–2025. J Bone Miner Res 22: 465–475.
29. Kenny AM, Prestwood KM (2000) Osteoporosis. Pathogenesis, diagnosis, and treatment in older adults. Rheum Dis Clin North Am 26: 569–591.
30. Ishijima M, Rittling SR, Yamashita T, Tsuji K, Kurosawa H, et al. (2001) Enhancement of osteoclastic bone resorption and suppression of osteoblastic bone formation in response to reduced mechanical stress do not occur in the absence of osteopontin. J Exp Med 193: 399–404.
31. Phillips JA, Almeida EA, Hill EL, Aguirre JI, Rivera MF, et al. (2008) Role for beta1 integrins in cortical osteocytes during acute musculoskeletal disuse. Matrix Biol 27: 609–618.
32. Litzenberger JB, Tang WJ, Castillo AB, Jacobs CR (2009) Deletion of beta 1 integrins from cortical osteocytes reduces load-induced bone formation Cellular and Molecular Bioengineering In press.
33. Praetorius HA, Spring KR (2003) Removal of the MDCK cell primary cilium abolishes flow sensing. Journal of Membrane Biology 191: 69–76.
34. Nonaka S, Shiratori H, Saijoh Y, Hamada H (2002) Determination of left-right patterning of the mouse embryo by artificial nodal flow. Nature 418: 96–99.
35. Xiao Z, Zhang S, Mahlios J, Zhou G, Magenheimer BS, et al. (2006) Cilia-like structures and polycystin-1 in osteoblasts/osteocytes and associated abnormalities in skeletogenesis and runx2 expression. Journal of Biological Chemistry 281: 30884–30895.
36. Wilson PD (2004) Polycystic kidney disease. N Engl J Med 350: 151–164.
37. May SR, Ashique AM, Karlen M, Wang B, Shen Y, et al. (2005) Loss of the retrograde motor for IFT disrupts localization of Smo to cilia and prevents the expression of both activator and repressor functions of Gli. Dev Biol 287: 378–389.
38. Lancaster MA, Schroth J, Gleeson JG Subcellular spatial regulation of canonical Wnt signalling at the primary cilium. Nat Cell Biol 13: 700–707.
39. Kwon RY, Temiyasathit S, Tummala P, Quah CC, Jacobs CR (2010) Primary cilium-dependent mechanosensing is mediated by adenylyl cyclase 6 and cyclic AMP in bone cells. FASEB J 24: 2859–2868.
40. McGlashan SR, Knight MM, Chowdhury TT, Joshi P, Jensen CG, et al. Mechanical loading modulates chondrocyte primary cilia incidence and length. Cell Biol Int 34: 441–446.
41. Song B, Haycraft CJ, Seo HS, Yoder BK, Serra R (2007) Development of the post-natal growth plate requires intraflagellar transport proteins. Dev Biol 305: 202–216.
42. Koyama E, Young B, Nagayama M, Shibukawa Y, Enomoto-Iwamoto M, et al. (2007) Conditional Kif3a ablation causes abnormal hedgehog signaling topography, growth plate dysfunction, and excessive bone and cartilage formation during mouse skeletogenesis. Development 134: 2159–2169.
43. Kondo S, Sato-Yoshitake R, Noda Y, Aizawa H, Nakata T, et al. (1994) KIF3A is a new microtubule-based anterograde motor in the nerve axon. J Cell Biol 125: 1095–1107.
44. Wiesner C, Faix J, Himmel M, Bentzien F, Linder S KIF5B and KIF3A/KIF3B kinesins drive MT1-MMP surface exposure, CD44 shedding, and extracellular matrix degradation in primary macrophages. Blood 116: 1559–1569.
45. Huang CJ, Huang CC, Chang CC Association of the testis-specific TRIM/RBCC protein RNF33/TRIM60 with the cytoplasmic motor proteins KIF3A and KIF3B. Mol Cell Biochem 360: 121–131.
46. Wang Y, McNamara LM, Schaffler MB, Weinbaum S (2008) Strain amplification and integrin based signaling in osteocytes. J Musculoskelet Neuronal Interact 8: 332–334.
47. Genetos DC, Kephart CJ, Zhang Y, Yellowley CE, Donahue HJ (2007) Oscillating fluid flow activation of gap junction hemichannels induces ATP release from MLO-Y4 osteocytes. J Cell Physiol 212: 207–214.
48. Duncan RL, Hruska KA (1994) Chronic, intermittent loading alters mechanosensitive channel characteristics in osteoblast-like cells. Am J Physiol 267: F909–916.
49. McGarry JG, Klein-Nulend J, Prendergast PJ (2005) The effect of cytoskeletal disruption on pulsatile fluid flow-induced nitric oxide and prostaglandin E-2

release in osteocytes and osteoblasts. Biochemical and Biophysical Research Communications 330: 341–348.
50. Soriano P (1999) Generalized lacZ expression with the ROSA26 Cre reporter strain. Nat Genet 21: 70–71.
51. Sheehan DC, Hrapchak BB (1980) Theory and Practice of Histotechnology. 2nd Edition ed. Columbus, OH: Batelle Press. pp 103–104.
52. Colnot C, Huang S, Helms J (2006) Analyzing the cellular contribution of bone marrow to fracture healing using bone marrow transplantation in mice. Biochem Biophys Res Commun 350: 557–561.
53. McLeod MJ (1980) Differential staining of cartilage and bone in whole mouse fetuses by alcian blue and alizarin red S. Teratology 22: 299–301.
54. Selby PB (1987) A rapid method for preparing high quality alizarin stained skeletons of adult mice. Stain Technol 62: 143–146.
55. Robling AG, Turner CH (2002) Mechanotransduction in bone: genetic effects on mechanosensitivity in mice. Bone 31: 562–569.

4

Isolation of Antiosteoporotic Compounds from Seeds of *Sophora japonica*

Hossam M. Abdallah[1,2], Ahmed M. Al-Abd[3,4], Gihan F. Asaad[3,5], Ashraf B. Abdel-Naim[4], Ali M. El-halawany[1,2]*

1 Department of Natural Products, Faculty of Pharmacy, King Abdulaziz University, Jeddah, Saudi Arabia, **2** Department of Pharmacognosy, Faculty of Pharmacy, Cairo University, Cairo, Egypt, **3** Pharmacology Department, Medical Division, National Research Center, Giza, Egypt, **4** Department of Pharmacology and Toxicology, Faculty of Pharmacy, King Abdulaziz University, Jeddah, Saudi Arabia, **5** Pharmacology Department, Faculty of Pharmacy, Jazan University, Jazan, Saudia Arabia

Abstract

Chemical investigation of *Sophora japonica* seeds resulted in the isolation of seven metabolites identified as: genistin (**1**), sophoricoside (**2**), sophorabioside (**3**), sophoraflavonoloside (**4**), genistein 7,4′-di-*O*-β-D-glucopyransoide (**5**), kaempferol 3-*O*-α–L-rhamnopyranosyl(1→6)β-D-glucopyranosyl(1→2)β-D-glucopyranoside (**6**) and rutin (**7**). Compounds **1**, **2** and **5** showed significant estrogenic proliferative effect in MCF-7 cell in sub-cytotoxic concentration range. Compounds **1** and **2** showed minimal cell membrane damaging effect using LDH leakage assay. Accordingly, compound **2** (sophoricoside, (SPH)) was selected for further *in-vivo* studies as a potential anti-osteoporosis agent. The anti-osteoporotic effect of SPH was assessed in ovarectomized (OVX) rats after oral administration (15 mg/kg and 30 mg/kg) for 45 days compared to estradiol (10 µg/kg) as a positive control. Only in a dose of 30 mg/kg, SPH regained the original mechanical bone hardness compared to normal non-osteoporotic group. However, SPH (15 mg/kg) significantly increased the level of alkaline phosphatase (ALP) to normal level. Treatment with SPH (30 mg/kg) increased the level of ALP to be higher than normal group. SPH (15 mg/kg) did not significantly increase the serum level of osteocalcin (OC) compared to OVX group. On the other hand, treatment with SPH (30 mg/kg) significantly increased the level of OC to 78% higher than normal non-ovarectomized animals group. In addition, SPH (15 mg/kg) decreased the bone resorption marker, acid phosphatase (ACP) to normal level and SPH (30 mg/kg) further diminished the level of serum ACP. Histopathologically, sophoricoside ameliorated the ovarectomy induced osteoporosis in a dose dependent manner. The drug showed thicker bony trabeculae, more osteoid, and more osteoblastic rimming compared to OVX group.

Editor: Jean-Marc A. Lobaccaro, Clermont Université, France

Funding: This project was funded by the Deanship of Scientific Research (DSR), King Abdulaziz University, Jeddah, under grant no. 208/166/1433. The authors, therefore, acknowledge with thanks DSR technical and financial support. The funders had no role in study design, data collection and analysis, decision to publish, or preparation of the manuscript.

Competing Interests: The co-author Ashraf B. Abdel-Naim is a PLOS ONE Editorial Board member. However, this does not alter the authors' adherence to PLOS ONE Editorial policies and criteria.

* E-mail: ali.elhalawany@pharma.cu.edu.eg

Introduction

According to the World Health Organization "Osteoporosis is a disease characterized by low bone mass and micro-architectural deterioration of bone tissues, leading to enhanced fragility and consequent increase in fracture risk that results in fractures with minimal trauma". Osteoporosis, a silent epidemic has become a chief health hazard in recent years, afflicting over 2000 million people worldwide [1]. Osteoporosis is associated with deficiency of ovarian hormone following menopause. A sharp decrease in ovarian estrogen production is the predominant cause of rapid, hormone-related bone loss after menopause [2] as a result of higher bone turnover, an imbalance between bone formation and bone resorption & net bone loss [3]. The common sites of fracture among postmenopausal women include the vertebrae, forearm and hip. The incidence of hip fractures & cost for treatment will rise in the future, unless successful prophylactic actions are taken [4].

In Saudi Arabia, the incidence of osteoporosis is common among postmenopausal women; it is often associated with early or late onset of menopause. It was found that osteoporosis is familiar (60%) among postmenopausal Saudi Arabian women [5,6].

Hormone replacement therapy (HRT) effectively ameliorates postmenopausal symptoms and lowers the risk for coronary heart disease and osteoporosis. However, HRT increases the risk of breast cancer and cardiovascular diseases. To overcome the wide range of side effects produced by HRT, there is an increasing demand for "backing to nature" which is considered to be healthier and safer for the treatment of osteoporosis. Phytoestrogens are plant-derived compounds that structurally or functionally mimic mammalian estrogens, and therefore are considered to play an important role in the prevention of cancers, heart disease, menopausal symptoms, and osteoporosis.

Recent reports indicate that phytoestrogens exert their effects in selective estrogen receptor modulators (SERMs) -like manner [7]. The plant food sources high in phytoestrogens are numerous and include soybeans, flaxseeds, and certain other fruits and vegetables rich in polyphenolic compounds.

Sophora japonica L. family Fabaceae, is a tree native to China and Korea. It is also named Japanese pagoda tree (Enju) or Chinese scholar tree. It has been used in Chinese traditional medicine as a haemostatic agent. Flavones from the buds and pericarp were discovered as haemostatic constituents [8,9]. Triterpenes, phospholipids, alkaloids, amino acids and fatty acids have been reported as the main chemical constituents of the seeds of this plant [10,11].

The naringinase-digested methanol extract of *S. japonica* seeds showed potent estrogen agonist activity due to its genistein and kaempferol contents [12]. Genistein from *S. japonica* was also reported to prevent osteoporosis [13]. Moreover, *in-vivo* studies have shown that *S. japonica* extracts prevented bone loss, partly by inhibiting osteoclastic activity [14]. Dichloromethane (DCM) of *S. japonica* fruit extract stimulated alkaline phosphatase activity and matrix mineralization. The DCM fraction also induced expression of osteoblast markers such as alkaline phosphatase, osterix, and osteocalcin in C3H10T1/2 cells and primary bone marrow cells [15].

In the present study the major phenolic compounds from *S. japonica* seed were isolated and their estrogenic activity was determined in MCF-7 cells. Compound that proved highest estrogenic proliferative activity was tested *in-vivo* for its osteoprotective effect in ovarectomized rats.

Results

The methanol extract of *S. japonica* seeds was partitioned with chloroform and the remaining water soluble portion was fractionated on a Diaion HP-20 column to afford 25%, 50%, and 100% methanol fractions. The 50% methanol fraction was purified on several silica gel, ODS and Sephadex LH-20 columns to produce seven compounds. The identification of isolated compounds was achieved systematically by trying the response of the isolated compounds to different spray reagents using thin layer chromatography (TLC) aiming to identify the nature of the compounds. ^{1}H NMR study was carried out for all compounds to, un-ambiguously, identify its structure. Compounds with more than one sugar moiety such as compounds **3–6** were further subjected to ^{13}C NMR measurement to clearly identify site of sugar attachment (Figure S1–S5). The identity of compounds was confirmed by comparing NMR data with previously reported ones as (Figure S1–S5, Table S1), genistin (**1**) [16], sophoricoside (**2**) [17], sophorabioside (**3**), sophoraflavonoloside (**4**), genistein 7,4'-di-*O*-*β*-D-glucopyransoide (**5**) [18], kaempferol 3-*O*-α-L-rhamnopyranosyl(1→6)*β*-D-glucopyranosyl(1→2)*β*-D-glucopyranoside (**6**) [19], and rutin (**7**) (Fig. 1). Purity of all isolated compounds was confirmed through HPLC analysis. The purity of compounds **4–6** was over 92%, while that of the remaining compounds was over 95% as indicated by their HPLC chromatograms (Figure S6).

The estrogenic/proliferative properties of compounds isolated from *S. japonica* in MCF-7 cell line

The proliferative effect in estrogen dependent MCF-7 cell line of the isolated compounds was tested. Sub-cytotoxic dose range with potential estrogenic proliferative effect of compounds under investigation was determined using trypan blue exclusion assay and further confirmed using LDH leakage assay.

Trypan blue positive cells was less than 50% after exposure to all compounds under investigation indicative of negative cytotoxic effect until 100 µM concentration. Exposure to 1 mM of compounds **3**, **4**, **6**, and **7** induced trypan staining in more than 50% of cells. On the other hand, exposure to compounds **1**, **2**, and **5** showed trypan blue positive cells less than 1% until 100 µM concentration; and accordingly these compounds can be considered the safest to cell integrity (Table 1).

Effect of compounds under investigation on the cell membrane integrity was further confirmed using more sensitive technique (LDH leakage assay). Exposure to 1 µM of compounds **3**, **4** and **6** induced 2.2, 2.6 and 2.8 folds LDH leakage that in the control group, respectively. The concentration of LDH in media was about 5 folds control group after exposure to 100 µM of compounds **3**, **4** and **6**. On the other hand, the amount of LDH in media over cells treated with concentrations less than 10 µM of compounds **1**, **2**, **5**, and **7** did not exceed double the concentration of LDH leakage in control group. These indicate the harmless effect of these compounds on cell membrane (Figure 2-A).

With respect to the proliferative effect in MCF-7 cell, compounds **3**, **4**, and **6** did not show any significant proliferation enhancement after 72 h of exposure to concentration range of 0.01 to 100 µM. The proliferative effect of compounds **1**, **2**, and **5** was significant in MCF-7 starting from a concentration of 0.01 µM (1.4, 1.5, and 1.2 folds, respectively); and most prominent at concentration of 0.1 µM showing 1.5, 1.6, and 1.3 folds, respectively (Figure 2-B). Based on the cytotoxicity profile, effect on membrane integrity and estrogenic proliferative activity; compound **2** (sophoricoside) was selected for further studies as a potential anti-osteoporosis agent *in-vivo*.

Anti-osteoporosis effect of sophoricoside *in-vivo*

The anti-osteoporosis effect of sophoricoside was investigated mechanically and biochemically in ovarectomized rats after oral administration (15 mg/kg and 30 mg/kg) for 45 days compared to estradiol (10 µg/kg). Mechanical hardness of femur bones was determined after applying longitudinal and vertical forces to the bone shaft and identifying the breaking point pressure.

Mechanically, the forces required to break the femur bones longitudinally and vertically were significantly decreased in response to ovarectomy to be 34% and 56% of the normal bone hardness, respectively. Treatment with E_2 (10 µg/kg) and low dose SPH (15 mg/kg) did not affect the bone hardness in response to longitudinal force; however high dose SPH (30 mg/kg) improved the bone hardness by 43.3% compared to OVX group. In other words, treatment with SPH (30 mg/kg) regained the original longitudinal bone hardness (Figure 3-A). On the other hand, treatment with E_2 (10 µg/kg), SPH (15 mg/g) and SPH (30 mg/kg) significantly improved bone hardness to vertical force by 89.3% and 97.4%, respectively compared to OVX group (Figure 3-B).

Osteoporosis was assessed biochemically by measuring the serum concentration of alkaline phosphatase (ALP) and osteocalcin (OC) as markers for bone formation. In addition, acid phosphatase (ACP) was measured as an indicator for bone resorption. Serum level of ALP was significantly decreased in OVX group indicative of osteoporosis. Treatment with E_2 significantly increased the level of ALP to above normal level. Treatment with sophoricoside (15 mg/kg) significantly increased the level of ALP and brought it to normal level. However, treatment with sophoricoside (30 mg/kg) increased the level of ALP to be higher than normal group (Figure 3- C).

Similar to ALP, Serum level of OC was significantly decreased to about half its original value in response to ovarectomy confirming the incidence of osteoporosis. Treatment with E_2 significantly increased the level of OC back to its normal level. Treatment with sophoricoside (15 mg/kg) did not significantly increase the serum level of OC compared to OVX group. However, treatment with sophoricoside (30 mg/kg) significantly increased the level of OC to 78% higher than normal group non-ovarectomized animals (Figure 3- D).

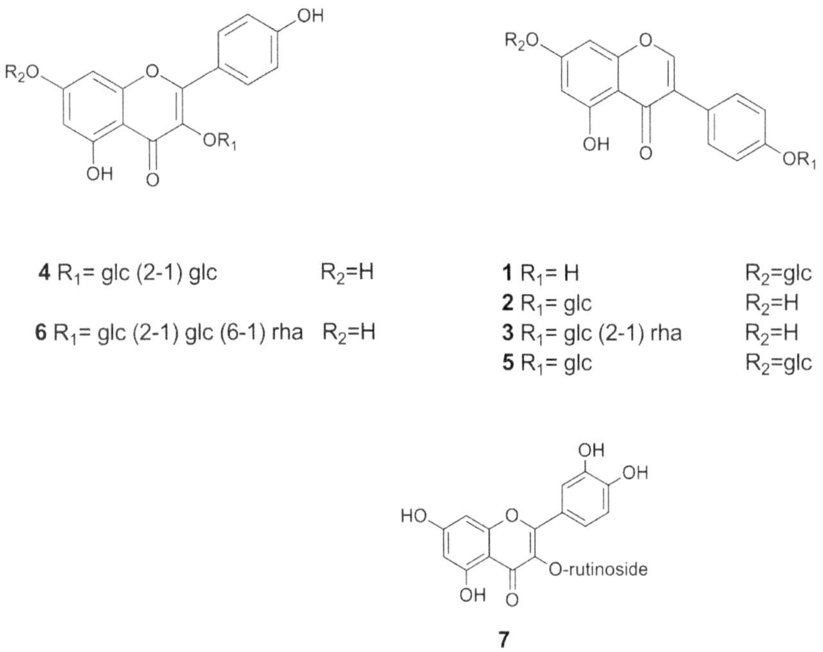

Figure 1. Chemical structure for compounds isolated from *Sophora japonica* seeds.

Serum level of ACP was significantly increased (60% compared to control group) in response to OVX indicating prominent hormone dependent bone resorption. ACP level was significantly depressed by E_2 treatment to reach 17.2% of OVX group level. Treatment with sophoricoside (15 mg/kg) significantly decreased the level of ACP and brought it to normal level. Surprisingly, treatment with sophoricoside (30 mg/kg) extensively decreased the level of ACP to be only 4.5% of OVX group level (Figure 3- E).

Histopathological assessment of the anti-osteoporosis effect of sophoricoside

The anti-osteoporotic effect of sophoricoside was confirmed pathologically. Histological pictures of femurs of normal animals showed intact, well-formed, dense bony trabeculae with osteoblastic rimming and average intervening bone marrow (Fig. 4-A). Ovarectomy resulted in prominent osteoporosis in OVX group manifested as thin and widely separated trabeculae with notched and eroded surfaces (Fig. 4-B). Estradiol partly reversed the osteoporosis status showing thicker bony trabeculae and more osteoid and osteoblastic rimming compared to OVX group (Fig. 4-C). Sophoricoside ameliorated the ovarectomy induced osteoporosis in a dose dependent manner. Femurs of animals treated with SPH (15 mg/kg) showed thicker bony trabeculae, more osteoid, and more osteoblastic rimming compared to OVX group (Fig. 4-D). Femurs of animals treated with higher dose of SPH (30 mg/kg) showed thicker bony trabeculae, higher osteoid activity with narrow bone marrow spaces compared to OVX group (Fig. 4-E).

Discussion

Osteoporosis is a major health problem particularly for post-menopause women due to hormonal deficiency [15]. The osteoprotective use of natural compounds with estrogenic activity enabled the avoidance of estrogen replacement therapy and its debilitating side effects [15]. Natural products with inherit nutritional value on top of estrogenic activity such as *S. japonica* represent an interesting nutraceutical alternative for osteoporosis [20–22]. In the current study, we examined the estrogenic proliferative activity of seven compounds isolated from *S. Japonica*

Table 1. Cytotoxicity assessment of compounds isolated from *S. Japonica* using trypan blue exclusion assay.

Cpd	Compound name	Percent dead cells				
		0.1 μM	1 μM	10 μM	100 μM	1 mM
1	Genistin	<1%	<1%	<1%	<1%	42.5±3.6%
2	Sophoricoside	<1%	<1%	<1%	<1%	39.2±2.8%
3	Sophorabicoside	<1%	<1%	2.4±0.2%	15.7±2.7%	63.9±5.1%
4	Sophoraflavonoloside	<1%	1.5±0.3%	8.3±2.6%	17.5±3.1%	74.2±7.4%
5	genistein glucoside	<1%	<1%	<1%	<1%	41.7±3.7%
6	kaempferol glucoside	2.6±0.8%	8.6±1.5%	14.8±3.6%	21.7±4.2%	87.3±5.1%
7	Rutin	<1%	<1%	6.8±2.15	14.3±3.1%	68.5±4.9%

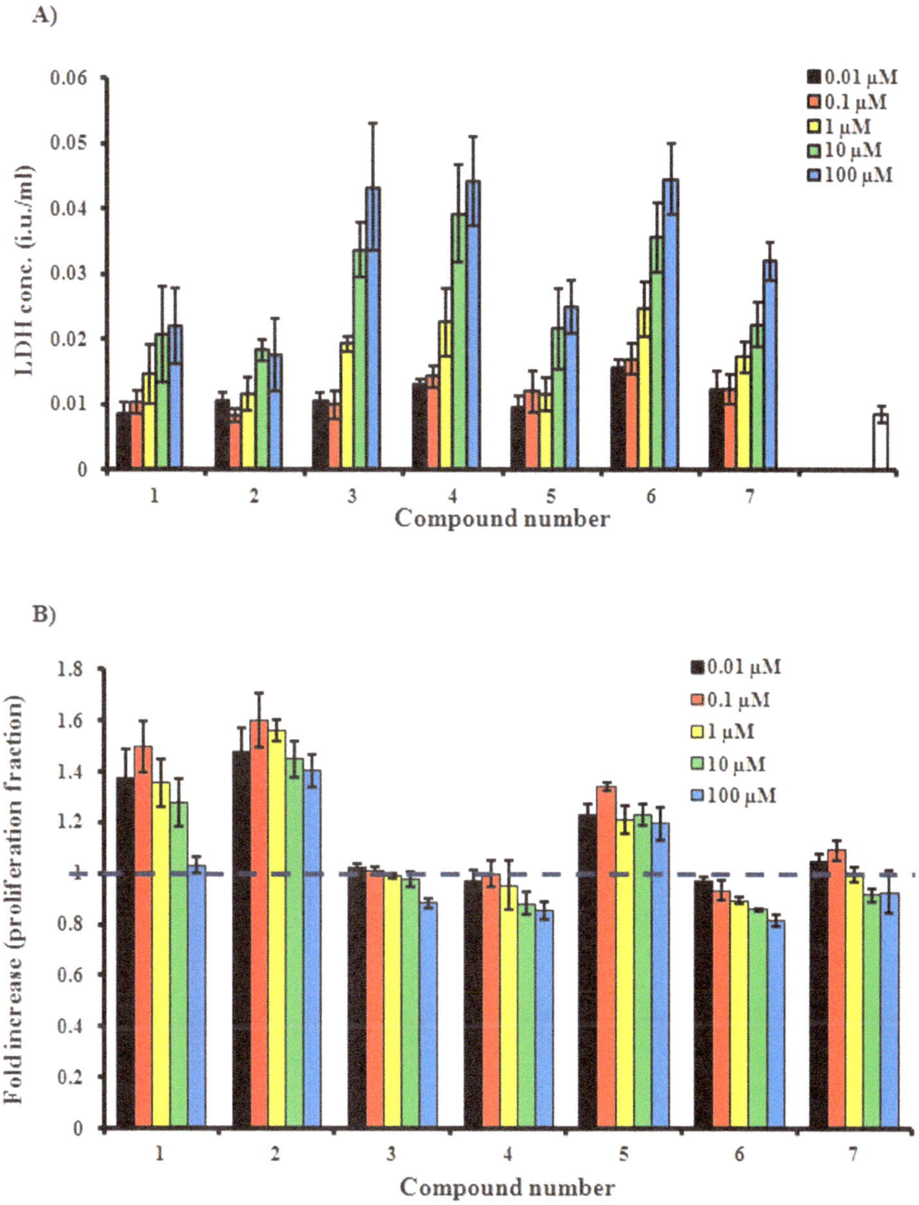

Figure 2. Assessing the estrogenic properties of compounds isolated from *S. japonica* in estrogen dependent MCF-7 cell line. Sub-cytotoxic concentrations of the isolated compounds were determined using LDH leakage assay (A); and proliferative effect was determined using SRB assay (B).

in the estrogen dependent MCF-7 cell line. The best candidate estrogenic compound (Sophoricoside) was further tested for potential osteo-protective activity using ovarectomized rat model.

In the current study, genistin, sophoricoside and genistein 7,4'-di-*O*-*β*-D-glucopyransoide showed significant proliferative activity in estrogen dependent MCF-7 cell line in a subcytotoxic concentration range. Sophoricoside which is highly abundant phytoestrogen in the methanolic extract of *S. Japonica* seeds [12] did not induce any tangible cell membrane damage up to 100 µM concentration. In a previous report, prominent anti-osteoporosis effect of dichloromethane extract of *S. Japonica* fruits was attributed to the high content of the genistein aglycone as evidenced by LC-MS analysis [15]. Sophoricoside which is another genistein glycoside, possess potent estrogenic activity as assessed in our previous work using yeast hybrid assay [12].

Herein, sophoricoside (15 mg/kg and 30 mg/kg) showed promising and dose dependent osteo-protective effect against ovarectomy induced osteoporosis rat model compared to estradiol. Sophoricoside improved the mechanical bone hardness in ovarectomized rats after treatment for 6 weeks. Sophoricoside (4–16 mg/kg for 4 weeks) improved the pathological picture of trabecular bones in ovarectomized rats in previous report [20]; however, herein both mechanical as well as pathological evidences are presented for the osteo-protective effect of sophoricoside. In addition, it was observed that sophoricoside induced significant elevation in the osteogenic biochemical markers such as serum alkaline phosphate and osteocalcin.

Osteo-protective effect of sophoricoside might be attributed to the resulting genistein after hydrolysis in GIT flora or directly to the parent compound *per se*. Therefore, the use of the total

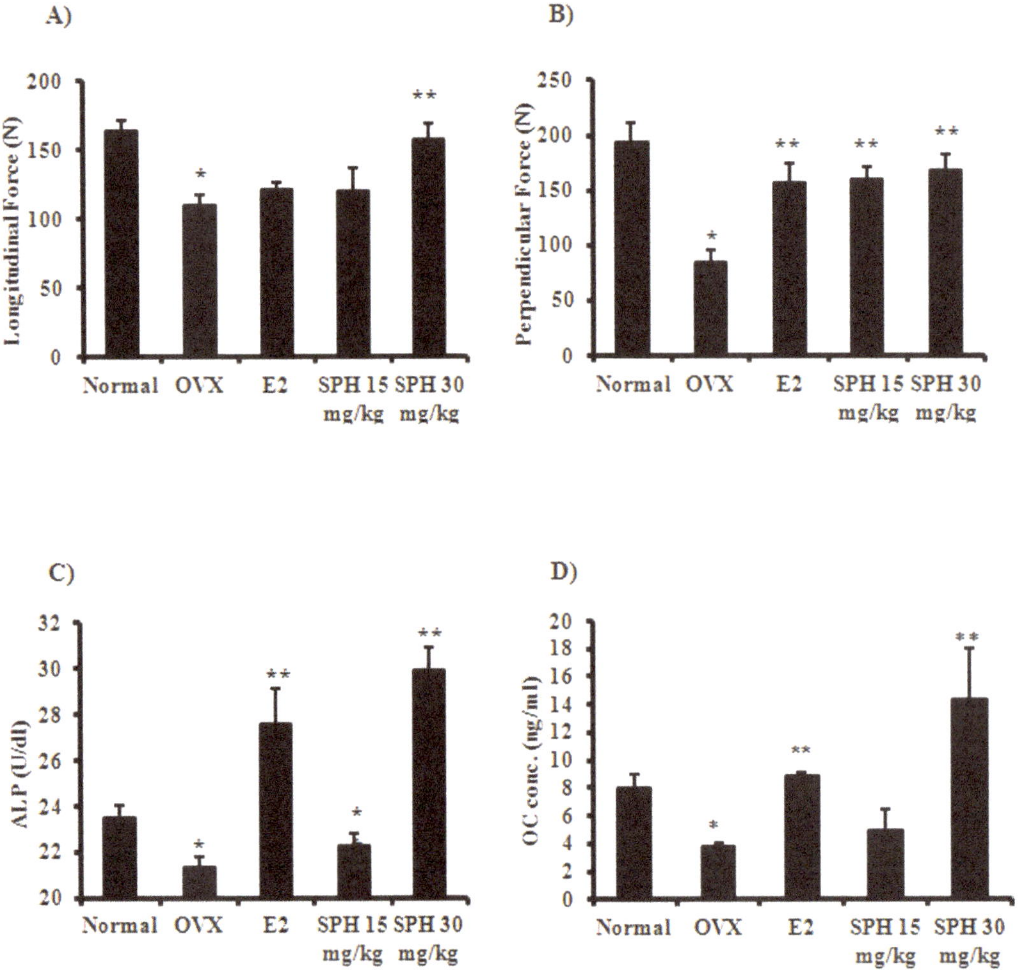

Figure 3. Mechanical and biochemical assessment for anti-osteoporosis effect of sophoricoside *in-vivo*. Ovariectomized rats were treated with SPH (15 mg/kg and 30 mg/kg) for 6 weeks and compared to E_2 treated animals (10 µg/kg) and sham-operation group. Mechanical hardness was evaluated using hardness tester along (A) and perpendicular (B) to femur bone shaft. Biochemical assessment of osteoporosis was evaluated by measuring serum alkaline phosphatase (C) and osteocalcin (D) at the end of treatment period.

alcoholic extract of *S. japonica* seeds could be as effective as sophoricoside due to its high content of geniestein-derived glycosides which will be transformed to genistein upon hydrolysis by GIT flora.

Materials and Methods

General

TLC was carried out on precoated Silica gel 60 F_{254} (0.25 mm, Merck) and RP-18 F_{254}S (0.25 mm, Merck Co., Dermstadt) and spots were detected under UV light or after spraying with anisaldehyde-H_2SO_4 reagent followed by heating. Column chromatography (CC) was carried out on (BW-820MH silica gel), Wakosil C-300 (40–64 µm) (Wako, Osaka, Japan), ODS DM 1020T (ODS, Fuji Silysia, Nagoya, Japan), Diaion HP-20 (Mitsubishi Kasei, Tokyo, Japan) and Sephadex LH-20 (Pharmacia Co.). Medium pressure liquid chromatography (MPLC) was performed on LiChroprep RP-18 and LiChroprep Si 60 (size A and B, Merck Co.). HPLC analysis was conducted on Agilent 1200 liquid chromatography equipped a photodiode array detector. A C18 reversed-phase packing column (4.5 mm×15 cm, 5 µm) were used for separation throughout this study.

Plant material

Seeds of *S. japonica* were collected from the ripe fruits cultivated in the Medicinal Plant Station of Faculty of Pharmacy, Cairo University during December 2012. Authentication of the plant was established by Ass. Prof. Dr. Sherif El-Khanagry, Agriculture Museum, El-Dokki, Cairo, Egypt. A Herbarium specimen (SJ-1023) was prepared and kept at the Herbarium of the Department of Natural Products and Alternative Medicine, Faculty of Pharmacy, King Abdulaziz University.

Extraction and isolation

The pulverized seeds of *S. japonica* (1300 g) were extracted with MeOH (1L x 3) at room temperature and the combined extract was evaporated in *vacuo*. The methanol extract (104 g) was suspended in MeOH and water and successively partitioned with hexane and chloroform to produce hexane (31 g) and chloroform (4 g) soluble fractions. The remaining aqueous layer was fractionated on a Diaion HP-20 column (60 cm×6 cm) stepwisely eluted with H_2O, 25%, 50% and 100% MeOH. The eluates were evaporated under vacuum to afford H_2O fraction (26 g), 25% MeOH fraction (8.5 g), 50% MeOH fraction (14 g) and 100% MeOH fraction 5.8 g. The 50% MeOH (12 g) was applied to a

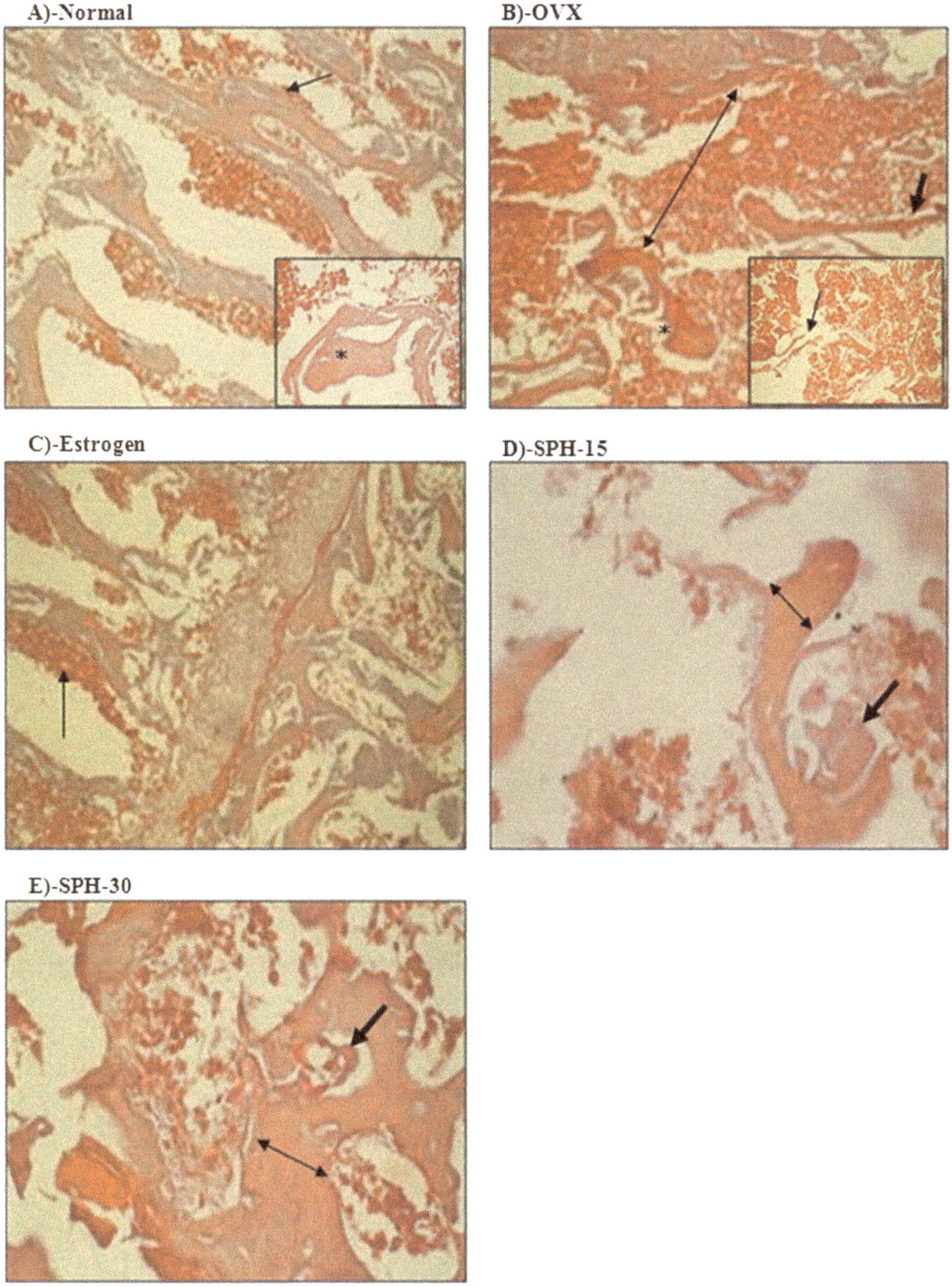

Figure 4. Histopathological assessment of the anti-osteoporosis effect of sophoricoside. Normal group (A) shows normal bony tissue with intact well-formed dense trabeculae (star in the inner panel) with osteoblastic rimming (arrow) and average intervening bone marrow. OVX group (B) showed scant, disconnected (arrow in inner panel), thin (arrow in the outer panel), and widely separated trabeculae (double-headed arrow in the outer panel) with eroded surface (star in the outer panel). Estrogen treated group (C) showed widely distributed osteoid and osteoblastic rimming (arrow). SPH-15 group (D) showed thick trabeculae (double-headed arrow), more osteoid, and osteoblastic activity (arrow). SPH-30 group (E) showed thick trabeculae (double-headed arrow), more osteoid and osteoblastic activity (arrow).

silica gel column (300 g silica) and gradienltly eluted with $CHCl_3$-MeOH-H_2O (9:1:0.1 v/v/v) to obtain 8 fractions. Fraction 3 (2 g) gave a yellow precipitate upon concentration, that was washed several times by chloroform-methanol to obtain compound **3** (193 mg). The supernatant of this fraction was purified on an MPLC RP-18 column (size A) using MeOH-H_2O (4:6 v/v) to afford compounds **1** (120 mg), and **2** (500 mg). Fraction 4 gave compound **4** (358 mg) upon crystallization from MeOH and the remaining supernatant was applied to an MPLC RP-18 column (size A) eluted with MeOH-H_2O (3:7 v/v) to get **7** (5 mg). Fraction 5 gave compound **5** (180 mg) by crystallization from MeOH-$CHCl_3$.Fraction 6 (1.5 g) was purified on a Sephadex LH-

20 column (30 cm×3 cm) eluted with MeOH-H_2O (1:1 v/v). Subfractions 17–30 of this column was combined together and applied to an MPLC RP-18 column (size A) eluted with MeOH-H_2O (3:7 v/v) to get compound **6** (37.4 mg). Purity of all compounds were analyzed using HPLC using a gradient elution (water – TFA, 0.1% v/v) to solvent B (acetonitrile), with a flow rate of 1.0 ml min

Chemicals and drugs

Sulfarhodamine B (SRB) and 17β-hydroxyesradiol were purchased from Sigma-Aldrich Chemical Company (St. Louis, MO, USA), RPMI-1640 media, fetal bovine serum and other cell culture materials were purchased from Euroclone (Milano, Italy). Urethane was purchased from Biobasic Inc. (Toronto, Canada). All other chemicals were of the highest available analytical grade.

Cell culture

Human estrogen dependent breast adenocarcinoma cells (MCF-7 cell line) were obtained from the Vacsera (Giza, Egypt). Cells were maintained in RPMI-1640 supplemented with 100 μg/mL streptomycin, 100 units/mL penicillin and 10% heat-inactivated fetal bovine serum in a humidified, 5% (v/v) CO_2 atmosphere at 37°C.

Cytotoxicity assessment

Cytotoxicity of compounds isolated from *S. Japonica* was tested in MCF-7 cells by trypan-blue exclusion assay. Briefly, exponentially growing cells were plated in 96-well plates. Cells were exposed to serial dilutions of isolated compounds for 2, 4, 7 and 10 days and the percent of trypan blue positive cells was determined in live culture [1,23].

Cell membrane integrity assessment

The influence of compounds isolated from *S. Japonica* against the cell membrane integrity was assessed in MCF-7 cells by LDH leakage assay [24]. Briefly, exponentially growing cells were plated in 6-well plates. Cells were exposed to serial concentrations of isolated compounds for 24 h and the LDH was determined in the culture media using colorimetric assay (Biosystems, Barcelona, Spain).

Proliferation assay

The proliferative effect of compounds isolated from *S. Japonica* was tested in MCF-7 cells by SRB assay as well. Briefly, exponentially growing cells were exposed to sub-cytotoxic concentrations of the isolated compounds for 72 h and subsequently stained with SRB solution for quantification [25,26].

Animals and animal treatment

Animal handling and treatment was approved by the bioethical and research committee of The National Research Center. Female Sprague Drawly rats (300 g weight) were acclimatized in the animal house facility of The National Research Center, Cairo, Egypt, for at least one week prior to experimentation. Animals were kept at 20±2°C and 65±10% relative humidity during the whole experiment. Standard food pellets and water were supplied *ad labium*. All experiments were performed between 8–10 A.M.

Osteoporosis was induced in rats by ovarectomy as previously described with minor modification [3]. Briefly, rats in the same menstrual phase were selected and confirmed by vaginal smear and underwent experimental ovarectomy. Animals were anesthetized by i.p. injection of urethane (1 g/kg). Surgical incision of about 5 mm was made in each of the hind dorsal flank regions of rats exposing the ovary and surrounding periovarian fat bed. Both fallopian tubes were suture-closed at the most distal end and both ovaries were surgically excised carefully. The incision was sutured and dressed with sterile povidone iodine solution. Sham operations were performed to animals of control groups. Animal were let for two weeks to recover from the surgical trauma. Then, animals were divided into 5 groups (n = 10 per group). Control group which was subjected to sham operation; OVX group was surgically ovarectomized and received saline vehicle daily. Estrogen group (E_2) was subjected to surgical ovarectomy and received 17β-estradiol (10 μg/kg) via i.p. injection daily; sophoricoside low dose group (SPH-15) was subjected to surgical ovarectomy and received sophoricoside (15 mg/kg) p.o. daily. Sophoricoside high dose group (SPH-30) was subjected to surgical ovarectomy and received sophoricoside (30 mg/kg) p.o. daily. All animals were allowed free access for food and water throughout the whole experiment (45 day). Blood samples were withdrawn by retro-orbital plexus puncture; and the serum was collected then animals were sacrificed by cervical dislocation. Both right and left femur bones were dissected immediately *post mortem*; left femurs were used to measure hardness; and the right femurs were fixed in buffered formalin solution (4%) for histological assessment.

Bone hardness assessment

To quantify the degree of osteoporosis, hardness of left femurs was measured using hardness tester (Erweka GmbH, Heusenstamm, Germany) as previously described with minor modification [27]. Briefly, left femurs were placed in the clamp assembly of the hardness tester in a vertical (n = 5) and horizontal (n = 5) positions to the force direction. Minimum force required to induce bone shaft fracture was recorded.

Serological evaluation of osteoporosis in-vivo

To assess the ossification process in response to treatment with sophoricoside, serum level of alkaline phosphatase (ALP), acid phophatase (ACP) and osteocalcin (OC) were measured. ALP and tartarate-resistant ACP were determined by direct HTS-ready colorimetric assay (Abcam, Cambridge, UK) [28]. Osteocalcin was determined using Uscan immunoassay ELISA Kit (Life Science Inc. Wuhan, China) according to the manufacturer's instructions [29].

Histological examination for rat lamellar bone tissue

Histological assessment for lamellar bone was performed according the lab routine protocol. Briefly, paraformaldhyde fixed tissues were decalcified by EDTA and embedded in paraffin wax. Cross vertical sections (5 μm) were obtained and after dewaxing and rehydration sections were stained with H&E.

Statistical analysis

Data are presented as mean ± SEM. Analysis of variance (ANOVA) with LSD post hoc test was used for testing the significance using SPSS for windows, version 17.0.0. $p<0.05$ was taken as a cut off value for significance.

Author Contributions

Conceived and designed the experiments: HMA AMA ABA AME. Performed the experiments: HMA AMA GFA AME. Analyzed the data: AMA AME. Contributed reagents/materials/analysis tools: HMA AMA. Wrote the paper: HMA AMA GFA AME.

References

1. Cowan JD, Von Hoff DD, Neuenefldt B, Mills LS GM, Clark GM (1984) Predictive value of trypan blue exclusion viability measurements for colony formation in a human tumor cloning assay. Canc Drug Del 1: 95–100.
2. Gruber HE, Ivey JL, Baylink DJ, Matthews M, Nelp WB, et al. (1984) Long-term calcitonin therapy in postmenopausal osteoporosis. Metabolism 33: 295–303.
3. Reddy NP, Lakshmana M (2005) Assessment of experimental osteoporosis using CT-scanning, quantitative X-ray analysis and impact test in calcium deficient ovariectomized rats. J Pharmacol Toxicol 52: 350–355.
4. Obrant KJ, Bengner U, Johnell O, Nilsson BE, Sernbo I (1989) Increasing age-adjusted risk of fragility fractures: a sign of increasing osteoporosis in successive generations? Calcif Tissue Int 44: 157–167.
5. Addar M, El Desouki M, Babay Z (2004) Correlates of age at menopause and osteoporosis in Saudi women. Clin Exp Obstet Gyn 32: 135–137.
6. Sadat-Ali M, Al-Habdan IM, Al-Mulhim FA, El-Hassan AY (2004) Bone mineral density among postmenopausal Saudi women. Saudi Med J 25: 1623–1625.
7. Brzezinski A, Debi A (1999) Phytoestrogens: the "natural" selective estrogen receptor modulators? Eur J Obstet Gyn R B 85: 47–51.
8. Ishida H, Umino T, Tsuji K, Kosuge T (1989) Studies on the anti-hemorrhagic substances in herbs classified as hemostatics in Chinese medicine. X. On hemostatic activities of the parched herbs for hemostatics]. Yakugaku zasshi 109: 179.
9. Tang Y, Lou F, Wang J, Zhuang S (2001) Four New Isoflavone Triglycosides from *Sophora japonica*. J Nat Prod 64: 1107–1110.
10. Grishkovets V, Gorbacheva L (1995) Triterpene glycosides of*Sophora japonica* seeds. Chem Nat Comp 31: 596–599.
11. Mukhamedova KS, Glushenkova A (1997) Phospholipids of ripeSophora japonica seeds. Chem Nat Comp 33: 445–448.
12. El-Halawany AM, Chung MH, Abdallah HM, Nishihara T, Hattori M (2010) Estrogenic activity of a naringinase-treated extract of *Sophora japonica* cultivated in Egypt. Pharm Biol 48: 177–181.
13. Wang Z, Sun J, Wang D, Xie Y, Wang S, et al. (2006) Pharmacological studies of the large-scaled purified genistein from Huaijiao *Sophora japonica* – Leguminosae) on anti-osteoporosis. Phytomedicine 13: 718–723.
14. Shim JG, Yeom SH, Kim HJ, Choi YW, Song KY, et al. (2005) Bone loss preventing effect of Sophorae Fructus on ovariectomized rats. Arch Pharm Res 28: 106–110.
15. Yoon H-J, Seo C-R, Kim M, Kim Y-J, Song N-J, et al. (2013) Dichloromethane extracts of *Sophora japonica* L. stimulate osteoblast differentiation in mesenchymal stem cells. Nutr Res 33: 1035–1062.
16. Mostafa K, Ahmed A, Ali A (2003) Chemical constituents and antidiabetic activity of *Trifolium alexandrinum* L. Bull Fac Pharm 41: 253–263.
17. Min B, Oh SR, Lee H-K, Takatsu K, Chang I-M, et al. (1999) Sophoricoside analogs as the IL-5 inhibitors from *Sophora japonica*. Planta Med 65: 408–412.
18. Watanabe K, Kinjo J, Nohara T (1993) Three new isoflavonoid glycosides from *Lupinus luteus* L.and *polyphyllus arboreus*. Chem Pharm Bull 41: 394–396.
19. Tang Y-P, Li Y-F, Hu J, Lou F-C (2002) Isolation and identification of antioxidants from *Sophora japonica*. J Asian Nat Prod Res 4: 123–128.
20. Du N, Xu Y, Chen WZ, Zhang FH (2003) [Effect of Sophoricoside on histomorphology of bone in ovariectomized rats]. Zhong Xi Yi Jie He Xue Bao 1: 44–46.
21. Jia TL, Wang HZ, Xie LP, Wang XY, Zhang RQ (2003) Daidzein enhances osteoblast growth that may be mediated by increased bone morphogenetic protein (BMP) production. Biochem Pharmacol 65: 709–715.
22. Shim JG, Yeom SH, Kim HJ, Choi YW, Lee DI, et al. (2005) Bone loss preventing effect of Sophorae Fructus on ovariectomized rats. Arch Pharm Res 28: 106–110.
23. Mahmoud AM, Al-Abd AM, Lightfoot DA, El-Shemy HA (2012) Anti-cancer characteristics of mevinolin against three different solid tumor cell lines was not solely p53-dependent. J Enzyme Inhib Med Chem 27: 673–679.
24. Phillips CA, Hughes DR, Huja SS (2009) Modifications of the lactate dehydrogenase assay, a histochemical determinant of osteocyte viability–A qualitative study. Acta Histochem 111: 166–171.
25. Skehan P, Storeng R, Scudiero D, Monks A, McMahon J, et al. (1990) New colorimetric cytotoxicity assay for anticancer-drug screening. J Natl Cancer I 82: 1107–1112.
26. Mosli HA, Tolba MF, Al-Abd AM, Abdel-Naim AB (2013) Catechol estrogens induce proliferation and malignant transformation in prostate epithelial cells. Toxicol Lett 220: 247–258.
27. Ko Y-J, Wu J-B, Ho H-Y, Lin W-C (2012) Antiosteoporotic activity of *Davallia formosana*. J Ethnopharmacol 139: 558–565.
28. Gerhardt W, Nielsen ML, Nielsen OV, Olsen J, Statland B (1974) Clinical evaluation of routine measurement of liver and bone alkaline phosphatases in human serum: Differential inhibition by l-phenylalanine and carbamide (urea) on the LKB 8600 reaction rate analyzer. Clin Chim Acta 53: 291–297.
29. Fu J, Muller D (1999) Simple, rapid enzyme-linked immunosorbent assay (ELISA) for the determination of rat osteocalcin. Calcif Tissue Int 64: 229–233.

5

Age-Related Adaptation of Bone-PDL-Tooth Complex: *Rattus-Norvegicus* as a Model System

Narita L. Leong[1], Jonathan M. Hurng[1], Sabra I. Djomehri[1], Stuart A. Gansky[2], Mark I. Ryder[3], Sunita P. Ho[1]*

1 Division of Biomaterials & Bioengineering, University of California San Francisco, San Francisco, California, United States of America, **2** Division of Oral Epidemiology & Dental Public Health, Department of Preventive and Restorative Dental Sciences, University of California San Francisco, San Francisco, California, United States of America, **3** Division of Periodontology, Department of Orofacial Sciences, University of California San Francisco, San Francisco, California, United States of America

Abstract

Functional loads on an organ induce tissue adaptations by converting mechanical energy into chemical energy at a cell-level. The transducing capacity of cells alters physico-chemical properties of tissues, developing a positive feedback commonly recognized as the form-function relationship. In this study, organ and tissue adaptations were mapped in the bone-tooth complex by identifying and correlating biomolecular expressions to physico-chemical properties in rats from 1.5 to 15 months. However, future research using hard and soft chow over relevant age groups would decouple the function related effects from aging affects. Progressive curvature in the distal root with increased root resorption was observed using micro X-ray computed tomography. Resorption was correlated to the increased activity of multinucleated osteoclasts on the distal side of the molars until 6 months using tartrate resistant acid phosphatase (TRAP). Interestingly, mononucleated TRAP positive cells within PDL vasculature were observed in older rats. Higher levels of glycosaminoglycans were identified at PDL-bone and PDL-cementum entheses using alcian blue stain. Decreasing biochemical gradients from coronal to apical zones, specifically biomolecules that can induce osteogenic (biglycan) and fibrogenic (fibromodulin, decorin) phenotypes, and PDL-specific negative regulator of mineralization (asporin) were observed using immunohistochemistry. Heterogeneous distribution of Ca and P in alveolar bone, and relatively lower contents at the entheses, were observed using energy dispersive X-ray analysis. No correlation between age and microhardness of alveolar bone (0.7±0.1 to 0.9±0.2 GPa) and cementum (0.6±0.1 to 0.8±0.3 GPa) was observed using a microindenter. However, hardness of cementum and alveolar bone at any given age were significantly different ($P<0.05$). These observations should be taken into account as baseline parameters, during development (1.5 to 4 months), growth (4 to 10 months), followed by a senescent phase (10 to 15 months), from which deviations due to experimentally induced perturbations can be effectively investigated.

Editor: Hani A. Awad, University of Rochester, United States of America

Funding: This work was supported by: NIH/NIDCR R01DE022032 (SPH), NIH/NIDCR R00 DE018212 (SPH) and NIH/NCRR 1S10RR026645 (SPH), Division of Bioengineering and Biomaterials, Department of Preventive and Restorative Dental Sciences, UCSF; The Praxis Fund and the Benjamin Dienstein Fund, Division of Periodontology, Department of Orofacial Sciences, UCSF. The funders had no role in study design, data collection and analysis, decision to publish, or preparation of the manuscript.

Competing Interests: The authors have declared that no competing interests exist.

* E-mail: sunita.ho@ucsf.edu

Introduction

The change in morphology or form of an organ throughout development, growth, and senescent phases of an organism, is mediated by genetic and epigenetic factors [1,2,3,4,5]. The inherited genetic influences dominate morphogenesis in pre-function, which then become basal to the epigenetic factors (for e.g. functional loads) that mediate organ adaptation over a prolonged time [5]. Prolonged time alters form-function behavior due to load-related changes at an organ level and strain-related events at a cellular level.

Cellular events are identified through genetic and protein expressions, which in turn promote physico-chemical changes in tissues. Physico-chemical changes include mineral formation or resorption, changes in elemental composition, and mechanical resistance of extracellular matrices of tissues. Collectively, these processes occur in several adjoining tissues of the load bearing joint and play a key role in maintaining its functional efficiency. Hence, over prolonged time, tissues adapt to functional demands to maintain mechanical efficiency of an organ [5,6]. However, adaptation over prolonged time also includes effects due to physiological aging of an organism. Acknowledging that aging is a science in and of itself, we present in this study the specific changes in biochemical and physico-chemical properties of the bone-tooth complex in younger, middle-aged, and older rats. This allows us to better understand the rat periodontium and its appropriateness as an animal model for various applications.

The bone-tooth organ in rats is extensively used as a model system to study the effects of various external perturbations, which include extraneous loads and disease states [7,8]. Systematic studies [9] at the cell, tissue, and organ levels [10] continue to be performed on rats because of the limited availability of whole human bone-tooth complexes. Examples include but are not limited to periodontal diseases (gingivitis, periodontitis) [11,12,13,14,15,16,17] and load-mediated effects (traumatic loads using orthodontic braces [7,18], over load using hyper-occlusion

[19] and disuse using hypo-occlusion [20], which parallel skeletal bone adaptation [21]. Despite all these studies, few age-related studies exist on the bone-tooth complex in humans or other model organisms [22,23,24]. Selection of appropriate animal age groups is imperative, as it plays an underlying role when investigating effects of experimental variables. This is because the effect of an experimental variable could be compounded or masked by innate age-related changes (i.e. injury in younger developing patients form minimal scar tissue, in contrast to the more extensive scar tissue formation in older patients). While younger animal models may still be undergoing the complex processes of development and maturation, those in the senescent phase may already be compromised by age associated diseases [25,26].

Age-related differences can also be translated into biochemical and physico-chemical changes, critical to accurate interpretation of experimental factors. These changes in part could be due to the varying response of the mechanosensory system and/or hormonal influences, both of which alter the mechanical efficiency of muscle, bone, and their respective interfaces [27]. There is evidence supporting the loss of functional efficiency in a joint with age due to an innate decrease in metabolic rate of cells within mineralized and soft tissues, as well as the soft-hard and hard-hard tissue interfaces [28,29,30,31,32,33]. To understand function-related changes, time-related functional adaptation of bone was intelligently delineated as modeling, compared to the innate remodeling [34,35,36] of tissues. Modeling dominates in growing rats, where gains in bone formation, strength, and mass were observed due to the dominance of muscle mass in shaping bone as functional units. However, from adulthood (i.e. load-bearing organs well into function), extraneous loads and significant deviations from physiological threshold limits could affect the form or shape of load bearing functional units [37]. Age-related changes in organ biomechanics, were related to the changes in PDL mechanical properties, turnover rate, PDL-width and density [38], along with increased cementum apposition [39]. However, the common denominator for all developed periodontal tissues is functional load. As a result, the rate of change in functional loads with age can alter the rate of mechanobiological events with age [40,41]. These mechanobiological events could manifest as biophysical changes within the load bearing bone, cementum and PDL in rats [42,43].

Markers to identify physico-chemical changes in load bearing tissues include varying distribution and relative contents of inorganic and organic constituents, as well as their resulting mechanical properties. It is well known that across mammalian species, the inorganic constituents in various forms of apatite [44,45,46] and organic constituents [47], such as proteoglycans (PGs), other noncollagenous proteins, and collagen, together affect tissue and interface mechanics [24,48]. Low and high molecular weight glycosaminoglycan (GAG) contents associated with small and large proteoglycans (PGs) were observed to decrease with age in the human periodontium [49], joint articular discs [50], bone [51], and cartilage [52]. In the rat, the amount of PGs decrease in the temporomandibular joint [53], brain [54], and skin [55], with no studies to our knowledge on the rat periodontium. A disproportionate amount of studies continue to be focused on the effects of disease and/or loading of the periodontium, but lack information on age-related changes in structure, chemical composition, and mechanical properties, all of which maintain the load bearing function of the periodontium [16,23,56,57,58,59]. The importance of mapping changes in tissues and organs with respect to time/age addresses the fact that the transducing capacity of cells alters the load bearing nature of tissues, developing a positive feedback, commonly recognized as the form-function relationship of an organ.

This investigation provides various insights at organ and tissue levels of a bone-tooth complex in animal models (i.e. the Sprague Dawley rat) with an increase in age. Specifically, three factors were considered: 1) the ongoing basal adaptation maintaining the tooth-bone complex, 2) changes inherent to the process of aging (providing a timeline from development, growth, through senescence) and 3) identification by mapping changes in biochemical and physico-chemical properties. The innate changes in tissues and organs need to be understood so that meaningful experimental results can be efficiently and accurately extrapolated to intended clinical problems. The results of this investigation set the stage for future studies on distinguishing age-related effects from function-related effects. Function-related effects can be better understood by correlating protein expressions and tissue related physico-chemical changes modulated by diet stiffness [42].

Results

2.1. Occlusal Wear and Morphology of the Root

Light micrographs complemented by micro x-ray computed tomography (MicroXCT) volumetric reconstructions (Fig. 1 and Fig. S2) illustrated structural changes in molars as rats aged. Although in occlusal function by 1.5 months, complete development marked by a closed root apex was not noted until the 4 month time point. From a functional perspective, occlusal wear preceded and continued after complete root formation, which occurred within the 1.5 to 4 month window (Fig. S2). In the reconstructed tomographs, the occlusal surfaces were designated as blue for wear and red for regions of highest contact. Similarly, cratered root surfaces were designated red to represent the density of root resorption. Morphology changes with age were confirmed by an increase in the size of the mandible (Fig. S1) [60] and dentition [61,62], but more interestingly by the mesial curving of the roots caused primarily by secondary cementum apposition (Fig. 1). Root morphology was characterized by the shape and overall root angle with respect to the occlusal plane. Roots in 1.5 month old rats were straight compared to 4 month old rats with mesial curving, and by 10 months the roots assumed a "J" shape (Fig. 1 and Fig. S2).

2.2. Structural Evaluation of the Bone-PDL-cementum Complex

The measured structural parameters were i) cementoenamel junction–alveolar bone crest (CEJ-ABC) distance and the radial widths of ii) primary cementum (PC), iii) secondary cementum (SC), iv) periodontal ligament space adjoining primary cementum (PDL-PC), v) periodontal ligament space adjoining secondary cementum (PDL-SC) (Fig. 2a). The CEJ-ABC distance increased with age (Figs. 1, 2b), a measure of decreasing bone height. Another observation was the loss of CEJ (Fig. 1) around 6 months in the form of a butt joint and the appearance of a gap CEJ [15,63] with further increase in age. Consistent with other observations [60,61,62], increasing cementum apposition, measured as radial width, particularly in SC was noted in rats from 14 to 500 days, (Fig. 2c). While PC spanned the majority of the coronal length in younger age groups, increasing SC deposition spanned the root length with age. Overall PDL-space demonstrated a gradual decrease after 1.5 months and an increase around 10 and 12 months (Fig. 2c). Significant differences (ANOVA $P<0.05$) in coronal PDL-PC width were observed until 10 months, while apical PDL-SC width differed significantly at 1.5 and 15 months (Fig. 2c). Cement lines in bone of younger rats

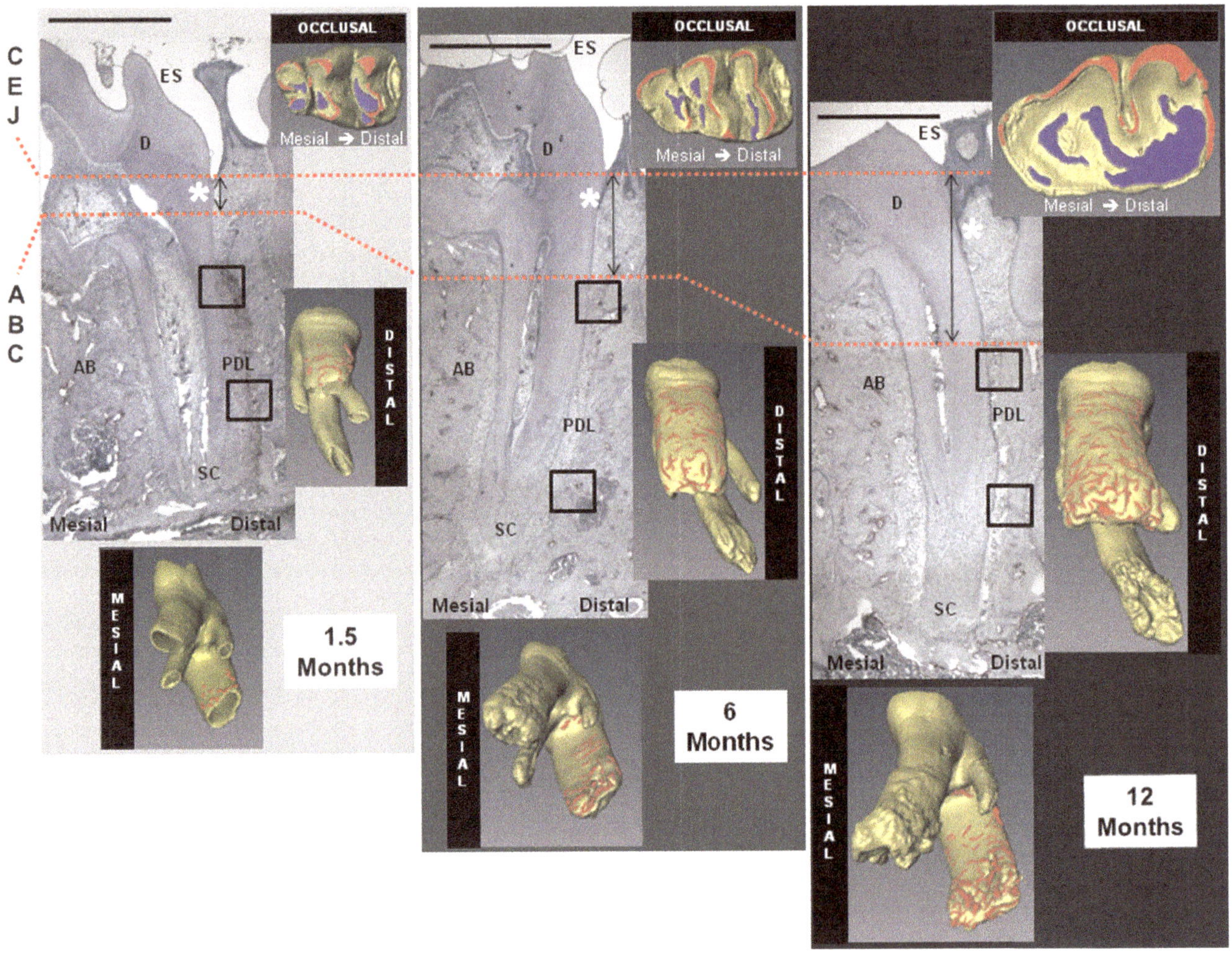

Figure 1. Morphological changes and anatomical locations within TRAP positive cells. Morphological changes were observed in histological sections and confirmed in three dimensional space using a MicroXCT (shown in insets comparing occlusal, distal, and mesial surfaces). The distal preference of TRAP positive cells and progressive mesial curving were observed. Anatomical structures include enamel space (ES), dentin (D), periodontal ligament (PDL), alveolar bone (AB), and secondary cementum (SC). TRAP stained micrographs at 4X magnification show first molar distal roots decreasing in osteoclast intensity and frequency with age. Representative coronal and apical TRAP positive areas in the encircled regions are enlarged in Figure 3. With age, a transition from CEJ to DGJ (demarcated by white asterisk) and increasing recession (CEJ-ABC distance represented by distance between dashed red lines) were observed. Scale bar = 1 millimeter. CEJ: cementoenamel junction; DGJ: dentin gingival junction; ABC: alveolar bone crest.

were observed more on the distal side, but became increasingly prominent on the mesial side with age (data not shown).

2.3. TRAP Histochemistry for Clastic Activity of Bone and Cementum

Bone, PDL and cementum within the complex form a continuum through interfaces, although often considered as discrete tissues. Resorption at the PDL-bone and PDL-cementum attachment sites was identified in all age groups with tartrate resistant acid phosphatase (TRAP) staining for positive mineral resorption cells on soft-hard interfaces observed on all molars (Figs. 1, 3). Quantification of TRAP positive cells confirmed distal preference. Mesial and distal sides were comparable in active resorption only in older 12–15 month age groups (Figs. 3c, 3d). Based on TRAP staining, PDL-cementum resorption was less frequent relative to that of PDL-bone resorption, but was observed in younger 1.5, 4, and 6 month old rats. Overall TRAP positive activity declined in staining intensity and number with age (Figs. 3a, 3b, Figs. S1, S2). Young rats exhibited multinucleated TRAP positive osteoclasts, whereas old rats predominantly contained mononucleated TRAP positive cells. Mononucleated TRAP positive cells were observed at the soft-hard tissue interfaces as well as endosteal and marrow spaces in interradicular and apical bone, including the PDL-space (Figs. 1, indicated by black arrows in 3a, 3b, Fig. S3). TRAP positive clastic activity was complemented by resorption pits observed in tomographies of the adjoining root surfaces (Fig. 1, Fig. S2). The complementary information supports preference of distal apical root resorption and diminishing region specificity with age.

2.4. Alcian Blue Staining for High and Low Molecular Weight Proteoglycans

Localization of alcian blue (Fig. 4) opposes TRAP positive staining (Figs. 1 and 3) in the younger 1.5 month age group. Alcian blue was consistently observed on the PDL-bone enthesis of the mesial and interradicular surfaces of the roots in younger rats

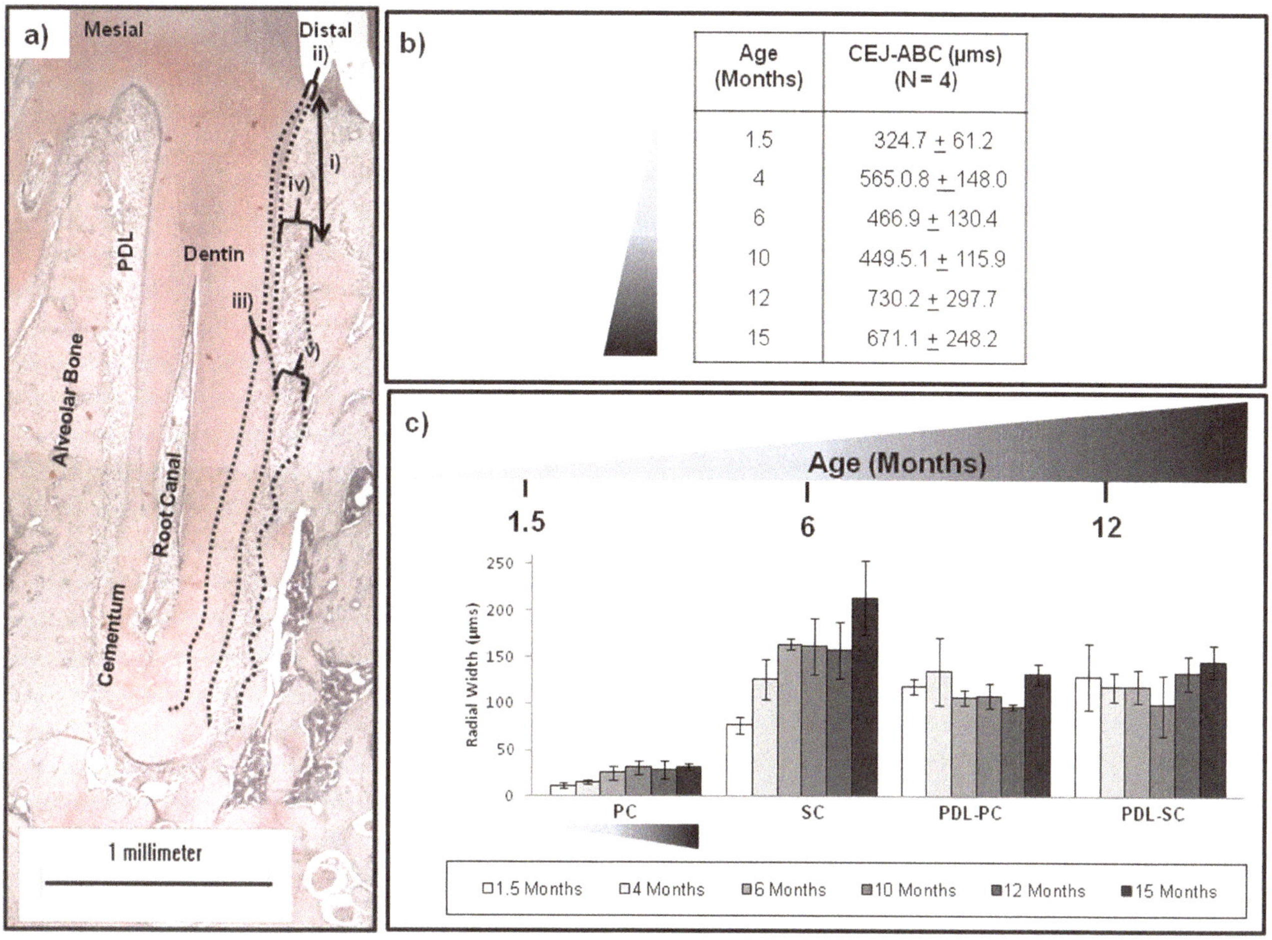

Age (Months)	CEJ-ABC (μms) (N = 4)
1.5	324.7 ± 61.2
4	565.0.8 ± 148.0
6	466.9 ± 130.4
10	449.5.1 ± 115.9
12	730.2 ± 297.7
15	671.1 ± 248.2

Figure 2. Histomorphometry as a function of age. a) Representative light micrograph of first molar distal root at 4X magnification illustrates histomorphometric parameters including i) CEJ-ABC distance, radial widths of: ii) primary cementum, iii) secondary cementum (SC), iv) PDL adjoining primary cementum (PDL-PC), and v) PDL adjoining secondary cementum (PDL-SC). Scale bar = 1 millimeter. b) The table illustrates increasing values of CEJ-ABC distance signifying recession with age. c) Plotted histomorphometric parameters as a function of age comparatively demonstrates increasing cementum and decreasing PDL trends with age.

(Fig. 4a, black arrows) with minimal stain at the distal PDL-bone complex. With age, alcian blue was predominantly found in the PDL-cementum entheses of the mesial, coronal, and interradicular root surfaces (Fig. 4b). Regardless of age, alcian blue staining was consistently found around the osteocytes in the alveolar bone, precementum (Fig. 4a, white arrows) and cementum dentin junction (Fig. 4a, asterisks). Increasing intensity of alcian blue stain in the younger groups (growth phase), decreasing intensity in the older groups (senescent phase), and no coronal-apical patterns were observed. Staining was also observed in dentin (mantle dentin, predentin), closest to the occlusal surface (not shown).

2.5. Immunostaining for SLRPs

Immunohistochemistry located biglycan (BGN), decorin (DCN), fibromodulin (FMOD), and asporin (ASPN) coronally, apically, and at the enthesis regions of PDL-cementum and PDL-bone (Fig. 5) with increasing age. Biglycan, decorin (Class I SLRPs), and fibromodulin (a Class II SLRP) were consistently located at these soft-hard interfaces, endosteal spaces, and vasculature independent of age. The exception was asporin, a leucine rich protein with a unique aspartate-rich N-terminus that is not a proteoglycan (PG) [64], and was confirmed to be specific to PDL in rats. A localization gradient in all SLRPs was observed with higher concentrations coronally relative to apical regions in both distal and mesial sides of all specimens in all age groups (Fig. 5b). Immunostaining for SLRPs other than asporin was also observed at the precementum layers (black arrow heads, inset in Fig. 5a), CDJ (black arrows in inset, Fig. 5a), predentin, and the transseptal fibers (asterisk, Fig. 5a) between any two molars. Shown in Figure 5a is immunostaining for BGN, which was observed to localize at the mesial side of the root across all age groups.

2.6. Scanning Electron Microscope

Back scattered electron mapping [65] on rat molars across age illustrated increased distribution of lighter and darker gray regions indicating heterogeneity owing to distributions of higher and lower atomic number (Z) elements in the alveolar bone of older rats (Figs. 6a, 6b). Observations were confirmed by point analyses using EDS elemental mapping of relative counts of calcium and phosphate, in which all age groups consistently demonstrated calcium and phosphate Kα1, Kα2, and Kβ1 lines in lighter areas (higher average Z; HZ in Figs. 6a and 6b) compared to corresponding lines in the darker areas (lower average Z; LZ in Figs. 6a and 6b) areas. EDS analyses demonstrated higher counts

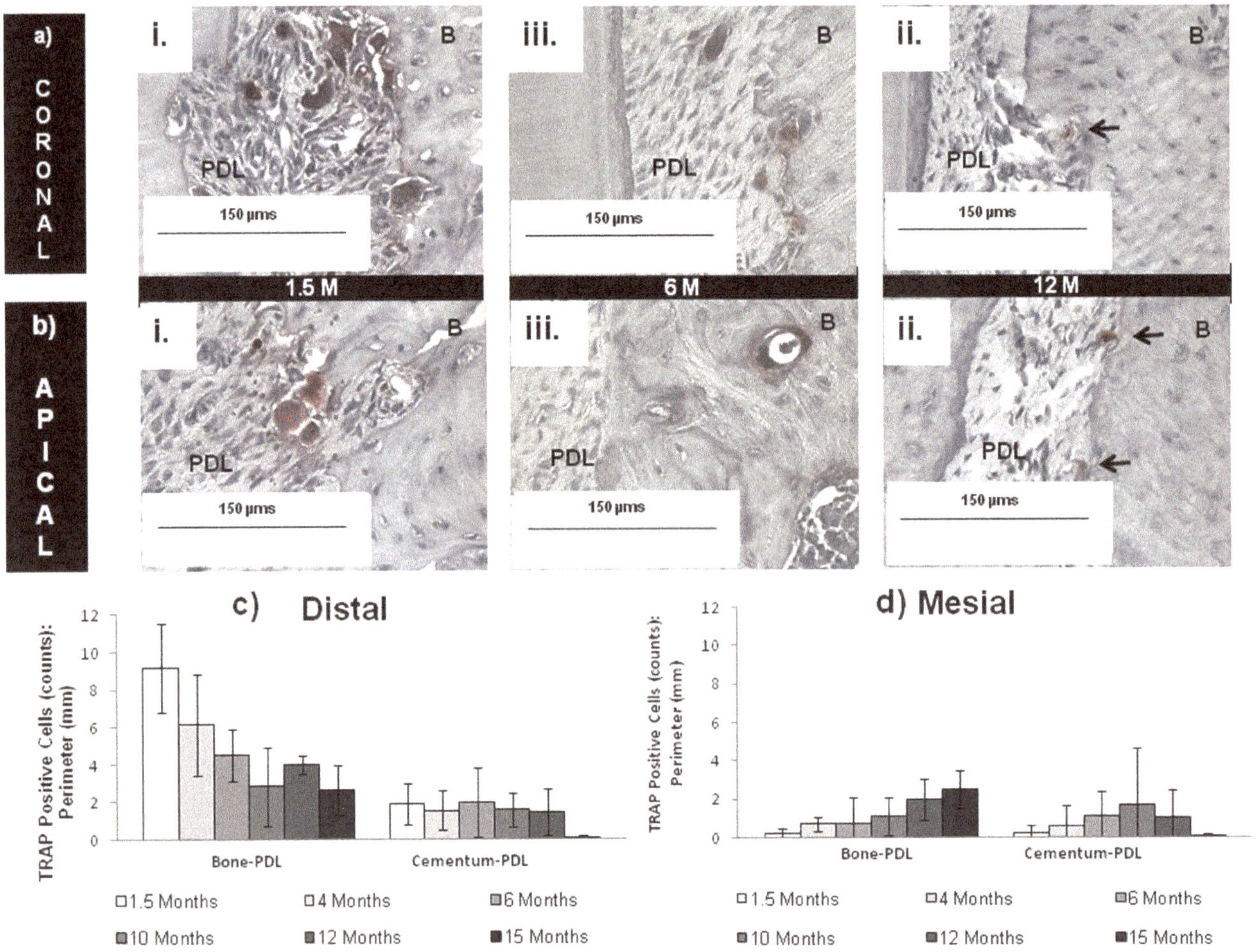

Figure 5. Regions of osteoclastic activity with age. Enlarged at 40X from encircled areas in Figure 1, TRAP localization is demonstrated across all age groups in a) coronal and b) apical regions. In young rats, resorption activity is represented by robust multinucleated pits (red staining) surrounded by several dark purple nuclei. In older rats mononucleated pits predominated with decreased intensity of red stain. Scale bar = 150 µm. Results show osteoclastic activity declined with increasing age in c) distal regions and d) increased in mesial regions.

of Ca and P in more mature and lighter layers of bone compared to newly laid bone near resorbed sites at PDL-bone enthesis (Fig. 6b). Standard SE images illustrated resorption sites with the presence of collagen fibers inserting on the distal side of bone at the PDL-bone enthesis (Figs. 6c, 6d, 6e) and into dentin at the tooth side.

2.7. Microhardness (see Appendix S1)

The Box-Tidwell non-linearity test [66] and linear regression test for association of mineral tissue hardness (cementum and bone; dependent variables) with age (independent variable) conducted via Statistics Online Computational Resource (SOCR) (http://www.socr.ucla.edu/) did not show a significant non-linear relationship between age and hardness of secondary cementum or alveolar bone (both $P = 0.94$). This implies that neither the hardness of bone nor that of cementum was non-linearly related to age of the organism. The linear regression test did not show a significant linear relationship between microhardness and age (both $P > 0.46$). Similarly the ANCOVA test of differences in material hardness (secondary cementum and alveolar bone) and age concluded no significant relationship (P of age = 0.194). However, a significant relationship between material and hardness (P of material = 0.007) at a specific age group was demonstrated, with point estimate of the difference of hardness = −0.105 and 95% confidence of −0.163 to −0.046. However this relationship was not modified by age (P of age*material = 0.880).

Discussion

This is the first cross-sectional study to map function related changes in structure, (bio)chemical composition, and mechanical properties, from which differential changes due to experimentally induced perturbations can be optimally addressed. The results of this study are discussed giving due consideration to Wolff's Law, continuous occlusal wear, and natural distal drift of rat molars [7,8,60,62,67,68,69]. Based on our observations, we speculate that each tissue's functional response is unique and the synchronization of individual physical and chemical properties could explain functional maintenance of the bone-PDL-cementum complex at an organ level.

Physical Changes at an Organ and Tissue Levels: MicroXCT and Histomorphometry

Macroscale changes due to overall growth of a root and adjacent bone adaptation within the bone-tooth fibrous joint

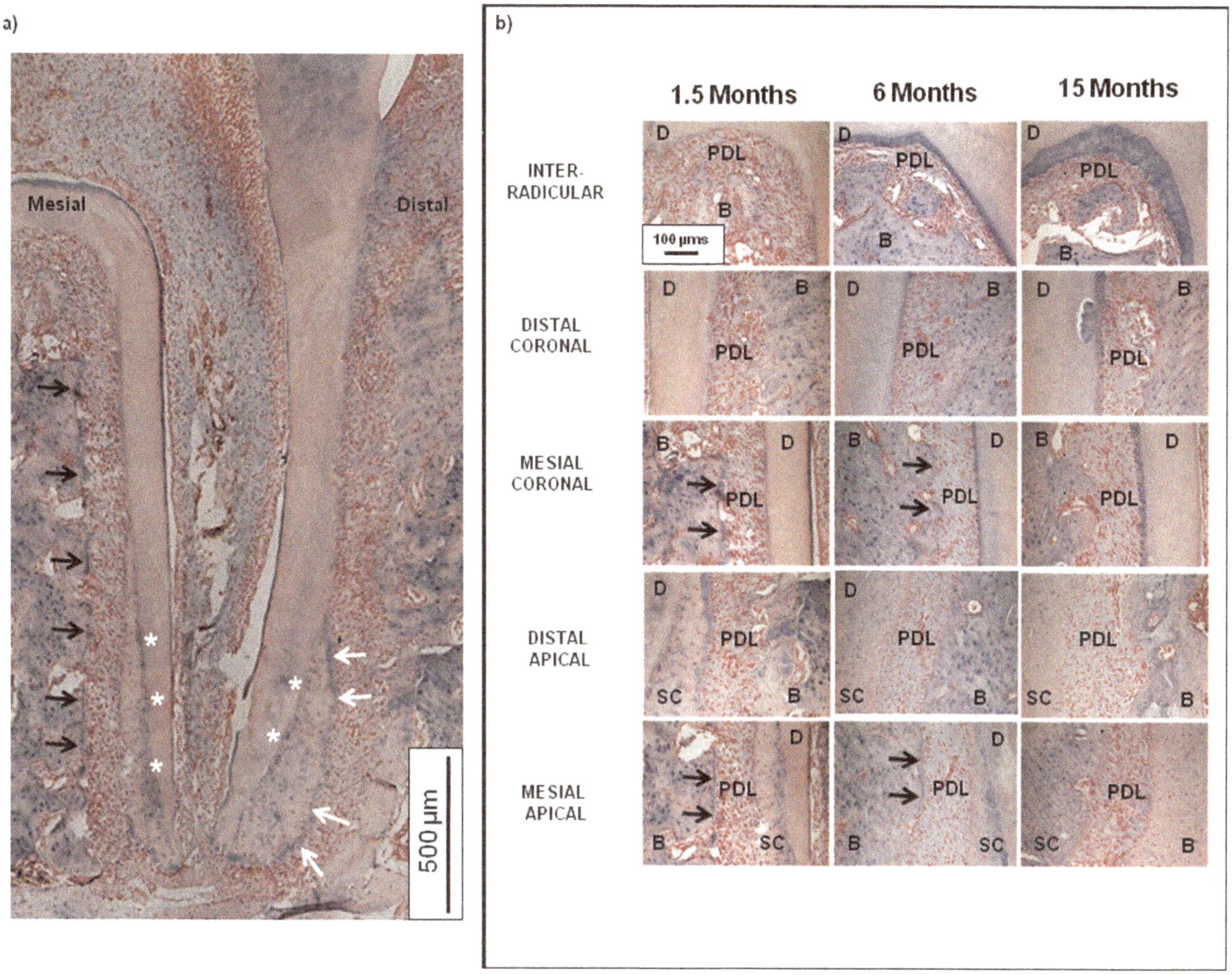

Figure 4. Localization of sulfated GAGs using alcian blue stain. a) Light micrographs at 10X of alcian blue with nuclear fast red counterstain indicates more sulfated GAGs on the mesial aspect as indicated by black arrows (shown here in a 1.5 month old rat), as well as around osteocytes in the alveolar bone, precementum (white arrows) and cementum dentin junction (white asterisks). We also observed staining to occur in dentin. Scale bars = 500 µm. b) Corresponding age-related changes at interradicular, coronal-apical, and mesial-distal entheses regions showed decreased alcian blue staining and lost mesial specificity with age (black arrows). Scale bars = 100 µm.

(Fig. 1, Fig. S2) were illustrated using MicroXCT. These changes can be related to functional loads, which act as stimuli to cells within various tissues and interfaces. Upon loading, molars pivot about the interradicular bone, which is considered as the natural fulcrum [70]. Age-related changes in muscle efficiency and occlusion [71] result in different chewing forces [72] over time. As a result, functional loads alone can cause tension, compression, shear and related mechanical strains within the fibrous matrix between the bone and tooth. The effect of matrix-related strains [21,73,74,75], and fluid flow (blood and interstitial fluid) [86,87] can be traced to changes in gene expressions of stem cells within the marrow space of the alveolar bone and blood vessels of the PDL. A good example is the origin of RANKL, a molecule involved in osteoclastogenesis, which can be traced from the vascularized PDL to bone marrow space containing stromal and hematopoietic stem cells [21,73]. As a result, histomorphometric changes of load-bearing tissues with time included increased radial width of cementum and increased bone recession (measured as the vertical distance between the CEJ and the ABC) (Fig. 2c). Observed trends are reflective of bone "carving," which would conceivably be due to functional adaptation [76,77] and in turn could alter tooth attachment (Fig. 2b) to bone (Fig. 6) to preserve optimal function space. Although age-related increases in cementum width and decreases in PDL-space were observed (Fig. 2), the combined radial widths of SC and PDL-SC remained a constant in younger rats 1.5 to 6 months and in older rats 12 to 15 months (ANOVA $P \leq 0.05$). The functional role of SC and PDL in load adaptation [15] provide the basis for considering the coupled PDL-cementum thickness in cooperative maintenance of the dynamic complex. Localized remodeling of bone is thought to dominate and allows for the uniform size increases in the growing periodontium between 1.5 to 4 months. When in function, modeling becomes more prevalent with complete secondary cementum formation and apposition from 4 to 15 months, simultaneously carving bone equivalent to tooth morphology as a result of functional stimuli.

Changes in function can be identified as compromised PDL attachment and closing of endosteal spaces in rats 12 to 15 months of age (Figs. 1, 3, 4). Generally, cement lines in bone increased, exhibiting a dominant lamellar-like pattern around endosteal and

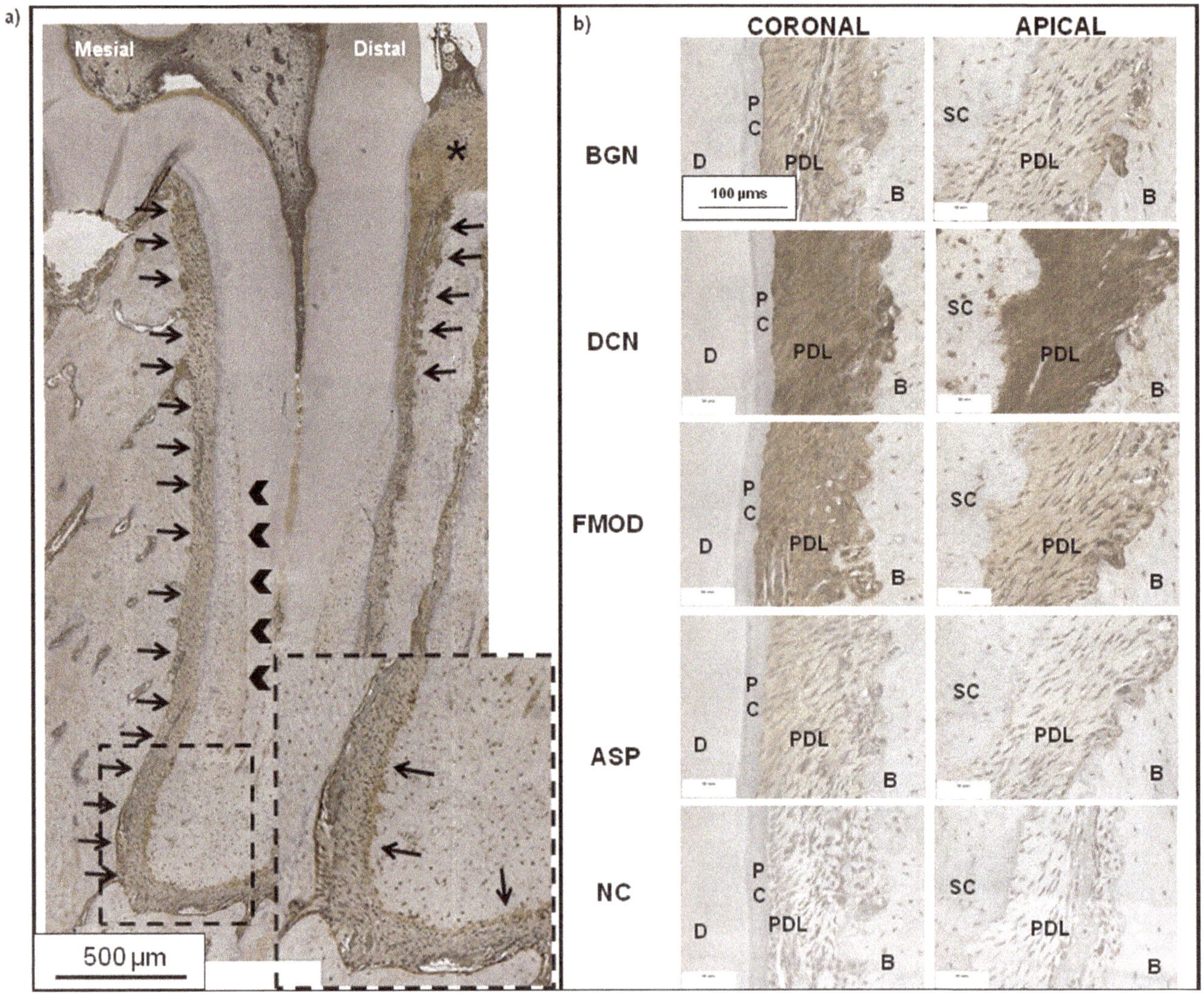

Figure 5. Immunohistochemical staining for identification of SLRPs. a) Light micrograph at 10X using immunohistochemical methods shows representative localization of SLRPs (biglycan expression in a 6 month old rat) counterstained with hematoxylin. Black arrows indicate localization at mesial PDL-bone enthesis spanning the root length as well as the coronal predominance. In addition localization was also observed in precementum layers (black arrow heads, in Fig. 5a) and at the CDJ (black arrow in inset, Fig. 5a), predentin, and the transseptal fibers (asterisk, Fig. 5a) between any two molars. Scale bars = 500 μm. b) Serially sectioned 60X light micrographs show immunohistochemical localization of SLRPs: biglycan (BGN), decorin (DCN), fibromodulin (FMOD), asporin (ASP), and negative controls (NC). Localization indicates more intense staining in coronal regions relative to apical regions across all age groups. All micrographs indicate regions where PDL meets primary bone (B) and primary cementum (PC) or secondary cementum (SC), with adjacent dentin (D). All Scale bars = 100 μm.

marrow spaces with age. The observed patterns can be associated with remodeling related events, which were identified in endocortical and marrow regions in aging rats [78]. Based on narrowing endosteal spaces in aging rats, it is plausible that changes in PDL-width, bone and root surface are related to changes in blood flow, supply of nutrients, and chemotactic factors responsible for turnover of tissues. Shaping of the alveolar socket or modeling at endocortical and marrow regions, compromised turnover rate of the PDL in aging rats [78,79], including changes in PDL-width, suggests the deterioration of PDL's mechanical integrity. However, it should be noted that observed increases in bone recession could be due to several factors. These include natural hair and food impaction, which stimulate local inflammation and bone recession. Conversely, heightened reception to hormones during the period of social maturation at 6 and 10 months (Fig. 2b) have been associated with a bone protective effect due to anabolic increases in rats at 4 months, with stabilization by 5–9 months [80].

Bone "carving" and resulting form of the socket, is functionally stimulated by clastic and blastic activities within the bony socket in which the tooth is suspended. Function related stimulation promotes bone modeling in addition to the physiological remodeling that is innate to most tissues within an organ [21,36,81]. This phenomena can be captured in the lifetime process of distal tooth-drift [67], and when combined with function, imposes a continuous tension-based mesial complex and a compression-based distal complex. Pre-strained functional complexes cause mineral formation on the mesial side in tension and mineral resorption on the distal side in compression. The mesial apposition of mineral, marked as stratified growth, and distal resorption of mineral, identified by its pitted border, continue to be illustrated through fluorochrome and TRAP

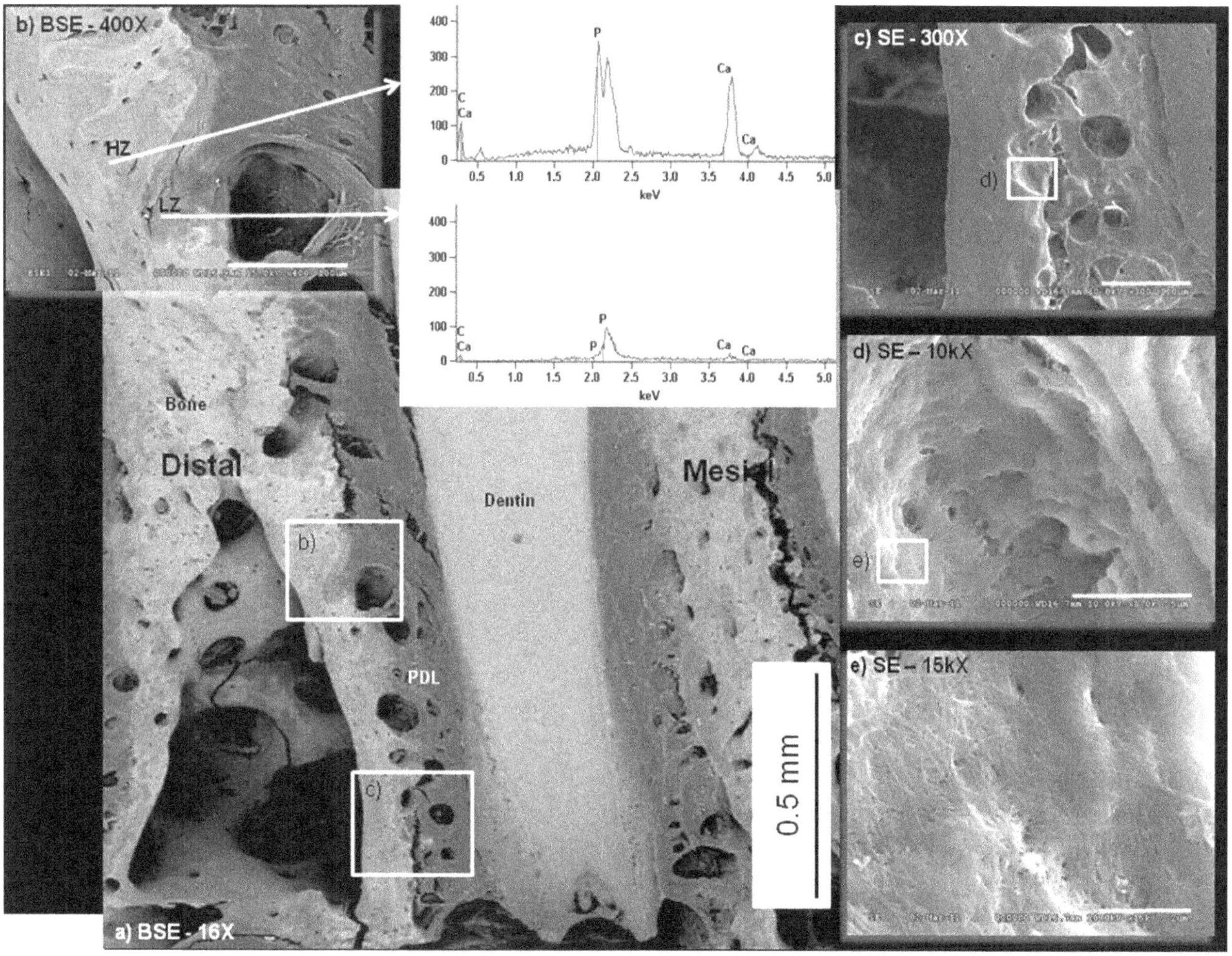

Figure 6. Elemental mapping using BSE and EDS. a) SEM in BSE mode indicated distribution of high and low Z elements of the periodontium. Scale Bar = 0.5 mm. b) Using SEM-BSE greatest heterogeneity is observed in the different layers of bone owing to different chemical compositions of bone during its turnover (i.e. remodeling or modeling). Scale Bar = 100 μm. Representative point shoot EDS demonstrate varying counts of Ca and P (Kα1, Kα2, and Kβ1 lines) within adjacent regions. SE mode indicates at length scales c) the enthesis region of PDL-bone with scale bar = 100 μm, d) the site of a resorption pit, which indicate the digested layers of bone with scale bar = 5 μm, and e) the exposed collagen fibers that help compose a mineralized matrix with scale bar = 4 μm.

analyses [23]. As previously delineated, our TRAP analysis embraces this logic appropriately, and can be seen as distal osteoclastic preference in regions of compression (Figs. 1, 3c, 3d, Fig. S2). However, with increasing age, no particular preference was observed with the distal resorption compared to that of the mesial formation (Figs. 3c, 3d). This observation can be argued with the predominance of mononucleated TRAP positive cells within PDL-space (Fig. 3a, 3b), indicative of a decline in osteoclastic maturation with age [82,83]. The αvβ3 integrin and vitronectin receptor, commonly expressed in platelets, has been implicated in successful fusion of mononucleated osteoclastic precursors [84]. Additionally, increased formation of advanced glycation end-products with age interferes with the integrin binding RGD sequence [85]. This, in addition to the narrowing of blood vessels and endosteal spaces, could explain the compromised mechanotransduction and the subsequent lack of cell-matrix interactions to promote maturation of a mononucleated osteoclast to a multinucleated osteoclast with age. Additionally, it is important to note that the varying numbers of mononucleated osteoclasts within the PDL support the theory of their hematopoetic origin and possibly reflect upon their declining presence and ability to migrate from the vasculature within PDL and bone with age.

Biochemical Changes at the Soft-hard Interface Levels in a Pre-strained Complex

It is proposed that formation and resorption related effects identified at the mesial and distal complexes are prompted by cellular activity equivalent to tension- and compression-strain gradients within respective complexes and at the soft-hard tissue interfaces. Mineral formation in a bone-tooth complex can be first identified at the osteoid and the precementum layers. However, based on our results, formation does not only occur at the interfaces. Mineral resorption related events also occur, but more specifically at the distal side complex. To better understand events responsible for formation and resorption of bone and cementum the localization of load resisting and dampening biochemical molecules, namely the higher molecular weight PGs using alcian blue, and lower molecular weights (i.e. SLRPs) using immunohistochemistry, were targeted. It is known that PGs in general are also responsible for water retention, fibrillogenesis, and the maintenance of tissue architecture and strain relieving properties (i.e. the scaffold upon which cell migration and mineralization occurs) [86]. Specifically, we identified PGs at the mesial and distal sites within the dynamic bone-tooth complex.

Biomolecules are also chemotactic agents that facilitate durotaxis, the stiffness dependent migration of cells [87]. The location and intensity of these biomolecules during development is dictated by genetic inheritance, but is predominantly governed by function when in growth. Regardless, in both development and growth, PGs are responsible for maintaining the organic matrix upon which mineral formation or resorption can occur. Moreover, this implies that in compressed regions, mineral resorbing molecules would be more dominant (Fig. 1), in contrast to tension regions that would contain more mineral forming molecules (Fig. 4a). In this study, biochemical events were mapped at a macroscale using alcian blue (Fig. 4) and more locally by identifying SLRP localization (Fig. 5). Interestingly, alcian blue stained sulfated GAGs were identified in newly formed bone sites (i.e. mesial trailing edge compared to the distal leading edge), as confirmed by others [88]. We also observed increasing gradients of sulfated GAGs on the mesial sides of PDL-bone and PDL-cementum sites, as indicated by alcian blue stains at these respective regions (Fig. 4). We observed GAG localization in regions of decreased osteoclastic activity by correlating alcian blue stain with TRAP positive stain (Figs. 3 and 4). With age, an increase in GAG localization was observed at PDL-PC, while decreases at PDL-SC and PDL-bone occurred until distal-mesial regions became comparable (Fig. 4). We hypothesize that these localizations can be related to increased tensile strains in the coronal portion of the bone-PDL-cementum complex and at the attachment sites. Increased strains can be attributed to changes in organic to inorganic ratios as a result of function related active mineral formation and resorption in bone and cementum with age [89]. Higher levels of tenascin and fibronectin, including other SLRPs noted in our study [89,90,91], were also identified at the attachment sites. Asporin was observed only within PDL, marking its innate nonmineralizing phenotype in maintaining the functional space necessary for adequate range of tooth motion within the bony socket. From these results it is conceivable, that should functional loads vary as a result of therapy (an alteration of compression and tension sites within the bone-tooth complex via orthodontics braces) [92], the generation of grossly altered biomolecules with mineralizing phenotypes (ankylosis) and mineral resorbing phenotypes are possible [93,94,95,96]. An analog in orthopedics is the age associated loss of cartilage and joint mobility under osteoarthritic conditions that are associated with decreases in asporin [97] and other proteoglycans. Other analogs include distraction osteogenesis, in which bone formation is stimulated through unidirectional forces on excised bone. These observations suggest that the synergistic nature of PGs on tension and compression-based matrices permit mineral formation or resorption related events due to function and is not limited solely to heredity. Additionally, these biochemical events could occur concomitantly, as seen by coronal-apical gradients and specifically at the attachment sites of PDL-bone and PDL-cementum, resulting in mineralization fronts as osteoid or precementum layers at the soft-hard tissue borders.

Physical and Chemical Changes using SEM-BSE-EDS

Newly formed layers of bone (i.e. mineralizing osteoid and precementum) contained lower counts of calcium (Ca) and phosphorus (P) compared to the older layers of bone [98] (Fig. 6). Formation of mineral on and at the strained attachment sites is a complex and systematic process, some of which can be marked by speciation of phosphate groups. This is because the phosphate (PO_4^{3-}) to pyrophosphate ($P_2O_7^{4-}$) ionic ratio increases as physiological aging progresses [99,100,101]. Modeling and/or remodeling related biomineralization events can also be mapped using SEM in backscattered electron [65] mode, along with electron dispersion X-ray spectroscopy (EDS). In this study we used complementary techniques of BSE and EDS to identify higher and lower Z elements within the dynamic tissue, bone, and less dynamic, cementum (Fig. 6) [102]. Lower Ca and P in the new bone compared to older bone at sites of modeling (Fig. 5) were observed. Despite the observed heterogeneity in bone regardless of age, it is important to note that differences in younger groups may be more related to inherited genetic factors (i.e. 1.5 months – which is closer still to development), and this most often is marked by the hypertrophic growth of cells indicated by higher metabolic activity [103].

Beyond the ongoing development in the 1.5 month age group, the increased heterogeneity observed in bone from 4 to 15 months could be due to functional loads. Moreover, growth related distal drift is dependent on functional loads (a decrease in rate of distal drift identified by lack of functional loads) [20,68,104,105]. As a result, we observed an increase in the number of "patchy areas" in bone, which could be due to increased differences in Ca and P contents (Figs. 6a, 6b) as a function of modeling and remodeling related events. This in turn could be necessary to maintain the functional integrity of bone (Fig. 6b) with age. At the bone-tooth organ level, we observed stratified bone formation parallel to the root length on the tension based mesial complex with lower Z (newer bone). Compression based distal complex, identified as the "leading" edge, was observed as higher Z content (older bone) and contained several resorption pits (Fig. 6c). Interestingly, PDL was attached to bone at these resorption sites, demonstrating no loss of attachment (Figs. 6d, 6e).

Hardness Changes Using Microindentation

The observed heterogeneity primarily in bone can be correlated to varying contents of Ca, P, and possibly other elements at certain regions, and stages of mineralization, as seen in SEM-BSE-EDS (Fig. 6). Microindentation was used to estimate hardness values representative of the tissue's bulk properties. Several hierarchical levels of organization and substructures, from crystal formation to crystal alignment within and around the fibril, to the packaging of fibrils into a fiber [45], can affect mechanical hardness. Interestingly, mechanical testing concluded no correlation between age and microhardness of AB and SC, but microhardness of AB was significantly different from SC (see Appendix S1). Based on these results, it is conceivable that the varying chemical disparities within the patches, number of patches, and the size of patches could provide similar hardness with age. As a result, hardness (H_k) values do not demonstrate the aging of mineralized tissues (Fig. 7) in rats. Without discriminating between new and mature bone, we pooled in the new and old bone hardness values and sampled alveolar bone as one material. Hence, it is likely that the effect of adaptation with age was not seen in hardness measurements. An engineering analogy is that different phases in a metal joined by grain boundaries could contribute to the overall functional integrity of the metal, but each phase has its own characteristic property. In the case of biological materials that are more organic based, microindentation, when conducted under dry (nonphysiological) conditions, could mask some of the innate energy absorbing characteristics of hygroscopic, organic

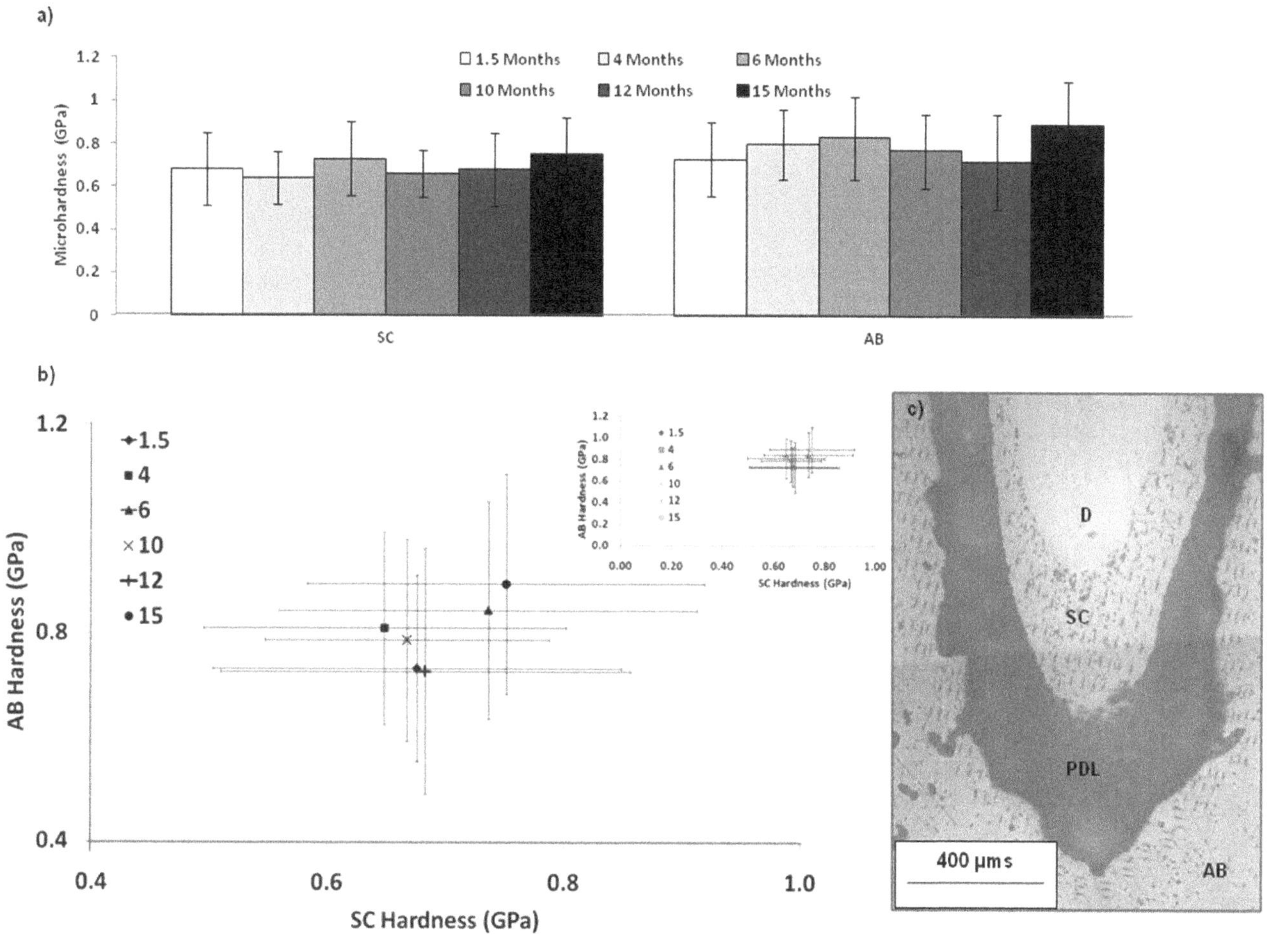

Figure 7. Hardness values for secondary cementum (SC) and alveolar bone (B) with age. a) Histogram shows average calculated Knoop hardness and standard deviation (GPa) values for SC and B. Values demonstrated no significant differences in both SC and B microhardness with age. b) Inset demonstrates original values plotted with reference to the origin. The main plot zooms into the clustered data set to demonstrate that the discrete points showed no relationship between SC and B with progression of age. c) Typical microindentation distribution and pattern conducted under dry conditions is shown at 10X.

components (i.e. GAGs, collagen) of mineralized tissues. Hence, the observed trends could be true and that only the relative differences between bone and cementum should be considered. For the same reason, a more accurate approximation can be made between AB and SC under wet (hydrated, physiological) conditions.

In summary, our results suggest that age-related physiological adaptations in organs should be taken into account, such that their use as a model can be streamlined and the effects of the intended experimental factors are accurately investigated. Specifically, we suggest that hard tissue modeling related studies in rats should not exceed 6 months. With increase in age, the adaptation in each tissue, whether they arise from evolutionarily inherent adaptations, physiological changes due to growth, or natural environmental insults, are accounted for throughout the organ system as a whole. Although each tissue's functional response is unique owing to its characteristic cellular and acellular components, the periodontium inherently adapts as a continuum in a synchronized fashion to maintain function. Despite nature's efficient design of the organ complex and its ability to continually withstand perturbations and functionally perform, the adaptive trend of its component tissues will be critical for future success in biomimetics. However, function-related effects should be decoupled from the effects of aging in future studies by modulating diet stiffness.

Materials and Methods

Ethics Statement

All animal housing, care, euthanasia, and tissue transfer protocols in this study were approved and complied with the guidelines of the Institutional Animal Care and Use Committee (IACUC) of the University of California, San Francisco and the National Institute of Health based on the IACUC Approval Number: AN083692-02.

The functional dentition of rats (1.5 months old, male, Sprague Dawley) [67] were taken as our starting time point, from which differential changes in properties will be discussed to illustrate adaptation. Experiments were performed on male Sprague-Dawley rats from six age groups: 1.5, 4, 6, 10, 12, and 15 months. Histomorphometry using hematoxylin and eosin (H&E) stained sections, alcian blue staining for sulfated glycosaminoglycans (GAGs), immunohistochemistry for small leucine rich proteins (SLRPs), and tartrate-resistant acid phosphatase (TRAP) [106] for osteoclast resorption was performed with n = 4 rats each from 1.5 to 15 month age groups using serial sections. The corresponding halves of the mandibles were used for microindentation studies. Another set of hemimandibles from all age groups (n = 3) were used for scanning electron microscopy (SEM), energy dispersive X-ray spectroscopy (EDS), and micro X-ray computed tomography (MicroXCT) analyses.

4.1. MicroXCT and Image Processing

Left hemimandibles from each age group were fixed in 4% paraformaldehyde (PFA) (Sigma-Aldrich, catalog P6148, St. Louis, MO), stored and imaged in 70% ethanol. Each specimen was scanned (MicroXCT-200, Xradia Inc., Pleasanton, CA) at 4X, 50 KVp, 140 µA, 2100 projections, binning 2, 7 second exposure time, and an angle sweep from −95° to 95°. At this magnification, isotropic voxel sizes were 5.5 µm with an image size of 1012 × 1012 µm. Each tomography was reconstructed using the TXM reconstructor software (Version 7.0.2817, Xradia Inc., Pleasanton, CA) to obtain DICOM image files for 3D image analysis using Visage Imaging Amira 5.3.3 (Visage Imaging, San Diego, California). Using an identical brightness and contrast threshold, root surfaces were constructed using the SurfaceGen module in Amira 5.3.3 (Visage Imaging, San Diego, CA).

4.2. Specimen Preparation for Histology

Hemimandibles were stored in 10% neutral buffered formalin for 4 days followed by end-stage decalcification using Cal-EX II decalcifying formalin solution (Fischer Scientific, Fair Lawn, NJ). The specimens were dehydrated with increasing concentrations of Flex 80%, 95%, and 100% alcohol (Richard-Allan Scientific, Kalamazoo, MI) before embedding in paraffin (Tissue Prep-II, Fisher Scientific, Fair Lawn, NJ) [107]. The paraffin blocks were sectioned on a rotary microtome (Reichert-Jung Biocut, Vienna, Austria) using disposable steel blades (TBFTM Inc., Shur/SharpTM, Fisher Scientific, Fair Lawn, NJ), deparaffinized with xylene, followed by rehydration with decreasing concentrations of 100%, 95%, and 80% Flex alcohols, and then stained with Hematoxylin Gill 3X (Fisher Scientific, Kalamazoo, MI) and Eosin Y Solution (Fisher Scientific, Kalamazoo, MI). For alcian blue and TRAP staining, a slight variation in specimen preparation involved tissue fixation with 4% PFA shaken overnight at room temperature and decalcified for 14 days with 0.5 M EDTA at pH 8.0. The distal root of the first mandibular molar in each rat was evaluated (see supplemental information).

4.3. Histomorphometry

Sagittal sections containing the maximum root length illustrating the cementoenamel junction and the pulp through the apical foramen were used for histomorphometry. Light microscopy (BX 51, Olympus America Inc., San Diego, CA), as shown in H&E stained sections of the cementum, PDL-space, and bone height of the first molar distal root complex were measured using Image-Pro Plus v6.0 data acquisition software (Media Cybernetics, Inc., Bethesda, MD). Image-Pro Plus v6.0's magnification/zoom function was utilized to accurately measure the mentioned parameters on the distal side. 20 measurements were taken for parameters along the coronal length of the root (i.e. primary cementum (PC) and PDL-PC), 20 measurements for apical parameters (i.e. secondary cementum (SC) and PDL-SC), and one measurement for the distance between the cementoenamel junction (CEJ) and alveolar bone crest (ABC), as an indicator of bone recession [77,108,109,110]. Thus, a total of 30 cementum-width and PDL-width respectively, and 1 CEJ-ABC measurements were made around the first molar along the coronal-apical length of the distal root of each specimen. Average measurements in coronal-apical regions of respective tissues for each distal root in each rat were determined. The resulting average values were used to test statistical significance among rat age groups using ANOVA with 95% confidence intervals ($P \leq 0.05$). Average values and standard deviations representative of each regional tissue for each age group were plotted.

4.4. TRAP Histochemistry for Osteoclasts

Deparaffinized serial sections were used for staining TRAP [111]. In brief, the method included treating the rehydrated specimens with 0.2 M acetate buffer, a solution of 0.2 M sodium acetate (Sigma Aldrich, catalog 52889, St. Louis, MO) and sodium tartrate dibasic dehydrate (Sigma Aldrich, catalog T6521, St. Louis, MO). After 20 minute incubation at room temperature, napthol AS-MX phosphate (Sigma, catalog N4875, St. Louis, MO) and fast red TR salt 1,5-napthalenedisulfonate salt (Sigma, F6760, St. Louis, MO) were added, followed by incubation at 37°C for 1 hour, with close monitoring under the microscope after the first half hour for bright red staining of osteoclastic activity. The stained sections were washed in deionized water and counterstained with Gill 3X hematoxylin (Fisher Scientific, Kalamazoo, MI) for subsequent examination under a light microscope. Distal and mesial side osteoclasts were manually counted along a measured PDL-bone and PDL-cementum perimeter using Image-Pro Plus v6.0 data acquisition software and its magnification/zoom function (Media Cybernetics, Inc., Bethesda, MD). Ratios of osteoclast count to perimeter per mesial-distal location [112], PDL-bone and PDL-cementum interfaces, were calculated across all age groups. These ratios were tested for statistical significance among age groups using ANOVA with 95% confidence intervals ($P \leq 0.05$). Additionally, average ratios and their standard deviations representative of regional osteoclastic density for each age group were plotted.

4.5. Alcian Blue Histochemistry for Sulfated GAGs

Deparrafinized serial sections were rehydrated in distilled water and stained in 1% alcian blue in 0.1 N hydrochloric acid at pH 1.0 for [illegible] minutes and then briefly rinsed in 0.1 N hydrochloric acid. Counterstaining with nuclear-fast red solution for 5 minutes was performed, followed by washing in distilled water. Dehydration with two changes each of 95% and >99% (absolute) ethyl alcohol, then deparaffinization in xylene was done before mounting the specimens. As a cationic copper containing dye, alcian blue has been widely used to stain the polyanionic sulfated GAGs at pH 1.0 [113].

4.6. Immunohistochemistry for SLRPs

Immunohistochemical localization of different SLRPs, specifically biglycan (BGN), decorin (DCN), fibromodulin (FMOD), and asporin (ASPN) within tissues and at the PDL-bone and PDL-cementum attachment sites (entheses) was performed. Followed by the same method for conventional histology, after rehydration of the deparaffinized sections, endogenous peroxidases were deactivated with 80% methanol and 0.6% H_2O_2. Further digestion for antigen retrieval was performed using a solution of 1 M Tris pH 7.4, 3 M sodium acetate pH 5.2, chondroitinase ABC (Seikagaku Biobusiness, catalog 100332) in 0.1% BSA, keratinase (Seikagaku Biobusiness, catalog 100810) in 0.1% BSA and ddH_2O in a humidified chamber at 37°C for 60 minutes. Sections were then blocked by incubation with 1% BSA and 1.5% rabbit serum in phosphate-buffered saline at 25°C for 30 minutes. Polyclonal antibodies kindly provided by Dr. Larry Fisher (NIDCR, National Institutes of Health) were added at a dilution of 1:50, 1:100, 1:100, and 1:20 for BGN, DCN, FMOD, and ASPN, respectively, in phosphate-buffered saline, and incubated overnight at 4°C. After washing, sections were incubated with Sigma mouse anti-rabbit IgG-HRP (catalog A2074, St. Louis, MO) at a dilution of 1:100 and then incubated at room temperature for 30 min. The sections were washed again and visualized with 3,3′-diaminobenzidine tetrachloride solution (Sigma, catalog D3939, St. Louis, MO) for immunoreaction sites. Sections were counterstained with Hematoxylin Gill 3x (Fisher Scientific, Kalamazoo, MI). Negative controls by substitution of only the primary antibody with unimmunized rabbit serum in blocking solution, while keeping other experimental steps identical, were also used for analysis.

4.7. SEM, BSE and EDS for Morphology, Distribution of Higher and Lower Atomic Weight Elements, and Overall Chemical Composition

Scanning electron microscopy (SEM) (Hitachi S-4300SE/N, Hitachi America) was performed to evaluate structural and chemical compositional differences at a tissue level near PDL-bone and PDL-cementum attachment sites, and in bone. Following microindentation, three samples each from the six study groups mounted in Buehler Epoxycure Resin (Buehler Ltd., Lake Bluff, IL) with surfaces polished to 1 µm using a diamond polishing suspension were coated with ~25Å thickness gold. Imaging was performed using SEM operating at 10 keV for secondary electron (SE), 10 keV for back-scattered electron, and 15 keV for electron dispersive spectroscopy (EDS) modes. SE was used for evaluation of structure of the bone-tooth complex, while BSE was used for comparing regional variations in atomic number (Z). Areas of lower and higher Z were further explored by point analysis using EDS to compare zones of lower and higher Ca and P contents. Elemental mapping was performed predominantly measuring the $K\alpha 1$, $K\alpha 2$, and $K\beta 1$ lines of calcium (orbital energy 3691.68, 3688.09, and 4012.7 eV, respectively) and phosphorus (orbital energy 2013.7, 2012.7, and 2139.1 eV, respectively) [114].

4.8. Mechanical Testing

Prior to indentation, hemimandibles (n = 4 per 6 age groups) were embedded in epoxy (Buehler, Lake Bluff, IL) and polished using carbide grit sizes 1200 and 2400 (Buehler Ltd., Lake Bluff, IL) followed by fine polishing using diamond suspension slurries in descending order from 6, 3, 1, to 0.25 µm (Buehler Ltd., Lake Bluff, IL). Microindentation was performed under dry conditions with a microindenter with a Knoop diamond tip (Buehler Ltd., Lake Bluff, IL) using a load of 10 gf, and the long diagonal of each Knoop indent was immediately measured with Image-Pro data-acquisition software (Media Cybernetics, Inc., Bethesda, MD) using a light microscope. The microhardness (H_K) was calculated with the following equation: $H_K = 0.014229P/D^2$ where P is the normal load in Newtons (N) and D (mm) the length of the long diagonal. Multiple rows of radially oriented indents were performed in secondary cementum and alveolar bone with approximately 3–5 indents per row. The distance between any two indents was chosen as per ASTM standards [115]. The mechanical properties of the first molar distal root from all groups were analyzed by first averaging the Knoop hardness values individually of bone and SC per rat. The resulting average values from each rat were used as representative hardness values for each rat within a group. Alveolar bone and SC of the first molar complex in each hemimandible were treated as separate tissues and as such, an average from all the indents of each tissue within each rat was evaluated. The resulting average values for each rat were used to test for statistical significant associations between age and hardness by performing a Box-Tidwell non-linearity test and linear regression test [66]. Additionally, the mean of the average hardness of bone and secondary cementum (representative hardness of bone and cementum in any given age group) was calculated and used to test for significant associations adjusting for age via analysis of covariance (ANCOVA) and simple regression analysis [116].

Supporting Information

Figure S1 Gross physical changes in hemimandible and molars with age: TOP: Changes in the growing rat molars from younger rats at 1.5, 4, and 6 months. BOTTOM: Changes in rat molars taken from older rats at 10 and 12 months. Both top and bottom rows have insets illustrating respective hemimandibles. Alignment with centimeter ruler shows in the molar view observable increases in occlusal wear and decreases in bone height with age. In the hemimandible inset view, widening of the first molar crown appears to cease at 0.3 cm at 4 months, while mandibles appear to cease at approximately 3.75 cm in length, around 6 months of age.

Figure S2 Mesial curving, occlusal wear, and resorption pits with age: MicroXCT reconstructed roots of 1.5, 6, and 12 month first mandibular molars are shown at various buccal, angled, lingual, and occlusal views. Mesial curving becomes prominent at 6 months, as seen in the buccal and angled buccal views. Occlusal wearing is significantly observed with age, especially in the 12 month old molar, as seen in the occlusal view. Buccal and lingual views best demonstrate discrepancies between mesial and distal roots in the first molar.

Figure S3 Osteoclastic activity with age: Enlarged at 40X from encircled areas in Figure 1, TRAP localization across all age groups in respective coronal and apical regions is shown. Resorption activity appears to be localized in multinucleated pits as indicated by the red stain surrounding several dark purple nuclei. Osteoclastic activity and multinucleated cells declined with increasing age regardless of region. Scale bar = 150 µm.

Acknowledgments

The authors would like to thank Adriane Joo, Ph.D., Department of Orofacial Sciences for her insight regarding TRAP staining, Linda Prentice for her expertise and the use of her rotary microtome, Kelly Ahern, Michael Matthes, Ph.D., and Professor Matthew LaVail, Department of Anatomy and Opthamology, Beckman Vision Center, UCSF School of Medicine for generously providing Sprague Dawley rats, Patrick Chuang for MicroXCT root reconstructions, Larry Fisher of NIDCR for his kind donation of antibodies for SLRP localization and the Lawrence Berkeley National Laboratory and their staff for the use of their SEM.

Author Contributions

Conceived and designed the experiments: NLL SAG MIR SPH. Performed the experiments: NLL JMH SID. Analyzed the data: NLL JMH SAG SPH. Contributed reagents/materials/analysis tools: MIR SPH. Wrote the paper: NLL SPH.

References

1. Robert L, Labat-Robert J (2000) Aging of connective tissues: from genetic to epigenetic mechanisms. Biogerontology 1: 123–131.
2. Fraga MF, Ballestar E, Paz MF, Ropero S, Setien F, et al. (2005) Epigenetic differences arise during the lifetime of monozygotic twins. Proc Natl Acad Sci U S A 102: 10604–10609.
3. Wang JH, Thampatty BP, Lin JS, Im HJ (2007) Mechanoregulation of gene expression in fibroblasts. Gene 391: 1–15.
4. Hayflick L (2007) Biological aging is no longer an unsolved problem. Ann N Y Acad Sci 1100: 1–13.
5. Carter DR, Beaupré GS (2001) Skeletal function and form : mechanobiology of skeletal development, aging, and regeneration. Cambridge; New York: Cambridge University Press. xii, 318 p.
6. Brinckmann P, Frobin W, Leivseth G (2002) Musculoskeletal biomechanics. Stuttgart; New York: Thieme. x, 243 p.
7. Ren Y, Maltha JC, Kuijpers-Jagtman AM (2004) The rat as a model for orthodontic tooth movement–a critical review and a proposed solution. Eur J Orthod 26: 483–490.
8. Klausen B (1991) Microbiological and immunological aspects of experimental periodontal disease in rats: a review article. J Periodontol 62: 59–73.
9. Struillou X, Boutigny H, Soueidan A, Layrolle P (2010) Experimental animal models in periodontology: a review. Open Dent J 4: 37–47.
10. Shimono M, Ishikawa T, Ishikawa H, Matsuzaki H, Hashimoto S, et al. (2003) Regulatory mechanisms of periodontal regeneration. Microsc Res Tech 60: 491–502.
11. Keles GG, Acikgoz G, Ayas B, Sakallioglu E, Firatli E (2005) Determination of systemically & locally induced periodontal defects in rats. Indian J Med Res 121: 176–184.
12. Ramamurthy NS, Xu JW, Bird J, Baxter A, Bhogal R, et al. (2002) Inhibition of alveolar bone loss by matrix metalloproteinase inhibitors in experimental periodontal disease. J Periodontal Res 37: 1–7.
13. Achong R, Nishimura I, Ramachandran H, Howell TH, Fiorellini JP, et al. (2003) Membrane type (MT) 1-matrix metalloproteinase (MMP) and MMP-2 expression in ligature-induced periodontitis in the rat. J Periodontol 74: 494–500.
14. Kuhr A, Popa-Wagner A, Schmoll H, Schwahn C, Kocher T (2004) Observations on experimental marginal periodontitis in rats. J Periodontal Res 39: 101–106.
15. Nanci A (2007) Ten Cate's oral histology : development, structure, and function. St. Louis, MO: Mosby, Inc., and affiliate of Elsevier Inc.
16. Klausen B, Sfintescu C, Evans RT (1991) Asymmetry in periodontal bone loss of gnotobiotic Sprague-Dawley rats. Arch Oral Biol 36: 685–687.
17. Ijuhin N (1988) Light and electron microscopic studies of experimentally-induced pathologic changes in the rat periodontal tissue. Adv Dent Res 2: 209–214.
18. King GJ, Keeling SD, McCoy EA, Ward TH (1991) Measuring dental drift and orthodontic tooth movement in response to various initial forces in adult rats. Am J Orthod Dentofacial Orthop 99: 456–465.
19. Goto KT, Kajiya H, Nemoto T, Tsutsumi T, Tsuzuki T, et al. (2011) Hyperocclusion stimulates osteoclastogenesis via CCL2 expression. J Dent Res 90: 793–798.
20. Fujita T, Montet X, Tanne K, Kiliaridis S (2009) Supraposition of unopposed molars in young and adult rats. Arch Oral Biol 54: 40–44.
21. Robling AG, Castillo AB, Turner CH (2006) Biomechanical and molecular regulation of bone remodeling. Annu Rev Biomed Eng 8: 455–498.
22. Wang L, Banu J, McMahan CA, Kalu DN (2001) Male rodent model of age-related bone loss in men. Bone 29: 141–148.
23. Misawa-Kageyama Y, Kageyama T, Moriyama K, Kurihara S, Yagasaki H, et al. (2007) Histomorphometric study on the effects of age on orthodontic tooth movement and alveolar bone turnover in rats. Eur J Oral Sci 115: 124–130.
24. Hall RC, Embery G (1997) The use of immunohistochemistry in understanding the structure and function of the extracellular matrix of dental tissues. Adv Dent Res 11: 478–486.
25. Buffenstein R, Edrey, Y. H, Larsen, L P (2008) Animal Models in Aging Research A Critical Examination. Sourcebook of Models for Biomedical Research. pp 499–506.
26. Baer MJ, Bosma JF, Ackerman JL (1983) The postnatal development of the rat skull. Ann Arbor: University of Michigan Press. xv, 432 p., 433 folded leaves of plates p.
27. Sievanen H (2005) Hormonal influences on the muscle-bone feedback system: a perspective. J Musculoskelet Neuronal Interact 5: 255–261.
28. Roholl PJ, Blauw E, Zurcher C, Dormans JA, Theuns HM (1994) Evidence for a diminished maturation of preosteoblasts into osteoblasts during aging in rats: an ultrastructural analysis. J Bone Miner Res 9: 355–366.
29. Hayflick L, Moorhead PS (1961) The serial cultivation of human diploid cell strains. Exp Cell Res 25: 585–621.
30. Barros EM, Rodrigues CJ, Rodrigues NR, Oliveira RP, Barros TE, et al. (2002) Aging of the elastic and collagen fibers in the human cervical interspinous ligaments. Spine J 2: 57–62.
31. Pereira Junior FJ, Lundh H, Westesson PL (1996) Age-related changes of the retrodiscal tissues in the temporomandibular joint. J Oral Maxillofac Surg 54: 55–61; discussion 61–52.
32. Klingsberg J, Butcher EO (1960) Comparative histology of age changes in oral tissues of rat, hamster, and monkey. J Dent Res 39: 158–169.
33. Baumhammers A, Stallard RE, Zander HA (1965) Remodeling of alveolar bone. J Periodontol 36: 439–442.
34. Frost HM (1964) Bone biodynamics. Boston: Little. xvi, 687 p.
35. Frost HM (1990) Skeletal structural adaptations to mechanical usage (SATMU): 1. Redefining Wolff's law: the bone modeling problem. Anat Rec 226: 403–413.
36. Roberts WE, Roberts JA, Epker BN, Burr DB, Hartsfield JK (2006) Remodeling of Mineralized Tissues, Part I: The Frost Legacy. Seminars In Orthodontics 12: 216–237.
37. Frost HM (1997) On our age-related bone loss: insights from a new paradigm. J Bone Miner Res 12: 1539–1546.
38. Komatsu K, Kanazashi M, Shimada A, Shibata T, Viidik A, et al. (2004) Effects of age on the stress-strain and stress-relaxation properties of the rat molar periodontal ligament. Arch Oral Biol 49: 817–824.
39. Louridis O, Bazopoulou-Kyrkanidou E, Demetriou N (1972) Age effect upon cementum width of albino rat: a histometric study. J Periodontol 43: 533–536.
40. Cao JJ, Kurimoto P, Boudignon B, Rosen C, Lima F, et al. (2007) Aging impairs IGF-I receptor activation and induces skeletal resistance to IGF-I. J Bone Miner Res 22: 1271–1279.
41. Donahue SW, Jacobs CR, Donahue HJ (2001) Flow-induced calcium oscillations in rat osteoblasts are age, loading frequency, and shear stress dependent. American Journal of Physiology Cell Physiology 281: C1635–1641.
42. Niver EL, Leong N, Greene J, Curtis D, Ryder MI, et al. (2011) Reduced functional loads alter the physical characteristics of the bone-periodontal ligament-cementum complex. J Periodontal Res.
43. Kingsmill VJ, Boyde A, Davis GR, Howell PG, Rawlinson SC (2010) Changes in bone mineral and matrix in response to a soft diet. J Dent Res 89: 510–514.
44. Posner AS, Harper RA, Muller SA, Menczel J (1965) Age changes in the crystal chemistry of bone apatite. Ann N Y Acad Sci 131: 737–742.
45. Weiner S, Wagner HD (1998) The Material Bone: Structure-Mechanical Function Relations. Annu Rev Mater Sci 28: 271–298.
46. Mann S (2001) Biomineralization : principles and concepts in bioinorganic materials chemistry. New York: Oxford University Press. xii, 198 p.
47. Bailey AJ (2001) Molecular mechanisms of ageing in connective tissues. Mech Ageing Dev 122: 735–755.
48. Ho SP, Yu B, Yun W, Marshall GW, Ryder MI, et al. (2009) Structure, chemical composition and mechanical properties of human and rat cementum and its interface with root dentin. Acta Biomater 5: 707–718.
49. Mariotti A (1993) The extracellular matrix of the periodontium: dynamic and interactive tissues. Periodontol 2000 3: 39–63.
50. Melrose J, Fuller ES, Roughley PJ, Smith MM, Kerr B, et al. (2008) Fragmentation of decorin, biglycan, lumican and keratocan is elevated in degenerate human meniscus, knee and hip articular cartilages compared with age-matched macroscopically normal and control tissues. Arthritis Res Ther 10: R79.
51. Grzesik WJ, Frazier CR, Shapiro JR, Sponseller PD, Robey PG, et al. (2002) Age-related changes in human bone proteoglycan structure. Impact of osteogenesis imperfecta. J Biol Chem 277: 43638–43647.
52. Roughley PJ (2006) The structure and function of cartilage proteoglycans. Eur Cell Mater 12: 92–101.
53. Okazaki J, Kamada A, Higuchi Y, Kanabayashi T, Sakaki T, et al. (1996) Age changes in the rat temporomandibular joint articular disc: a biochemical study on glycosaminoglycan content. J Oral Rehabil 23: 536–540.
54. Jenkins HG, Bachelard HS (1988) Developmental and age-related changes in rat brain glycosaminoglycans. J Neurochem 51: 1634–1640.
55. Ito Y, Takeuchi J, Yamamoto K, Hashizume Y, Sato T, et al. (2001) Age differences in immunohistochemical localizations of large proteoglycan, PG-M/versican, and small proteoglycan, decorin, in the dermis of rats. Experimental Animals 50: 159–166.
56. Meikle MC (2006) The tissue, cellular, and molecular regulation of orthodontic tooth movement: 100 years after Carl Sandstedt. Eur J Orthod 28: 221–240.
57. Shimizu N, Yamaguchi M, Uesu K, Goseki T, Abiko Y (2000) Stimulation of prostaglandin E2 and interleukin-1beta production from old rat periodontal ligament cells subjected to mechanical stress. J Gerontol A Biol Sci Med Sci 55: B489–495.
58. Bridges T, King G, Mohammed A (1988) The effect of age on tooth movement and mineral density in the alveolar tissues of the rat. Am J Orthod Dentofacial Orthop 93: 245–250.
59. Ren Y, Maltha JC, Liem RS, Stokroos I, Kuijpers-Jagtman AM (2008) Age-dependent external root resorption during tooth movement in rats. Acta Odontol Scand 66: 93–98.
60. Spence JM (1940) Method of Studying the Skull Development of the Living Rat by Serial Cephalometric Roentgenograms. The Angle Orthodontist X: 127–139.
61. Hoffman MMaS, I (1940) Quantitative Studies in the Development of the Rat Molar. Presented Before the American Association of Orthodontists. pp 854–874.
62. Applebaum E (1947) Development of rat molar crowns and jaws. J Dent Res 26: 73–78.

63. Ho SP, Senkyrikova P, Marshall GW, Yun W, Wang Y, et al. (2009) Structure, chemical composition and mechanical properties of coronal cementum in human deciduous molars. Dent Mater 25: 1195–1204.
64. Royce PM, Steinmann BU (2002) Connective tissue and it heritable disorders : molecular, genetic, and medical aspects. New York: Wiley-Liss. xvii, 1201 p.
65. Afonso L, Bandaru H, Rathod A, Badheka A, Ali Kizilbash M, et al. (2011) Prevalence, determinants, and clinical significance of cardiac troponin-I elevation in individuals admitted for a hypertensive emergency. J Clin Hypertens (Greenwich) 13: 551–556.
66. Box GEP, Tidwell PW (1962) Transformation of the Independent Variables. United States: American Statistical Association and American Society for Quality. 531–550 p.
67. Schneider BJ, Meyer J (1965) Experimental Studies on the Interrelations of Condylar Growth and Alveolar Bone Formation. Angle Orthod 35: 187–199.
68. Sicher H, Weinmann JP (1944) Bone Growth and Physiologic Tooth Movement. American journal of orthodontics and oral surgery 30: C109.
69. Enlow DH (1967) Morphogenic interpretation of cephalometric data. J Dent Res 46: 1209.
70. Chattah NL-T, Shahar R, Weiner S (2009) Design Strategy of Minipig Molars Using Electronic Speckle Pattern Interferometry: Comparison of Deformation under Load between the Tooth-Mandible Complex and the Isolated Tooth. Advanced Materials 21: 413–418.
71. Nishijima K, Kuwahara S, Ohno T, Miyaishi O, Ito Y, et al. (2009) Occlusal tooth wear in male F344/N rats with aging. Arch Gerontol Geriatr 48: 178–181.
72. Bani D, Bani T, Bergamini M (1999) Morphologic and biochemical changes of the masseter muscles induced by occlusal wear: studies in a rat model. J Dent Res 78: 1735–1744.
73. Robling AG, Turner CH (2009) Mechanical signaling for bone modeling and remodeling. Crit Rev Eukaryot Gene Expr 19: 319–338.
74. Ingber DE (2006) Cellular mechanotransduction: putting all the pieces together again. FASEB J 20: 811–827.
75. Ingber DE (2004) The mechanochemical basis of cell and tissue regulation. Mech Chem Biosyst 1: 53–68.
76. Oehmke MJ, Schramm CR, Knolle E, Frickey N, Bernhart T, et al. (2004) Age-dependent changes of the periodontal ligament in rats. Microsc Res Tech 63: 198–202.
77. Klausen B, Evans RT, Sfintescu C (1989) Two complementary methods of assessing periodontal bone level in rats. Scand J Dent Res 97: 494–499.
78. Frost HM, Jee WS (1992) On the rat model of human osteopenias and osteoporoses. Bone Miner 18: 227–236.
79. Saffar JL, Lasfargues JJ, Cherruau M (1997) Alveolar bone and the alveolar process: the socket that is never stable. Periodontol 2000 13: 76–90.
80. Ghanadian R, Lewis JG, Chisholm GD (1975) Serum testosterone and dihydrotestosterone changes with age in rat. Steroids 25: 753–762.
81. Frost HM (1987) Bone "mass" and the "mechanostat": a proposal. Anat Rec 219: 1–9.
82. Arai F, Miyamoto T, Ohneda O, Inada T, Sudo T, et al. (1999) Commitment and differentiation of osteoclast precursor cells by the sequential expression of c-Fms and receptor activator of nuclear factor kappaB (RANK) receptors. Journal of Experimental Medicine 190: 1741–1754.
83. Boyle WJ, Simonet WS, Lacey DL (2003) Osteoclast differentiation and activation. Nature 423: 337–342.
84. Boissy P, Machuca I, Pfaff M, Ficheux D, Jurdic P (1998) Aggregation of mononucleated precursors triggers cell surface expression of alphavbeta3 integrin, essential to formation of osteoclast-like multinucleated cells. J Cell Sci 111 (Pt 17): 2563–2574.
85. Paul RG, Bailey AJ (1999) The effect of advanced glycation end-product formation upon cell-matrix interactions. International Journal of Biochemistry and Cell Biology 31: 653–660.
86. Iozzo RV, Murdoch AD (1996) Proteoglycans of the extracellular environment: clues from the gene and protein side offer novel perspectives in molecular diversity and function. FASEB J 10: 598–614.
87. Carter SB (1967) Haptotaxis and the mechanism of cell motility. Nature 213: 256–260.
88. Takagi M, Maeno M, Kagami A, Takahashi Y, Otsuka K (1991) Biochemical and immunocytochemical characterization of mineral binding proteoglycans in rat bone. J Histochem Cytochem 39: 41–50.
89. Qian L, Todo M, Morita Y, Matsushita Y, Koyano K (2009) Deformation analysis of the periodontium considering the viscoelasticity of the periodontal ligament. Dental Materials 25: 1285–1292.
90. Lukinmaa PL, Mackie EJ, Thesleff I (1991) Immunohistochemical localization of the matrix glycoproteins–tenascin and the ED-sequence-containing form of cellular fibronectin–in human permanent teeth and periodontal ligament. J Dent Res 70: 19–26.
91. McCulloch CA, Lekic P, McKee MD (2000) Role of physical forces in regulating the form and function of the periodontal ligament. Periodontol 2000 24: 56–72.
92. Krishnan V, Davidovitch Z (2006) Cellular, molecular, and tissue-level reactions to orthodontic force. Am J Orthod Dentofacial Orthop 129: 469 e461–432.
93. Santra M, Mann DM, Mercer EW, Skorski T, Calabretta B, et al. (1997) Ectopic expression of decorin protein core causes a generalized growth suppression in neoplastic cells of various histogenetic origin and requires endogenous p21, an inhibitor of cyclin-dependent kinases. J Clin Invest 100: 149–157.
94. Hakkinen L, Strassburger S, Kahari VM, Scott PG, Eichstetter I, et al. (2000) A role for decorin in the structural organization of periodontal ligament. Lab Invest 80: 1869–1880.
95. Nakamura Y, Tanaka T, Noda K, Shimpo S, Oikawa T, et al. (2003) Calcification of degenerating tissues in the periodontal ligament during tooth movement. J Periodontal Res 38: 343–350.
96. Nakamura Y, Noda K, Shimoda S, Oikawa T, Arai C, et al. (2008) Time-lapse observation of rat periodontal ligament during function and tooth movement, using microcomputed tomography. Eur J Orthod 30: 320–326.
97. Yamada S, Tomoeda M, Ozawa Y, Yoneda S, Terashima Y, et al. (2007) PLAP-1/asporin, a novel negative regulator of periodontal ligament mineralization. J Biol Chem 282: 23070–23080.
98. Goldberg M, Septier D, Lecolle S, Chardin H, Quintana MA, et al. (1995) Dental mineralization. International Journal of Developmental Biology 39: 93–110.
99. Groeneveld MC, Everts V, Beertsen W (1995) Alkaline phosphatase activity in the periodontal ligament and gingiva of the rat molar: its relation to cementum formation. J Dent Res 74: 1374–1381.
100. Foster BL, Nagatomo KJ, Bamashmous SO, Tompkins KA, Fong H, et al. (2011) The Progressive Ankylosis Protein Regulates Cementum Apposition and Extracellular Matrix Composition. Cells Tissues Organs.
101. Whyte MP (1994) Hypophosphatasia and the role of alkaline phosphatase in skeletal mineralization. Endocrine Reviews 15: 439–461.
102. Foster BL, Popowics TE, Fong HK, Somerman MJ (2007) Advances in defining regulators of cementum development and periodontal regeneration. Current Topics in Developmental Biology 78: 47–126.
103. Hayflick L (1970) Aging under glass. Exp Gerontol 5: 291–303.
104. Luan X, Diekwisch TG (2007) Vienna-Chicago: the cultural transformation of the model system of the un-opposed molar. Bioessays 29: 819–830.
105. Holliday S, Schneider B, Galang MT, Fukui T, Yamane A, et al. (2005) Bones, teeth, and genes: a genomic homage to Harry Sicher's "Axial Movement of Teeth". World J Orthod 6: 61–70.
106. Weiner JP, Tucker AM, Collins AM, Fakhraei H, Lieberman R, et al. (1998) The development of a risk-adjusted capitation payment system: the Maryland Medicaid model. J Ambul Care Manage 21: 29–52.
107. Ho SP, Kurylo MP, Fong TK, Lee SS, Wagner HD, et al. (2010) The biomechanical characteristics of the bone-periodontal ligament-cementum complex. Biomaterials 31: 6635–6646.
108. Guggenheim B, Schroeder HE (1974) Reactions in the periodontium to continuous antigenic stimulation in sensitized gnotobiotic rats. Infect Immun 10: 565–577.
109. Crawford JM, Taubman MA, Smith DJ (1978) The natural history of periodontal bone loss in germfree and gnotobiotic rats infected with periodontopathic microorganisms. J Periodontal Res 13: 316–325.
110. Arai K, Tanaka S, Yamamoto-Sawamura T, Sone K, Miyaishi O, et al. (2005) Aging changes in the periodontal bone of F344/N rat. Archives of Gerontology and Geriatrics 40: 225–229.
111. Erlebacher A, Derynck R (1996) Increased expression of TGF-beta 2 in osteoblasts results in an osteoporosis-like phenotype. J Cell Biol 132: 195–210.
112. Sawyer A, Lott P, Titrud J, McDonald J (2003) Quantification of tartrate resistant acid phosphatase distribution in mouse tibiae using image analysis. Biotechnic and Histochemistry 78: 271–278.
113. Pedlar J (1979) Histochemistry of glycosaminoglycans in the skin and oral mucosa of the rat. Arch Oral Biol 24: 777–786.
114. Thompson A, Kirz, J, Attwood DT, Gullikson EM, Howells MR, et al. (2009) Center for X-Ray Optics and Advanced Light Source X-ray Data Booklet. In: Energy USDo, ed. Third ed. Berkeley: Lawrence Berkeley National Laboratory. 9 p.
115. ASTM E384 - Standard Test Method for Knoop and Vickers Hardness of Materials. West Conshohocken, PA: American Standard for Testing Materials International p.399.
116. Edwards AL (1979) Multiple regression and the analysis of variance and covariance. A series of books in psychology. New York, NY, US: W.H. Freeman/Times Books/Holt & Co. 221 p.

6

Computationally-Optimized Bone Mechanical Modeling from High-Resolution Structural Images

Jeremy F. Magland*, Ning Zhang, Chamith S. Rajapakse, Felix W. Wehrli

Laboratory for Structural NMR Imaging, Department of Radiology, University of Pennsylvania Medical Center, Philadelphia, Pennsylvania, United States of America

Abstract

Image-based mechanical modeling of the complex micro-structure of human bone has shown promise as a non-invasive method for characterizing bone strength and fracture risk *in vivo*. In particular, elastic moduli obtained from image-derived micro-finite element (μFE) simulations have been shown to correlate well with results obtained by mechanical testing of cadaveric bone. However, most existing large-scale finite-element simulation programs require significant computing resources, which hamper their use in common laboratory and clinical environments. In this work, we theoretically derive and computationally evaluate the resources needed to perform such simulations (in terms of computer memory and computation time), which are dependent on the number of finite elements in the image-derived bone model. A detailed description of our approach is provided, which is specifically optimized for μFE modeling of the complex three-dimensional architecture of trabecular bone. Our implementation includes domain decomposition for parallel computing, a novel stopping criterion, and a system for speeding up convergence by pre-iterating on coarser grids. The performance of the system is demonstrated on a dual quad-core Xeon 3.16 GHz CPUs equipped with 40 GB of RAM. Models of distal tibia derived from 3D in-vivo MR images in a patient comprising 200,000 elements required less than 30 seconds to converge (and 40 MB RAM). To illustrate the system's potential for large-scale μFE simulations, axial stiffness was estimated from high-resolution micro-CT images of a voxel array of 90 million elements comprising the human proximal femur in seven hours CPU time. In conclusion, the system described should enable image-based finite-element bone simulations in practical computation times on high-end desktop computers with applications to laboratory studies and clinical imaging.

Editor: Xiaoyuan Chen, NIH, United States of America

Funding: This work was supported by National Institutes of Health grants R01 AR55647, R01 AR55356 and K25 AR 060283. The funders had no role in study design, data collection and analysis, decision to publish, or preparation of the manuscript.

Competing Interests: The authors have declared that no competing interests exist.

* E-mail: Jeremy.Magland@gmail.com

Introduction

Large-scale finite-element simulations of complex physical systems (e.g. involving 10 million or more finite elements) are being used increasingly in many areas of science, engineering, biomedical and clinical research and industry [1,2,3,4]. However, most existing large-scale finite-element simulation programs require significant computing resources, which may hamper their use in common laboratory and clinical environments. The development of computationally efficient finite-element solvers for targeted applications is therefore of great interest.

Image-based micro-finite-element (μFE) modeling on the basis of high-resolution medical images has shown promise as a technique for mechanical characterization of the complex micro-structure of bone. Both magnetic resonance (MR) and peripheral high-resolution computed tomography (HR-pQCT) have already demonstrated the ability to monitor alterations in bone mechanical properties resulting from disease progression or drug intervention [5,6] or for assessment of fracture risk [7,8]. FE analyses at multiple scales from macro- to micro-structure have also been proposed as possible means to provide insight into failure mechanisms [9].

Bone is classified into two structural types: cortical and trabecular. Both types of bone remodel throughout human life, with old bone being resorbed and new bone being deposited. Remodeling controls the reshaping or replacement of bone during growth and following injury, and generally occurs in response to changes in functional demands of mechanical loading [10]. Perturbation in bone mineral homeostasis, e.g. due to hormone loss following menopause [11,12] or extended exposure to microgravity [13] causes a remodeling imbalance with greater rate of resorption than new bone formation, resulting in structural and mechanical impairment of the skeleton due to architectural deterioration along with net loss of trabecular and cortical bone [14,15,16]. The above scenario is characteristic of the etiology of osteoporosis, a condition that leads to increased risk of fracture.

High-resolution image-based μFE analysis is able to simulate the effects of mechanical loading of bone, thus providing insight into the relationship between bone microarchitecture and bone strength. Excellent agreement has been noted between biomechanical compression tests and μFE-derived elastic moduli based on images acquired at high spatial resolution [17,18,19]. Unlike direct mechanical testing, the gold standard for determining bone mechanical competence, image-based μFE modeling is nondestructive and is hence feasible *in vivo* [6,20].

Human trabecular bone is a complex network of interconnected plates and struts on the order of 100–150 μm thickness [15] whereas the macroscopic scale of bone is on the order of centimeters or even tens of centimeters. The computational demands (in terms of RAM and CPU) can therefore be enormous for accurate high-resolution simulation of even a portion of the bone (such as the vertebrae, distal radius or proximal femur–locations of high fracture incidence). For example, FE simulation of a single human vertebral body would require around 185 million elements at an element size (and thus image voxel size) of 30 μm. While such resolution is far beyond any in-vivo imaging modality's capability, the potential to predict bone mechanical properties on the basis of lower-resolution in vivo images, is of significant clinical interest [6,20]. Under the best of circumstances *in vivo* MRI and CT currently yield an effective resolution on the order of 100–200 μm at selected skeletal locations [20,21,22] in practical scan times (MRI) and acceptable radiation dose (CT), which typically reduces data size to 10 million elements or less. However, it is conceivable that pre-processing of the images to higher apparent resolution via interpolation techniques such as subvoxel processing [23] or zero filling in Fourier space [24] may significantly enhance accuracy in the prediction of the bone's mechanical behavior, but would also significantly increase data array size. Although not addressed in this paper, simulations in the nonlinear regime increase computational demands by an order of magnitude or more, and are thus impractical unless computational efficiency is substantially augmented.

Here, we investigate the feasibility of large-scale FE simulations (performed on desktop personal computers) and describe an optimized FE solver designed for high-resolution image-based computational bone mechanics of systems with 10–100 million elements within the constraints of standard workstations in minutes to hours. These advances are achieved through algorithmic improvements involving effective memory usage, accelerated convergence and parallelization. Critical to these endeavors is a reduction in the number of iterations required toward convergence of the solution. We show that this goal can be achieved by starting iteration on coarser grids (i.e. using larger size thereby reducing the number of elements). Further we describe an iteration procedure that enables a more effective estimate of the relative error in total stress, accurately indicating when to halt the conjugate gradient iterations. Lastly, we show that significant speed enhancements can be achieved by making efficient usage of the available processors through parallelization of the computing tasks. The performance of the FE solver is illustrated with applications to human specimen micro-CT and in vivo high-resolution MR images as input into the model to estimate stiffness and failure load.

Materials and Methods

Definition of the linear system

Image-based estimation of macroscopic mechanical properties of bone involves (a) defining the image-derived structural bone model (b) simulating the induced macroscopic strain by applying appropriate boundary conditions, (c) solving for the resulting equilibrium displacements throughout the structure, and (d) computing stiffness from macroscopic stress/strain ratios. In the linear elastic regime (which we assume throughout), local stress and strain are linearly related by Hooke's Law:

$$\sigma = C\varepsilon, \tag{1}$$

where

$$\sigma = [\sigma_{xx} \quad \sigma_{yy} \quad \sigma_{zz} \quad \sigma_{yz} \quad \sigma_{zx} \quad \sigma_{xy}]^T$$

and

$$\varepsilon = [\varepsilon_{xx} \quad \varepsilon_{yy} \quad \varepsilon_{zz} \quad \varepsilon_{yz} \quad \varepsilon_{zx} \quad \varepsilon_{xy}]^T$$

are the local stress and strain vectors, respectively, and $C=(C_{ij})$ is the 6×6 stiffness matrix for the material. In the case of isotropic material, the stiffness matrix takes the form

$$C = \frac{E}{(1-\nu)(1-2\nu)} \begin{bmatrix} 1-\nu & \nu & \nu & 0 & 0 & 0 \\ \nu & 1-\nu & \nu & 0 & 0 & 0 \\ \nu & \nu & 1-\nu & 0 & 0 & 0 \\ 0 & 0 & 0 & \frac{1-2\nu}{2} & 0 & 0 \\ 0 & 0 & 0 & 0 & \frac{1-2\nu}{2} & 0 \\ 0 & 0 & 0 & 0 & 0 & \frac{1-2\nu}{2} \end{bmatrix}, \tag{2}$$

where E is Young's modulus and ν is Poisson's ratio. Here, for trabecular bone, we assume $\nu = 0.3$, and $E = 15\,\mathrm{GPa}\cdot BVF$, where BVF represents the voxel-wise bone- volume fraction (see [25] for MR or [26] for CT). Even though on a microscopic scale the bone material modulus is not isotropic [27,28], for most applications the assumption of voxel-wise isotropy is warranted.

Following [29], we let each 3D image voxel represent a single hexahedral (brick) element in our finite element model. By assuming a tri-linear displacement field within each brick element, the microscopic Hooke's law defines a linear relationship between the vertex displacements $\vec{u}^{(B)}_{i,j,k}$ and the induced vertex forces $\vec{F}^{(B)}_{i,j,k}$ ($i,j,k = 0,1$ are the coordinate indices). The superscript "(B)" indicates that this is the force acting on the vertex by a single element, and is therefore only one component of the total force at the vertex. The method for determining the precise relationship between induced vertex forces and displacements for a single element is described in Appendix S1. This relationship can be expressed as

$$\vec{F}^{(B)} = C_{\mathrm{kernel}}\vec{u}^{(B)}, \tag{3}$$

where C_{kernel} is a 24×24 kernel matrix. The total force at a vertex v in the direction d, denoted by $F(v,d)$, is the sum of all forces at v (in direction d) induced by the brick elements containing v.

Simulation of applied strain (step (b) above) involves application of boundary conditions of the form:

$$u(v,d) = c_{v,d}, \tag{4}$$

where $u(v,d)$ is the displacement of the vertex v in the direction d at selected vertex locations (usually on a boundary surface of the image volume). The condition of force equilibrium (step (c)) can then be expressed as

$$F(v,d) = 0, \tag{5}$$

at all free vertex/direction pairs (i.e., those without applied boundary conditions). Therefore, the number of equations in this linear system is equal to N_v, the number of free (displacement) variables. The (macroscopic) linear system for the force can be expressed as

$$AU = B, \tag{6}$$

where A is a sparse $N_v \times N_v$ matrix referred to as the *macroscopic stiffness matrix* and U are the displacements at all free vertex/direction pairs. The right-hand side, B is defined according to the applied boundary conditions. The central (and most time-consuming) step in the mechanical modeling procedure is to solve this linear system (6).

Conjugate gradient iteration

Because the microscopic stiffness matrix C (e.g. Equation (2)) is symmetric, one can show that the macroscopic stiffness matrix A is positive definite (this condition is equivalent to the total energy always being nonnegative, for any vertex displacement configuration). We may therefore use the preconditioned conjugate-gradient (PCG) algorithm to solve equation (6) [30,31]. Because we will subsequently refer to the details of this algorithm, the processing steps are outlined below for the conjugate gradient procedure.

Algorithm 1. Conjugate Gradient Algorithm

Step 0: Select an initial displacement configuration u_0, compute the residual r_0 and set the initial search direction (for simplicity we leave out the preconditioner in this description):

$$r_0 = B - Au_0$$

$$p_0 = r_0.$$

Set $n := 0$.

Step 1: Compute $q_n = Ap_n$.

Step 2: Compute $\alpha_n = \frac{\langle r_n, r_n \rangle}{\langle p_n, q_n \rangle}$ (where $\langle a, b \rangle$ stands for inner product of two vectors a, b), and then compute the new displacement and residual vectors.

$$u_{n+1} = u_n + \alpha_n p_n$$

$$r_{n+1} = r_n - \alpha_n q_n$$

Step 3: Compute $\beta_n = \frac{\langle r_{n+1}, r_{n+1} \rangle}{\langle r_n, r_n \rangle}$ and then compute the new search direction:

$$p_{n+1} = \beta_n p_n + r_{n+1}.$$

Step 4: If within error tolerance, stop. Otherwise increment $n := n+1$ and return to Step 1.

Memory usage estimation

Even when using a memory-efficient sparse-matrix storage scheme, construction of the $N_v \times N_v$ sparse matrix A is highly memory-intensive as compared with the element-by-element (EBE) approach [32,33]. Because each vertex has up to *27* neighbor vertices (including itself), a single row of the matrix can have up to 81 non-zero entries (three displacement directions for each vertex), requiring storage of up to (81 entries per variable)x(4 bytes per entry) = 324 bytes per free variable (this is even neglecting memory required to store the entry locations). Throughout this paper, we empirically estimate the number of variables as approximately 4 times the number of elements, $N_v \approx 4N_e$, where N_e is the number of elements (note: if bone were to occupy the entire volume of the image, this ratio would equal 3, but accounting for boundary vertices, this ratio tends to be closer to 4). Therefore, the full-matrix method (i.e. storing A using an efficient sparse matrix scheme) requires up to 1,296 bytes per element for matrix storage alone.

In contrast, the EBE method demands substantially less memory, since only the *BVF* scaling factor and vertex indices need to be stored for each element. The key assumption is that the *24×24* kernel matrix (C_{kernel}) is identical (up to BVF scaling factor) at all elements. However, there is a tradeoff in terms of computation time. With the sparse matrix construction method, each matrix multiplication (Step 1 in the CG algorithm) involves up to $81N_v$ multiplication operations, compared with $24 \times 24N_e$ for the EBE approach. Assuming $N_v \approx 4N_e$ as above, this suggests that EBE would be slower by a factor of around 1.8. However, the true ratio for comparing the two methods may differ depending on the efficiency of the sparse matrix multiplication algorithm, and the actual average number of entries per row (recall that 81 is an upper estimate). Nevertheless, the significant memory savings of the EBE technique generally outweighs the modest loss in iteration speed.

Table 1 shows a breakdown of the total theoretical memory usage for the EBE technique. In addition to bone-volume fraction (1 byte per element), 24 variable indices must be stored at each brick element (8 vertices×3 directions per vertex). Assuming 32-bit integers are used for storing indices, this requires 24×4 = 96 bytes per element. However, if variables are stored sequentially according to 4-dimensional coordinates (three spatial and one direction, with direction as the inner iteration), then only one sixth of these variable indices need to be stored by the element, because other indices can be obtained by offsetting the base indices. Thus only 16 bytes per element are required for variable indices. The bulk of memory usage (≈80 bytes per element) is required by the five CG vectors: displacement (u), residual (r), search direction (p), search direction multiplied by A ($q = Ap$), and the vector storing the Jacobi preconditioner. Finally, we need to store the variable index lookup map, so that vertex-variable indices can be related to locations on the original image grid. This requires 4 bytes per

Table 1. Estimated memory usage by number of elements.

	Expected Memory Usage: Element-by-Element Method
Bone-volume fraction map	(1 byte)×N_e
Element vertex-variable indices	(16 bytes)×N_e
Five vectors in the conjugate gradient algorithm: u, r, p, q, +preconditioner	(4 bytes)×N_v×5≈(80 bytes)×N_e
Variable index lookup map	(4 bytes)×$N_xN_yN_z$≈(32 bytes)×N_e
Total	**≈(130 bytes)×N_e**

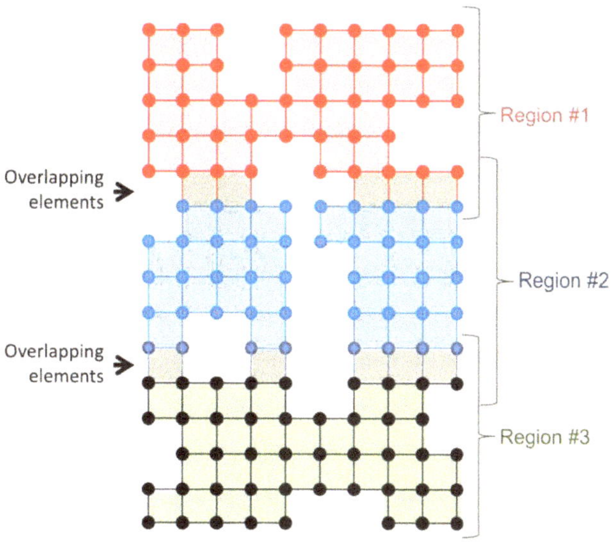

Figure 1. Two-dimensional representation of the finite element model, with each point representing a vertex or node in the system. Parallel computing requires additional memory allocation since vertices located at the interfaces between sub-regions must be stored twice.

image vertex, or at most 32 bytes per element (assuming at least 1/8 of image voxels are occupied by positive bone volume fraction).

As described below, parallel computing requires allocation of additional memory since data located at the interface between sub-regions must be duplicated between multiple processor threads (see Figure 1). Assuming that the structure is split into sub-regions along the Z-direction (inferior-superior direction in most cases), the formula for the fraction of overhead is given by $\frac{2(K-1)}{N_z+1}$ where K is the number of threads (or number of sub-regions) and N_z is the number of voxels along the Z direction. For example, if $K = 8$ threads are used and $N_z = 100$, then the overhead would be around 14%, for an expected memory usage of around **150 bytes per element**.

Parallel processing

To make use of multiple processors for speeding up the simulation, it is necessary to divide the workload among the processors [34]. Ideally, with perfect distribution of computations, total simulation time will be reduced by a factor equal to the number of processors. However, as with memory usage estimates, we need to consider the cost of additional computations performed on the interfaces between sub-regions. Below is a parallelized version of the PCG algorithm. Within each sub-region, we distinguish between *inner* and *outer* vertices according to the color-coding of Figure 1. For example, the blue vertices are the inner vertices of Region #2, whereas this region also contains two rows of outer vertices (red and black).

Algorithm 2 (below) has been reorganized (compare with Algorithm 1) in order to facilitate parallel computing. Steps 1a, 1b, and 3a can all be implemented independently within each sub-region. On the other hand, steps 2 and 3b involve interaction between sub-regions. Fortunately, 2 and 3b do not require significant computation time as compared with the remainder of the algorithm. Therefore, we can expect to achieve close to a K-fold speedup. Toward this end, the sub-regions should be chosen so that the vertices are distributed as uniformly as possible. In the present implementation, we chose the sub-region bounding planes to be parallel to one another, and optimize their positions so that each sub-region has an approximately equal share of vertices.

Algorithm 2. Parallelized Conjugate Gradient Algorithm

Step 0: Select an initial displacement configuration u_0, compute the residual r_0 and set the initial search direction (for simplicity we leave out the preconditioner):

$$r_0 = B - Au_0$$

$$p_0 = r_0.$$

Set $n := 0$.

Divide the volume into K sub-regions $S_1, \ldots, S_k$ (as shown in Figure 1), where K is the number of processing threads. The choice of sub-regions should be load-balancing (e.g. using the technique described below).

Step 1a: For each sub-region, compute $q_n = Ap_n$ on the inner vertices.

Step 1b: For each sub-region S_k, compute the following partial inner products

$$\langle r_n, r_n \rangle_{I_k}, \langle r_n, q_n \rangle_{I_k}, \langle p_n, q_n \rangle_{I_k}, \langle q_n, q_n \rangle_{I_k}$$

where

$$\langle v, w \rangle_{I_k} = \sum_{m \in I_k} v_m w_m$$

And the sum is computed over the inner vertex indices I_k of the subregion S_k.

Step 2: Compute the full inner-products $\langle r_n, r_n \rangle$, $\langle r_n, q_n \rangle$, $\langle p_n, q_n \rangle$, $\langle q_n, q_n \rangle$ by summing over the partial inner products from step 1b in the following manner:

$$\langle v, w \rangle = \sum_{k=1}^{K} \langle v, w \rangle_{I_k}.$$

Then, compute $\alpha_n = \frac{\langle r_n, r_n \rangle}{\langle p_n, q_n \rangle}$.

$$\beta_n = \frac{\langle r_{n+1}, r_{n+1} \rangle}{\langle r_n, r_n \rangle} = 1 + 2\frac{\langle r_n, q_n \rangle}{\langle p_n, q_n \rangle} + \frac{\langle r_n, r_n \rangle \langle q_n, q_n \rangle}{\langle p_n, q_n \rangle^2}.$$

Step 3a: For each sub-region, compute the new displacement on all (inner and outer) vertices

$$u_{n+1} = u_n + \alpha_n p_n$$

and compute the new residual and search direction vectors on the inner vertices only:

$$r_{n+1} = r_n - \alpha_n q_n$$

$$p_{n+1} = \beta_n p_n + r_{n+1}.$$

Step 3b: For each sub-region, update p_{n+1} on the outer vertices by retrieving the information from the inner vertices of neighboring sub-regions.

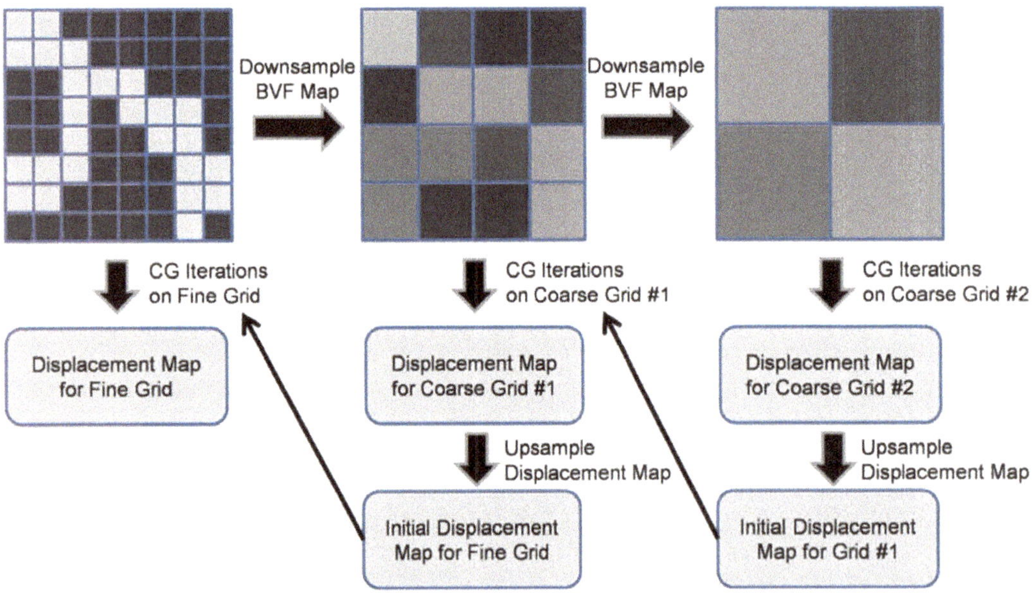

Figure 2. Total simulation time can be significantly decreased by performing initial iterations on coarser grids prior to solving the system on the original (fine) grid. Since the solution obtained at the coarser scale is already close to the final solution, fewer iterations are required at the finest scale.

Step 4: If within error tolerance, stop. Otherwise increment $n := n+1$ and go to Step 1.

Convergence criterion

Traditionally, the magnitude of the residual vector r_n, is used to determine when to halt the conjugate gradient iteration procedure. However, the direct quantity of interest is the computed total stress (as a function of applied strain), and we are therefore most interested in how closely this computed value at each iteration is to its converged (i.e., "true") value. Here we describe a method for estimating the relative error in this total stress in order to more accurately determine when to halt the conjugate gradient iterations.

Let S_n be the computed total stress after the n_{th} iteration. We assume that, after a finite number of iterations, S_n will converge approximately exponentially to its (unknown) true value S_∞ according to

$$S_n \approx S_\infty + ae^{-bn}.$$

Taking the log of the absolute derivative, with respect to n, we get

$$\log|S'_n| \approx \log|a| + \log|b| - bn,$$

which is a linear function of n. Therefore, by performing a linear fit to $\log|S'_n|$(for n indexing, say, the 30 most recent iterations), we can estimate a and b, and then use these to estimate the relative error:

$$E_n = \frac{|S_\infty - S_n|}{S_\infty} \approx \frac{ae^{-bn}}{S_n}.$$

In this study we used finite differences to estimate the absolute derivative of S_n.

Pre-iteration on coarser grids (PICG)

To further reduce the total simulation time, a pre-iteration on coarser grids (PICG) approach was applied (which is similar to the multilevel method [35]). Instead of running simulation directly on the original grid, we first perform simulations on a sequence of coarser grids, obtained by downsampling from the original (fine) grid, as illustrated in Figure 2. Starting from the coarsest grid, displacements obtained on each grid (for, say grid #2) were utilized as the initial displacements to CG iteration on the next grid (grid #1 in this case). This method significantly speeds up simulation since solutions obtained on coarser grids progressively approach the final solution. An overview of the entire problem-solving pipeline is provided in Figure 3, including image pre-processing, application of boundary conditions, pre-iteration on course grids, and parallelized conjugate gradient iteration.

Experiments

To estimate actual memory usage and computation time as a function of the number of elements, fourteen sub-volumes of various sizes were extracted from a single 3D μCT image of a cadaver specimen of the human distal tibia (25 μm isotropic voxel size) and processed via simulated compression tests as described above. The simulation sizes for each sub-volume ranged between 1 and 75 million elements, corresponding to a range of 4.6 to 290 million variables for the linear systems. These were processed using 1, 2, 4, and 8 threads of execution.

In-vivo MR image data of the distal tibia of a postmenopausal woman previously acquired with a 3D fast spin-echo sequence [36] at $137 \times 137 \times 410 \mu m^3$ resolution as part of an ongoing study to evaluate the effect of treatment with antiresorptive drugs were subjected to μFE analysis as described previously. The patient had been treated with zoledronic acid (Reclast^{TM}) and was examined at the start of intervention(baseline) and re-examined 12 months thereafter. Mechanical analysis was performed on both data sets (after mutual registration [37]) to evaluate the potential of the method to detect a possible improvement in the bone's mechanical

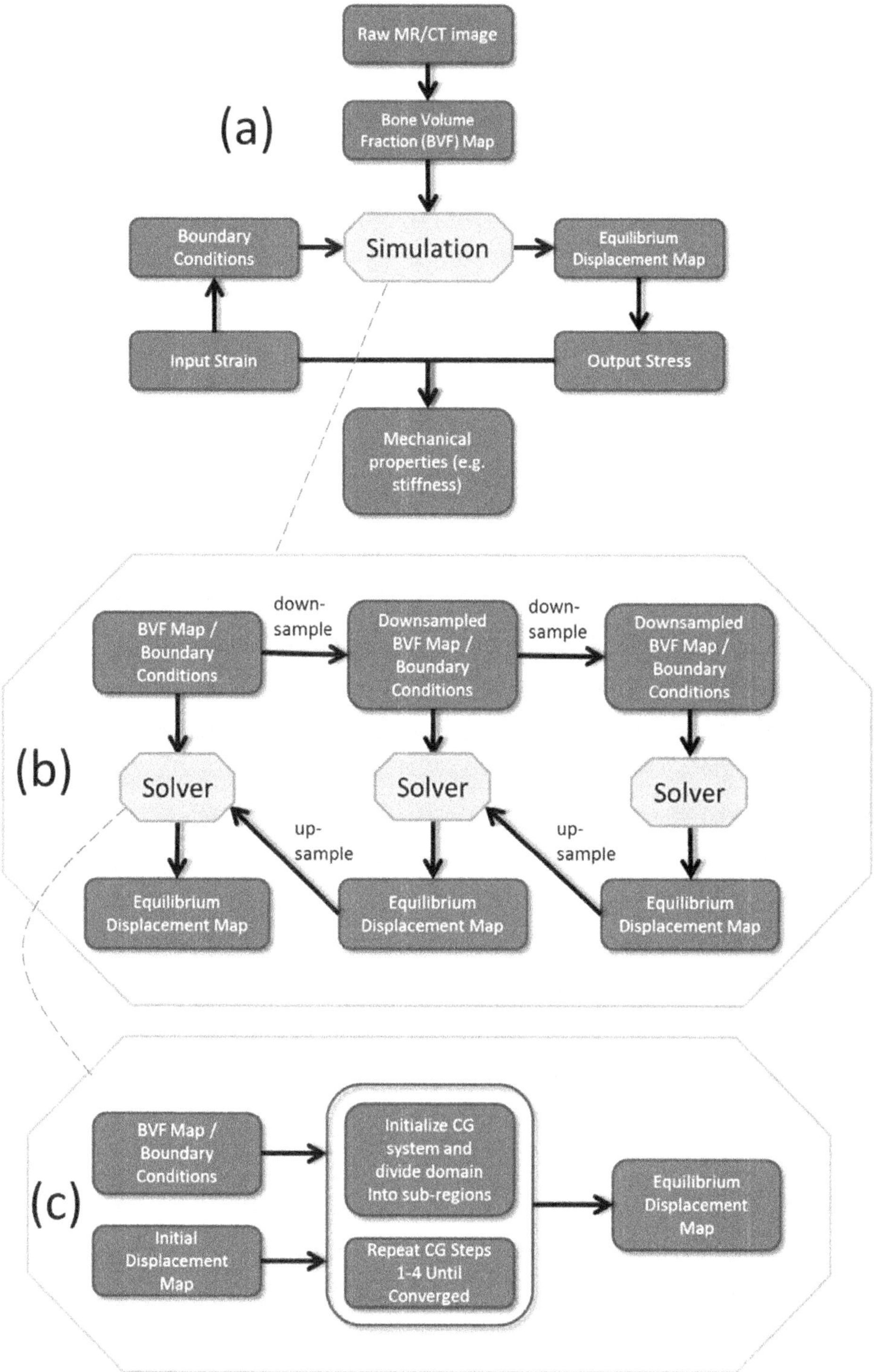

Figure 3. Flow diagram for the processing pipeline. (a) Mechanical properties for the image-based finite-element model are obtained via the relationship between simulated input strain (applied boundary conditions) and resulting simulated stress, computed from the equilibrium displacement map. (b) The equilibrium displacement map is obtained using a series of parallelized conjugate gradient solvers (c) applied at a series of resolutions (pre-iteration on courser grids).

competence in response to drug intervention. Structural parameters known to affect bone strength (e.g. bone volume fraction (BVF) and trabecular thickness) were evaluated at the two time-points as well.

In an additional experiment designed to evaluate the performance of the algorithm for processing of very large data sets, the proximal end of an intact human proximal femur was studied. The specimen was imaged by μCT on an X5000 industrial X-ray

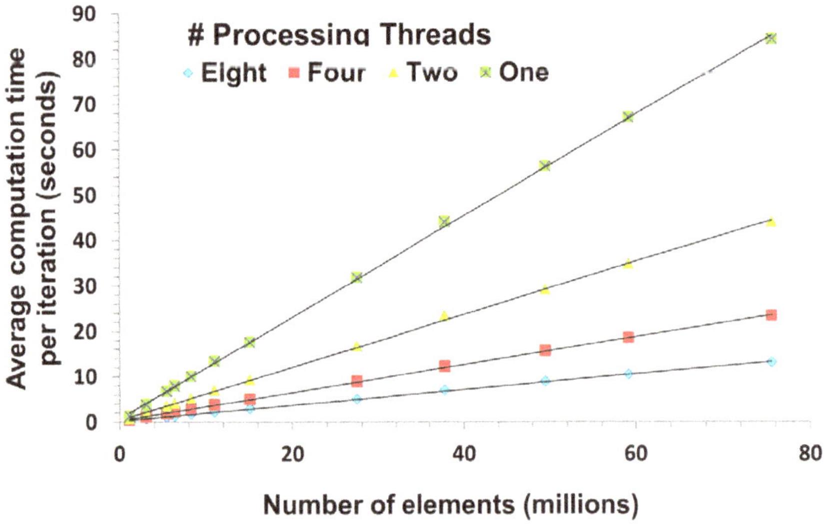

Figure 4. Memory usage (GB) versus number of elements (millions) for µFE simulations on sub-volumes of a single µCT image using a single thread and eight threads. The total number of elements in the µFE models ranged from 1 to 75 million. Symbols represent experimental data points, straight lines are best fits.

inspection system (North Star Imaging, Rogers, MN) at an isotropic voxel size of 45 µm. The reconstructed images were then digitally stitched together to produce a single 3D volumetric image of matrix size 2444×1115×1770. The µFE solver was utilized to simulate compression applied to the top surface of the femoral head through a fictitious cap encompassing the top region of the femoral head (to mimic force transmitted through the acetabulum).

All simulations were performed on a laboratory desktop computer (dual quad core Xeon 3.16 GHz CPUs equipped with 40 GB of RAM).

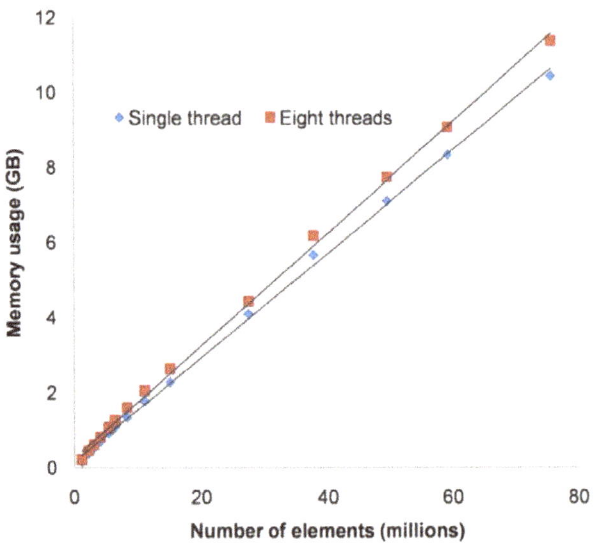

Figure 5. Average time per iteration (seconds) versus number of elements (millions) for running µFE simulations on sub-volumes of a single µCT image using one, two, four, and eight threads respectively. Symbols represent experimental data points, straight lines are best fits. Linear relationships were found in all cases with *$R^2 \geq 0.998$.*

Results

Memory usage

Figure 4 provides the results of the memory usage experiments, showing the actual memory allocation during the conjugate gradient iterations as a linear function of the number of elements. The slopes suggest that 138 bytes per element are required for a single thread and 149 bytes per element when using eight threads. This is somewhat higher than the theoretical expectation of 130 bytes per element (single thread), partly because when estimating the theoretical expectation, approximations were made between number of elements, number of variables and the product of dimensions. These data suggest that on a system with 4 GB of RAM, we can expect to be able to simulate a system with ~20 million elements, whereas 100 million elements would be possible on a computer with 16 GB of RAM.

Table 2. Total number of iterations to reach 1% accuracy estimated with and without using the PICG approach in µFE simulations on sub-volumes with different number of elements.

	Without PICG	With PICG ('4 2 1')
One-million-element data set	224	88
Three-million-element data set	448	232
Six-million-element data set	459	240
Eight-million-element data set	476	235
Eleven-million-element data set	475	344
Twenty-seven-million-element data set	594	333
Forty-nine-million-element data set	598	317
Seventy-five-million-element data set	603	295

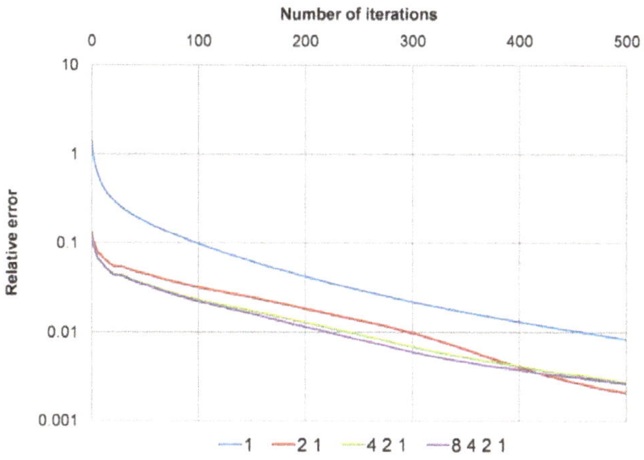

Figure 6. Plots of the "true" relative errors on the finest grid obtained after using four different combinations of pre-iteration on coarser grids: '1', '2 1', '4 2 1', and '8 4 2 1'. E.g., '4 2 1' means running simulations on data sets downsampled from the original data set by a factor of 4 and 2 sequentially, and then running simulations on the original data set. The combination '4 2 1' achieves the same accuracy as the more time-consuming combination, '8 4 2 1'.

Computation time

Figure 5 displays plots of average computation time per iteration versus number of elements for running μFE simulations on sub-volumes of a single μCT image using different numbers of threads: one, two, four, and eight. A speedup factor of 6.5 was observed when comparing eight processor threads to a single thread, compared with an ideal speedup factor of 8. The discrepancy is caused partly by interface communications between threads as well as the ~1–2% non-parallel part within each iteration, as described in the Methods. If 600 iterations are required based on the analysis above, then 2.2 hours would be needed to run a simulation on a data set with seventy-five million elements (using 8 threads). Furthermore, if applying the pre-iteration on coarser grids (PICG) approach, the total number of iterations on the finest grid could be reduced to 295 (see Table 2). Thus, approximately 1.3 hours (including computation time spent on the coarser grids) would be needed to run the same simulation in this context.

In Figure 6, the true relative errors (on the finest grid) obtained from using six different combinations of coarser grids in the PICG approach are plotted. For simulations on the coarser grids 200 iterations were used, whereas 500 iterations were used in simulation on the finest grid (the objective was to determine the true converged value, and then to retrospectively study the rate of convergence). As can be seen in Figure 6 the combination '4 2 1' achieves the same accuracy as the more time-consuming combination '8 4 2 1'.

Figure 7 provides a comparison of the true relative errors (on the finest grid) obtained using a different number of iterations on the downsampled grids using the combination '4 2 1', which was shown in Figure 6 to be optimal. To achieve 1% accuracy, around 200 iterations were needed on the finest grid when running 200 iterations on each of the coarser grids, while almost 400 iterations were needed on the finest grid when running 12 iterations on those coarser grids. Therefore the combination '4 2 1' was used in all subsequent experiments, with 200 iterations on the coarser grids.

In addition to the experimental results in terms of computation time using the authors' algorithms and programs, comparisons in computational performance with data reported in the literature are summarized in Table 3.

Convergence criterion

Figures 8a and b show comparisons of different convergence criteria (in log scale) using two experiments (compression simulations on sub-volumes of the μCT image with 1 and 3 million elements respectively). The estimated relative error was obtained from applying the log-derivative approach as described in the Method Section; the scaled residual was obtained from scaling the ratio between the L_2 norm of the residual from each iteration and the L_2 norm of the right hand side of Eq. (6), which is equivalent to the ratio between the residual in the net force from each iteration and the force imposed on the boundary surfaces;

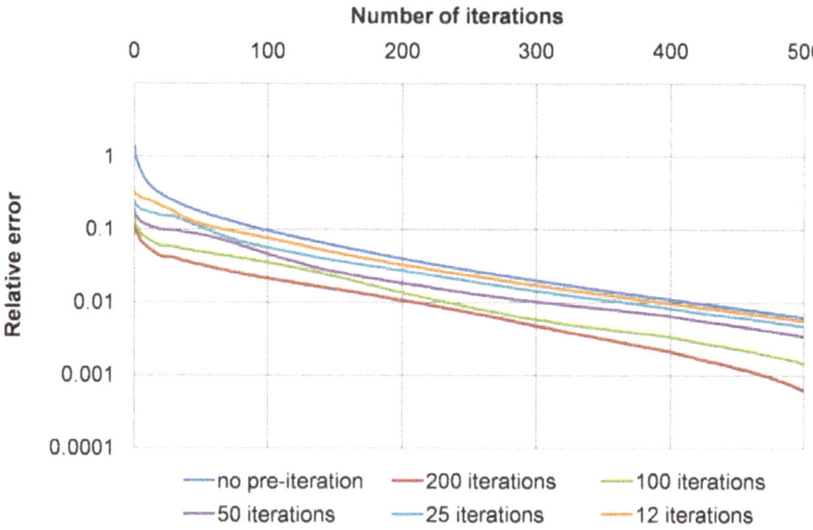

Figure 7. Comparisons of the true relative errors on the finest grid obtained from running different number of iterations (200: red; 100: green; 50: purple; 25: blue; 12: orange) on all coarser grids in the combination strategy '4 2 1'. Using 200 iterations on each coarser grid reduced the total number of iterations on the finest grid to around 200 compared to around 400 when using no pre-iteration for a 1% accuracy.

Table 3. Comparisons in computational performance with literature-reported data.

Ref.	Year	Anatomic Location	Number of Elements (million)	Number of Processors	FE Solver	Computer Type	Comp. Time/Million Elements
[29]	1995	N/A	0.35	not reported	N/A	Supercomputer	12 h
[43]	2003	Femur	96	30	N/A	SGI-Origin2000	260.4cpuh
[43]	2003	Femur	33	16	N/A	SGI-Origin3800	606.1cpuh
[40]	2004	N/A	135	4000	Olympus	IBM SP Power3	~25.2 s
[44]	2006	N/A	≤2.7	not reported	Olympus	Cray-Dell PowerEdge Xeon cluster parallel supercomputer	4.5 h**
[45]	2007	N/A	5.44	256	ParFE	Cray XT3	10.8 s
[46]	2008	N/A	247.73	1024	ParFE	Cray XT3	2.9 s
[47]	2009	radius & tibia	8	not reported	Scanco	Workstation	45 m
[30]	2010	N/A	~375*	8192	ParFE	IBM Blue Gene	~3.6 s*
[39]	2011	Radius	2	not reported	Scanco	N/A	1.5 h
[39]	2011	Tibia	5	not reported	Scanco	N/A	1 h
	2011	**Tibia**	**0.2**	**8**	**FESBI**	**desktop computer**	**4.52 m**
	2011	**Femur**	**90.3**	**8**	**FESBI**	**desktop computer**	**2.25 m**

Note: numbers marked with.
*are approximations based on reported number of degrees of freedom; numbers with.
are approximated averages; **the last two rows (bold) are performance results from the authors' software. Although difficult to compare different methodologies (with varying parameters, etc), these numbers are accurate to the best of the authors' knowledge.

and the true relative error was obtained using $\frac{\|x - x_{true}\|}{\|x_{true}\|}$, where x is the computed solution (the primary stress in our case) from each iteration and x_{true} is the true solution obtained from running many more iterations than needed.

Retrospectively tested, the estimated relative error has similar trends as the true relative error while the scaled residual does not. Furthermore, the estimated relative error is accurate to within a factor of at most two of the true relative error and tends to be increasingly accurate as the iteration number increases.

Table 2 lists the total numbers of iterations required to achieve around 1% accuracy of the true solution (the "infinitely converged" solution) for data sets with different numbers of elements. Results with and without applying the PICG approach are given, showing that using PICG reduces the total number of iterations required to reach a 1% accuracy by a factor of ~2. Based on our experimental results (see Figures 6 and 7), the combination strategy '4 2 1' was utilized here in the PICG approach.

Applications to trabecular bone mechanics

Simulated axial compression tests of the 7T MRI patient image data for the two 3D data sets described in the Methods section (baseline and 12-month follow-up) contained approximately 0.2 million elements taking 27 seconds to converge. Measured bone-volume fraction, trabecular thickness and axial stiffness were found to have increased over the course of the one-year treatment period. BVF had increased from 7.4 to 8.7%; trabecular thickness from 99.5 to 102.4 μm; and axial stiffness from 247 to 293 MPa. Figure 9 displays mutually registered parametric strain energy maps at the two time-points. The images at the two time-points show remarkable similarity indicative of relatively small remodeling changes (Figures 9b and f) which, however, appear to have significant mechanical consequences as suggested by the 19% increase in predicted stiffness. We also notice a rather unequal loading pattern exhibiting greater strain medially than laterally at least in the anterior region displayed in Figures 9d and f.

In an additional experiment designed to evaluate the performance of the algorithm for processing of very large data sets, the proximal end of an intact human proximal femur was studied. A sample slice of the simulated strain-energy map in coronal view is given in Figure 10. The total number of elements in the μFE model for the downsampled data was 90.3 million and the total time for solving the resultant linear system was 6.0 hours on the desktop computer (as described in the Methods) using parallel computing with eight threads. The PICG approach was also applied for comparison. Because of the large size of the femur data, a combination '32 16 8 4 2 1' was utilized where a total of 200 iterations were performed on simulations based on the coarse grids, thereby reducing total computation time to 2.3 hours.

Discussion

We have conceived and implemented substantially improved algorithms yielding a computationally efficient program for large-scale finite-element simulations of bone mechanics on the basis of μMR and μCT images. The work's primary goal was to enable the performance of such simulations on desktop computers within practical computation times. Three key factors for improving efficiency were investigated: memory usage, computation time and convergence criteria.

The implementation of the EBE approach [32,33] avoids storing the entire linear system thereby greatly reducing memory usage. The theoretical memory savings (from using EBE), was estimated in this work as a factor of 10, agreeing well with the estimate of a factor of 9 from [38]. A row-by-row (RBR) approach was also proposed in [38], but based on numerical examples, the RBR approach appears to use as much as 35% more memory than the EBE approach.

Thus far, computational constraints on desktop computers limited image-based FE analyses of bone structure networks to

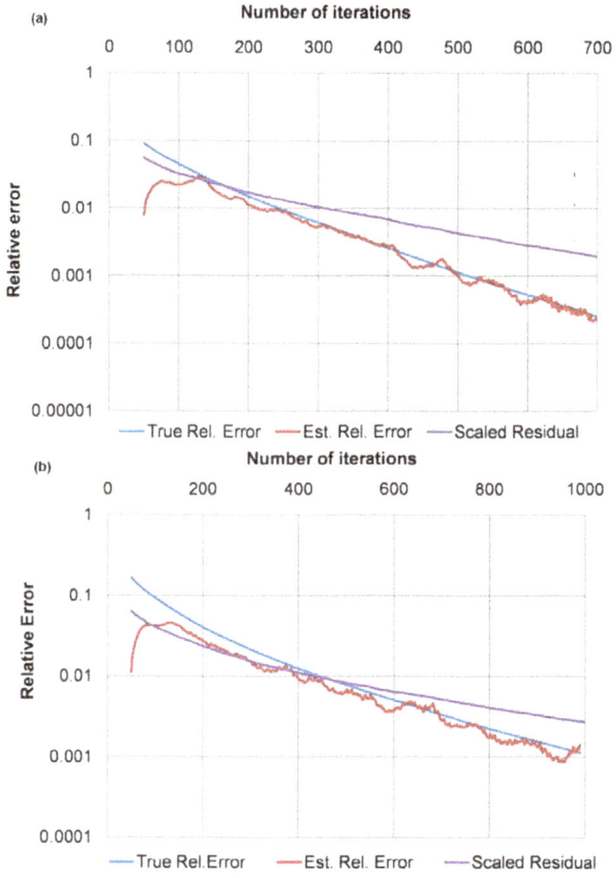

Figure 8. Convergence criteria comparisons. (a) in example 1, the estimated relative error (red) has almost the same trend as the true relative error (blue), whereas the scaled residual (purple) deviates substantially; (b) the estimated relative error (red) in example 2 also better approximates to the true relative error (blue) than the scaled residual (purple).

models with relatively small numbers of finite elements. Simulation of a distal tibia model with 5 million elements, for example, typically takes around 5 hours as reported in recent work [39]. With the enhanced FE algorithms detailed in the present work, a bone structure model of this complexity can be solved in 9 minutes to achieve 1% estimated accuracy in the output parameter.

Large-scale FE simulations of trabecular bone networks have previously been performed on highly scalable, implicitly parallel, one-of-a-kind supercomputers. For example, Adams et al. in 2004 solved a FE model of a vertebral body with 135 million elements using an ASCI White supercomputer consisting of 292 computer nodes [40]. A recent study reported solving FE systems with up to about 1.5 billion unknowns (~375 million elements) within half an hour using 8192 cores of the Blue Gene/L supercomputer at IBM T.J. [30]. Our current desktop FE implementation can achieve a comparable task consisting of a system with 135 million elements in approximately 6 hours utilizing 20 GB of memory. Currently, with our 8-core laboratory computer is equipped with 40 GB of memory, we project a maximum solvable system size of around 266 million elements in ~13 hours. To the best of the authors' knowledge, solving of such large-scale models of trabecular bone networks on a single desktop computer has not previously been feasible.

We compared the computation time achievable by the present work against literature-reported values (see Table 3). It is to be noted that the majority of the work reported therein has been performed on large-scale computer clusters, with hundreds to thousands of processors using canned software packages. While one to two orders slower than such computers, our system far outperforms desktop-based systems currently in use. Furthermore, the present program has been designed from scratch to optimally handle bone structural images in terms of its I/O capabilities and its computational efficiency is achieved with a mere eight cores of a standard, readily available, desktop computer. With simulation times on the order of minutes for typical array sizes for in vivo images on the order of 1–2 million elements, on-line computation as part of the image reconstruction and processing pipeline now has become practical. The system makes simulations on very large arrays such as those resulting from whole-bone μCT images feasible, which previously required access to supercomputers.

Parallel programming on desktop computers is becoming increasingly attractive with the availability of multi-core computers systems. With the trend of continually increasing the number of cores on a single computer (e.g. 16 or 32 cores), even larger FE systems than those demonstrated here can be expected to be solved on desktop systems in the near future without the need for supercomputers with the algorithmic optimizations described in this work. In some situations, computation time could be further reduced by adapting the present methodology to graphics processing unit (GPU) computing (substantially increasing the parallelization factor). However, at present, the available RAM on a GPU is often limited to around 1 GB, precluding simulations involving more than around 10 million elements.

Comparison of computation times reported by different studies is often not straightforward because convergence criteria are not explicitly stated. The magnitude of the residual at a given iteration is widely used to decide when to stop the simulation. However, since the residual is computed as an internal step while solving the linear system of equations, it is not directly reflective of the magnitude of error in the output parameter (stiffness, for example) at a given FE iteration. To overcome these limitations, a novel convergence criterion was adopted in our FE implementation, which indicates how close the computed stiffness value at each iteration is to the "true" value. For this study, a 1% error in stiffness was used as a convergence criterion. Our experiments suggest that the total number of iterations needed using the new convergence criterion is closer to the actual requirement than that estimated using other convergence criteria, for instance, estimations based on (relative/scaled) residual. With the PICG approach the total number of iterations has been shown to decrease from 485±125 (without PICG) to 260±83.

Compared to general-purpose FE software, the computational infrastructure described here provides a number of advantages for the target application of high-resolution image-based bone biomechanics. First, an integrated interface is provided to directly import raw medical images (including k-space) data for analysis, thereby eliminating the need for additional file conversion software. Second, since the FE model is generated by one-to-one mapping of image voxels into finite elements, the mechanical estimates are not influenced by differences in various mesh-generation methods, which are also computationally demanding for large systems [41]. Third, the program can operate in the binary as well as gray-scale mode, customized for generating FE models on the basis of high-resolution (e.g. micro-CT) and in-vivo (e.g. MR or CT) images of bone to account for partial volume mixing, or regional variations in attenuation coefficients.

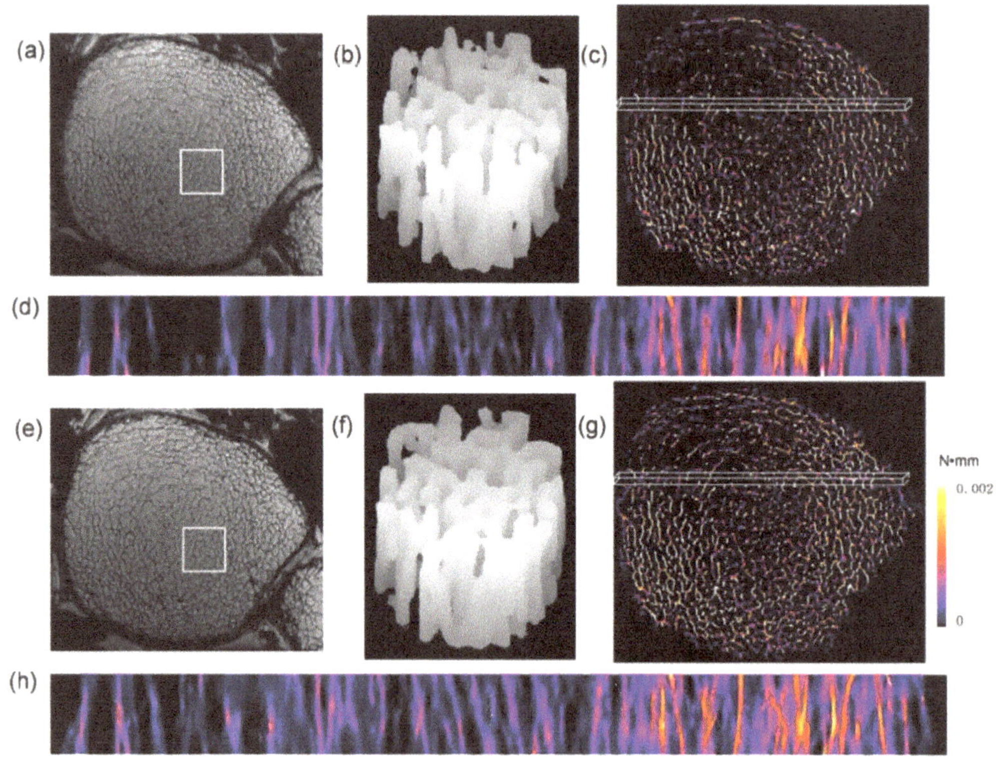

Figure 9. Structural MR images and resulting strain energy maps from two 3D data sets taken at 7T field strength at the left distal femur in a patient treated with zoledronic acid (Reclast^{TM}) for a period of 12 months. a, e) cross-sectional images from stack of contiguous slices at baseline and after 12 months of treatment; b, f) volume-renderings of square-shaped sub-regions (7.8×7.8×3.7 mm^3) indicated in images a and e, highlighting structural similarity at the two time-points; d, h) longitudinal projections of strain-energy data displayed for a thin slab (1.1×37.7×3.7 mm^3) in the anterior region indicated in c and g.

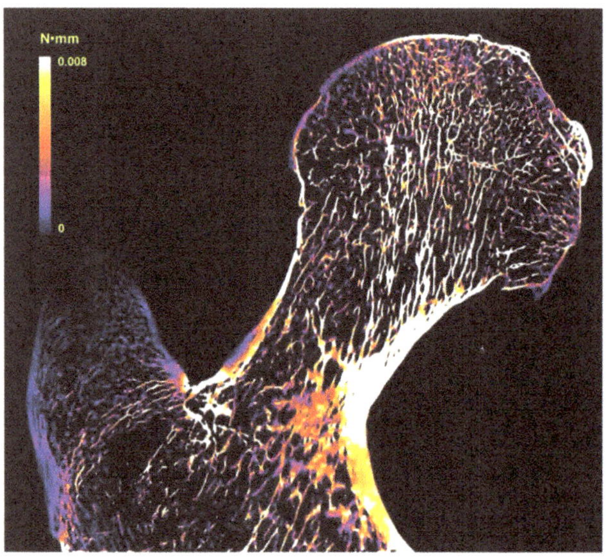

Figure 10. Sample slice of simulated strain-energy map of a human femur in coronal view. To simulate a compression along the z-axis, a 1% strain was applied to the top surface of the femoral head. For details see text.

Some limitations of the present work are noted. So far, we have confined the analysis presented here to the linear elastic regime, although nonlinear FE modeling can provide additional information on bone's failure mechanisms [42]. We expect that the substantial improvements in speed and resource utilization achieved under the present work will make nonlinear analysis feasible within clinically acceptable computation time limits. Nonlinear analysis typically entails application of a series of incremental strains with each step involving solution of a linear system. Therefore, the present methodology may substantially improve the efficiency of non-linear analyses. We project that nonlinear analysis on an in-vivo MRI data set on the order of one million elements could be tackled within an hour or at least in the time needed currently with commercial desktop based systems for linear analysis.

In conclusion, the desktop computer based FE approach detailed here enables computational biomechanics of bone, previously confined to research studies, in clinical settings.

Acknowledgments

The authors would like to thank Dr. Alexander Wright and Dr. Yusuf Bhagat of the Laboratory for Structural NMR Imaging for providing experimental data, and Dr. Michael Wald for providing software to do volume rendering.

Author Contributions

Conceived and designed the experiments: JM NZ CR FW. Performed the experiments: JM NZ. Analyzed the data: JM NZ. Contributed reagents/materials/analysis tools: JM. Wrote the paper: JM NZ CR FW.

References

1. Mcculloch A, Waldman L, Rogers J, Guccione J (1992) Large-Scale Finite-Element Analysis of the Beating Heart. Critical Reviews in Biomedical Engineering 20: 427–449.
2. Hou TY, Wu XH (1997) A multiscale finite element method for elliptic problems in composite materials and porous media. Journal of Computational Physics 134: 169–189.
3. Van Rietbergen B, Muller R, Ulrich D, Ruegsegger P, Huiskes R (1999) Tissue stresses and strain in trabeculae of a canine proximal femur can be quantified from computer reconstructions. J Biomech 32: 443–451.
4. Danilov S, Kivman G, Schroter J (2004) A finite-element ocean model: principles and evaluation. Ocean Modelling 6: 125–150.
5. Zhang XH, Liu XS, Vasilic B, Wehrli FW, Benito M, et al. (2008) In vivo microMRI-based finite element and morphological analyses of tibial trabecular bone in eugonadal and hypogonadal men before and after testosterone treatment. J Bone Miner Res 23: 1426–1434.
6. Wehrli FW, Rajapakse CS, Magland JF, Snyder PJ (2010) Mechanical implications of estrogen supplementation in early postmenopausal women. J Bone Miner Res 25: 1406–1414.
7. Silva MJ, Keaveny TM, Hayes WC (1998) Computed tomography-based finite element analysis predicts failure loads and fracture patterns for vertebral sections. J Orthop Res 16: 300–308.
8. Vilayphiou N, Boutroy S, Sornay-rendu E, Van rietbergen B, Munoz F, et al. (2010) Finite element analysis performed on radius and tibia HR-pQCT images and fragility fractures at all sites in postmenopausal women. Bone 46: 1030–1037.
9. Podshivalov L, Fischer A, Bar-Yoseph PZ (2011) 3D hierarchical geometric modeling and multiscale FE analysis as a base for individualized medical diagnosis of bone structure. Bone 48: 693–703.
10. Jaworski ZFG (1987) Physiology and pathology of bone remodeling. Cellular basis of bone structure in health and in osteoporosis. Orthopedic Clinics of North America 12: 485.
11. Recker R, Lappe J, Davies KM, Heaney R (2004) Bone remodeling increases substantially in the years after menopause and remains increased in older osteoporosis patients. J Bone Miner Res 19: 1628–1633.
12. Muller R (2004) Long-term prediction of three-dimensional bone architecture in simulations of pre-, peri- and post-menopausal microstructural bone remodeling. Osteoporos Int.
13. Vico L, Chappard D, Palle S, Bakulin AV, Novikov VE, et al. (1988) Trabecular bone remodeling after seven days of weightlessness exposure (BIOCOSMOS 1667). Am J Physiol 255: R243–247.
14. Saha PK, Wald MJ, Radin A, Wehrli FW (2005) Predicting mechanical competence of trabecular bone using 3D tensor-scale-based parameters. Proc SPIE 5746: 12.
15. Wehrli FW (2007) Structural and functional assessment of trabecular and cortical bone by micro magnetic resonance imaging. J Magn Reson Imaging 25: 390–409.
16. Zikan V, Tyblova M, Raska I, Michalska D, Luchavova M (2011) Bone Health in Patients with Multiple Sclerosis Treated with Low Dose Glucocorticoids. Osteoporosis International 22: 391–391.
17. Ulrich D, Hildebrand T, Van Rietbergen B, Muller R, Ruegsegger P (1997) The quality of trabecular bone evaluated with micro-computed tomography, FEA and mechanical testing. Stud Health Technol Inform 40: 97–112.
18. Ladd AJ, Kinney JH, Haupt DL, Goldstein SA (1998) Finite-element modeling of trabecular bone: comparison with mechanical testing and determination of tissue modulus. J Orthop Res 16: 622–628.
19. Kabel J, van Rietbergen B, Dalstra M, Odgaard A, Huiskes R (1999) The role of an effective isotropic tissue modulus in the elastic properties of cancellous bone. J Biomech 32: 673–680.
20. Boutroy S, Van Rietbergen B, Sornay-Rendu E, Munoz F, Bouxsein ML, et al. (2008) Finite element analysis based on in vivo HR-pQCT images of the distal radius is associated with wrist fracture in postmenopausal women. J Bone Miner Res 23: 392–399.
21. Wehrli FW, Hwang SN, Ma J, Song HK, Ford JC, et al. (1998) Cancellous bone volume and structure in the forearm: noninvasive assessment with MR microimaging and image processing [published erratum appears in Radiology 1998 Jun;207(3):833]. Radiology 206: 347–357.
22. Boutry N, Cortet B, Dubois P, Marchandise X, Cotten A (2003) Trabecular bone structure of the calcaneus: preliminary in vivo MR imaging assessment in men with osteoporosis. Radiology 227: 708–717.
23. Hwang SN, Wehrli FW (2002) Subvoxel Processing: A Method for reducing partial volume blurring with application to in vivo MR images of trabecular bone. Magnetic Resonance in Medicine 47: 948–957.
24. Magland JF, Wehrli FW (2008) Trabecular bone structure analysis in the limited spatial resolution regime of in vivo MRI. Acad Radiol 15: 1482–1493.
25. Rajapakse CS, Magland JF, Wald MJ, Liu XS, Zhang XH, et al. (2010) Computational biomechanics of the distal tibia from high-resolution MR and micro-CT images. Bone 47: 556–563.
26. Macneil JA, Boyd SK (2008) Bone strength at the distal radius can be estimated from high-resolution peripheral quantitative computed tomography and the finite element method. Bone 42: 1203–1213.
27. Dempster WT, Liddicoat RT (1952) Compact bone as a non-isotropic material. American Journal of Anatomy 91: 32.
28. Goulet RW, Goldstein SA, Ciarelli MJ, Kuhn JL, Brown MB, et al. (1994) The relationship between the structural and orthogonal compressive properties of trabecular bone. Journal of Biomechanics 27: 375–389.
29. van Rietbergen B, Weinans H, Huiskes R, Odgaard A (1995) A new method to determine trabecular bone elastic properties and loading using micromechanical finite-element models. Journal of Biomechanics 28: 69–81.
30. Bekas C, Curioni A, Arbenz P, Flaig C, Van Lenthe GH, et al. (2010) Extreme scalability challenges in micro finite element simulations of human bone. Concurrency and Computation: Practice and Experience 22: 2282–2296.
31. Saad Y, Saad Y (1996) Iterative methods for sparse linear systems: PWS Pub. Co.
32. Hughes TJR, Levit I, Winget J (1983) An Element-by-Element Solution Algorithm for Problems of Structural and Solid Mechanics. Computer Methods in Applied Mechanics and Engineering 36: 241–254.
33. Hughes TJR, Ferencz RM, Hallquist JO (1987) Large-Scale Vectorized Implicit Calculations in Solid Mechanics on a Cray X-Mp/48 Utilizing Ebe Preconditioned Conjugate Gradients. Computer Methods in Applied Mechanics and Engineering 61: 215–248.
34. Hendrickson B, Leland R, Plimpton S (1993) An E cient Parallel Algorithm for Matrix-Vector Multiplication. Sandia Report SAND92-2765, Sandia National Lab, Albuquerque, NM 87185.
35. Teng SH (1999) Coarsening, sampling, and smoothing: Elements of the multilevel method. Algorithms for Parallel Processing 105: 247–276.
36. Magland JF, Rajapakse CS, Wright AC, Acciavatti R, Wehrli FW (2010) 3D fast spin echo with out-of-slab cancellation: a technique for high-resolution structural imaging of trabecular bone at 7 Tesla. Magn Reson Med 63: 719–727.
37. Magland JF, Jones CE, Leonard MB, Wehrli FW (2009) Retrospective 3D registration of trabecular bone MR images for longitudinal studies. J Magn Reson Imaging 29: 118–126.
38. VanRietbergen B, Weinans H, Huiskes R, Polman BJW (1996) Computational strategies for iterative solutions of large FEM applications employing voxel data. International Journal for Numerical Methods in Engineering 39: 2743–2767.
39. Vilayphiou N, Boutroy S, Szulc P, Van Rietbergen B, Munoz F, et al. (2011) Finite element analysis performed on radius and tibia HR pQCT images and fragility fractures at all sites in men. Journal of Bone and Mineral Research 26: 965–973.
40. Adams MF, Bayraktar HH, Keaveny TM, Papadopoulos P (2004) Ultrascalable implicit finite element analyses in solid mechanics with over a half a billion degrees of freedom. ACM/IEEE Proceedings of SC2004: High Performance Networking and Computing. 34 p.
41. Bern M, Eppstein D (1992) Mesh generation and optimal triangulation. Computing in Euclidean geometry 1: 23–90.
42. Bevill G, Keaveny TM (2009) Trabecular bone strength predictions using finite element analysis of micro-scale images at limited spatial resolution. Bone 44: 579–584.
43. Zienkiewicz OC, Taylor RL, Zhu JZ The Finite Element Method: Its Basis and Fundamentals, Sixth Edition: Butterworth-Heinemann.
44. Van Rietbergen B, Huiskes R, Eckstein F, Ruegsegger P (2003) Trabecular bone tissue strains in the healthy and osteoporotic human femur. J Bone Miner Res 18: 1781–1788.
45. Bevill G, Eswaran SK, Gupta A, Papadopoulos P, Keaveny TM (2006) Influence of bone volume fraction and architecture on computed large-deformation failure mechanisms in human trabecular bone. Bone 39: 1218–1225.
46. Arbenz P, van Lenthe G, Mennel U, Muller R, Sala M (2007) Multi-level μ-finite element analysis for human bone structures. Applied Parallel Computing State of the Art in Scientific Computing. pp 240–250.
47. Arbenz P, Van Lenthe GH, Mennel U, Muller R, Sala M (2008) A Scalable Multi-level Preconditioner for Matrix-Free μ-Finite Element Analysis of Human Bone Structures. Numerical Methods in Engineering. 21 p.
48. Dalzell N, Kaptoge S, Morris N, Berthier A, Koller B, et al. (2009) Bone micro-architecture and determinants of strength in the radius and tibia: age-related changes in a population-based study of normal adults measured with high-resolution pQCT. Osteoporosis international 20: 1683–1694.

7

Heterogeneous Glycation of Cancellous Bone and Its Association with Bone Quality and Fragility

Lamya Karim[¤], **Deepak Vashishth***

Center for Biotechnology and Interdisciplinary Studies, Department of Biomedical Engineering, Rensselaer Polytechnic Institute, Troy, New York, United States of America

Abstract

Non-enzymatic glycation (NEG) and enzymatic biochemical processes create crosslinks that modify the extracellular matrix (ECM) and affect the turnover of bone tissue. Because NEG affects turnover and turnover at the local level affects microarchitecture and formation and removal of microdamage, we hypothesized that NEG in cancellous bone is heterogeneous and accounts partly for the contribution of microarchitecture and microdamage on bone fragility. Human trabecular bone cores from 23 donors were subjected to compression tests. Mechanically tested cores as well as an additional 19 cores were stained with lead-uranyl acetate and imaged to determine microarchitecture and measure microdamage. Post-yield mechanical properties were measured and damaged trabeculae were extracted from a subset of specimens and characterized for the morphology of induced microdamage. Tested specimens and extracted trabeculae were quantified for enzymatic and non-enzymatic crosslink content using a colorimetric assay and Ultra-high Performance Liquid Chromatography (UPLC). Results show that an increase in enzymatic crosslinks was beneficial for bone where they were associated with increased toughness and decreased microdamage. Conversely, bone with increased NEG required less strain to reach failure and were less tough. NEG heterogeneously modified trabecular microarchitecture where high amounts of NEG crosslinks were found in trabecular rods and with the mechanically deleterious form of microdamage (linear microcracks). The extent of NEG in tibial cancellous bone was the dominant predictor of bone fragility and was associated with changes in microarchitecture and microdamage.

Editor: Sudha Agarwal, Ohio State University, United States of America

Funding: The study was supported by United States National Institutes of Health grants AG20618 and T32GM067545. We acknowledge National Disease Research Interchange for providing human tissue with support from NIH grant 5 U42 RR006042 (www.nih.gov). The funders had no role in study design, data collection and analysis, decision to publish, or preparation of the manuscript.

Competing Interests: The authors have declared that no competing interests exist.

* E-mail: vashid@rpi.edu

¤ Current address: Center for Advanced Orthopaedic Studies, Beth Israel Deaconess Medical Center, Boston, Massachusetts, United States of America

Introduction

Age-related bone fracture is a major health problem that can result in disability and substantial medical care costs [1]. Low bone mass or bone mineral density (BMD) is considered the key factor in determining loss of bone strength and increased fracture risk [2,3]. However, studies demonstrate that decreased bone mass alone is not sufficient to cause a fracture [4–6]. Therefore, other factors such as changes in bone quality [7] may also be key determinants of fracture risk. Bone quality can be altered by several features including changes in the extracellular matrix (ECM) and microarchitecture, which interact under applied loading to influence microdamage formation that can contribute to bone's mechanical properties [7,8].

Bone's ECM components undergo numerous biochemical changes with aging. Any changes in these constituents can detrimentally alter the mechanical behavior of bone and explain the increased fracture incidence in the aging population [5]. In particular, type I collagen is susceptible to both enzymatic and non-enzymatic biochemical changes [9]. Both pathways yield crosslinks, but they affect bone's mechanical properties differently. Enzymatic processes produce pyridinium crosslinks (e.g. pyridinoline [Pyd], deoxypyridinoline [Dpd]) [10,11], which are necessary for the maturation and mechanical integrity of collagen. On the other hand, non-enzymatic glycation creates advanced glycation end products (AGEs) [9,12,13]. Glycation-induced crosslinks are inversely related to bone toughness [14] and specific AGEs such as pentosidine explain up to 23% of the variation in bone fracture toughness [15]. However, since pentosidine is only a single component of the total fluorescent AGE content in bone, pentosidine measurement may not be fully illustrative of the overall influence of glycation on bone fragility [16,17]. AGE accumulation has been shown to reduce osteoclastic bone resorption and lead to reduced turnover [18]. Because turnover affects formation and removal of microdamage and the local microarchitecture, AGEs may act through reduced turnover and influence other measures of bone quality associated with bone fragility.

To date, two studies have been conducted on the effect of crosslinks on trabecular microarchitecture [19,20] and only a single study has explored the effects of non-enzymatic glycation on microdamage formation [21]. These three components of bone quality may interact with each other and determine the magnitude of bone fragility, but their relative influence on each other is currently unknown. For example, both microarchitecture and bone matrix composition may interact with applied loading to influence microdamage formation and determine mechanical properties, which illustrate bone's ability to resist fracture [22–24].

More importantly, it has been recently shown that the presence of rod-like trabeculae, characteristic of osteoporotic bone, makes cancellous bone more susceptible to form harmful microdamage [25–27]. However, no information is available on the extent of non-enzymatic glycation and microdamage formation within single trabeculae. This information can help determine if NEG in cancellous bone is heterogeneous and explain the matrix-based mechanism through which cancellous bone transitions into a fragile and weak structure.

Thus, the goal of this study was to determine whether the trabecular microarchitecture of cancellous bone is heterogeneously modified by NEG, and whether AGEs are associated with changes in microarchitecture and microdamage and predict the fracture properties of cancellous bone. To pursue this goal, cancellous bone specimens from adult human tibiae were subjected to compression tests and then quantified for microarchitecture, microdamage, and the extent of non-enzymatic glycation. Extracted trabeculae were characterized for microdamage and quantified for AGEs.

Methods

Specimen Collection

42 cancellous bone cores (7.5 mm diameter, 10.5 mm length) were obtained from tibial plateaus of male (n = 24) and female (n = 18) human donors ranging from age 18 to 97 (average 59.3±22.1). None of the donors were diagnosed with osteoarthritis, and they were also certified to be free of bone metabolic diseases, HIV, and hepatitis B (National Disease Research Interchange and International Institute for the Advancement of Medicine). All specimens were stored in −80°C in saline soaked gauze until use.

Microarchitecture and Microdamage Analysis

Each specimen was scanned using micro-computed tomography (Scanco Medical AG) at 17.5 micron voxel resolution to obtain the following parameters: volumetric bone mineral density (BMD), bone volume fraction (BV/TV), connectivity density (Conn.D), structure model index (SMI), trabecular number (Tb.N), trabecular thickness (Tb.Th), and trabecular separation (Tb.Sp). Thresholds used to evaluate specimens were determined empirically based on 2D evaluations of a subset of samples.

Mechanical data was collected for a subset of the bone cores chosen at random (male n = 11, female n = 12, age range = 18–97, average 60.1±23.1). Uniaxial unconfined compression tests to post-yield (1.1%) apparent-level strain were performed using established protocols [28–30]. The mechanical testing was conducted at 37°C in physiological saline using a Bionix 858 servo-hydraulic testing system (MTS) with TestStar II software. An extensometer (MTS) was used for strain data collection. Stress-strain data were used to determine several mechanical parameters including elastic modulus, yield point (using the 0.2% offset method), ultimate point (determined as the point of maximum load), post-yield strain (determined as the difference between ultimate strain and yield strain), post-yield strain energy, and toughness [28,29,31].

All bone cores were stained using a recently developed technique allowing for the non-invasive measurement of microdamage through micro-computed tomography. The cores were cleaned of excess blood, fat, and marrow, and stained in a lead-uranyl acetate solution containing an equal mixture of 20% lead acetate in 70% acetone and 8% uranyl acetate in 70% acetone for 2 weeks, followed by a 1 week submersion in 1% ammonium sulfide in acetone [21,32,33].

After staining, the cores were scanned via micro-computed tomography with the same parameters used previously. Microdamage was characterized in a central 8 mm^3 cubic region. The ratio of damaged volume to bone volume was calculated to quantify microdamage [21]. This same ratio was also determined in the region of minimum BV/TV since that region offers a more accurate prediction of bone fragility compared to overall BV/TV [34]. The minimum BV/TV region was obtained by dividing the 8 mm^3 cubic region into four equally sized volumes and then selecting the volume with the smallest BV/TV value [27].

19 individual damaged trabeculae were extracted from a subset of specimens chosen randomly using a random number generator function in Microsoft Excel (male n = 10, female n = 9). These specimens ranged in age from 18 to 97 (average 53.8±25.1). Each trabecula was imaged via microCT using the above-specified parameters. The ratio of damaged surface area to damaged bone volume was calculated to characterize the morphology of microdamage where higher values indicate more crack-like microdamage and lower values indicate more diffuse-like microdamage [21,27].

Specimen Preparation for Crosslink Analysis of Bone Cores and Damaged Trabeculae

Individual trabeculae, analyzed for microdamage, were lyophilized overnight using a freeze dry system (Labconco). They were then hydrolyzed in 6N hydrochloric acid for 20 hours at 110°C. Hydrosylates were centrifuged for 30 minutes at 13000 rpm at 4°C to remove any debris. Centrifuged hydrosylates were stored at −80°C in complete darkness until use. A bone slice (7.5 mm diameter, 1 mm thickness) obtained from each of the 42 bone cores, was also hydrolyzed and stored in the same fashion. Collagen quality and purity obtained through this method of hydrolysis has been previously confirmed in our laboratory via sodium dodecyl sulfate-polyacrylamide gel electrophoresis [35]. Also, work done in our laboratory has verified that there is no difference in non-enzymatic glycation content measured in bone with and without lead-uranyl acetate stain.

Measurement of Total Fluorescent AGEs

The fluorescence was measured for quinine standards (stock: 10 µg/mL quinine per 0.1 N sulfuric acid) and hydrosylates from individual trabeculae and bone slices at 360/460 nm excitation/emission using an Infinite 200 microplate reader (Tecan). Chloramine-T, 3.15 M perchloric acid, and p-dimethylaminobenzaldehyde solutions were all made immediately before use. Chloramine-T was added to hydroxyproline standards (stock: 2000 µg/mL L-hydroxyproline per 0.001 N HCl) and sample hydrosylates. The resulting solution was then incubated at room temperature for 20 minutes to oxidize hydroxyproline. To quench chloramine-T, 3.15 M perchloric acid was added and incubated for 5 minutes at room temperature. Finally, the p-dimethylaminobenzaldehyde solution was added and incubated for 20 minutes at 60°C. All standards and samples were cooled in darkness for 5 minutes. The absorbance was measured at 570 nm using a microplate reader. Collagen content was calculated based on the hydroxyproline quantity measured [36]. Total fluorescent AGEs were quantified in terms of unit quinine per unit collagen. Individual trabeculae were quantified for total fluorescent AGEs only, while bone slices from whole bone cores were quantified for both total fluorescent AGEs as well as specific collagen crosslinks as described in the next section.

Measurement of Pyd, Dpd, and Pentosidine

The hydrosylate from each bone slice was divided in two parts and each part was used to measure collagen content or crosslinks by Ultra-high Performance Liquid Chromatography (UPLC, Waters). A hydroxyproline kit (BioRad) was used for hydroxyproline quantification. A Pyd/Dpd calibrator (Quidel) and pentosidine stock (kindly donated by Dr. Vincent Monnier's group from Case Western Reserve University) were used as standards for Pyd, Dpd, and pentosidine quantification using recently developed methods [35]. This technique has been validated where the coefficient of variation for the intra-assay and inter-assay for Pyd, Dpd, and pentosidine were all ≤2% [35]. All separations were performed for standards and each specimen hydrosylate (Figure 1). Separations for hydroxyproline quantification were completed at 60°C with a flow rate of 0.5 mL/min (detector: 471 nm). For crosslink quantification, separations were achieved at 40°C with a flow rate of 0.667 mL/min (Pyd and Dpd at 297/395 nm excitation/emission, pentosidine at 335/385 nm excitation/emission). Collagen content was calculated based on the measured hydroxyproline content [36]. All crosslink quantities were normalized to the amount of collagen.

Statistical Analysis

Outliers were determined as points beyond two standard deviations of the mean and were removed from analysis. Non-parametric statistical tests were used for all measures taken in whole bone specimens because Kolmogorov-Smirnov normality tests determined that several data sets were not normally distributed. Spearman correlations were run between enzymatic crosslink content (Pyd/Dpd), measures of non-enzymatic glycation (AGEs and pentosidine), microarchitecture, and microdamage for all specimens. These measures were also tested for correlation with mechanical parameters measured in the subset of 23 specimens. Forward stepwise regression tests were conducted for mechanical properties in order to determine significantly influential variables. Since data sets were normally distributed for individual trabeculae, Pearson correlations were run between SMI and the ratio of damaged surface area to damaged volume as well as between SMI and total fluorescent AGE content for each trabecula. The power to detect correlations was approximately 87%. All statistical tests were performed using SigmaStat version 2.03 (SPSS).

Results

Pentosidine content and total fluorescent AGEs were positively correlated ($r = 0.40$, $p < 0.05$) at the level of bone cores. However, they both showed different magnitudes of association with microarchitecture, microdamage, and mechanical properties (Table 1). Highly glycated samples had more trabecular rods than plates (higher SMI) and also contained more microdamage. Mechanical measures related to bone's fracture resistance (yield strain, ultimate strain, and toughness) deteriorated in samples with high levels of non-enzymatic glycation (Table 1, Figure 2).

In addition their relationships with the extent of non-enzymatic glycation, microarchitecture and microdamage were also associated with each other. We found that with increases in microdamage quantity, there was deterioration in microarchitecture on both the global level and region of minimum BV/TV (Table 2). Also, although several measures of microarchitecture, namely BV/TV and Conn.D, had some association with bone's mechanical properties (Figure 3), microdamage showed a trend towards significance with yield and ultimate strain (Table 2).

At the level of individual trabeculae, there were relationships between microarchitecture (SMI) and microdamage content. An increase in the amount of crack-like microdamage (high ratio of damaged surface area to damaged volume) was associated with an increase in SMI (i.e. increase in the relative proportion of trabecular rods over plates) ($r = 0.48$, $p < 0.05$). Trabeculae containing crack-like microdamage were more glycated than trabeculae containing diffuse-like damage ($r = 0.49$, $p < 0.05$).

Two other major variables, donor age and BMD, were associated with several properties but did not directly correlate with mechanical parameters. Pentosidine ($r = 0.44$, $p < 0.01$), but not total fluorescent AGE content ($r = 0.20$, $p = 0.27$), increased with age. Also, microdamage content at a global level increased ($r = 0.31$, $p = 0.06$) increased with age. Age had no significant relationship with microarchitecture. On the other hand, BMD was positively correlated with BV/TV ($r = 0.26$, $p = 0.10$) and Tb.Th ($r = 0.42$, $p < 0.01$). However, BMD had no relationship with microdamage or non-enzymatic glycation content.

There was no relationship between enzymatic crosslinks and age or BMD. Pyd/Dpd was negatively associated with pentosidine ($r = -0.27$, $p = 0.054$), but not with total fluorescent AGEs. Additionally, increased Pyd/Dpd was associated with increased bone toughness and decreased microdamage content (Table 1). Pyd/Dpd was also associated with several microarchitectural properties (Table 1).

Forward stepwise regression tests to predict yield strain ($p < 0.05$), ultimate strain ($p < 0.05$), and toughness ($p < 0.05$) as dependent variables using all significant properties as independent variables showed that, regardless of the numerous existing interrelationships, the extent of non-enzymatic glycation (total fluorescent AGEs or pentosidine) was the only significant predictive variable of mechanical properties.

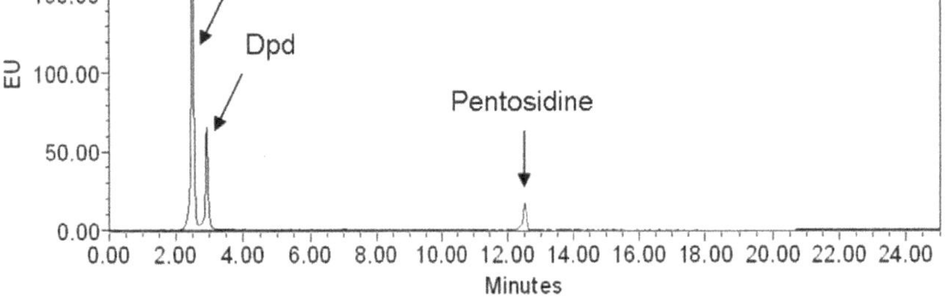

Figure 1. Schematic of UPLC chromatogram. Eluted peak areas were used for quantification of Pyd, Dpd, and pentosidine.

Table 1. Relationships between crosslink content and mechanical properties, microarchitecture, and microdamage content.

		Total fluorescent AGEs	Pentosidine	Pyd/Dpd
		[ng Quinine/mg collagen]	**[mmol/mol collagen]**	**[mg/μmol]**
Mechanical properties	**Elastic modulus [N/mm²]**	0.13 (NS)	0.13 (NS)	0.29 (NS)
	Yield stress [N/mm2]	0.01 (NS)	−0.17 (NS)	0.28 (NS)
	Yield strain	**0.54 (<0.01)**	**0.46 (<0.05)**	−0.45 (NS)
	Ultimate stress [N/mm2]	−0.03 (NS)	−0.21 (NS)	0.32 (NS)
	Ultimate strain	**0.38 (=0.09)**	**0.44 (<0.05)**	−0.36 (NS)
	Toughness [mJ/mm³]	**−0.39 (=0.08)**	−0.25 (NS)	**0.49 (=0.06)**
Microarchitecture	**BV/TV**	0.06 (NS)	−0.14 (NS)	**0.38 (<0.05)**
	Conn/D [1/mm³]	0.21 (NS)	−0.02 (NS)	**0.43 (<0.05)**
	SMI	**0.54 (<0.01)**	**0.38 (<0.05)**	−0.29 (=0.11)
	Tb.N [1/mm]	0.29 (NS)	−0.11 (NS)	**0.57 (<0.01)**
	Tb.Th [mm]	0.03 (NS)	0.09 (NS)	**0.35 (<0.05)**
	Tb.Sp [mm]	0.27 (NS)	0.22 (NS)	**−0.56 (<0.01)**
Microdamage content	**Global level**	0.26 (NS)	**0.35 (=0.054)**	**−0.39 (<0.05)**
	Region of minimum BV/TV	**0.43 (<0.05)**	**0.55 (<0.01)**	−0.20 (NS)

Data is presented as the Spearman correlation coefficient with the p-value in parentheses. NS = not significant. Variables showing significance (p<0.05 but <0.10) are shown in bold.

Discussion

Non-enzymatic glycation has been shown to deteriorate bone's mechanical parameters, but its distribution within cancellous bone and the extent of its influence on fracture in comparison to other changes in bone quality remains unclear [14,28,37,38]. Our goal was to determine if microarchitecture of cancellous bone is heterogeneously modified by NEG, and if AGEs predict the fracture properties of cancellous bone and correlate with changes in microarchitecture and microdamage.

In contrast to AGEs, pentosidine is more commonly used as a marker of NEG in bone [16,28,37]. However, it is not known whether measurement of pentosidine is adequate to illustrate the effects of non-enzymatic glycation on the mechanical integrity of bone [15]. Our results show that pentosidine explained 40% of the variance in bulk fluorescent AGE content and comprises only a portion of total fluorescent AGEs. Unlike age-dependence of pentosidine concentration [15,39], our data indicated that total fluorescent AGEs in human tibial cancellous bone do not follow this trend and may therefore, contribute differently to the overall influence of non-enzymatic glycation. Moreover, unlike pentosidine, our data illustrated that AGE content predicted bone toughness. Thus, pentosidine alone does not represent the collective effects of all AGEs on bone fracture.

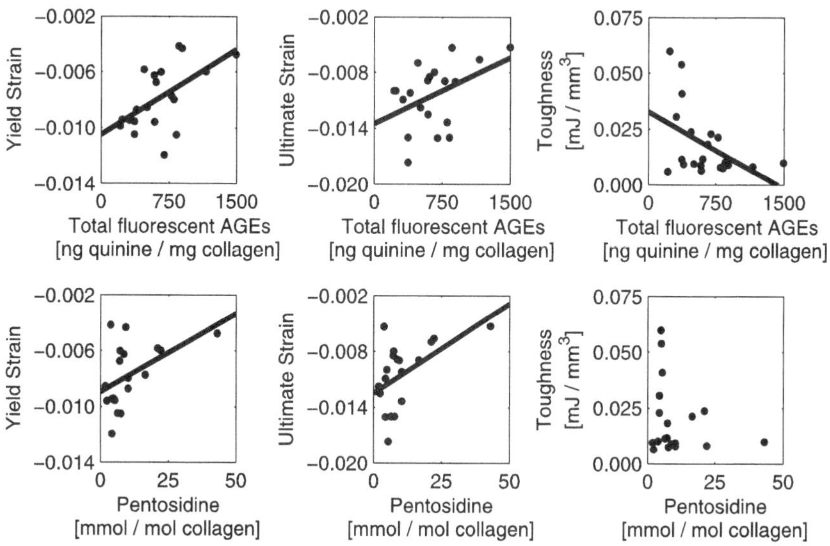

Figure 2. Mechanical properties versus NEG crosslinks. Graphical data for several mechanical parameters versus total fluorescent AGEs (top) and pentosidine (bottom) are shown.

Table 2. Relationships between microdamage content, mechanical properties, and microarchitecture.

		Microdamage content	Microdamage content
		Global level	Region of minimum BV/TV
Mechanical properties	Elastic modulus [N/mm^2]	−0.09 (NS)	0.00 (NS)
	Yield stress [N/mm2]	−0.37 (NS)	−0.34 (NS)
	Yield strain	**0.41 (=0.08)**	0.37 (NS)
	Ultimate stress [N/mm2]	−0.39 (NS)	**−0.39 (=0.09)**
	Ultimate strain	0.38 (NS)	0.29 (NS)
	Toughness [mJ/mm^3]	−0.06 (NS)	0.10 (NS)
Microarchitecture	BV/TV	**−0.37 (<0.05)**	**−0.33 (<0.05)**
	Conn/D [1/mm^3]	**−0.34 (<0.05)**	−0.19 (NS)
	SMI	**0.30 (=0.08)**	**0.38 (<0.05)**
	Tb.N [1/mm]	**−0.43 (<0.01)**	**−0.31 (=0.07)**
	Tb.Th [mm]	−0.16 (NS)	0.00 (NS)
	Tb.Sp [mm]	**0.50 (<0.01)**	**0.42 (<0.05)**

Data is presented as the Spearman correlation coefficient with the p-value in parentheses. NS = not significant. Variables showing significance ($p<0.05$ but <0.10) are shown in bold.

To date, only two studies have investigated the effect of crosslinking on trabecular microarchitecture. Microarchitecture is known to interact with applied loading at multiple length scales [20,23] and form in vivo microdamage of distinct morphologies, which reflect the quality and fracture resistance of bone matrix [40]. However, one of these two studies was limited to quantification of enzymatic crosslinks while using 2D histomorphometric methods for microarchitectural imaging [19]. The other more recent work included measurement of non-enzymatic crosslinks and used 3D microCT imaging methods; however, it measured only pentosidine [20].

Out of all microarchitectural variables, our study found that increased glycation showed a strong positive correlation only with SMI. SMI illustrates the prevalence of rods and plates in a trabecular network where an increase in SMI illustrates a transition from plate-like to rod-like trabecular structure. AGEs may cause an alteration in turnover and, as a result, affect the microarchitecture. In particular, the inside of trabeculae is composed of older bone tissue that is sandwiched between trabecular packets. Working with cortical bone, we have demonstrated that older bone tissue contains higher AGE levels including pentosidine in comparison to younger bone tissue [41]. This evidence, combined with previous results showing a negative relationship between AGEs and in vitro bone resorption by osteoclasts [18], and between AGEs and bone turnover [37], strongly suggests that rods would contain more AGEs than plates, as was found in our study. Therefore, non-enzymatic glycation may act via the reduced propensity of osteoclastic resorption to retain fragile trabecular rods in the structural network.

Since the accumulation of AGEs increases bone fragility, the high glycation level in rod-like trabeculae may further weaken the cylindrical structures, which are already prone to bending and buckling [42]. Consistent with this notion, we found that the rod-like trabeculae are indeed more prone to producing crack-like microdamage (Figure 4), which may further contribute to the failure of trabecular rods than plates.

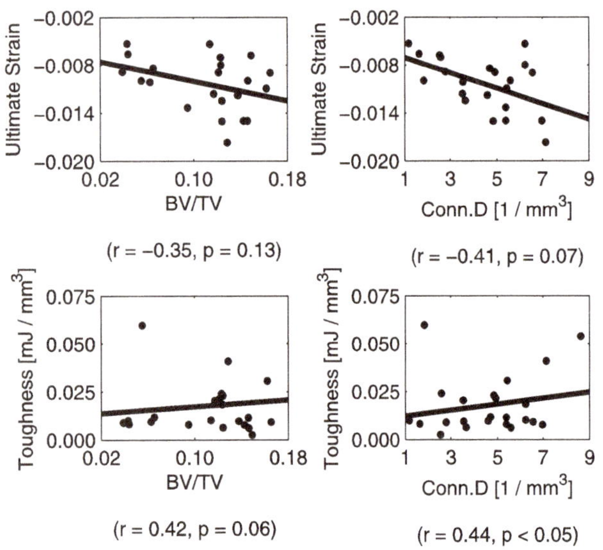

Figure 3. Mechanical properties versus microarchitecture. Several microarchitectural properties were correlated with cancellous bone's mechanical parameters.

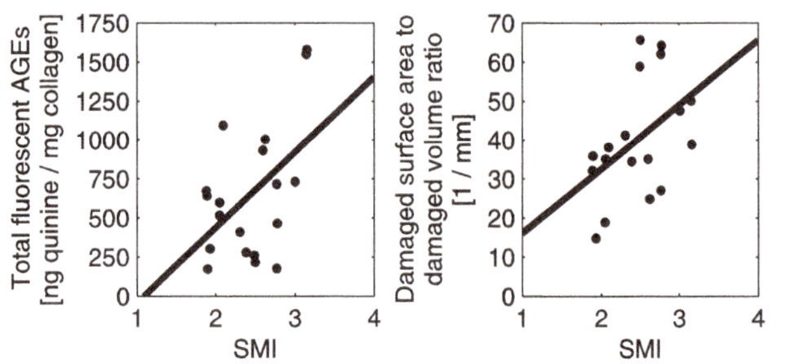

Figure 4. NEG influences microdamage morphology. (Left) Higher NEG levels exist in rod-like trabeculae compared to plate-like trabeculae. (Right) Also, rod-like trabeculae are prone to producing more crack-like microdamage.

A recent study established that in vitro induced non-enzymatic glycation affects mechanical properties along with alterations in microdamage [21], but this study was done in a single donor. To improve on this previous work, our project explored in vivo glycation in 42 donors with a wide age and BV/TV range and investigated the relationship of non-enzymatic glycation with changes in microdamage and microarchitecture. Similar to previous findings, we found that rod-like trabeculae in a weakened microstructure are conducive to increased formation of microdamage [21], and that glycation altered the extent of accumulated microdamage in bone.

AGEs, microarchitecture, and microdamage are therefore all interrelated to bone's mechanical properties, and show relationships with yield strain, ultimate strain, and toughness in our study. Furthermore, measures of non-enzymatic glycation are also correlated to microarchitectural variables, microdamage content, and mechanical properties. Due to the host of interrelated factors, it was necessary to establish the leading variables that influence mechanical properties. Although microdamage was associated with microarchitecture, and microarchitecture was directly correlated with mechanical parameters, our forward stepwise regression analysis indicated that the extent of glycation was the only dominant predictor. Unlike previous results on cancellous bone [2,43], we did not find correlations between microdamage content and mechanical properties in cancellous bone. These differences between our and previous studies may indicate that the effect of bone quality measures including microdamage may be site specific, and microdamage may have a greater influence on the fracture of low density vertebral bone. Further work is necessary to explain such differences.

Measurement of enzymatic crosslinks is critical because they are also determinants of bone quality [44,45] and may positively affect bone's mechanical strength [46]. In particular, the Pyd/Dpd ratio is illustrative of collagen maturity since both of these crosslinks provide the fibers with strength and stability [47,48]. A previous study, in which the relationship between enzymatic crosslinks and bone strength was investigated, showed that high Pyd/Dpd bone was stronger than low Pyd/Dpd bone [49]. Here, we found that high Pyd/Dpd bone was tougher than low Pyd/Dpd bone. Additionally, high Pyd/Dpd was less glycated, had more favorable microarchitecture, and contained less microdamage than low Pyd/Dpd bone. Our results reconfirm that enzymatic crosslinking in bone is a favorable process.

Our data should be considered in light of a limitation. 1–2 data points, associated with high amount of pentosidine, leverage the magnitude of association between pentosidine and mechanical properties (i.e. yield strain, Figure 2). Because removal of these points was not statistically justifiable, these points remained in our final analyses. A previous study on human cancellous bone also showed several donors with high pentosidine levels (beyond 40 mmol pentosidine per mol collagen) similar to the higher values seen in our work [50]. However, in order to further clarify the relationship between non-enzymatic glycation and mechanical properties, future work should consider inclusion of more samples with high pentosidine concentrations, associated with advanced age [39], diabetes [51–52] and anti-resorptive treatments [37].

In conclusion, we found that non-enzymatic glycation heterogeneously modified cancellous bone's trabecular microarchitecture where high amounts of AGEs were found in trabecular rods and with linear microcracks. We found that the extent of NEG in human tibial cancellous bone was the dominant predictor of bone fragility and was associated with changes in microdamage and microarchitecture.

Acknowledgments

We would like to thank the Imaging Core Facility at the Center for Biotechnology and Interdisciplinary Studies at Rensselaer Polytechnic Institute for use of the microCT, Dr. Simon Tang for help with the lead-uranyl acetate staining protocol, and Dr. Grazyna Sroga for help with the UPLC protocol.

Author Contributions

Conceived and designed the experiments: LK DV. Performed the experiments: LK. Analyzed the data: LK. Contributed reagents/materials/analysis tools: LK DV. Wrote the paper: LK DV.

References

1. Johnell O, Kanis JA (2006) An estimate of the worldwide prevalence and disability associated with osteoporotic fractures. Osteoporos Int 17: 1726–1733.
2. Burr DB, Forwood MR, Fyhrie DP, Martin RB, Schaffler MB, et al. (1997) Bone microdamage and skeletal fragility in osteoporotic and stress fractures. J Bone Miner Res 12: 6–15.
3. Chevalley T, Bonjour JP, Ferrari S, Rizzoli R (2011) Pubertal timing and body mass index gain from birth to maturity in relation with femoral neck BMD and distal tibia microstructure in healthy female subjects. Osteoporos Int. In press.
4. Hui SL, Johnston CC, Jr., Slemenda CW (1988) Age and bone mass as predictors of fracture in a prospective study. J Clin Invest 81: 1804–1809.
5. Singer BR, McLauchlan GJ, Robinson CM, Christie J (1998) Epidemiology of fractures in 15,000 adults: the influence of age and gender. J Bone Joint Surg 80: 243–248.
6. Schuit S, van Der Klift M, Weel AE, de Laet CE, Burger H, et al. (2004) Fracture incidence and association with bone mineral density in elderly men and women: the Rotterdam Study. Bone 34: 195–202.
7. Vashishth D (2005) Age-dependent biomechanical modifications in bone. Crit Rev Eukaryot Gene Expr 15: 343–358.
8. Felsenberg D, Boonen S (2005) The bone quality framework: determinants of bone strength and their interrelationships, and implications for osteoporosis management. Clin Ther 27: 1–11.
9. Bailey AJ, Paul RG, Knott L (1998) Mechanisms of maturation and ageing of collagen. Mech Ageing Dev 106: 1–56.
10. Robins SP, Duncan A, Wilson N, Evans BJ (1996) Standardization of pyridinium crosslinks, pyridinoline and deoxypyridinoline, for use as biochemical markers of collagen degradation. Clin Chem 42: 1621–1626.
11. Knott L, Bailey AJ (1998) Collagen cross-links in mineralizing tissues: a review of their chemistry, function, and clinical relevance. Bone 22: 181–187.
12. Paul RG, Bailey AJ (1996) Glycation of collagen: the basis of its central role in the late complications of ageing and diabetes. Int J Biochem Cell Biol 28: 1297–1310.
13. Ahmed N, Argirov OK, Minhas HS, Cordeiro CAA, Thornalley PJ (2002) Assay of advanced glycation endproducts (AGEs): surveying AGEs by chromatographic assay with derivatization by 6-aminoquinolyl-N- hydroxysuccinimidyl-carbamate and application to N-carboxymethyl-lysine-and N-(1-carboxyethyl)-lysine-modified albumin. Biochem J 364: 1–14.
14. Vashishth D, Gibson GJ, Khoury JI, Schaffler MB, Kimura J, et al. (2001) Influence of nonenzymatic glycation on biomechanical properties of cortical bone. Bone 28: 195–201.
15. Wang X, Shen X, Li X, Agrawal CM (2002) Age-related changes in the collagen network and toughness of bone. Bone 31: 1–7.
16. Hernandez CJ, van Der Ham F, Tang SY, Baumbach BM, Hwu PB, et al. (2005) Trabecular microfracture and the influence of pyridinium and non-enzymatic glycation-mediated collagen cross-links. Bone 37: 825–832.
17. Knott L, Whitehead CC, Fleming RH, Bailey AJ (1995) Biochemical changes in the collagenous matrix of osteoporotic avian bone. Biochem J 310: 1045–1051.
18. Valcourt U, Merle B, Gineyts E, Viguet-Carrin S, Delmas PD, et al. (2007) Non-enzymatic glycation of bone collagen modifies osteoclastic activity and differentiation. J Biol Chem 282: 5691–5703.
19. Banse X, Devogelaer JP, Lafosse A, Sims TJ, Grynpas M, et al. (2002) Cross-link Profile of Bone Collagen Correlates With Structural Organization of Trabeculae. Bone 31: 70–76.
20. Viguet-Carrin S, Follet H, Gineyts E, Roux JP, Munoz F, et al. (2010) Association between collagen cross-links and trabecular microarchitecture properties of human vertebral bone. Bone 46: 342–347.
21. Tang SY, Vashishth D (2010) Non-enzymatic glycation alters microdamage formation in human cancellous bone. Bone 46: 148–154.
22. Wenzel TE, Schaffler MB, Fyhrie DP (1996) In vivo trabecular microcracks in human vertebral bone. Bone 19: 89–95.
23. Vashishth D (2007) Hierarchy of Bone Microdamage at Multiple Length Scales. Int J Fatigue 29: 1024–1033.

24. Schaffler MB, Choi K, Milgrom C (1995) Aging and matrix microdamage accumulation in human compact bone. Bone 17: 521–525.
25. Liu S, Sajda P, Saha PK, Wehrli FW, Bevill G, et al. (2008) Complete Volumetric Decomposition of Individual Trabecular Plates and Rods and Its Morphological Correlations With Anisotropic Elastic Moduli in Human Trabecular Bone. J Bone Miner Res 23: 223–235.
26. Shi X, Liu XS, Wang X, Guo XE, Niebur GL (2010) Effects of trabecular type and orientation on microdamage susceptibility in trabecular bone. Bone 46: 1260–1266.
27. Karim L, Vashishth D (2011) Role of trabecular microarchitecture in the formation, accumulation, and morphology of microdamage in human cancellous bone. J Orthop Res 29: 1739–1744.
28. Tang SY, Zeenath U, Vashishth D (2007) Effects of non-enzymatic glycation on cancellous bone fragility. Bone 40: 1144–1151.
29. Keaveny TM, Pinilla TP, Crawford RP, Kopperdahl DL, Lou A (1997) Systematic and random errors in compression testing of trabecular bone. J Orthop Res 15: 101–110.
30. Fyhrie DP, Vashishth D (2000) Bone stiffness predicts strength similarly for human vertebral cancellous bone in compression and for cortical bone in tension. Bone 26: 169–173.
31. Kuster MS, Wood GA, Stachowiak GW, Gachter A (1997) Joint load considerations in total knee replacement. J Bone Joint Surg 79: 109–113.
32. Schaffler MB, Pitchford WC, Choi K, Riddle JM (1994) Examination of compact bone microdamage using back-scattered electron microscopy. Bone 15: 483–488.
33. Tang SY, Vashishth D (2007) A non-invasive in vitro technique for the three-dimensional quantification of microdamage in trabecular bone. Bone 40: 1259–1264.
34. Nazarian A, Stauber M, Zurakowski D, Snyder BD, Muller R (2006) The interaction of microstructure and volume fraction in predicting failure in cancellous bone. Bone 39: 1196–1202.
35. Sroga GE, Vashishth D (2011) UPLC methodology for identification and quantitation of naturally fluorescent crosslinks in proteins: a study of bone collagen. J Chromatogr B. In press.
36. Gross J (1958) Studies on the formation of collagen. I. Properties and fractionation of neutral salt extracts of normal guinea pig connective tissue. J Exp Med 107: 247–263.
37. Tang SY, Allen MR, Phipps R, Burr DB, Vashishth D (2009) Changes in non-enzymatic glycation and its association with altered mechanical properties following 1-year treatment with risedronate or alendronate. Osteoporos Int 20: 887–894.
38. Viguet-Carrin S, Roux JP, Arlot ME, Merabet Z, Leeming DJ, et al. (2006) Contribution of the advanced glycation end product pentosidine and of maturation of type I collagen to compressive biomechanical properties of human lumbar vertebrae. J Bone Miner Res 39: 1073–1079.
39. Odetti P, Rossi S, Monacelli F, Poggi A, Cirnigliaro M, et al. (2005) Advanced glycation end products and bone loss during aging. Ann NY Acad Sci 1043: 710–717.
40. Vashishth D, Behiri JC, Bonfield W (1997) Crack growth resistance in cortical bone: concept of microcrack toughening. J Biomech 30: 763–769.
41. Sroga GE, Karim L, Colon W, Vashishth D (2011) Biochemical characterization of major bone-matrix proteins using nanoscale-size bone samples and proteomics methodology. Mol Cell Proteomics 10: M110.006718.
42. Parfitt AM (2002) High bone turnover is intrinsically harmful: two paths to a similar conclusion. The Parfitt view. J Bone Miner Res 17: 1558–1559.
43. Fazzalari NL, Forwood MR, Smith K, Manthey BA, Herreen P (1998) Assessment of cancellous bone quality in severe osteoarthrosis: bone mineral density, mechanics, and microdamage. Bone 22: 381–388.
44. Paschalis EP, Verdelis K, Doty SB, Boskey AL, Mendelsohn R, et al. (2001) Spectroscopic characterization of collagen cross-links in bone. J Bone Miner Res 16: 1821–1828.
45. Paschalis EP, Shane E, Lyritis G, Skarantavos G, Mendelsohn R, et al. (2004) Bone fragility and collagen cross-links. J Bone Miner Res 19: 2000–2004.
46. Rath NC, Balog JM, Huff WE, Huff GR, Kulkarni GB, et al. (1999) Comparative differences in the composition and biomechanical properties of tibiae of seven- and seventy-two-week-old male and female broiler breeder chickens. Poult Sci 78: 1232–1239.
47. Allen MJ (2003) Biochemical markers of bone metabolism in animals: uses and limitations. Vet Clin Path 32: 101–113.
48. Viguet-Carrin S, Garnero P, Delmas PD (2006) The role of collagen in bone strength. Osteoporos Int 17: 319–336.
49. Banse X, Sims TJ, Bailey AJ (2002) Mechanical Properties of Adult Vertebral Cancellous Bone: Correlation With Collagen Intermolecular Cross-Links. J Bone Miner Res 17: 1621–1628.
50. Saito M, Fujii K, Marumo K (2006) Degree of mineralization-related collagen crosslinking in the femoral neck cancellous bone in cases of hip fracture and controls. Calcif Tissue Int 79: 160–168.
51. Silva MJ, Brodt MD, Lynch MA, McKenzie JA, Tanouye KM, et al. (2009) Type 1 diabetes in young rats leads to progressive trabecular bone loss, cessation of cortical bone growth, and diminished whole bone strength and fatigue life. J Bone Miner Res 24: 1618–1627.
52. Schwartz AV, Garnero P, Hillier TA, Sellmeyer DE, Strotmeyer ES, et al. (2009) Pentosidine and increased fracture risk in older adults with type 2 diabetes. J Clin Endocrinol Metab 94: 2380–2386.

8

Tibial Loading Increases Osteogenic Gene Expression and Cortical Bone Volume in Mature and Middle-Aged Mice

Matthew J. Silva[1,2]*, Michael D. Brodt[1], Michelle A. Lynch[1], Abby L. Stephens[1,2], Daniel J. Wood[1], Roberto Civitelli[3]

1 Department of Orthopaedic Surgery, Washington University, St. Louis, Missouri, United States of America, 2 Department of Biomedical Engineering, Washington University, St. Louis, Missouri, United States of America, 3 Department of Internal Medicine, Washington University, St. Louis, Missouri, United States of America

Abstract

There are conflicting data on whether age reduces the response of the skeleton to mechanical stimuli. We examined this question in female BALB/c mice of different ages, ranging from young to middle-aged (2, 4, 7, 12 months). We first assessed markers of bone turnover in control (non-loaded) mice. Serum osteocalcin and CTX declined significantly from 2 to 4 months ($p<0.001$). There were similar age-related declines in tibial mRNA expression of osteoblast- and osteoclast-related genes, most notably in late osteoblast/matrix genes. For example, *Col1a1* expression declined 90% from 2 to 7 months ($p<0.001$). We then assessed tibial responses to mechanical loading using age-specific forces to produce similar peak strains (-1300 $\mu\varepsilon$ endocortical; -2350 $\mu\varepsilon$ periosteal). Axial tibial compression was applied to the right leg for 60 cycles/day on alternate days for 1 or 6 weeks. qPCR after 1 week revealed no effect of loading in young (2-month) mice, but significant increases in osteoblast/matrix genes in older mice. For example, in 12-month old mice *Col1a1* was increased 6-fold in loaded tibias vs. controls ($p=0.001$). In vivo microCT after 6 weeks revealed that loaded tibias in each age group had greater cortical bone volume (BV) than contralateral control tibias ($p<0.05$), due to relative periosteal expansion. The loading-induced increase in cortical BV was greatest in 4-month old mice (+13%; $p<0.05$ vs. other ages). In summary, non-loaded female BALB/c mice exhibit an age-related decline in measures related to bone formation. Yet when subjected to tibial compression, mice from 2–12 months have an increase in cortical bone volume. Older mice respond with an upregulation of osteoblast/matrix genes, which increase to levels comparable to young mice. We conclude that mechanical loading of the tibia is anabolic for cortical bone in young and middle-aged female BALB/c mice.

Editor: Brenda Smith, Oklahoma State University, United States of America

Funding: This work was supported by NIH/NIAMS (www.niams.nih.gov) grants R01AR047867 and P30AR057235 (Washington University Musculoskeletal Research Center). The funders had no role in study design, data collection and analysis, decision to publish, or preparation of the manuscript.

Competing Interests: The authors have declared that no competing interests exist.

* E-mail: silvam@wustl.edu

Introduction

Mechanical loading is a powerful anabolic stimulus for bone. Methods to deliver increased mechanical loading to the skeleton represent a non-pharmacological strategy with potential to treat age-related osteoporosis [1]. For this strategy to be effective, the ability of the skeleton to respond to mechanical stimuli must persist with aging.

There is a lack of consensus on skeletal mechanoresponsiveness and aging. Exercise studies of young and aged rodents have demonstrated either reduced responsiveness in aged animals [2,3], no difference between ages [4,5,6], or enhanced responsiveness in aged animals [7,8]. Several studies that used extrinsic loading (e.g., tibial bending) reported reduced cortical responsiveness in aged turkeys [9], rats [10] and mice [11] compared to younger animals. In contrast, we recently reported no loss of cortical bone responsiveness in aged (22 month) mice compared to young-adult (7 month) mice subjected to 1 week of axial tibial compression [12].

The studies cited above on mechanoresponsiveness and aging focused on changes in bone mass or bone formation rate. A number of recent studies have described upregulation of osteogenic genes following loading in young animals [13,14,15]. To date there have been no reports on whether age affects loading-induced changes in expression of genes related to bone formation. Studies at the molecular level may clarify the role, if any, that age plays in the response of the skeleton to mechanical loading.

Our objective was to follow up on our previous study that used axial tibial compression in young-adult and aged mice [12], and to focus on short-term molecular and longer-term structural effects. Because we observed no decline in responsiveness from 7 to 22 months, we asked if a decline might occur earlier in the lifespan. In addition, we asked if age affected the upregulation of osteogenic genes following loading. Therefore, we compared responses to axial tibial compression in mice of different ages, ranging from young to middle-aged (2–12 months). We applied age-specific forces to produce similar values of peak strain. We assessed markers of bone turnover in non-loaded control mice, and then assessed bone responses to loading using molecular (quantitative RT-PCR) and structural (in vivo microCT) outcomes.

Results

Markers of bone formation are diminished with maturation

Based on cross-sectional analysis of control mice at different ages, serum markers of bone formation (osteocalcin) and resorption (CTX) declined significantly from 2 to 4 months age ($p<0.001$; Figure 1). Osteocalcin further declined from 7 to 12 months age, although this difference did not reach statistical significance ($p<0.10$). CTX did not change after 4 months.

Similarly, analysis of tibial mRNA revealed declines from 2 to 4 months age in the expression of many osteoblast- and osteoclast-related genes (Figure 2). The clearest pattern was in the osteoblast and matrix genes *Osx*, *Alp*, *Col1a1*, *Bsp* and *Bglap*, which declined from 35–65% from 2 to 4 months ($p<0.01$). Expression of *Osx*, *Col1a1* and *Bglap* declined from 4 to 7 months, although these differences did not reach statistical significance ($p<0.10$); there were no further changes from 7 to 12 months. The *Rankl/Opg* ratio, an important factor for osteoclastogenesis, and the osteoclast activity gene *Ctsk* also declined from 2 to 4 months ($p<0.01$), but not thereafter. In contrast, the bone morphogen *Bmp2* and the early osteoblast transcription factor *Runx2* did not change from 2 to 4 months age. *Bmp2* did decrease modestly from 2 to 7 months ($p<0.05$), but then increased from 7 to12 months ($p<0.001$), the only gene that showed such a pattern. *Runx2* showed no clear pattern with age. In summary, nearly all systemic and local measures of bone turnover declined significantly from 2 to 4 months age; there were only marginal changes after 4 months.

1 week of tibial loading increases expression of bone formation genes in older mice

The right legs of mice were subjected to tibial compression on alternate days for 1 week followed by gene expression analysis of right (loaded) and left (contralateral control) tibias (Figure 3). Age-specific forces were applied to produce similar peak strains (approx. $-1300\ \mu\varepsilon$ endocortical; $-2350\ \mu\varepsilon$ periosteal). Expression of seven of nine genes examined (all but *Runx2* and *Ctsk*) was higher in loaded tibias vs. controls ($p<0.05$; Figure 4). Expression of five of these seven genes depended significantly on age or had a significant age-load interaction ($p<0.05$). Specifically, at 2 months age, there were no significant differences between loaded and control bones; at 4 and 7 months, expression of *Col1a1* and *Bglap* were greater in loaded than control bones ($p<0.05$); at 12 months, *Osx*, *Alp*, *Col1a1*, *Bsp*, and *Bglap* were greater in loaded than control bones ($p<0.005$). The largest differences between loaded and control occurred in the 12-month group for the osteoblast/matrix genes *Col1a1* (up 6.2 fold) and *Bglap* (up 4.4 fold).

Comparisons of gene expression in contralateral control bones from loaded mice of different ages revealed similar findings as for the baseline controls, i.e., the expression of *Osx*, *Alp*, *Col1a1* and *Bglap* were lower at older ages ($p<0.05$; Figure 4). For example, at 12 months the expression of *Col1a1* was 8.4-fold less than at 2 months, while the expression of *Bglap* was 5.9-fold less. In contrast, in loaded tibias the relative expression of genes did not vary significantly with age, with the exception of *Bglap* which was 2.2-fold lower at 7 months than at 2 months ($p=0.011$). Thus, age-related differences in expression of osteoblast/matrix genes that were observed in control bones were largely not observed in bones after 1 week of tibial compression.

6 weeks of tibial compression increases cortical bone volume at all ages

The right legs of mice were subjected to tibial compression on alternate days for 6 weeks (Figure 3). Again, age-specific forces were applied to produce similar peak strains (approx. $-1300\ \mu\varepsilon$ endocortical; $-2350\ \mu\varepsilon$ periosteal). MicroCT scans of the mid-diaphysis at the 6-week timepoint revealed that loaded tibias in each age group had significantly greater cortical bone volume (BV) than contralateral control tibias ($p<0.05$; Figure 5; Table 1). This difference between loaded and control tibias was due to a significant increase in cortical BV with time in loaded tibias from each age group, while BV in control tibias either decreased slightly (4, 12 month groups) or did not change (2, 7 month groups). The increase in cortical BV of loaded tibias from baseline to 6 weeks was significantly greater in the 4-month group (+13%) compared to other age groups ($p<0.05$). Analysis of medullary volume (MV) and total volume (TV) indicated that the mechanism of increase in cortical BV was increased TV (i.e., periosteal expansion) in the 4, 7 and 12 month groups, and prevention of decreased TV (i.e., periosteal maintenance) in the 2 month group. Thus, tibial compression increased cortical bone volume by relative expansion of the periosteal margin in all age groups.

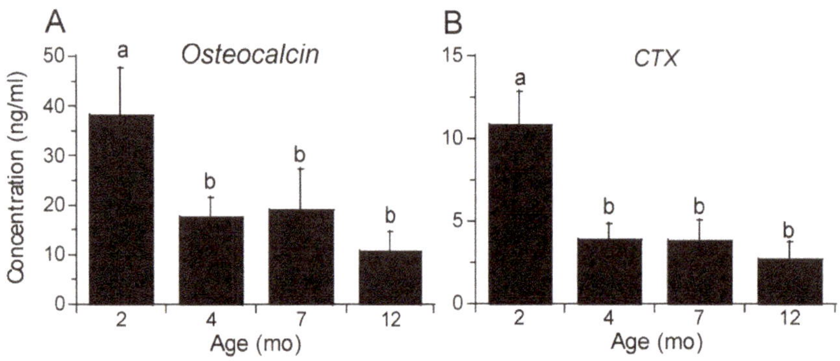

Figure 1. Systemic bone turnover decreases with age. Serum was collected from baseline control (non-loaded) mice of four different ages, and indices of bone turnover were measured by ELISA. (a) Osteocalcin, a marker of bone formation, and (b) carboxyl-terminal collagen cross-links (CTX), a marker of bone resorption, declined significantly with age. ($n=8$; mean $\pm$ SD; a,b: groups with no common letters are significantly different, $p<0.05$).

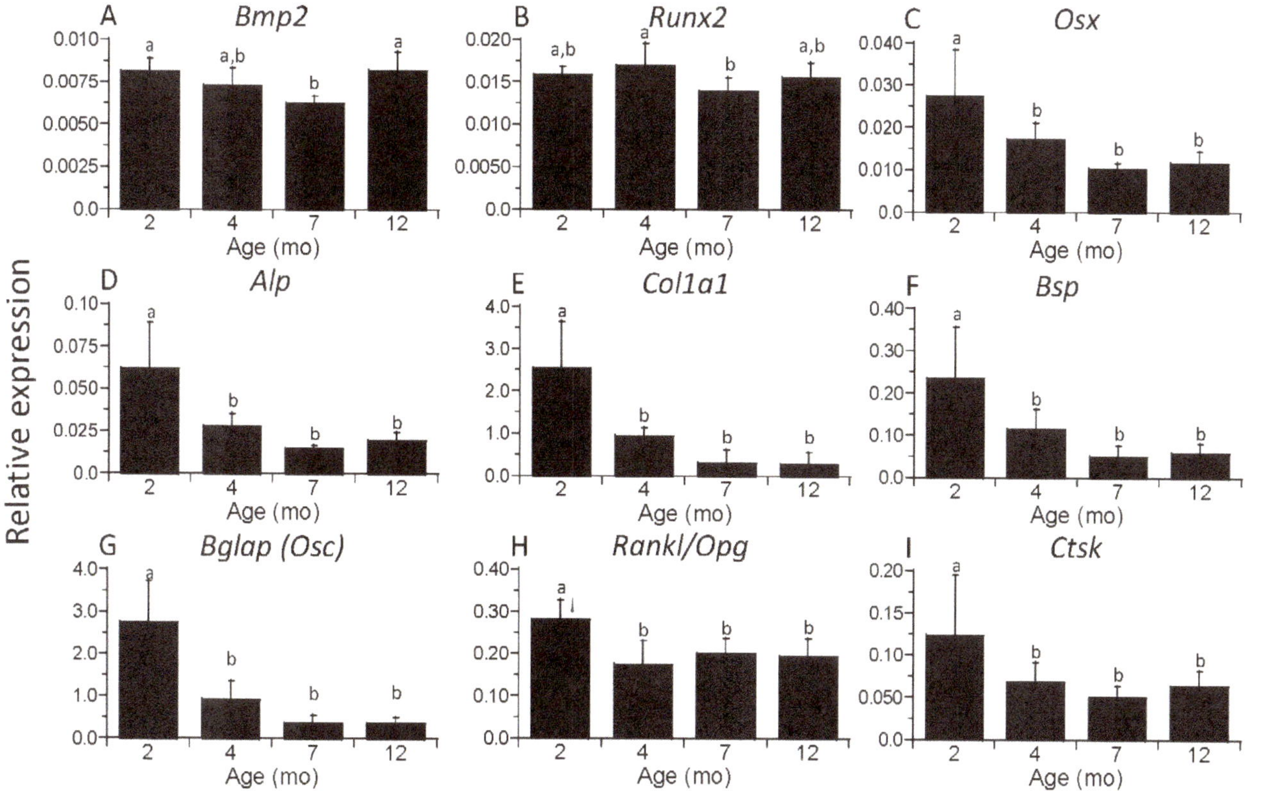

Figure 2. Expression of bone genes is age dependent. mRNA was isolated from the tibia of baseline, non-loaded control mice of four different ages, quantified by real-time RT-PCR and expressed relative to the housekeeping gene *cyclophilin*. Expression of most osteoblast- and matrix-related genes was age-dependent, with significant declines from 2 to 4 months. Expression of osteoclast-related genes also declined from 2 to 4 months but not thereafter. (n = 7–8; mean ± SD; a,b: groups with no common letters are significantly different, $p<0.05$).

6 weeks of tibial compression decreases trabecular BV/TV in 4, 7 and 12 month mice

MicroCT scans of the proximal tibial metaphysis revealed that loaded tibias in the 4- and 7-month age groups had lower trabecular bone volume fraction (BV/TV) than control tibias at the 6-week timepoint ($p<0.05$; Figure 6; Table 2). In the 4–12 month age groups, both loaded and control tibias had reduced BV/TV with time ($p<0.05$), but loaded tibias lost significantly more BV/TV than controls ($p<0.05$). There were no changes with time in tibial BV/TV of 2-month old mice. Thus, in contrast to its anabolic effect on diaphyseal cortical bone, tibial compression had a catabolic effect on metaphyseal trabecular bone in older mice.

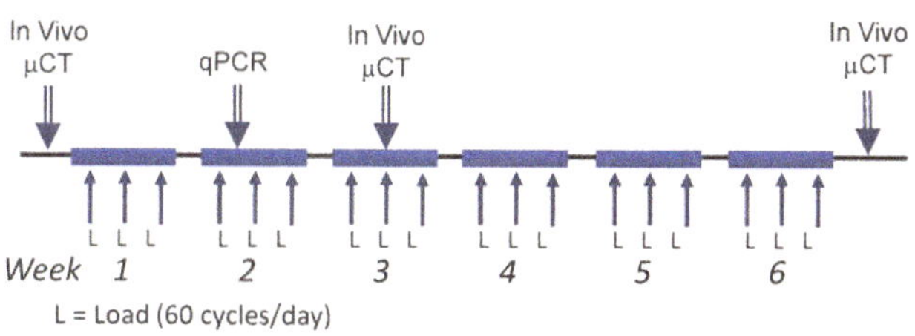

Figure 3. Study timeline. Mice were loaded 3 days/wk.

Discussion

We assessed the response to skeletal loading in female BALB/c mice in the age range from youth to middle age. We determined that systemic and local markers of bone turnover in non-loaded control animals decline significantly with maturation (i.e., from 2 to 4 months); with further aging there were only non-significant trends for modest decline in bone formation markers. One week of skeletal loading by axial tibial compression increased the relative expression of osteoblast/matrix genes in older mice, offsetting some of the age-related decline. Six weeks of loading led to increased cortical bone volume by relative periosteal expansion in all age groups (2, 4, 7, 12 months). In contrast, 6 weeks of loading decreased trabecular bone volume in 4–12 month old mice. Taken together these findings indicate that, despite an age-related decline in expression of some osteogenic genes, skeletal loading can increase cortical bone volume in mice from youth to middle age.

The age-related declines in systemic and local markers of bone formation that we find in female BALB/c mice are consistent with the limited available data from other inbred mouse strains. We observed a sharp decline in serum osteocalcin from 2 to 4 months and a trend for further decline from 7 to 12 months. Others have studied C57Bl/6 and C3H/He mice and reported that serum osteocalcin declines from 1 to 3 [16] and 3 to 12 months [17], and serum alkaline phosphatase declines from 1 to 8 months age [18]. At the bone level, we also observed significant declines in expression of osteoblast and bone matrix genes from 2 to 4 months age, with trends for further decline from 4 to 7 months. Others have reported significant decreases in osteocalcin [19] and

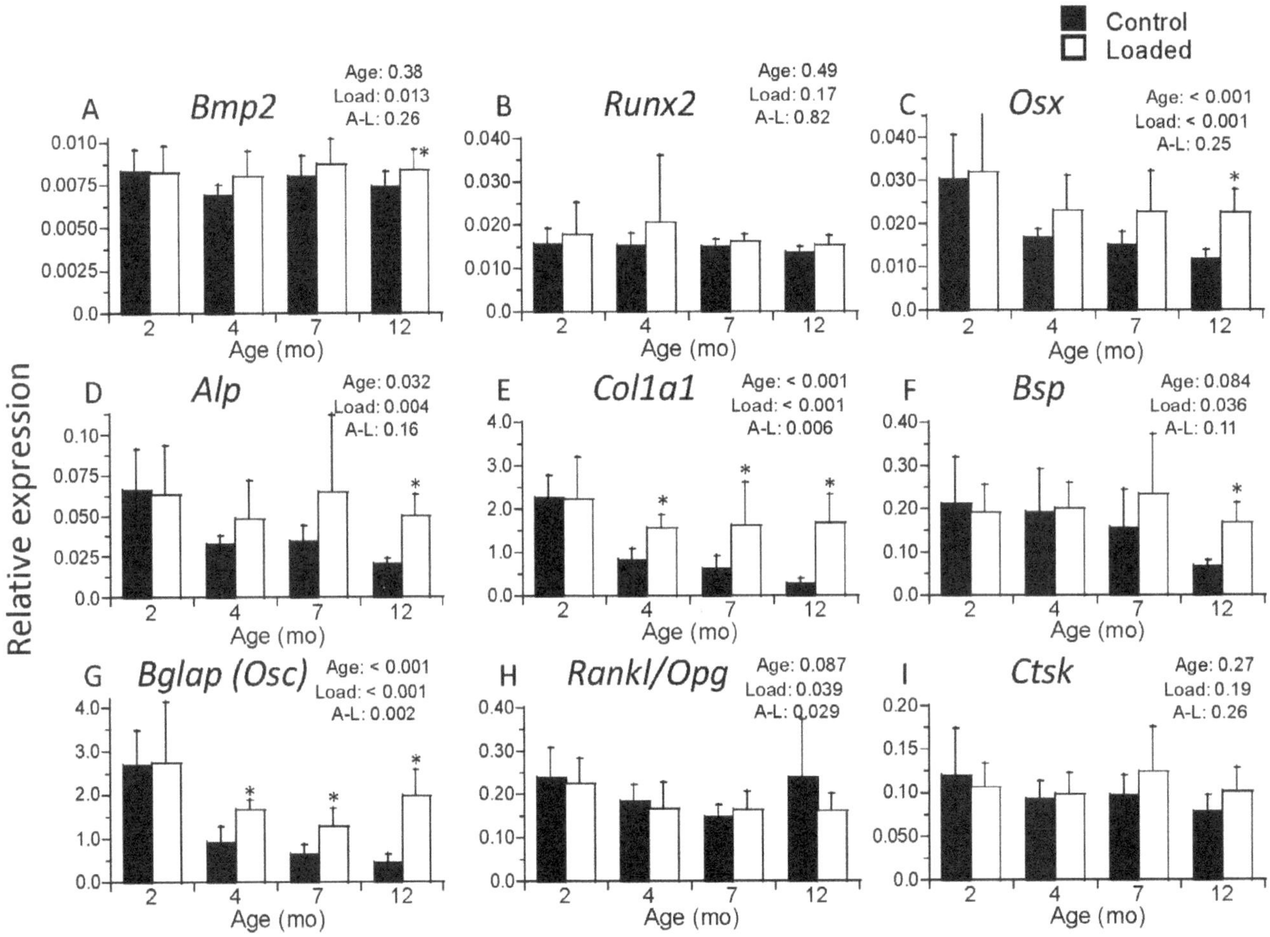

Figure 4. Mechanical loading upregulates bone genes in older mice. Bilateral tibias (left, Control; right, Loaded) were harvested after 1 week of unilateral mechanical loading. mRNA was isolated, quantified by real-time RT-PCR, normalized to the housekeeping gene *cyclophilin*, and then expressed as fold difference of loaded relative to control. There were no significant differences between loaded and control limbs at 2 months age. However, with increasing age there was an increase in relative expression of osteoblast and bone matrix genes in loaded versus control limbs. (n = 7–8; mean ± SD; p-values for Age, Load and Age-Load interaction are from 2-factor ANOVA; * loaded different from control, $p<0.05$).

alkaline phosphatase [18] activity in mouse bones from 1 to 3 months age. In addition, from 1 to 6 to 24 months age, tibial *Col1a1* and *Alp* expression declined in C57Bl/6 mice [20]. We previously noted a modest decline in cortical and trabecular bone formation rates from 7 to 22 months age in BALB/c mice [21]. (Mice in that study were subjected to sham or whole-body vibration loading; the age-related decline in bone formation rates was noted at the periosteal surface of the tibial diaphysis, and the trabecular bone in the proximal tibia and is based on data from all groups pooled, as there was no effect of vibrational loading.) Similarly, Ferguson et al. reported that cortical bone formation in C57Bl/6 mice declines sharply from 1 to 5 months, and beyond 5 months age there is no consistent fluorochrome labeling [22]. In summary, the available data indicate that bone formation in mice declines significantly from youth to middle age.

We detected significant increases in expression of osteoblast and bone matrix genes in loaded compared to control bones 1 week after the start of loading, most notably in older mice. This finding is consistent with reports describing increases in similar genes at 3–12 day timepoints in other loading models in mice [23] and rats [13,14]. Somewhat unexpectedly, we did not observe increased expression in loaded bones from 2-month old mice, whereas the greatest loading effects were observed in 12-month old mice. Others have reported that tibial bending in 2-month old C57Bl/6 mice led to increased expression of osteoblast-related genes [23], although the mechanical strain applied in that study was much greater than the current study (tensile gage-site strain ~3500 vs. ~1500 $\mu\varepsilon$). One possible reason for the lack of a gene expression response to loading in 2-month old mice is because the baseline levels of expression were already high. Perhaps an even greater stimulus is required to enhance gene expression in bones from young animals or under other conditions of high baseline activity. Importantly, in older mice loading increased the expression of genes related to bone formation, effectively offsetting much of their age-related decline.

Mechanical loading significantly increased cortical bone volume at all ages. The greatest effect occurred at 4-months, where the increase in cortical BV was approximately twice as great as at other ages (Fig. 5). This contrasts the gene expression results which indicated that the 12-month group was the most responsive to loading. The reason for this inconsistency is unclear. It may simply reflect the different timepoints for gene expression (1 week) versus cortical bone volume (3 and 6 weeks) measurements. It is also possible that loading triggers non-transcriptional events that influence bone accrual. Regardless, our results suggest that the

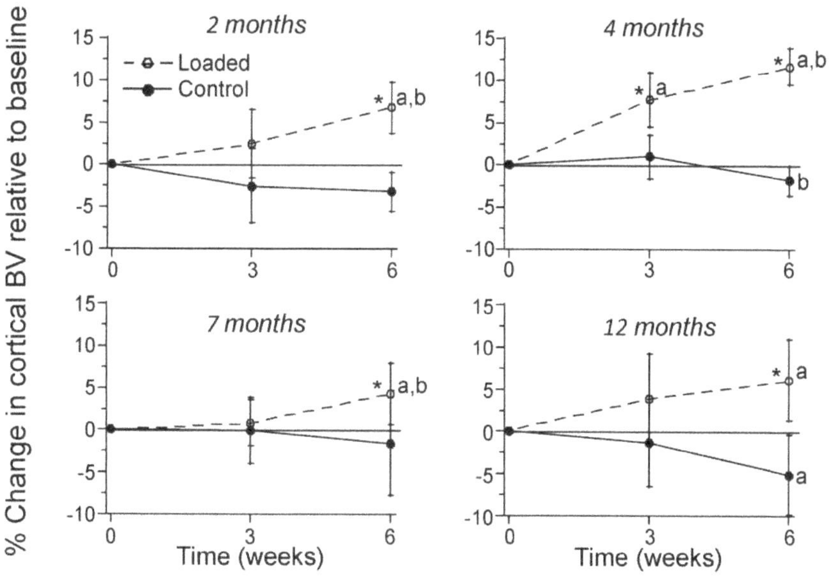

Figure 5. Mechanical loading increases cortical bone volume in all age groups. Cortical bone volume (BV) was assessed at the mid-diaphysis of loaded and contralateral control limbs using in vivo microCT at study baseline (0 weeks), middle (3 weeks) and end (6 weeks). Percent change was computed relative to the value at baseline. Cortical BV increased regardless of age in legs subjected to axial tibial compression. In each age group, significant temporal increases were observed in loaded tibias but not in contralateral controls. (n = 7–9; mean ± SD; * loaded different from control; a: different from 0 weeks; b: different from 3 weeks, $p<0.05$).

magnitude of the gene expression response at one particular time may not be a good predictor of the eventual increase in bone mass.

We observed some bone loss in control limbs, which suggests a negative systemic effect of loading. Cortical BV declined in non-loaded limbs from 4- and 12-month groups, while trabecular bone declined in non-loaded limbs from 4-, 7- and 12-month groups. Because we did not include an age-matched control group we cannot determine if this loss was simply the result of normal changes over the 6-week duration of our study. Data from non-loaded female BALB/c mice obtained at different ages indicate

Table 1. Cortical bone volume and density from in vivo microCT scans at baseline, middle and end of 6-week loading period.

Outcome	Age	Left (Control)			Right (Loaded)		
		0 wk	3 wk	6 wk	0 wk	3 wk	6 wk
Bone Volume (mm^3)	2 month (n = 7)	0.419±0.015	0.408±0.023	0.405±0.013	$0.411^{*}\pm0.012$	0.420±0.019	$0.438^{*ab}\pm0.019$
Medullary Volume (mm^3)		0.278±0.016	$0.257^{a}\pm0.017$	$0.216^{ab}\pm0.007$	0.291±0.036	$0.251^{a}\pm0.030$	$0.238^{*a}\pm0.024$
Total Volume (mm^3)		0.697±0.023	$0.666^{a}\pm0.031$	$0.622^{ab}\pm0.016$	0.702±0.045	0.672±0.036	$0.677^{*}\pm0.040$
TMD (mg HA/cm^3)		1040±16	$1078^{a}\pm27$	$1125^{ab}\pm12$	1037±27	$1084^{a}\pm16$	$1126^{ab}\pm6$
Bone Volume (mm^3)	4 month (n = 8)	0.457±0.032	0.461±0.032	$0.448^{b}\pm0.033$	0.455±0.030	$0.489^{*a}\pm0.019$	$0.508^{*ab}\pm0.031$
Medullary Volume (mm^3)		0.232±0.030	0.234±0.032	0.226±0.035	0.223±0.037	0.239±0.037	$0.250^{a}\pm0.042$
Total Volume (mm^3)		0.688±0.058	0.695±0.062	0.674±0.064	0.678±0.062	$0.728^{a}\pm0.050$	$0.758^{*ab}\pm0.069$
TMD (mg HA/cm^3)		1123±17	$1145^{a}\pm16$	$1167^{ab}\pm12$	1136±13	$1151^{a}\pm14$	$1175^{ab}\pm12$
Bone Volume (mm^3)	7 month (n = 9)	0.466±0.029	0.465±0.020	0.458±0.030	0.466±0.036	0.469±0.026	$0.485^{*ab}\pm0.026$
Medullary Volume (mm^3)		0.202±0.031	0.200±0.022	0.198±0.023	0.212±0.034	$0.220^{*}\pm0.032$	$0.219^{*}\pm0.028$
Total Volume (mm^3)		0.668±0.056	0.665±0.037	0.656±0.040	0.678±0.061	0.689±0.053	$0.705^{*ab}\pm0.049$
TMD (mg HA/cm^3)		1164±12	1173±17	1162±42	1170±17	$1184^{*a}\pm10$	$1184^{a}\pm16$
Bone Volume (mm^3)	12 month (n = 7)	0.474±0.035	0.467±0.031	$0.449^{a}\pm0.022$	0.471±0.017	0.488±0.020	$0.499^{*a}\pm0.016$
Medullary Volume (mm^3)		0.201±0.012	$0.213^{a}\pm0.019$	$0.215^{a}\pm0.023$	0.205±0.014	0.216±0.017	$0.228^{a}\pm0.010$
Total Volume (mm^3)		0.674±0.042	0.680±0.035	0.664±0.041	0.676±0.025	0.704±0.033	$0.727^{*a}\pm0.022$
TMD (mg HA/cm^3)		1195±16	1183±20	1182±26	1198±10	$1209^{*a}\pm10$	$1206^{*}\pm8$

mean ± SD;
*Right different from Left;
[a]: different from 0 wk;
[b]: different from 3 wk; $p<0.05$.

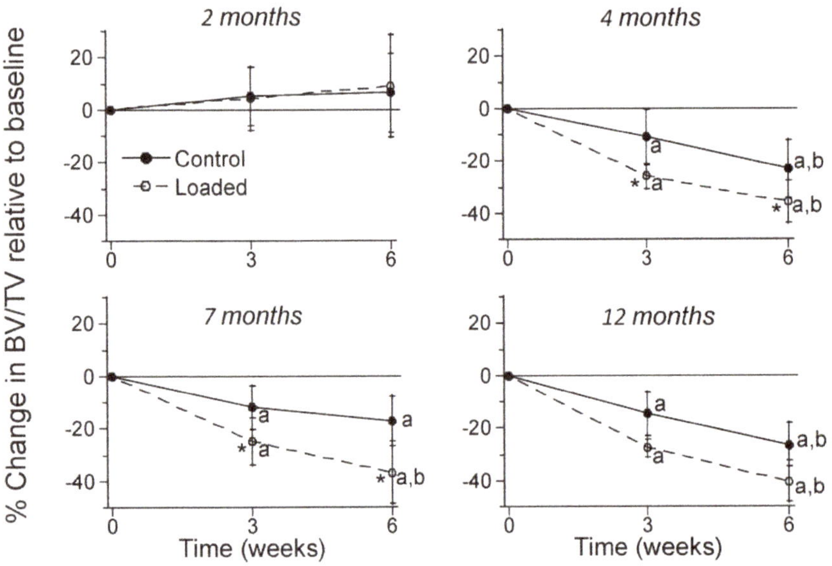

Figure 6. Mechanical loading decreases trabecular bone volume in older mice. Trabecular bone volume fraction (BV/TV) decreased in legs of 4, 7 and 12 month old mice subjected to axial tibial compression. BV/TV was assessed in the proximal tibias of loaded and contralateral control limbs using in vivo microCT at the study baseline (0 weeks), middle (3 weeks) and end (6 weeks). Percent change in BV/TV was computed relative to the value at baseline. Significant temporal decreases were observed in mice aged 4, 7 and 12 months, with greater declines in loaded limbs than controls. (n = 7–9; mean ± SD; * loaded different from control; a: change in BV/TV is different from 0 weeks; b: change in BV/TV is different from 3 weeks, $p<0.05$).

that cortical bone is not normally lost during growth and maturation, although tibial trabecular BV/TV does decline progressively after 4-months age [24]. Ongoing studies are addressing the issue of systemic effects in our loading protocol.

Our tibial compression loading protocol was not anabolic for *trabecular* bone at the proximal tibial metaphysis, despite being anabolic for *cortical* bone at the mid-diaphysis. Loading did not cause a change in trabecular BV/TV in 2-month old mice, and

Table 2. Trabecular bone microstructure and density from in vivo microCT scans at baseline, middle and end of 6-week loading period.

Outcome	Age	Left (Control)			Right (Loaded)		
		0 wk	**3 wk**	**6 wk**	**0 wk**	**3 wk**	**6 wk**
BV/TV (mm^3/mm^3)	2 month (n = 8)	0.233±0.034	0.245±0.041	0.248±0.044	0.229±0.031	0.238±0.034	0.250±0.057
Tb.Th (mm)		0.060±0.003	0.063^{a}±0.004	0.064^{a}±0.004	0.057^{*}±0.003	0.062^{a}±0.004	0.067^{*ab}±0.003
Tb.N (1/mm)		5.8±0.5	5.8±0.4	5.5^{ab}±0.5	5.9±0.5	5.8±0.3	5.5±0.7
vBMD (mg HA/cm^3)		212±19	221±25	222±27	208±19	217±22	226±38
BV/TV (mm^3/mm^3)	4 month (n = 8)	0.294±0.041	0.262^{a}±0.049	0.227^{ab}±0.052	0.291±0.027	0.216^{*a}±0.027	0.189^{*ab}±0.038
Tb.Th (mm)		0.069±0.003	0.068±0.003	0.068±0.004	0.066^{*}±0.003	0.059^{*a}±0.003	0.063^{*b}±0.005
Tb.N (1/mm)		6.4±0.7	5.8^{a}±0.6	5.0^{ab}±0.7	6.3±0.3	5.4^{a}±0.2	5.0^{ab}±0.3
vBMD (mg HA/cm^3)		250±21	232^{a}±30	214^{ab}±34	253±16	205^{*a}±16	189^{*ab}±24
BV/TV (mm^3/mm^3)	7 month (n = 9)	0.231±0.019	0.203^{a}±0.029	0.191^{a}±0.031	0.237±0.023	0.178^{*a}±0.029	0.149^{*ab}±0.029
Tb.Th (mm)		0.067±0.002	0.066±0.006	0.066±0.006	0.068±0.004	0.060±0.006^{*a}	0.059^{*a}±0.003
Tb.N (1/mm)		4.9±0.3	4.6^{a}±0.4	4.3^{ab}±0.3	4.8±0.5	4.5±0.4	4.2^{a}±0.4
vBMD (mg HA/cm^3)		215±11	198^{a}±18	189^{a}±21	220±15	179^{*a}±19	158^{*ab}±19
BV/TV (mm^3/mm^3)	12 month (n = 7)	0.220±0.032	0.189^{a}±0.039	0.163^{ab}±0.037	0.277±0.146	0.202^{a}±0.111	0.172^{ab}±0.116
Tb.Th (mm)		0.073±0.004	0.070±0.002	0.070±0.005	0.089±0.044	0.073±0.028	0.070^{a}±0.022
Tb.N (1/mm)		4.0±0.7	4.0±0.4	3.7^{ab}±0.4	4.2±0.8	3.9^{a}±0.6	3.8^{a}±0.7
vBMD (mg HA/cm^3)		207±20	187^{a}±27	168^{ab}±26	250±107	196^{a}±79	173^{a}±77

mean ± SD;
*Right different from Left;
[a]: different from 0 wk 0;
[b]: different from 3 wk; $p<0.05$.

caused a significant decrease in 4-, 7- and 12-month mice. This finding confirms our recent results using the same loading protocol in 7- and 22-month old male BALB/c mice [12]. In contrast, there are several reports of increased trabecular BV/TV after tibial compression in growing [25,26] and mature C57Bl/6 mice [27,28]. We rule out trabecular microfracture as a cause of bone loss in our study, as microCT scans from the current study and histological examination of samples in a previous study revealed no evidence of microfracture [12]. We can not rule out more subtle forms of microdamage, as we have not stained samples to look for microcracks or diffuse damage. Recent unpublished data from our lab indicate that mouse strain and loading history are factors in the loss of trabecular bone we observed. Briefly, C57Bl/6 mice subjected to the same loading history used in the current study did not lose trabecular bone, indicating that different inbred strains respond differently, perhaps due to differences in baseline trabecular BV/TV (BALB/c ~0.25; C57Bl/6 ~0.15 [25,26,28]). Moreover, when we used a loading protocol that has been used by other groups (1200 cycles/day; 4 Hz) [26,27], we observed increased trabecular bone volume. Additional studies are needed to confirm these preliminary findings and determine their underlying basis.

Returning to our main question: Does the aging skeleton lose its ability to respond to mechanical loading? Our current view is that there is a partial, but not complete loss of cortical mechanoresponsiveness with aging. The 4-month old mice here added the greatest amount of cortical bone, suggesting that there is an age when the skeleton most efficiently converts mechanical stimuli into increased bone mass. In support of this view, several previous studies found that loading protocols that were potently anabolic in younger animals stimulated little to no response in older animals [9,10,11]. On the other hand, a number of studies (including the present one) have found that declines in mechanoresponsiveness with aging are more modest and that aged animals maintain an ability to respond robustly to loading. Kesavan et al. [23] reported no difference in anabolic responses to tibial bending between 2-, 4- and 9-month old mice (both C57Bl/6 and C3H/He). In a recent study, we observed that tibial compression stimulated equal or greater cortical bone responses in 22-month old BALB/c mice compared to 7-month old mice [12]. Moreover, several (though not all [2,3]) exercise studies in rodents reported that the skeletal benefits of exercise are not limited by age [4,5,6,7,8]. For example, 12 weeks of daily treadmill running [8] and 8 weeks of daily jumping [5] each produced significant increases in bone mass in 2-year old rats. Critically, there is no proven mechanistic basis to support a loss of mechanoresponsiveness with age. On the one hand, there are reports of decreased osteocyte number with aging [29,30], which might lead to diminished mechanotransduction. On the other hand, in vitro studies have reported little or no cell autonomous decline in mechanoresponsiveness with aging [31,32,33]. In summary, there is increasing evidence that the aging skeleton maintains its ability to respond positively to loading.

One strength of our study was the use of longitudinal assessment of bone using in vivo microCT. Because 6 weeks is a relatively long duration for a loading study, we anticipated changes in bone structure would be detectable by microCT. For this reason we elected not to use histomorphometry to measure traditional dynamic indices of bone formation. This limits our ability to make strong conclusions about endocortical vs. periosteal responses. Although we do not express our data as rates of volume change, this could be done using any two timepoints from the microCT data (Tables 1, 2). Also, because we expressed changes relative to baseline (Figures 5,6) we are able to state whether there was bone loss or gain, not just a relative benefit of loading. Therefore, we chose not to report relative differences (loaded – control); data analysis based on relative differences did not lead to any change in our conclusions (data not shown).

Our study had several limitations. First, we analyzed only a single timepoint for gene expression and focused on osteoblast/matrix genes rather than early response genes or signaling pathways. Peak rates of bone formation occur 5–8 days after a single bout of loading [34]. Thus, the 1-week timepoint was selected to reflect the cumulative effects of the first three loading sessions, when expression of osteoblast/matrix genes should be relatively high. Analysis of bones after 6 weeks of loading showed few differences in expression between loaded and control tibias (data not shown), suggesting that the tibia had accommodated to the loading stimulus. A second limitation is the homogenization of the entire tibia (bone plus marrow) for qPCR analysis. This approach does not allow for evaluation of local differences. Thus, our qPCR analysis does not clarify the differences in the metaphyseal and diaphyseal sites seen by microCT. Another limitation is the use of a single loading force for each age group, chosen to provide an equivalent local strain stimulus. This "strain matching" strategy is standard for animal studies of mechanoresponsiveness, although it may not reflect the overall mechanical stimulus at the organ level. One way to offset this limitation in future studies is to use a "force matching" approach in addition to "strain matching". Based on the strain approach, we determined that the 7-month group required a lower force than the 4- or 12-month groups to produce an equivalent local strain magnitude (Table 3). Although this is not what we expected, Lynch et al. observed a similar phenomenon in C57Bl/6 mice [26,27]: they applied 11.5 N force to produce 1200 microstrain at the tibial mid-shaft in 2.5-month old mice, but applied only 5.9 N to produce the same strain in 6-month mice. We note that the 7-month group in our study had the smallest value of total volume (TV; Table 1) which may have contributed to the lower overall stiffness. We further suggest that age-related differences in curvature along the length of the tibia alter the force-strain relationships, although we did not assess curvature in this study. Another limitation related to loading was the use of a constant force rate (48 N/sec), which resulted in different strain rates between groups. The estimated strain rates (based on a peak of 1300 $\mu\varepsilon$) would have ranged from 5700 to 8300 $\mu\varepsilon$/s. These differences in strain rates may have contributed to variability in response, although we note that the most responsive group (4 month) had the second lowest strain rate (6250 $\mu\varepsilon$/s).

In summary, there is a normal age-related decline in markers of bone formation in female BALB/c mice. Despite this decline, mice from 2–22 months [12] have an anabolic cortical response to tibial compression. Current data indicate that maturing mice (4 month) are more responsive to loading than mice at other ages. Older mice respond with a marked upregulation of osteoblast and bone matrix genes, which increase to levels comparable to young, growing mice. We conclude that mechanical loading can be anabolic for cortical bone in older mice despite lower baseline bone formation.

Materials and Methods

Ethics Statement

The research described in this study involving animals is in compliance with all applicable Federal regulations and University and sponsoring agency policies and procedures. The study was approved by the Washington University Animal Studies Committee (protocol number 20080258).

Table 3. Average strain values (microstrain, με) for the applied forces used for in vivo tibial compression.

Age (mo)	Force (N)	Gage Site	Max Periosteal: Tension	Max Endocortical: Tension	Min Periosteal: Compression	Min Endocortical: Compression
2	−7.5	1290	1540	1080	−2200	−1340
4	−10	1340	1520	1030	−2320	−1270
7	−8.5	1480	1690	1040	−2490	−1390
12	−11	1510	1720	1050	−2520	−1390

Strains were measured at gage site; values at other sites obtained by linear interpolation of measured value based on cross-sectional geometry; shaded cells indicate target values.

Animals

Female BALB/cBy mice were purchased from the National Institute of Aging (NIA, Bethesda, MD, USA) aged mouse colony at four different ages. BALB/c mice have an intermediate bone mass compared to "low bone mass" C57Bl/6 and "high bone mass" C3H/He inbred strains [35]. They exhibit similar age-related changes in bone structure and density as C57Bl/6 mice [24], and they have an anabolic cortical bone response to tibial compression [12]. Age groups were selected to represent four life stages [36]: growing (2 month), maturing (4 month), mature (7 month), and middle-aged (12 month). After arrival mice were housed for 1–2 week before experimental use. Animals were housed 4–5 per cage with unlimited mouse food and water and were exposed to a 12:12 hour light:dark cycle. Some mice were used as baseline controls, and others were subjected to axial tibial compression.

Baseline controls

Serum markers of bone turnover and tibial gene expression were assessed using a set of 32 baseline control (non-loaded) mice (2, 4, 7, 12 months age; n = 8/group). Food was withdrawn 6 hr before death. Mice were anesthetized (i.p. ketamine [100 mg/kg] and xylazine [10 mg/kg]), and cardiac puncture was performed; mice died by exsanguination. Blood samples were centrifuged (8000 rpm, 5 min) and the serum stored (−80°C) until later use. The central portion (~60–75%) of each tibia was harvested within 8 min of death, flash frozen in liquid nitrogen, and stored (−80°C) until RNA isolation.

Serum markers of bone turnover were assessed using kits. Osteocalcin (Mouse Osteocalcin EIA Kit; Biomedical Technologies Inc., Stoughton, MA, USA) was used as a marker of bone formation, while the c-terminal cross-linking telopeptide of type I collagen (CTX) (RatLaps™ EIA; Immunodiagnostics Systems Inc., Fountain Hills, AZ, USA) was used as a marker of resorption.

Gene expression

The central portion of the tibias from both baseline control mice and 1-week loaded mice (see below) was used for quantitative gene expression by real-time reverse transcriptase polymerase chain reaction (qRT-PCR) using a previously described protocol [37]. Samples included cortical bone and marrow. Briefly, each sample was placed in a liquid nitrogen-cooled stainless steel flask along with a steel ball and shaken until pulverized (Micro-Dismembrator, B. Braun Biotech Inc.). The sample was then stabilized using TRIzol (Invitrogen, Carlsbad, CA, USA), and DNA and proteins were precipitated out of solution using chloroform (Sigma, Saint Louis, MO, USA) and phase lock gel tube (PLG-heavy, Eppendorf). The RNA was further purified using the RNeasy Mini Kit (Qiagen, Germantown MD, USA). The purity and concentration of the isolated RNA was determined using a spectrophotometer (Nanodrop 2000, Thermo Scientific, Wilmington, DE, USA). 1 μg of purified RNA was used to synthesize cDNA using random primers and superscript III reverse transcriptase (Invitrogen). qRT-PCR reactions were carried out using 20 μl of final volume and 40 cycles of denaturing and annealing/elongation (7500 Real-Time PCR System, Applied Biosystems, Foster City, CA, USA). SYBR green (Applied Biosystems) was used as a reporter agent and the cycle number to threshold (CT) was determined using the manufacturer's software. Nine genes were assessed: *Bmp2*, *Runx2*, *Osx*, *Alp*, *Col1a1*, *Bsp*, *Bglap*, *Rankl*, *Opg* and *Ctsk*. (See Table S1 for primer information.) Expression levels were normalized relative to the expression of the housekeeping gene cyclophillin (*Cyclo*). We confirmed that *Cyclo* expression did not differ between age groups or between loaded vs. control legs ($p>0.05$). For baseline controls, values are presented as fold-difference relative to *Cyclo* ($2^{-\Delta CT}$). For 1-week loaded tibias, values are presented as fold-difference relative to contralateral control ($2^{-\Delta\Delta CT}$).

Force-strain analysis

A set of 22 mice was used to determine the axial force that produced peak tibial strains of approximately1100 με tension and −1300 με compression on the endocortical surface at the mid-diaphysis. This was done for each age group (2, 4, 7, 12 months age; n = 5–6/group). These values of strain were chosen to match the intermediate loading level used in our previous study, where we also used endocortical strain as our target [12]. Briefly, each mouse was euthanized by CO_2 asphyxiation and a single element strain gage (FLK-1-11-1L, Texas Measurements, College Station, TX, USA) was applied to the antero-medial periosteal surface at the approximate site of peak tensile strain, 5 mm proximal to the distal tibio-fibular junction. The tibia was then loaded (waveform description below) to peak forces of 4 to 14 N (2 N increments) and strain was recorded. Relationships between peak force vs. peak gage-site strain were determined by linear regression. Strain values at the gage site were linearly interpolated to values at the sites of peak tension and compression on the endocortical surface based on dimensions obtained from microCT scans of the tibia with gage attached, a method we used previously [12,38]. The compressive force values that produced the target strains were: 7.5, 10.0, 8.5 and 11.0 N for 2, 4, 7 and 12 month old mice, respectively. The measured periosteal strain, and the estimated periosteal and endocortical strains engendered by these forces are listed in Table 3.

In vivo loading

Responses to in vivo loading were assessed in tibias from a total of 63 mice from four age groups (2, 4, 7, 12 months). Axial tibial compression is a non-invasive method to stimulate bone formation in mice [39,40]. As described [12], mice were anesthetized (2% isofluorane) and their right lower legs subjected to axial compression for 60 cycles/day using a rest-inserted protocol (preload: 0.5 N; triangle waveform with loading/unloading rate: 48 N/sec; rest between cycles: 10 sec) applied using a materials testing system (Dynamite 8841, Instron, Norwood, MA, USA). The peak force was age-specific, as described above. Mice were loaded for 3 days/week (Mon/Wed/Fri). For gene expression by qPCR, a set of mice (n = 7–8/age group) were loaded for four sessions (Mon/Wed/Fri/Mon) and euthanized 24 h after the last loading session (Figure 3). For structural analysis by in vivo microCT, a set of mice (n = 7–9/age group) were loaded 18 times over 6 weeks (Figure 3). The left leg served as a non-loaded, contralateral control. After each loading session, mice received buprenorphine (0.1 mg/kg i.m.) and were returned to their cages and allowed unrestricted activity. A 6-week duration has been used in some previous studies [25], and was chosen to allow sufficient time for structural changes in cortical and trabecular bone to occur. In our previous study [12], we observed decreased metaphyseal trabecular BV/TV after 1 week of tibial compression, despite increased cortical bone formation at the mid-diaphysis. We reasoned that this response may have been transient, and that a 6-week duration would provide an assessment of structural effects at equilibrium.

In vivo microCT

In vivo microCT was used to assess bone structure at three timepoints (baseline, middle, end) (Figure 3). The baseline scans were performed on the Thurs or Fri before the first loading session; the middle scans were performed on the Tue or Wed in the 3rd week of loading; the end scans were performed on the Mon or Tue after the last loading session. Mice were anesthetized (2–3% isofluorane) and each leg scanned separately (70 kV, 114 μA, medium resolution, 21 μm voxel, 100 msec integration; VivaCT40, Scanco, Brüttisellen, Switzerland). The scanner was calibrated weekly against a hydroxyapative (HA) mineral phantom; density is expressed as mg HA/cm^3. The leg was positioned parallel to the z-axis of the scanner so that scan slices were in the transverse plane. Diaphyseal scans were obtained over a ~0.6 mm region located 5.0 mm proximal to the distal tibio-fibular junction, and metaphyseal scans obtained over a ~2.0 mm region at the proximal metaphysis. To determine cortical parameters, 30 diaphyseal slices (0.63 mm length) were analyzed. The periosteal margin was defined using hand drawn contours, followed by a simple threshold to segment bone from non-bone (sigma = 0, support = 0, lower/upper threshold = 180/1000 = 332 mg HA/cm^3, peel iteration = 0). Cortical outcomes included total volume inside the periosteal margin (TV; this is the 3D analog to periosteal area in 2D), bone volume (BV; the 3D analog to cortical area in 2D), medullary volume and tissue mineral density (TMD). To determine trabecular parameters, the distal-most slice containing any remnant of growth plate was visualized and 30 slices (0.63 mm length) below this slice were analyzed. The endosteal margin was defined using hand drawn contours followed by thresholding (same parameters as cortical, except peel iteration = 4). Standard outcomes for the metaphysis included trabecular BV/TV, Tb.N, Tb.Th, Tb.Sp, and volumetric BMD. Studies in our lab have shown excellent intra- and inter-operator repeatability using the above protocols (intraclass correlation coefficients >0.90).

Statistical analysis

Effects of age and loading were assessed by analysis of variance (ANOVA; Statview 5.0, SAS Institute, Cary, NC, USA), followed by Tukey-Kramer multiple comparison tests (2 vs. 4 vs. 7 vs. 12 months) or paired t-tests (loaded vs. non-loaded) if overall ANOVA effects (or interactions) were significant ($p<0.05$). For baseline controls, effects of age were assessed by one-factor ANOVA. For loaded mice, effects of age and loading were assessed by two-factor ANOVA; in addition, relative data (loaded minus non-loaded; 6-week minus baseline) for microCT outcomes were analyzed by one-factor ANOVA, while temporal changes were assessed by repeated measures ANOVA.

Supporting Information

Table S1 Primers were either purchased as prescribed sequences from IDT and then validated, or purchased as proven primer sets from Qiagen.

Acknowledgments

We thank Marcus Watkins for assistance with primer selection and qPCR, and Tarpit Patel for assistant with microCT scanning and analysis.

Author Contributions

Conceived and designed the experiments: MJS MDB MAL RC. Performed the experiments: MDB MAL ALS DJW. Analyzed the data: MJS MDB MAL ALS. Wrote the paper: MJS. Manuscript review: MDB MAL ALS DJW RC.

References

1. Ozcivici E, Luu YK, Adler B, Qin YX, Rubin J, et al. (2010) Mechanical signals as anabolic agents in bone. Nat Rev Rheumatol 6: 50–59.
2. Hoshi A, Watanabe H, Chiba M, Inaba Y (1998) Effects of exercise at different ages on bone density and mechanical properties of femoral bone of aged mice. Tohoku J Exp Med 185: 15–24.
3. Silbermann M, Bar-Shira-Maymon B, Coleman R, Reznick A, Weisman Y, et al. (1990) Long-term physical exercise retards trabecular bone loss in lumbar vertebrae of aging female mice. Calcif Tiss Int 46: 80–93.
4. Raab DM, Smith EL, Crenshaw TD, Thomas DP (1990) Bone mechanical properties after exercise training in young and old rats. J Appl Physiol 68: 130–134.
5. Umemura Y, Ishiko T, Tsujimoto H, Miura H, Mokushi N, et al. (1995) Effects of jump training on bone hypertrophy in young and old rats. Int J Sports Med 16: 364–367.
6. Jarvinen TL, Pajamaki I, Sievanen H, Vuohelainen T, Tuukkanen J, et al. (2003) Femoral neck response to exercise and subsequent deconditioning in young and adult rats. J Bone Miner Res 18: 1292–1299.
7. Buhl KM, Jacobs CR, Turner RT, Evans GL, Farrell PA, et al. (2001) Aged bone displays an increased responsiveness to low-intensity resistance exercise. J Appl Physiol 90: 1359–1364.
8. Leppanen OV, Sievanen H, Jokihaara J, Pajamaki I, Kannus P, et al. (2008) Pathogenesis of age-related osteoporosis: impaired mechano-responsiveness of bone is not the culprit. PLoS ONE 3: e2540.
9. Rubin CT, Bain SD, McCleod KJ (1992) Suppression of osteogenic response in the aging skeleton. Calcif Tiss Int 50: 306–313.
10. Turner CH, Takano Y, Owan I (1995) Aging changes mechanical loading thresholds for bone formation in rats. J Bone Miner Res 10: 1544–1549.
11. Srinivasan S, Agans SC, King KA, Moy NY, Poliachik SL, et al. (2003) Enabling bone formation in the aged skeleton via rest-inserted mechanical loading. Bone 33: 946–955.
12. Brodt MD, Silva MJ (2010) Aged mice have enhanced endocortical response and normal periosteal response compared to young-adult mice following 1 week of axial tibial compression. J Bone Miner Res 25: 2006–2015.
13. McKenzie JA, Silva MJ (2011) Comparing histological, vascular and molecular responses associated with woven and lamellar bone formation induced by mechanical loading in the rat ulna. Bone 48: 250–258.
14. Mantila Roosa SM, Liu Y, Turner CH (2011) Gene expression patterns in bone following mechanical loading. J Bone Miner Res 26: 100–112.

15. Zaman G, Saxon LK, Sunters A, Hilton H, Underhill P, et al. (2010) Loading-related regulation of gene expression in bone in the contexts of estrogen deficiency, lack of estrogen receptor alpha and disuse. Bone 46: 628–642.
16. Li X, Srivastava AK, Gu W, Masinde G, Mohan S, et al. (2002) Opposing changes in osteocalcin levels in bone vs serum during the acquisition of peak bone density in C3H/HeJ and C57BL/6J mice. Calcif Tissue Int 71: 416–420.
17. Hamrick MW, Ding KH, Pennington C, Chao YJ, Wu YD, et al. (2006) Age-related loss of muscle mass and bone strength in mice is associated with a decline in physical activity and serum leptin. Bone 39: 845–853.
18. Dimai HP, Linkhart TA, Linkhart SG, Donahue LR, Beamer WG, et al. (1998) Alkaline phosphatase levels and osteoprogenitor cell numbers suggest bone formation may contribute to peak bone density differences between two inbred strains of mice. Bone 22: 211–216.
19. Frenkel B, Capparelli C, Van Auken M, Baran D, Bryan J, et al. (1997) Activity of the osteocalcin promoter in skeletal sites of transgenic mice and during osteoblast differentiation in bone marrow-derived stromal cell cultures: effects of age and sex. Endocrinology 138: 2109–2116.
20. Cao J, Venton L, Sakata T, Halloran BP (2003) Expression of RANKL and OPG correlates with age-related bone loss in male C57BL/6 mice. J Bone Miner Res 18: 270–277.
21. Lynch MA, Brodt MD, Silva MJ (2010) Skeletal effects of whole-body vibration in adult and aged mice. J Orthop Res 28: 241–247.
22. Ferguson VL, Ayers RA, Bateman TA, Simske SJ (2003) Bone development and age-related bone loss in male C57BL/6J mice. Bone 33: 387–398.
23. Kesavan C, Mohan S, Oberholtzer S, Wergedal JE, Baylink DJ (2005) Mechanical loading-induced gene expression and BMD changes are different in two inbred mouse strains. J Appl Physiol 99: 1951–1957.
24. Willinghamm MD, Brodt MD, Lee KL, Stephens AL, Ye J, et al. (2010) Age-related changes in bone structure and strength in female and male BALB/c mice. Calcif Tissue Int 86: 470–483.
25. Fritton JC, Myers ER, Wright TM, van der Meulen MC (2008) Bone mass is preserved and cancellous architecture altered due to cyclic loading of the mouse tibia after orchidectomy. J Bone Miner Res 23: 663–671.
26. Lynch ME, Main RP, Xu Q, Walsh DJ, Schaffler MB, et al. (2010) Cancellous bone adaptation to tibial compression is not sex dependent in growing mice. J Appl Physiol 109: 685–691.
27. Lynch ME, Main RP, Xu Q, Schmicker TL, Schaffler MB, et al. (2011) Tibial compression is anabolic in the adult mouse skeleton despite reduced responsiveness with aging. Bone 49: 439–446.
28. Sugiyama T, Saxon LK, Zaman G, Moustafa A, Sunters A, et al. (2008) Mechanical loading enhances the anabolic effects of intermittent parathyroid hormone (1–34) on trabecular and cortical bone in mice. Bone 43: 238–248.
29. Busse B, Djonic D, Milovanovic P, Hahn M, Puschel K, et al. (2010) Decrease in the osteocyte lacunar density accompanied by hypermineralized lacunar occlusion reveals failure and delay of remodeling in aged human bone. Aging Cell 9: 1065–1075.
30. Vashishth D, Verborgt O, Divine G, Schaffler MB, Fyhrie DP (2000) Decline in osteocyte lacunar density in human cortical bone is associated with accumulation of microcracks with age. Bone 26: 375–380.
31. Klein-Nulend J, Sterck JGH, Semeins CM, Lips P, Joldersma M, et al. (2002) Donor age and mechanosensitivity of human bone cells. Osteoporosis Int 13: 137–146.
32. Donahue SW, Jacobs CR, Donahue HJ (2001) Flow-induced calcium oscillations in rat osteoblasts are age, loading frequency, and shear stress dependent. Am J Physiol Cell Physiol 281: C1635–1641.
33. Sterck JG, Klein-Nulend J, Lips P, Burger EH (1998) Response of normal and osteoporotic human bone cells to mechanical stress in vitro. Am J Physiol 274: E1113–1120.
34. Forwood MR, Turner CH (1994) The response of rat tibiae to incremental bouts of mechanical loading: a quantum concept for bone formation. Bone 15: 603–609.
35. Beamer WG, Donahue LR, Rosen CJ, Baylink DJ (1996) Genetic variability in adult bone density among inbred strains of mice. Bone 18: 397–403.
36. Flurkey K, Currer JM, Harrison DE (2007) Mouse models in aging research. In: Fox JG, Barthold SW, Davisson MT, Newcomer CE, Quimby FW, et al., editor. The mouse in biomedical research. 2nd ed. Burlington: Academic Press. pp 637–672.
37. Kotiya AA, Bayly PV, Silva MJ (2011) Short-term low-strain vibration enhances chemo-transport yet does not stimulate osteogenic gene expression or cortical bone formation in adult mice. Bone 48: 468–475.
38. Silva MJ, Brodt MD, Hucker WJ (2005) Finite element analysis of the mouse tibia: Estimating endocortical strain during three-point bending in SAMP6 osteoporotic mice. Anat Rec A Discov Mol Cell Evol Biol 283A: 380–390.
39. De Souza RL, Matsuura M, Eckstein F, Rawlinson SC, Lanyon LE, et al. (2005) Non-invasive axial loading of mouse tibiae increases cortical bone formation and modifies trabecular organization: a new model to study cortical and cancellous compartments in a single loaded element. Bone 37: 810–818.
40. Fritton JC, Myers ER, Wright TM, van der Meulen MC (2005) Loading induces site-specific increases in mineral content assessed by microcomputed tomography of the mouse tibia. Bone 36: 1030–1038.

9

Generic Rules of Mechano-Regulation Combined with Subject Specific Loading Conditions Can Explain Bone Adaptation after THA

Tomasz D. Szwedowski[⁹], **William R. Taylor**[*⁹], **Markus O. Heller**[⁹], **Carsten Perka**, **Michael Müller**, **Georg N. Duda**

Julius Wolff Institute (JWI), Center for Musculoskeletal Surgery (CMSC), Center for Sports Science and Sports Medicine Berlin (CSSB), Charité – Universitätsmedizin Berlin, Berlin, Germany

Abstract

Bone adaptation after total hip arthroplasty is associated with the change in internal load environment, and can result in compromised bone stock, which presents a considerable challenge should a revision procedure be required. Under the assumption of a generic mechano-regulatory algorithm for governing bone adaptation, the aim of this study was to understand the contribution of subject specific loading conditions towards explaining the local periprosthetic remodelling variations in patients. CT scans of 3 consecutive THA patients were obtained and used for the construction of subject specific finite element models using verified musculoskeletal loading and physiological boundary conditions. Using either strain energy density or equivalent strain as mechano-transduction signals, predictions of bone adaptation were compared to DEXA derived BMD changes from 7 days to 12 months post-implantation. Individual changes in BMD of up to 33.6% were observed within the 12 month follow-up period, together with considerable inter-patient variability of up to 26%. Estimates of bone adaptation using equivalent strain and balanced loading conditions led to the best agreement with *in vivo* measured BMD, with RMS errors of only 3.9%, 7.3% and 7.3% for the individual subjects, compared to errors of over 10% when the loading conditions were simplified. This study provides evidence that subject specific loading conditions and physiological boundary constraints are essential for explaining inter-patient variations in bone adaptation patterns. This improved knowledge of the rules governing the adaptation of bone following THA helps towards understanding the interplay between mechanics and biology for better identifying patients at risk of excessive or problematic periprosthetic bone atrophy.

Editor: Ryan Keith Roeder, University of Notre Dame, United States of America

Funding: This work was financially supported by Zimmer Orthopaedics Inc. (Warsaw, Indiana, United States of America) and the Deutsche Forschungsgemeinschaft DFG SFB 760. The funders had no role in study design, data collection and analysis, decision to publish, or preparation of the manuscript.

Competing Interests: The authors have the following conflicts: The study was partially funded by Zimmer GmbH, but this does not alter the authors' adherence to all the PLoS ONE policies on sharing data and materials.

* E-mail: bill.taylor@charite.de

⁹ These authors contributed equally to this work.

Introduction

Periprosthetic bone loss continues to be a burden after total hip arthroplasty (THA) and exhibits substantial inter-patient variability in clinical radiographic measures [1–5]. Periprosthetic bone mineral density (BMD) changes are associated with the internal load distribution, where the local bone is thought to adapt to the requirements of loading and function [5–8]. Abrupt changes to the internal loading environment, such as after the implantation of a joint endoprosthesis, lead to a short term adaptation of the bone, resulting in periprosthetic bone atrophy in regions that become unloaded. Such bone loss is believed to influence THA longevity by undermining implant fixation and contributing to the risk of aseptic loosening [9,10]. The resulting compromised bone stock presents a considerable challenge should a revision procedure be required [11–13].

Although the mechanisms dictating individual patterns of bone adaptation are thought to be mechanically driven, the rules governing these processes remains unclear. To establish these rules of tissue adaptation, a number of computational models have been developed that aim to predict the changes in periprosthetic bone [14–24]. Such predictions of bone adaptation generally rely on models of the interplay between mechanics and biology [25], in which an increase in local loading leads to net bone deposition, while decreased loading results in bone loss, in order to return to customary physiological load levels within the tissue. Previous investigations have predominantly used changes in strain energy density (SED) following THA [9,14,22,26,27] as a remodelling signal to induce bone mineral changes. The choice of strain energy density was reasoned as being an indirect measure that represents a simplified index for bone gain or bone loss [14,15]. However, an investigation comparing the adaptation driven by different mechanical remodelling signals did not show strain energy density to be superior against the outcome of animal experiments *in vivo* [17].

In addition to animal experiments, determination of the accuracy and validity of remodelling algorithms in clinical THA cohorts has relied upon comparisons against averaged longitudinal measurements [22,23]. Such generic comparisons have partially achieved good agreement with RMS errors of approximately 5% [23] against cohort averaged DEXA measurements. However, these comparisons could not account for excessive trochanteric resorption [22] and predictions of less net resorption than occurred *in vivo* was observed in Gruen zones 1 and 2 [23]. Whilst the rules of mechanically regulated bone remodelling in such models have therefore been able to describe the general patterns of periprosthetic adaptation, they fail to explain the mechano-biological aetiology of the individual variations. Such discrepancies are generally thought to be guided by biological adaptive capacity, where it has been widely considered that the genome, proteome and secretome drive the patient specific response. In this study, we want to analyse to what degree mechanical specificity alone can explain the patient specific variations observed. If such individual adaptation is indeed related to subject specific musculoskeletal loading conditions, then next to genetic pre-disposition and molecular biological pathways, the patient specific intrinsic physical constraints [28–30] have to be taken into account if biological adaptation processes are to be successfully characterised.

Currently, the mechanisms of tissue adaptation following e.g. an abrupt change to the loading conditions after THA, are not well understood. Under the assumption of a generic mechano-regulatory algorithm for governing bone adaptation, the aim of this study was to understand the contribution of subject specific loading conditions towards explaining the local periprosthetic remodelling variations in patients.

Methods

Subjects and DEXA acquisition

Finite element models for predictions of bone adaptation were constructed for 3 consecutive patients who underwent a primary elective total hip arthroplasty, receiving an uncemented Zimmer Alloclassic® stem and Allofit® Pressfit- cup (Zimmer®, Warsaw, IN, USA) from the identical surgical team. The study was approved by the local ethics committee, and after providing written informed consent to participate, each of the three patients (2 female, 1 male, aged 68.7±2.3) received a three joint CT scan (hip, knee, ankle) that included the entire femur, both pre- and post-operatively (GE Centricity, 0.5 mm pixel size, slice thickness of 1 and 5 mm respectively). In addition, radiographic (DEXA) measurements were performed on each patient at 7 days and 12 months after surgery, and changes in BMD were determined within each Gruen zone.

Finite element models

Pre-operative femoral bone geometry was reconstructed using automated statistical shape modelling techniques (ZIB Amira, Zuse Institute Berlin) [31] with manual correction if necessary. Post-operative femoral geometry, specifically including the location of the resection plane and implant position, was determined from the post-operative CT scan. The triangulated surface reconstructions (intact, post-operative and implant) were converted into NURBS surface representations and anatomic landmarks were determined using the methods of Heller and co-workers (2001) (Geomagic Studio 10, Geomagic Inc., Triangle Park, NC). Virtual implantation and resection of the intact femoral head was performed using Boolean operations on the parametric representations of the femur, implant and resection plane (NX 3.0, Siemens PLN, Köln, DE).

The post-operative femur and implant assembly, that inherently included the anatomy of the intact femur, was then meshed using parabolic tetrahedral finite elements (MSC Patran 2008, MSC Software Corp., Santa Ana, CA) using a global mesh seed of 3.5 mm with a local refinement in areas of high detail (Figure 1). The mesh contained all solids required to construct both the intact and implanted models from the single assembly, allowing mesh congruency in regions common to the intact and implanted femurs, thus facilitating direct mapping of mechanical signals between the models. All models accounted for non-linear geometric effects (Abaqus 6.7-1, Dassault Systèmes, France).

Material Properties

A calibration phantom (Model #13002 Mindways Software, Inc., CA, USA) was placed under the thigh during all pre-operative CT scans, which allowed transformation of the CT values (in Hounsfeld units) into an apparent bone density. These average local densities were geometrically mapped onto each finite element of the femur model. Elastic modulus was then determined for each element by scaling the apparent density according to an established empirical relationship: $E = 15.1\ \rho^{2.25}$ [32]. All materials were modelled as linear elastic isotropic assuming a Poisson's ratio of 0.3.

Individual Loading and Mechanical Boundary Conditions

Two sets of different musculoskeletal loading conditions were applied to each patient model and were classified as either simplified or complex. In the simplified loading scenario a reduced set of musculoskeletal loads (Figure 2). was applied to both the pre- and post-operative models according to published data from Heller and co-workers [33]. The musculoskeletal forces were

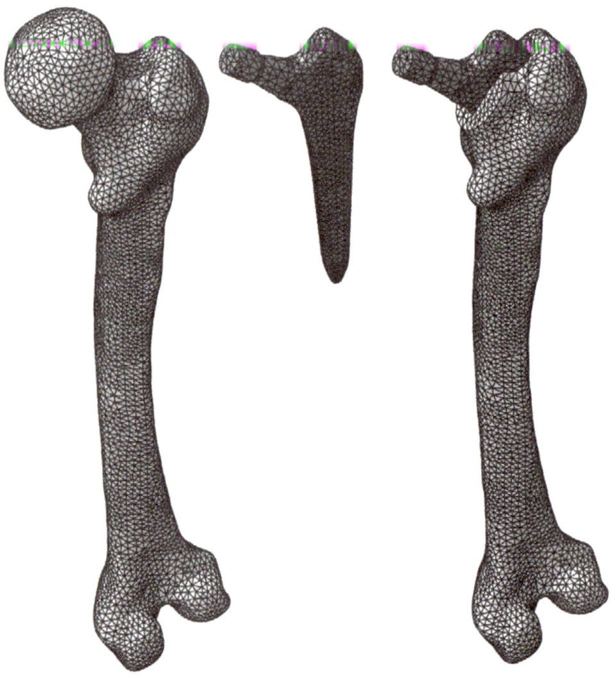

Figure 1. Schematic showing the intact femur (left), implant (centre) and implanted femur (right) meshes, consisting of approximately 80,000 second order tetrahedral elements.

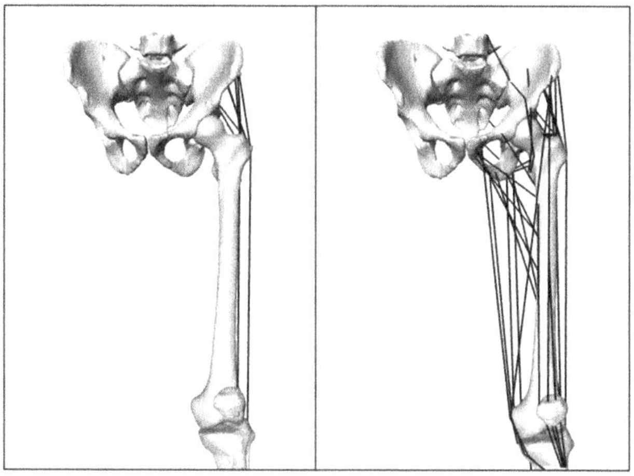

Figure 2. Simplified (left) and complex (right) musculoskeletal models used in the determination of subject specific muscle and joint loading. The simplified loading employs only the musculature that acts over the trochanteric region.

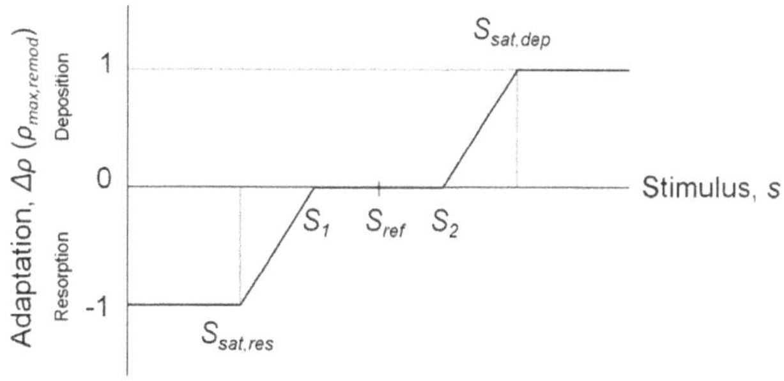

Figure 3. Mechanostat remodelling scheme. Change in the local density of bone for each time step, $\Delta\rho$, was governed by the local stimulus (s) according to the following rules:

$$If\quad s \leq S_{sat,dep} \qquad \Delta\rho = -\rho_{\max,re\,mod}$$

$$If\quad S_1 \geq s > S_{sat,res} \quad \Delta\rho = \frac{-(S_1 - s)}{(S_1 - S_{sat,res})}$$

$$If\quad S_1 \geq s \geq S_2 \qquad \Delta\rho = 0$$

$$If\quad S_{sat,dep} > s \geq S_2 \quad \Delta\rho = \frac{(s - S_2)}{(S_{sat,dep} - S_2)}$$

$$If\quad s \geq S_{sat,dep} \qquad \Delta\rho = \rho_{\max,re\,mod}$$

where $S_{sat,dep}$ and $S_{sat,res}$ were the stimuli at which deposition and resorption saturation occurred respectively, and S_1 and S_2 defined the limits of the lazy zone. $\rho_{\max,re\,mod}$ was the maximum rate of change of density for each of the remodelling steps.

scaled to each patient's body weight and the femur was fully constrained at the mid-diaphysis.

For the complex loading scenario, the intact and implanted hip, knee and ankle centres, femoral neck axis and femoral shaft axis were determined and used to transform all reconstructions into a local femoral coordinate system. Musculoskeletal loading was determined for each patient for both the intact anatomy and the implanted femur configurations using a previously validated musculoskeletal model [34,35]. This analysis accounted for subject specific anatomy/implantation (femoral antetorsion, caput-collum-diaphyseal angle (CCD) angle, neck length, limb length, limb alignment), as well as muscle origins and insertions (Figure 2). The forces corresponding to maximum joint loading (20% gait cycle) for the intact and implanted anatomies were then applied to the respective models.

Bone Remodelling Algorithms

Bone remodelling was governed according to a tri-linear curve [9] that possessed a 'lazy zone' in which net bone apposition and deposition rates remained in equilibrium, while increased loads stimulated local bone deposition and unloading resulted in local bone resorption (Figure 3). In a first step, the equivalent strain $\varepsilon_{\text{equivalent}} = \sqrt{\varepsilon_{ij}\varepsilon_{ij}}$ was employed as the mechanical remodelling signal for establishing the reference (intact pre-operative) loading conditions. This signal for the implanted model was then compared with the intact model and the course of remodelling simulated using an iterative adaptive bone remodelling algorithm. The lazy zone (S_1 & S_2) was specified as ± 100 με relative to the intact element-specific equivalent strain [16]. Remodelling proceeded in an iterative fashion, where a reduction in mechanical remodelling signal relative to the intact situation stimulated a decrease in element density and vice versa with a maximum change per iteration (saturation level) when the signal difference was 2000 με or more. Mechanical remodelling signal deviations of between 100 ($S_{sat,res}$) and 2000 με ($S_{sat,dep}$) from the reference signal resulted in a linear change in remodelling to a maximum rate or (saturation) of density change. A parametric study was performed to identify the remodelling rate (saturation) for which 25 iterations successfully reached remodelling equilibrium (all elements < 15% of max remodelling). To compare remodelling signals, a similar iterative model was investigated using strain energy density (SED) to drive the adaptive changes.

Post-processing

For comparison against DEXA measurements, the bone mineral densities for each finite element were sampled onto a regular grid and projected to simulate a 2D DEXA image. The bone mineral content contained within each Gruen Zone was then computed and normalized against the projected area (area BMD) that included only bone and excluded regions coincident with the implant. The ability of the various models to predict the clinical changes in BMD due to adaptation from the post-op to the 1 year follow-up time point was determined by evaluating the RMS error between the predicted and measured BMD changes for each Gruen zone.

Results

Over the course of the investigation, none of the patients experienced postoperative complications. The 3 patients exhibited periprosthetic bone atrophy of −8.1, −18.4 and −16.9% 12 months postoperatively, as measured using DEXA and averaged over 7 Gruen zones. All three patients exhibited atrophy in the most proximal regions (Gruen zones 1 and 7), ranging from −9.2 to −17.2% and −15.9 to −33.6% respectively (Figure 4).

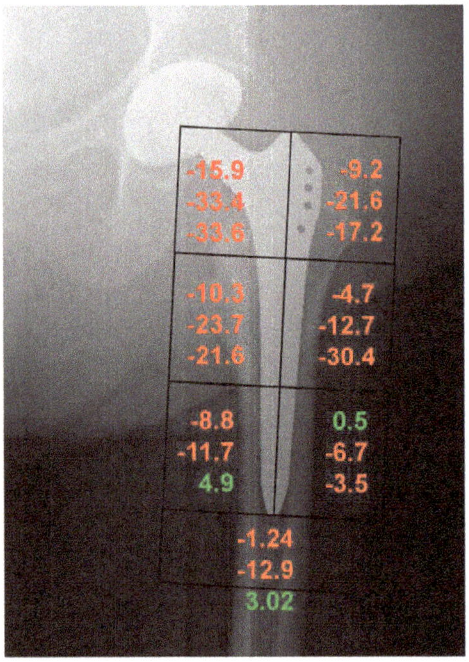

Figure 4. Summary of clinically measured changes in BMD from 7 days to 12 months after surgery. Values are presented for each patient as the percentage change relative to the 7 days postoperative BMD.

The corresponding FE models demonstrated average BMD changes (from 7 days to 12 months after implantation) of −7.5, −18.1 and −15.5% relative to the immediate postoperative BMD for the 3 patients respectively. Individual Gruen zone specific changes measured using DEXA were then compared to the subject specific FEA predictions, and exhibited considerable variation across patients and also as a consequence of loading conditions and mechano-regulation were observed (Figure 5).

For all three subjects, FEA predictions of the bone adaptation within each Gruen Zone demonstrated that mechano-regulation based on equivalent strain and that incorporated the complex musculoskeletal loading conditions (including physiological boundary constraints) resulted in the best agreement with the clinical DEXA measurements (Figure 5). The mean RMS error for the 3 patients was 6.2% while the patient specific RMS errors were 3.9%, 7.3% and 7.3% (Table 1). Adaptation based on equivalent strain with simplified loading conditions, rather than loading conditions that included the full anatomical complexity, reduced the levels of agreement with DEXA measurements to 10.7% overall. The overall best and worst case predictions on a patient and Gruen zone level were: equivalent strain and complex loading (best: 0.4%, worst: 16.0%), equivalent strain with simplified loading (0.4%, 28.1%), SED with complex loading (0.9%, 42.3%), and SED with simplified loading (0.3%, 84.4%) (Figure 5).

SED based predictions with complex loading had an average RMS error of 20%, which increased to 23.4% under simplified loading conditions. Individually (Table 1): subject 1 exhibited little change in agreement (complex loading; 12.3%, simplified loading; 12.6%), subject 2 showed an overall improvement of 21.1%, while subject 3 exhibited a reduction in agreement with complex loading (−11.6%).

In general, the three patient models exhibited unloading in the lower trochanteric region (Gruen zones 1 and 2), and a localized increase in loading directly adjacent to the implant in the proximal lateral region (Gruen zone 1). These patterns correspond to atrophy and bone densification respectively in the trabecular region (Figure 6). Additionally, patterns of unloading of the calcar region (Gruen zone 7) and an increase in loading at the tip of the implant (Gruen zone 4) corresponded to regions of atrophy and densification respectively. Regions of net bone atrophy and deposition exhibited similarities between the two signal types in the complex loading environment, but the application of simplified loading conditions led to more locally varied adaptation patterns.

Discussion

Bone loss following THA is well documented and frequently associated with changes in the mechanical environment. A detailed understanding of the rules that governing bone adaptation as well as the influence of subject specific factors is, however, lacking. In this study, we assumed that generic mechano-regulatory rules govern bone adaptation and then evaluated the contribution of subject specific anatomy and loading conditions towards explaining the local periprosthetic remodelling variations in 3 patients. The results of this study suggest that while generic rules of mechano-regulation can indeed estimate the broad patterns of periprosthetic bone adaptation observed *in vivo*, knowledge of the subject specific anatomy and loading conditions is indeed required before local variations in bone mineral changes can be discriminated.

This study has demonstrated that considerations regarding balanced musculoskeletal loading conditions [36] that enforce physiological deformation patterns [29,36] play a critical role for accurate predictions of periprosthetic bone adaptation. It is known that subtle changes to a subject's anatomy can play a critical role the internal loading conditions [37]. It therefore becomes apparent that simplified loading assumptions that have been predominantly employed in periprosthetic femoral remodelling studies, may not capture the complex balanced, subject specific loading conditions [36], and therefore enforce non-physiological deformation constraints [29]. Simplified loading conditions therefore seem limited in their ability to contribute towards understanding the underlying mechanisms that control the subject specific maintenance of bone stock [21].

In our study, 3 patients were observed over 12 months, resulting in average *in vivo* Gruen zone BMD changes of approximately −14.5%, with an RMS error of 6.2%. These results demonstrated that by considering detailed, subject specific loading conditions, the highly variable *in vivo* BMD outcomes of our three patients were all well predicted using our techniques (Figure 4). Importantly, the patient group displayed variations in periprosthetic bone adaptation patterns with average BMD changes ranging between −8.1 and −18.0%, with considerable inter-patient variation between the Gruen zones, and these variations could be explained in the models. Here, the equivalent strain based predictions and complex musculoskeletal loading conditions derived from subject specific analyses were accurate to within the magnitude of error observed in longitudinal DEXA measurements [38]. Although the study by Turner and co-workers [23] has suggested good agreement (5% RMS error) between longitudinal BMD changes and remodelling predictions based on equivalent strain, these predictions were assessed against cohort averaged values of bone remodelling, where local variations between and within individuals become obscured.

This study was able to compare the outcome of equivalent strain or SED mechano-regulation, and specifically how abrupt changes in the stimulus that result from implantation dictate predictions of

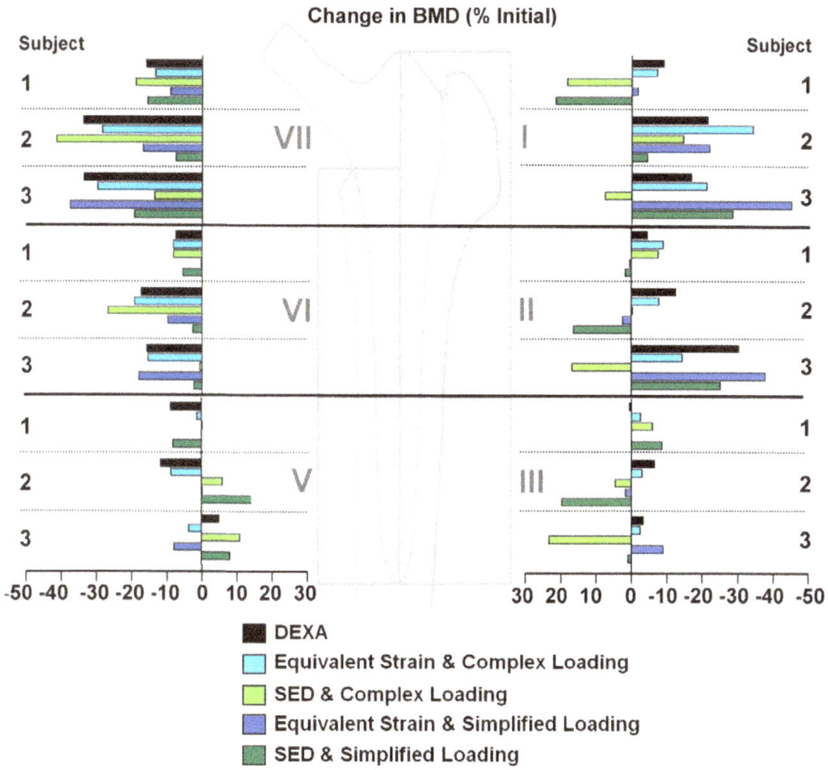

Figure 5. Comparison of change in BMD (% from initial) measured using DEXA against the adaptation signal based predictions of BMD. Also shown is the effect of simplified versus complex musculoskeletal loads depicted as the total change in the BMD of individual Gruen Zones.

periprosthetic bone remodelling (Figure 6). The changes in the signals (Figure 5) indicated that an unloading occurred most prominently in: 1. the calcar region (Gruen zone 7) and 2. the proximal lateral regions (Gruen zones 1 and 2), with localized increases adjacent to the implant. These changes were associated with decreases in BMD in the same general locations, reflecting clinical observations [3,38] with the notable exception in some cases that densification adjacent to the implant occurred in Gruen zone 1. Since these local phenomena appear to be due to boundary effects at the bone-implant interface, more detailed models that incorporate such interactions may be required before a more complete understanding of the local load transfer mechanisms across this interface can be reliably achieved.

Table 1. The root mean square (RMS) error (%) values for subject specific comparisons between the 12 month *in vivo* DEXA measurement and model variations that include equivalent strain and strain energy density based remodelling and their combinations with simplified and complete balanced musculoskeletal loading conditions.

RMS error (%)	Subject 1	2	3	Mean
Equivalent Strain & Simplified Loading	6.6	13.1	12.4	10.7
Equivalent Strain & Complex Loading	3.9	7.3	7.3	6.2
SED & Simplified Loading	12.6	39.8	17.8	23.4
SED & Complex Loading	12.3	18.7	29.4	20.2

The results of this study have demonstrated a better agreement between longitudinal clinical radiographic measurements and computational bone remodelling predictions based on equivalent strain than those based on SED [9,14,26,39] as the mechano-regulatory signal. This result is supported by previous work predicting experimentally observed adaptation patterns in a turkey ulna model [16] that did not find SED to be superior to other mechanical signals. Although these studies have contributed towards instilling confidence in the 'mechanostat' model of bone adaptation [40,41], individual specific patterns and their dependence on musculoskeletal forces, including implantation, have never been demonstrated. Equivalent strain as an alternative to SED was first used by Taylor an co-workers [17] and Turner and co-workers [23] based on work by Stülpner and co-workers [42] and derived from Mikic and Carter [43]. The rationale was that although bone adaptation stimuli could be based on stress or strain, strain was a parameter most likely detectable by bone. Furthermore, in the study of Kerner and co-workers [22], the SED mechanical signal was suggested to be responsible for resorption of the lesser trochanteric region, a result deemed clinically unrealistic. The results presented in this current study indicate that SED consistently invokes a proportionally larger change after implantation and exhibits larger local signal gradients than equivalent strain (Figure 6). This is likely related to the fact that SED is proportional to the square of the strain and therefore more sensitive to the changes in pre- to post-op signal.

For the first time this work considered the effect of physiological boundary conditions that enforce realistic femoral deformation

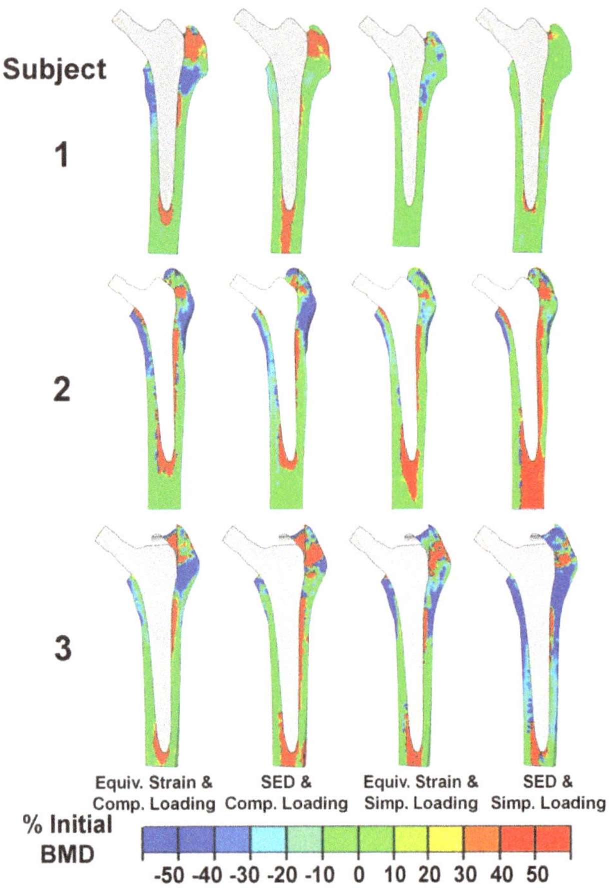

Figure 6. Percentage change in BMD distribution due to adaptation predicted using equivalent strain and strain energy density signals, as well as due to loading conditions, from the implanted to 12 months post-op situation.

patterns [29] and therefore internal loading conditions on predictions of bone adaptation. Additionally, in this study, the muscle and joint contact forces were taken from a musculoskeletal model [33,35] that had previously been validated against forces measured *in vivo* using instrumented telemetric hip implants [44]. Musculoskeletal loading in this study was adapted to the patients' geometry, where the musculoskeletal force predictions took into account the hip joint anatomy both before and after implantation. Patient specific gait patterns, however, were not included in this study, where kinematics were assumed to be the same both before and after implantation. The role of including subject specific gait patterns and external ground reaction forces might alter the characteristics of load estimations. Although not available in this study, one elegant approach for differentiating the impact of periprosthetic stress-shielding from global changes in limb loading, could be to normalise the proximal BMD to a reference BMD taken at a location well distal to the stem tip (sufficiently below Gruen Zone IV) pre- and post-operatively [45].

This investigation was able to achieve good agreement with DEXA BMD measurements despite certain limitations. DEXA can only produce a two dimensional projection that inherently reduces the amount of information available regarding the distribution of BMD. The third dimension is partially preserved in the operation of planar summation, but the spatial distribution is partially obscured. DEXA measurements also obscure information in regions that are coincident with the implant, and simplification into individual Gruen zone values further reduces the local specificity. However, in this study, DEXA allowed a quantitative and reproducible comparison for determining the adaptation of bone at multiple locations for longitudinal assessment of BMD in these subjects.

In summary, this study has demonstrated in three THA patients that under the assumption of generic bone adaptation rules, the variability in bone remodelling patterns between individuals can only be predicted when subject specific anatomy and loading conditions are taken into consideration. Additionally, this study has shown that mechano-regulation driven by an equivalent strain signal can produce good estimations of bone tissue adaptation. Here, the high level of agreement against clinical measurements using these techniques establishes a foundation for examining the variation in individual BMD adaptation patterns. This improved knowledge of the rules governing the adaptation of bone following the abrupt mechanical changes that occur due to the implantation of a prosthesis helps towards understanding the interplay between mechanics and biology for better identification of patients at risk of excessive or problematic periprosthetic bone atrophy.

Acknowledgments

The authors would like to thank Andrew Speirs and Adam Henderson for their contribution to the modelling techniques, as well as Annette Bowitz and Anne Zergiebel for the clinical administrative support.

Author Contributions

Conceived and designed the experiments: MH WT GD CP MM. Performed the experiments: MM TS. Analyzed the data: TS WT MH. Contributed reagents/materials/analysis tools: TS WT MH. Wrote the paper: GD WT MH TS CP.

References

1. Engh CA, McGovern TF, Schmidt LM (1993) Roentgenographic densitometry of bone adjacent to a femoral prosthesis. Clin Orthop Relat Res. pp 177–190.
2. Smart RC, Barbagallo S, Slater GL, Kuo RS, Butler SP, et al. (1996) Measurement of periprosthetic bone density in hip arthroplasty using dual-energy x-ray absorptiometry. Reproducibility of measurements. J Arthroplasty 11: 445–452.
3. Kiratli BJ, Heiner JP, McBeath AA, Wilson MA (1992) Determination of bone mineral density by dual x-ray absorptiometry in patients with uncemented total hip arthroplasty. J Orthop Res 10: 836–844.
4. Kiratli BJ, Checovich MM, McBeath AA, Wilson MA, Heiner JP (1996) Measurement of bone mineral density by dual-energy x-ray absorptiometry in patients with the Wisconsin hip, an uncemented femoral stem. J Arthroplasty 11: 184–193.
5. Perka C, Heller M, Wilke K, Taylor WR, Haas NP, et al. (2005) Surgical approach influences periprosthetic femoral bone density. Clin Orthop Relat Res 432: 153–159.
6. Rubin CT, Lanyon LE (1987) Kappa Delta Award paper. Osteoregulatory nature of mechanical stimuli: function as a determinant for adaptive remodeling in bone. J Orthop Res 5: 300–310.
7. Wolff J (2010) The classic: on the theory of fracture healing. 1873. Clin Orthop Relat Res 468: 1052–1055.
8. Wolff J (2010) The classic: on the inner architecture of bones and its importance for bone growth. 1870. Clin Orthop Relat Res 468: 1056–1065.
9. Huiskes R (1993) Stress shielding and bone resorption in THA: clinical versus computer-simulation studies. Acta Orthop Belg 59 Suppl 1: 118–129.
10. Sumner DR, Galante JO (1992) Determinants of stress shielding: design versus materials versus interface. Clin Orthop Relat Res. pp 202–212.
11. Dunbar MJ, Blackley HR, Bourne RB (2001) Osteolysis of the femur: principles of management. Instr Course Lect 50: 197–209.
12. Rosenbaum TG, Bloebaum RD, Ashrafi S, Lester DK (2006) Ambulatory activities maintain cortical bone after total hip arthroplasty. Clin Orthop Relat Res 450: 129–137.

13. Wilkinson JM, Hamer AJ, Rogers A, Stockley I, Eastell R (2003) Bone mineral density and biochemical markers of bone turnover in aseptic loosening after total hip arthroplasty. J Orthop Res 21: 691–696.
14. Huiskes R (1987) Finite element analysis of acetabular reconstruction. Noncemented threaded cups. Acta Orthop Scand 58: 620–625.
15. Schmitz MJ, Clift SE, Taylor WR, Hertig D, Warner MD, et al. (2004) Investigating the effect of remodelling signal type on the finite element based predictions of bone remodelling around the thrust plate prosthesis: a patient-specific comparison. Proc Inst Mech Eng H 218: 417–424.
16. Taylor WR, Ploeg H, Hertig D, Warner MD, Clift SE (2004) Bone remodelling of a proximal femur with the thrust plate prosthesis: an in vitro case. Comput Methods Biomech Biomed Engin 7: 131–137.
17. Taylor WR, Warner MD, Clift SE (2003) Finite element prediction of endosteal and periosteal bone remodelling in the turkey ulna: effect of remodelling signal and dead-zone definition. Proc Inst Mech Eng H 217: 349–356.
18. Weinans H, Huiskes R, van Rietbergen B, Sumner DR, Turner TM, et al. (1993) Adaptive bone remodeling around bonded noncemented total hip arthroplasty: a comparison between animal experiments and computer simulation. J Orthop Res 11: 500–513.
19. Van Rietbergen B, Huiskes R, Weinans H, Sumner DR, Turner TM, et al. (1993) ESB Research Award 1992. The mechanism of bone remodeling and resorption around press-fitted THA stems. J Biomech 26: 369–382.
20. Huiskes R, van Rietbergen B (1995) Preclinical testing of total hip stems. The effects of coating placement. Clin Orthop Relat Res. pp 64–76.
21. Bitsakos C, Kerner J, Fisher I, Amis AA (2005) The effect of muscle loading on the simulation of bone remodelling in the proximal femur. J Biomech 38: 133–139.
22. Kerner J, Huiskes R, van Lenthe GH, Weinans H, van Rietbergen B, et al. (1999) Correlation between pre-operative periprosthetic bone density and post-operative bone loss in THA can be explained by strain-adaptive remodelling. J Biomech 32: 695–703.
23. Turner AW, Gillies RM, Sekel R, Morris P, Bruce W, et al. (2005) Computational bone remodelling simulations and comparisons with DEXA results. J Orthop Res 23: 705–712.
24. Scannell PT, Prendergast PJ (2009) Cortical and interfacial bone changes around a non-cemented hip implant: simulations using a combined strain/damage remodelling algorithm. Med Eng Phys 31: 477–488.
25. Epari DR, Taylor WR, Heller MO, Duda GN (2006) Mechanical conditions in the initial phase of bone healing. Clin Biomech (Bristol, Avon) 21: 646–655.
26. Huiskes R, Weinans H, Dalstra M (1989) Adaptive bone remodeling and biomechanical design considerations for noncemented total hip arthroplasty. Orthopedics 12: 1255–1267.
27. Huiskes R, Weinans H, Grootenboer HJ, Dalstra M, Fudala B, et al. (1987) Adaptive bone-remodeling theory applied to prosthetic-design analysis. J Biomech 20: 1135–1150.
28. Kleemann RU, Heller MO, Stoeckle U, Taylor WR, Duda GN (2003) THA loading arising from increased femoral anteversion and offset may lead to critical cement stresses. J Orthop Res 21: 767–774.
29. Speirs AD, Heller MO, Duda GN, Taylor WR (2007) Physiologically based boundary conditions in finite element modelling. J Biomech 40: 2318–2323.
30. Speirs AD, Heller MO, Taylor WR, Duda GN, Perka C (2007) Influence of changes in stem positioning on femoral loading after THR using a short-stemmed hip implant. Clin Biomech (Bristol, Avon) 22: 431–439.
31. Kainmueller D, Lamecker H, Zachow S, Hege HC (2009) An articulated statistical shape model for accurate hip joint segmentation. Conf Proc IEEE Eng Med Biol Soc 2009: 6345–6351.
32. Les CM, Keyak JH, Stover SM, Taylor KT, Kaneps AJ (1994) Estimation of material properties in the equine metacarpus with use of quantitative computed tomography. J Orthop Res 12: 822–833.
33. Heller MO, Bergmann G, Kassi JP, Claes L, Haas NP, et al. (2005) Determination of muscle loading at the hip joint for use in pre-clinical testing. J Biomech 38: 1155–1163.
34. Heller MO, Bergmann G, Deuretzbacher G, Durselen L, Pohl M, et al. (2001) Musculo-skeletal loading conditions at the hip during walking and stair climbing. J Biomech 34: 883–893.
35. Taylor WR, Heller MO, Bergmann G, Duda GN (2004) Tibio-femoral loading during human gait and stair climbing. J Orthop Res 22: 625–632.
36. Duda GN, Heller M, Albinger J, Schulz O, Schneider E, et al. (1998) Influence of muscle forces on femoral strain distribution. J Biomech 31: 841–846.
37. Heller MO, Taylor WR, Perka C, Duda GN (2003) The influence of alignment on the musculo-skeletal loading conditions at the knee. Langenbecks Arch Surg 388: 291–297.
38. Kilgus DJ, Shimaoka EE, Tipton JS, Eberle RW (1993) Dual-energy X-ray absorptiometry measurement of bone mineral density around porous-coated cementless femoral implants. Methods and preliminary results. J Bone Joint Surg Br 75: 279–287.
39. Huiskes R, Weinans H, van Rietbergen B (1992) The relationship between stress shielding and bone resorption around total hip stems and the effects of flexible materials. Clin Orthop Relat Res. pp 124–134.
40. Frost HM (1987) Bone "mass" and the "mechanostat": a proposal. Anat Rec 219: 1–9.
41. Frost HM (2003) Bone's mechanostat: a 2003 update. Anat Rec A Discov Mol Cell Evol Biol 275: 1081–1101.
42. Stulpner MA, Reddy BD, Starke GR, Spirakis A (1997) A three-dimensional finite analysis of adaptive remodelling in the proximal femur. J Biomech 30: 1063–1066.
43. Mikic B, Carter DR (1995) Bone strain gage data and theoretical models of functional adaptation. J Biomech 28: 465–469.
44. Bergmann G, Deuretzbacher G, Heller M, Graichen F, Rohlmann A, et al. (2001) Hip contact forces and gait patterns from routine activities. J Biomech 34: 859–871.
45. Bryan JM, Sumner DR, Hurwitz DE, Tompkins GS, Andriacchi TP, et al. (1996) Altered load history affects periprosthetic bone loss following cementless total hip arthroplasty. J Orthop Res 14: 762–768.

10

Lrp5 Is Not Required for the Proliferative Response of Osteoblasts to Strain but Regulates Proliferation and Apoptosis in a Cell Autonomous Manner

Behzad Javaheri[1]*, Andrew Sunters[2], Gul Zaman[2], Rosemary F. L. Suswillo[2], Leanne K. Saxon[2], Lance E. Lanyon[2], Joanna S. Price[3]

1 Department of Oral Biology, UMKC School of Dentistry, Kansas City, Missouri, United States of America, **2** Department of Veterinary Basic Sciences, The Royal Veterinary College, Royal College Street, London, United Kingdom, **3** Bristol Veterinary School, Langford House, Langford, Bristol, United Kingdom

Abstract

Although Lrp5 is known to be an important contributor to the mechanisms regulating bone mass, its precise role remains unclear. The aim of this study was to establish whether mutations in *Lrp5* are associated with differences in the growth and/ or apoptosis of osteoblast-like cells and their proliferative response to mechanical strain *in vitro*. Primary osteoblast-like cells were derived from cortical bone of adult mice lacking functional *Lrp5* (*Lrp5*$^{-/-}$), those heterozygous for the human G171V High Bone Mass (HBM) mutation (*LRP5*^{G171V}) and their WT littermates (WT_{Lrp5}, WT_{HBM}). Osteoblast proliferation over time was significantly higher in cultures of cells from *LRP5*^{G171V} mice compared to their WT_{HBM} littermates, and lower in *Lrp5*$^{-/-}$ cells. Cells from female *LRP5*^{G171V} mice grew more rapidly than those from males, whereas cells from female *Lrp5*$^{-/-}$ mice grew more slowly than those from males. Apoptosis induced by serum withdrawal was significantly higher in cultures from *Lrp5*$^{-/-}$ mice than in those from WT_{HBM} or *LRP5*^{G171V} mice. Exposure to a single short period of dynamic mechanical strain was associated with a significant increase in cell number but this response was unaffected by genotype which also did not change the 'threshold' at which cells responded to strain. In conclusion, the data presented here suggest that *Lrp5* loss and gain of function mutations result in cell-autonomous alterations in osteoblast proliferation and apoptosis but do not alter the proliferative response of osteoblasts to mechanical strain *in vitro*.

Editor: Pierre J. Marie, Inserm U606 and University Paris Diderot, France

Funding: This work was supported by the Biotechnology and Biological Sciences Research Council (BBSRC) and the Wellcome Trust. The funders had no role in study design, data collection and analysis, decision to publish, or preparation of the manuscript.

Competing Interests: The authors have declared that no competing interests exist.

* E-mail: javaherib@umkc.edu

Introduction

Normal bone homeostasis is achieved by balancing the number and activity of bone forming osteoblasts and bone resorbing osteoclasts. In the adult skeleton the mechanical strain engendered within the bone tissue by the activities of normal life acts as a stimulus to regulate this osteoblast/osteoclast balance, thereby controlling bone mass and architecture such that the skeleton is of sufficient strength to withstand the loads placed upon it without damage. There is compelling evidence that the co-ordinated activities of many different signalling pathways function to control osteoblast number and activity both basally and in response to mechanical strain [1]. One such pathway is the Wnt pathway. Engagement of the Wnt ligand with the receptor complex comprising of Frizzled and *Lrp5/6* stimulates activation of the canonical (involving β-catenin activation) and planar cell polarity pathways. Indeed Wnt signalling has been implicated in the regulation of mesenchymal precursor commitment to the osteoblast lineage [2,3], osteoblast proliferation [4,5], terminal differentiation [6] and apoptosis [7–9]. Humans with an inactivating mutation in the *Lrp5* Wnt co-receptor gene have reduced bone mass [6,10,11], whilst individuals with an activating mutation (the G171V mutation) have correspondingly higher than normal bone mass [12–14]. Experimental models such as *Lrp5* knockout mice [4] or mice expressing human *LRP5* transgene containing the G171V activating mutation (*LRP5*^{G171V}) [7] generally recapitulate the situation in humans and have low and high bone mass respectively.

Sawakami *et al.*, (2006) provided *in vivo* evidence that the Wnt pathway may play a role in mediating bone's adaptive response to loading, by demonstrating that mice lacking functional *LRP5* have an impaired cortical bone response to ulna loading [15]. In a recent study that analysed multiple bone responses to graded strains we also demonstrated that absence of *Lrp5* activity due to the *Lrp5*$^{-/-}$ mutation reduces the osteogenic effects of loading in male (but not female) mice, whilst the presence of the *LRP5*^{G171V} mutated gene was associated with increased mechano-responsiveness [16]. However, this study supported only a limited gender-related role for LRP5 function in mediating bone's adaptive response to mechanical loading *in vivo*.

Given that *Lrp5* status *in vivo* impacts basal and mechanically influenced bone mass, we sought to investigate *in vitro* whether primary long-bone-derived osteoblast like cells derived from both the *Lrp5*$^{-/-}$ or *LRP5*^{G171V} mice displayed cell autonomous differences in their basal growth and apoptosis rates that could explain these physiological phenotypes. We also measured proliferation in these cells following exposure to mechanical strain in order to determine whether *Lrp5* functionality regulated the magnitude of the strain-related response and/or altered the 'threshold' at which a proliferative response to strain was engendered.

Materials and Methods

Ethics statement

The genetic background of *LRP5*^{G171V} and *Lrp5*$^{-/-}$ is the mouse strain C57BL/6 (Charles River Laboratories, Margate, Kent, U.K). *LRP5*^{G171V} transgenic and *Lrp5*$^{-/-}$ mice were a gift from Babij *et al.*, (2003) and Kato *et al.*, (2002) respectively [4,7]. Mice from both colonies were housed up to 5 per cage in polypropylene cages with wood chip and paper bedding and provided standard mouse chow and water ad libitum. Weaners up to 8 weeks of age were fed a standard rodent breeding diet and thereafter a standard rodent maintenance diet (Special Diet Services, South Witham, UK). All of the procedures conducted in the facility were carried out in accordance with the UK Animals Act (Scientific Procedures) 1986 under a UK Government Home Office project license number PIL70/6350, reviewed and approved by the Royal Veterinary College Local Ethical Review Committee (London, UK).

Cell extraction

At 19 weeks of age, *LRP5*^{G171V} and *Lrp5*$^{-/-}$ mice and their WT littermates (WT$_{HBM}$ and WT$_{Lrp5}$) were euthanized by means of cervical dislocation. Primary osteoblast-like cells were isolated from femur, radii, ulnae and humerus as described previously [17]. The osteoblast-like cells were maintained in Dulbecco's minimal essential medium (DMEM) without phenol-red, 2 mM L-glutamine (Life Technologies Ltd.), 100 U/ml penicillin (Life Technologies Ltd.), and 100 µg/ml streptomycin (Invitrogen Ltd, Paisley, Scotland, UK (Life Technologies Ltd.) supplemented with 10% heat-inactivated foetal calf serum (FCS) (LabTech International, East Sussex, UK) and were incubated at 37°C in a humidified 5% CO2 incubator. Only first passage cells (P1) were used.

Cell proliferation rates

Primary osteoblast-like cells isolated from female and male LRP5^{G171V} and Lrp5$^{-/-}$ mice and their WT littermates and experiments were repeated three times (2 mice of each gender and genotype were used). The cells were seeded evenly onto custom-made sterile, tissue culture-treated plastic strips (66 mm×22 mm) (Nunc, Dossel, Germany) at a density of 100,000 cells/strip. Four strips were incubated together in quadriPERM 4-well plates (Greiner Bio-One, Stonehouse, UK) in DMEM supplemented with 10% FCS. Cells were fixed for 10 minutes in absolute ice-cold MeOH (VWR International) 2, 4, 6 and 8 days after seeding followed by one wash with PBS. To quantify cell number, cells were stained with propidium iodide (INCYTO, Seoul, South Korea) and counted using a Microchip Type Automatic Cell Counter according to the manufacturer's instructions (INCYTO, Seoul, South Korea).

TUNEL staining

For each experiment and each experimental group, primary osteoblast-like cells were extracted from the femur, humerus, radius and ulna of one 19 week old mouse. These studies were repeated 3 times and thus included 3 mice per group. 20,000 first passage primary osteoblast-like cells derived from female and male *Lrp5*$^{-/-}$, *LRP5*^{G171V} and WT$_{HBM}$ mice were seeded onto 24-multiwell plates (16 mm in diameter) and cultured in DMEM supplemented with 10% FCS. Six wells per treatment group were used. After 72 hours the cells were washed twice with serum free DMEM and thereafter were incubated with fresh DMEM containing 0.1%, 2.5% or 10% FCS. After 48 hours the cells were fixed with 4% paraformaldehyde. Nuclear DNA fragmentation as a measure of apoptosis was evaluated by the terminal deoxynucleotidyl transferase-mediated dUTP nick-end labelling (TUNEL) method using DeadEnd Fluorometric TUNEL System (Promega, Madison, WI) according to the manufacturer's protocol. Vectashield mounting medium with DAPI (Vector Laboratories) was used for the counterstaining of nuclei. Nuclear TUNEL positive cells were judged to be apoptotic. Total cell number and the percentage of TUNEL positive cells were determined in 5 microscopic fields per well at 10× magnification. The fields were photographed using a Leica Q550IW fluorescent microscope with a DC 500 Leica digital camera and cells were counted from the computer screen with the assistance of the Leica Qwin computer programme (Leica, Solms, Germany).

Cell proliferation in response to mechanical strain

Primary osteoblast-like cells isolated from female and male LRP5^{G171V} and *Lrp5*$^{-/-}$ mice and their WT littermates were seeded onto custom-made sterile, tissue culture-treated plastic strips (Nunc, Dossel, Germany) at a density of 100,000 cells/strip (3 mice of each gender and genotype were used and experiments were repeated three times). Four strips were used per condition and were incubated together in quadriPERM 4-well plates (Greiner Bio-One, Stonehouse, UK) maintained in DMEM containing 10% FCS for 5 days. Mechanical strain was applied using a loading jig that applies four-point bending to each strip with minimal fluid perturbation as described previously [17]. Cells were subjected to a single period of 600 cycles of four-point-bending at a frequency of 1 Hz. This generated a peak strain of 2500, 2900 or 3400 µε. Following strain treatment the strips and media were replaced into the 4-well plates and incubated for 48 hours. Control strips were placed in wells of the loading apparatus and subjected to similar perturbation of surrounding media as experienced by the strained strips. However, these strips were not subjected to bending and thus the cells that were plated onto them were not subjected to strain. Cells were stained with propidium iodide (INCYTO, Seoul, South Korea) and counted using a Microchip Type Automatic Cell Counter according to the manufacturer's instructions (INCYTO, Seoul, South Korea).

Statistical Analysis

Statistical significance was determined by a 2-tailed unpaired Student's t-test or one way analysis of variance (ANOVA) followed by the post hoc (Bonferroni) multiple comparisons between treatment groups using SPSS statistics package version 16 for Windows (SPSS, Chicago, IL, USA). The mixed model analysis was performed using SAS system v9.0 (SAS Institute, Cary, NC, USA). Cell doubling time were calculated using GraphPad Prism v5.0 software for Windows (GraphPad Software Inc., San Diego, CA) by nonlinear regression (exponential growth equation) analysis. Least significant difference was determined and $p<0.05$ considered statistically significant. Data displayed as mean ± SEM.

Results

Osteoblast proliferation over time *in vitro*

Primary osteoblast-like cells extracted from the long bones of female and male *LRP5*^{G171V} and *Lrp5*$^{-/-}$ mice and their WT littermates were cultured for 2, 4, 6 or 8 days (Fig. 1). There was a main effect of genotype ($p<0.001$) and time in culture on cell number ($p<0.001$). The post-hoc analysis showed that cells from $LRP5^{G171V}$ mice proliferated faster than cells from the WT_{HBM} littermates ($p<0.001$), whereas cells from $Lrp5^{-/-}$ mice proliferated more slowly than cells from WT_{Lrp5} littermates. A gender and genotype interaction was detected ($p<0.001$) together with interaction between gender, genotype and time ($p<0.001$). The post-hoc analysis also showed that cells from female $LRP5^{G171V}$ mice grew faster than cells from male $LRP5^{G171V}$, male and female WT_{HBM} and male and female $Lrp5^{-/-}$ mice ($p<0.001$). Furthermore, female $Lrp5^{-/-}$ cells proliferated more slowly compared to male $Lrp5^{-/-}$ cells ($p<0.001$). Doubling time calculated from the regression analysis of each genotype is shown in table 1.

TUNEL staining of cells exposed to serum depletion

Having observed that cells from different genotypes of mice proliferated at different rates, we sought to establish whether this reflected a difference in the rate of apoptosis. Significantly higher levels of TUNEL stained cells were observed in cultures from $Lrp5^{-/-}$ mice compared to cultures from WT_{HBM} and $LRP5^{G171V}$ mice ($p<0.001$) (Fig. 2). In contrast, the percentage of TUNEL stained cells from $LRP5^{G171V}$ mice was significantly lower compared to $Lrp5^{-/-}$ and WT_{HBM} cells ($p<0.001$). There was an effect of gender, genotype and serum concentration on percentage of TUNEL stained cells ($p<0.001$) and an interaction between genotype and serum concentration was also detected ($p<0.001$). In 0.1 and 2.5% serum the percentage of TUNEL positive osteoblast-like cells was significantly higher in cultures of female and male $Lrp5^{-/-}$ mice compared to cultures of female and male WT_{HBM} and $LRP5^{G171V}$ cells ($p<0.001$ and $p<0.01$ respectively). Similar to the situation in 0.1 and 2.5% serum, the percentage of TUNEL positive cells in 10% serum was significantly higher in cultures of female and male $Lrp5^{-/-}$ cells compared to female and male WT_{HBM} and $LRP5^{G171V}$ cells ($p<0.05$). Gender related differences in the percentage of TUNEL positive cells were also observed within each genotype; in 2.5% and 10% serum the percentage of TUNEL positive cells was higher in cultures of male WT_{HBM} cells compared to cultures of female WT_{HBM} cells ($p<0.05$) and no gender differences in TUNEL positive cells was observed in 0.1% serum. In contrast, in 2.5% serum the percentage of TUNEL positive cells was higher in cultures of female $Lrp5^{-/-}$ cells compared to cultures of male $Lrp5^{-/-}$ cells ($p<0.01$) and no gender differences in 0.1% and 10% was observed.

Table 1. Cell population doubling time of primary osteoblast-like cells derived from female and male $Lrp5^{-/-}$, $LRP5^{G171V}$ and their WT littermates.

Genotype	Double time (days)
Female WT_{HBM}	3.42
Male WT_{HBM}	3.26
Female WT_{Lrp5}	3.26
Male WT_{Lrp5}	3.36
Female $LRP5^{G171V}$	2.52
Male $LRP5^{G171V}$	2.96
Female $Lrp5^{-/-}$	−4.34
Male $Lrp5^{-/-}$	4.14

Doubling time in days between 2 and 8 days of culture of primary osteoblast-like cells isolated from female and male $Lrp5^{-/-}$, $LRP5^{G171V}$ and their WT littermates. Cell doubling time were calculated using GraphPad Prism v5.0 software for Windows (GraphPad Software Inc., San Diego, CA) by nonlinear regression (exponential growth equation) analysis.

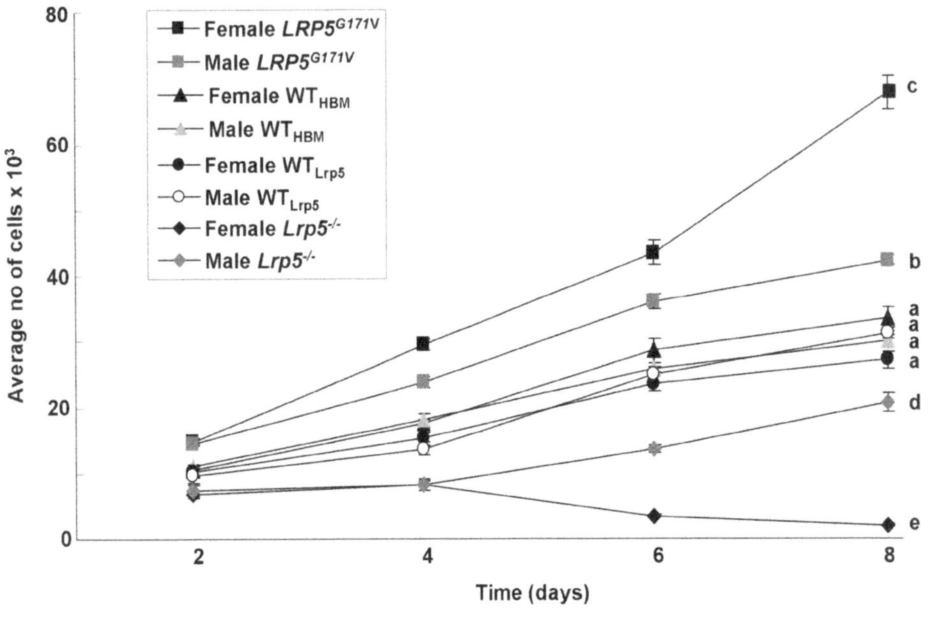

Figure 1. Proliferation of primary osteoblast-like cells derived from female and male $LRP5^{G171V}$ and $Lrp5^{-/-}$ mice and their WT littermates. Osteoblast-like cells were cultured over 8 days and were fixed in absolute ice-cold MeOH on day 2, 4, 6 and 8. Cell's nuclei were stained using propidium iodide and counted using Microchip Type Automatic Cell Counter machine. Results are the mean ± SEM of three independent experiments. N = 4. Groups with the same letter are not significantly different. b vs. a = $P<0.001$. a + b vs. c = $P<0.001$.

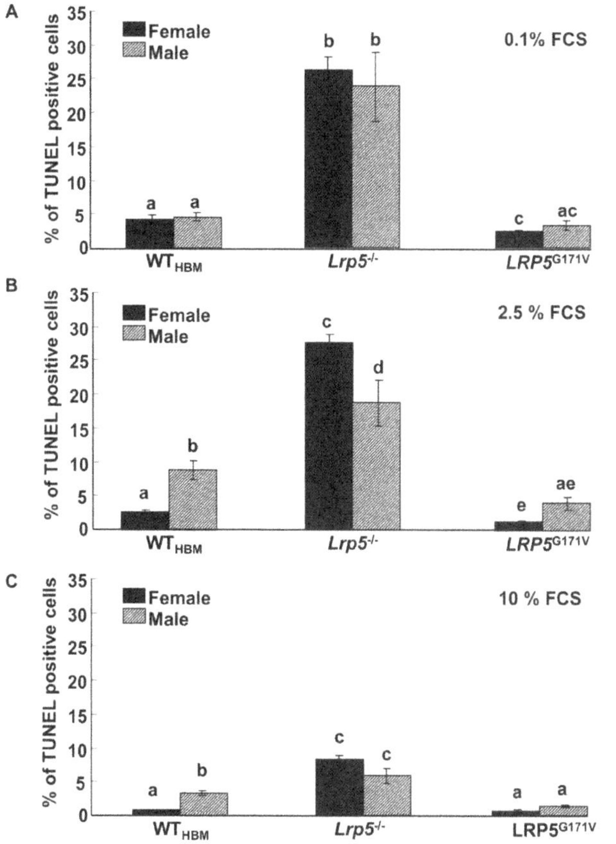

Figure 2. Percentage of apoptosis in osteoblast-like cells 48 hours after treatment with 0.1% (A), 2.5% (B) and 10% (C) serum. The TUNEL staining was used to determine the percentage of apoptotic cells in primary osteoblast-like cells derived from male and female WT$_{HBM}$, *Lrp5*$^{-/-}$ and *LRP5*^{G171V} mice. Results are mean ± SEM of three independent experiments. Groups with the same letter are not significantly different.

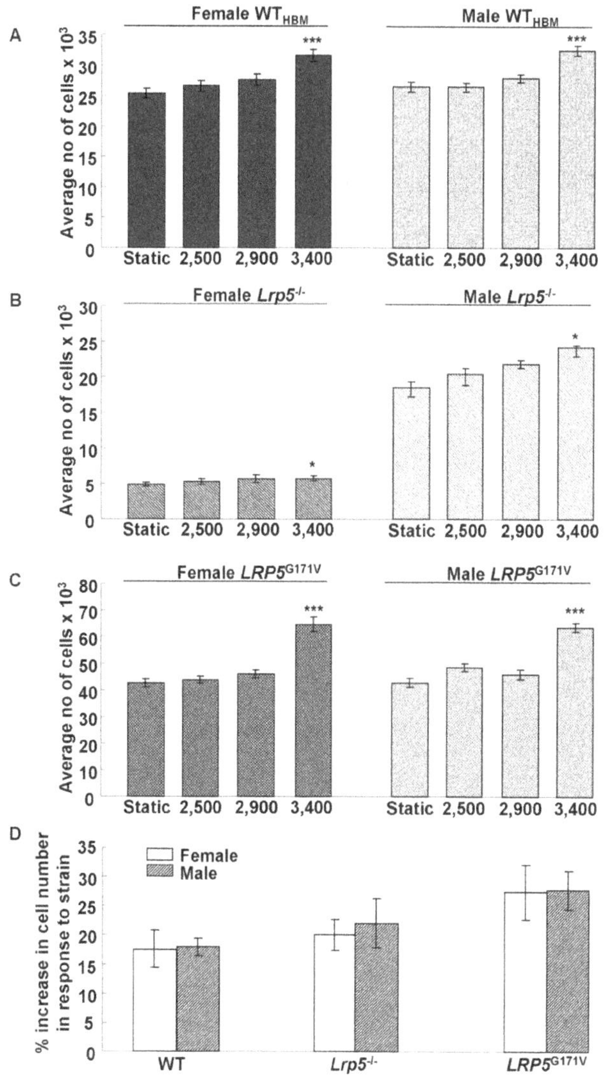

Figure 3. Effects of 2500, 2900 and 3400 με on proliferation of primary osteoblast-like cells derived from female and male WT (A), *Lrp5*$^{-/-}$ (B) and *LRP5*^{G171V} (C) mice. Changes in absolute number of cells between static and strain of both genotypes and genders are shown. Results are mean ± SEM of three independent experiments. Experiments were repeated 3 times. No significant differences at 2500 and 2900 με were observed. ***$p<0.001$ and *$p<0.05$ compared with the static control within the gender. (D) The effects of 3400 με on proliferation of primary osteoblast-like cells derived from female and male *LRP5*^{G171V} and *Lrp5*$^{-/-}$ mice and their WT littermates. Percentage differences between static and strain of both genotypes and genders are shown. Results are the mean ± SEM of three independent experiments. Experiments were repeated 3 times. There were no significant differences between groups.

Osteoblast proliferation in response to mechanical strain *in vitro*

The proliferative response of osteoblast-like cells cultured from each gender and genotype of mice to different magnitudes of mechanical strain is shown in figure 3. All groups showed no response at 2,500 με and 2,900 με however, for each gender and genotype ($p<0.001$) a significant increase in cell number was detected at 3,400 με (Figs. 3A, B and C). We also calculated the percentage increase in cell number between the control (static) and strained groups and found no significant differences between female and male or *LRP5*^{G171V}, *Lrp5*$^{-/-}$ and WT cells (Fig. 3D).

Mixed model analysis showed a main effect of gender ($p<0.001$), genotype ($p<0.001$) and strain ($p<0.001$) on cell number. A genotype and strain interaction was detected ($p<0.006$) and an interaction between gender, genotype and strain ($p<0.001$). As described previously, the number of cells in static control cultures of female and male *LRP5*^{G171V} cells was significantly higher than in *Lrp5*$^{-/-}$ and WT$_{HBM}$ cultures. This reflects significant differences in basal proliferation between *LRP5*^{G171V}, *Lrp5*$^{-/-}$ and WT cells (Fig. 1).

Discussion

LRP5 plays a role in osteoblast proliferation

The key finding from this study was that absence of *Lrp5* function in osteoblastic cells derived from the cortical bone of adult mice was associated with decreased proliferation as evidenced by an increase in cell population doubling time compared with WT$_{Lrp5}$ cells *in vitro*. Conversely, presence of the *LRP5*^{G171V} mutation in osteoblastic cells was associated with increased proliferation compared with *Lrp5*$^{-/-}$ and WT cells. Cell population doubling times were comparable in the cultures of female and male WT_{HBM} and WT_{Lrp5} cells, suggesting that WT cells from both backgrounds have a similar proliferation rate. These findings provide evidence that the presence of functional *LRP5* protein plays an important role in the regulation of osteoblast proliferation, which is in broad agreement with previous studies [4,6].

These results are not consistent with those of Yadav *et al.*, (2009) who observed no significant differences between the proliferation of *Lrp5*$^{-/-}$ and WT_{Lrp5} osteoblast-like cells [18]. However, differences between our two studies could potentially explain these apparently contrasting observations. The first relates to the site of origin of the cells; the study described here used osteoblast-like cells derived from long bones, whereas Yadav *et al*, (2009) used calvarial derived osteoblast-like cells. Several years ago our group demonstrated that osteoblastic cells from long bones and calvariae respond differently to a strain-related stimulus [19]. More recently another study confirmed that primary osteoblast-like cells derived from calvariae or long bones are both phenotypically different in vitro and also are significantly different at the level of gene expression [20]. Second, the age of animals was very different in the two studies; Yadav *et al* (2009) derived osteoblast-like cells from new born mice whereas cells from adult (19 week old) mice were used in the present study. Because pre-osteoblasts and osteoblasts from young humans and animals proliferate more rapidly than cells from older animals [21–29], this potentially could 'mask' the effect on proliferation of the loss of *Lrp5*. It must also be considered that the long-term loss of *Lrp5* (from birth to 19 weeks of age) has different effects to loss of the gene during development only. Kato *et al.*, (2002) demonstrated that bone formation was normal in *Lrp5*$^{-/-}$ mice at 17.5 days post coitum and at birth there was only a subtle delay in osteogenesis. However, the ossification defect in these mice became more pronounced with age and reflected a defect in osteoblast proliferation. Finally, different promoters were used in the two studies. The *LRP5*^{G171V} mice used for the present study were generated by Babij *et al*, (2003) using the 3.6 kb fragment of the collagen type 1 promoter to drive the expression of the transgene in pre-osteoblasts and osteoblasts, with minimal to no expression in other cell types [30,31]. In contrast, Yadav *et al.*, (2009) used the 2.3 kb collagen type I promoter –cre to replace one copy of the endogenous murine *Lrp5* gene with one copy of *Lrp5* carrying the high bone mass G171V mutation. This generated mice with one WT and one G171V allele, rather than two WT and one G171V allele as used here. The 2.3 kb promoter driving *Cre* expression is activated later in the osteoblast differentiation pathway than the 3.6 kb promoter, and is thus active in more mature osteoblasts [30].

We have also found that the effect of *Lrp5* mutations on osteoblast proliferation was more pronounced in cells from female mice, such that *Lrp5* gain of function stimulated whilst *Lrp5* loss of function impaired proliferation. We have previously shown that ERα is required for β-catenin function in response to strain and it is now apparent that this is mediated, at least in part, by the non-genomic signalling effects of ER involved with IGFIR's action [32,33]. This suggests that there are gender differences in LRP5-β-catenin signalling in osteoblasts, with females being more affected by changes in its activity because of potential interactions with the E2/ERα IGF-I signalling pathways. Interestingly, it has been shown that bone marrow stromal cells isolated from young women express higher levels of the ER and the ERR target gene Wnt11. Conversely, male BMSCs express higher levels of Wnt 16, which has two isoforms associated with either senescence or proliferation [34,35].

LRP5 is involved in osteoblast apoptosis

Having demonstrated differences in proliferation of cells from different genotypes, we studied the effect of *LRP5* mutations on TUNEL staining which showed that loss of *LRP5* function increased apoptosis in primary osteoblast-like cells from *Lrp5*$^{-/-}$ mice. This result suggest that the low bone mass phenotype observed *in vivo* may reflect, at least in part, high levels of apoptosis in the bone cells of these mice. This finding is in agreement with a previous *in vitro* study in which apoptosis in calvarial-derived osteoblast-like cells from *Lrp5*$^{-/-}$ mice was shown to be higher compared to WT cells [9]. However, our data is not in agreement with a previous *in vivo* study by Kato *et al.*, (2002), in which no difference in osteoblast apoptosis rates were observed in calvarial sections from *Lrp5*$^{-/-}$ mice. The *LRP5* G171V mutation seems to provide some protection against apoptosis induced by serum depletion however, the effect of this mutation on osteoblast apoptosis does not appear to be as significant as the loss of *LRP5* function. Notwithstanding, our findings support the idea that *LRP5* is a critical component in the regulation of bone cell apoptosis [7–9,36,37].

LRP5 is not required for the proliferative response of osteoblasts to strain

One of the effects of mechanical strain is to stimulate proliferation of cells that are, or will become, osteoblasts [38–47]. In the studies reported here neither absence of *LRP5* function nor the presence of the *LRP5*^{G171V} mutation altered the proliferative response of cortical derived primary osteoblast-like cells to mechanical strain *in vitro*. These data are in agreement with two recent *in vitro* studies which suggested that the strain-induced activation of β-catenin does not require *LRP5* [33,48,49], although a previous *in vivo* study had shown that the loading response was abolished in mice lacking *LRP5* [15].

Neither did the *Lrp5*$^{-/-}$ or the *LRP5*^{G171V} mutation alter the 'minimum effective strain' at which strain engendered a proliferative response, thus our findings are not consistent with *in vivo* evidence that a lower strain threshold is sufficient to induce cortical bone formation in *LRP5*^{G171V} mice [50,51]. We have also recently demonstrated that the increased load-induced osteogenesis in the cortical and cancellous bone of mice with the *LRP5*^{G171V} mutation is more pronounced in females than males [16]. One possible explanation for the apparent differences between our *in vitro* data and *in vivo* findings is that *LRP5* mutations may alter the strain responsiveness in osteocytes rather than osteoblasts. For example, differences in responses to fluid flow shear stress have been reported in osteocytes versus osteoblasts [49,52,53]. Our *in vitro* model includes osteoblasts with little or no osteocytic component and so does not replicate the complex context of cortical bone.

In conclusion, we have provided data to demonstrate that in cortical bone-derived primary osteoblast-like cells from adult mice, *LRP5* is an integral component of the signalling pathways that regulate cell proliferation and apoptosis. However, it is not required for the proliferative response of these cells to mechanical strain. The intrinsically higher rate of proliferation and reduced apoptosis observed in the *LRP5*^{G171V} osteoblastic cells may result in an increased amount of new bone being formed which would partially explain the high bone mass seen in individuals with this mutation.

Acknowledgments

The authors are grateful to Dr. Mark Johnson (UMKC, Kansas City, USA) for his insightful comments.

Author Contributions

Conceived and designed the experiments: BJ AS GZ LKS LEL JSP. Performed the experiments: BJ RFLS. Analyzed the data: BJ AS GZ LEL JSP. Contributed reagents/materials/analysis tools: LEL JSP. Wrote the paper: BJ AS LEL JSP.

References

1. Ehrlich PJ, Lanyon LE (2002) Mechanical strain and bone cell function: a review. Osteoporos Int 13: 688–700.
2. Bennett CN, Longo KA, Wright WS, Suva LJ, Lane TF, et al. (2005) Regulation of osteoblastogenesis and bone mass by Wnt10b. Proc Natl Acad Sci U S A 102: 3324–3329.
3. Day TF, Guo X, Garrett-Beal L, Yang Y (2005) Wnt/beta-catenin signaling in mesenchymal progenitors controls osteoblast and chondrocyte differentiation during vertebrate skeletogenesis. Dev Cell 8: 739–750.
4. Kato M, Patel MS, Levasseur R, Lobov I, Chang BH, et al. (2002) Cbfa1-independent decrease in osteoblast proliferation, osteopenia, and persistent embryonic eye vascularization in mice deficient in Lrp5, a Wnt coreceptor. J Cell Biol 157: 303–314.
5. Krishnan V, Bryant HU, Macdougald OA (2006) Regulation of bone mass by Wnt signaling. J Clin Invest 116: 1202–1209.
6. Gong Y, Slee RB, Fukai N, Rawadi G, Roman-Roman S, et al. (2001) LDL receptor-related protein 5 (LRP5) affects bone accrual and eye development. Cell 107: 513–523.
7. Babij P, Zhao W, Small C, Kharode Y, Yaworsky PJ, et al. (2003) High bone mass in mice expressing a mutant LRP5 gene. J Bone Miner Res 18: 960–974.
8. Bodine PV, Zhao W, Kharode YP, Bex FJ, Lambert AJ, et al. (2004) The Wnt antagonist secreted frizzled-related protein-1 is a negative regulator of trabecular bone formation in adult mice. Mol Endocrinol 18: 1222–1237.
9. Clement-Lacroix P, Ai M, Morvan F, Roman-Roman S, Vayssiere B, et al. (2005) Lrp5-independent activation of Wnt signaling by lithium chloride increases bone formation and bone mass in mice. Proc Natl Acad Sci U S A 102: 17406–17411.
10. Frontali M, Stomeo C, Dallapiccola B (1985) Osteoporosis-pseudoglioma syndrome: report of three affected sibs and an overview. American Journal of Medical Genetics 22: 35–47.
11. Gong Y, Vikkula M, Boon L, Liu J, Beighton P, et al. (1996) Osteoporosis-pseudoglioma syndrome, a disorder affecting skeletal strength and vision, is assigned to chromosome region 11q12–13. Am J Hum Genet 59: 146–151.
12. Boyden LM, Mao J, Belsky J, Mitzner L, Farhi A, et al. (2002) High bone density due to a mutation in LDL-receptor-related protein 5. N Engl J Med 346: 1513–1521.
13. Little RD, Carulli JP, Del Mastro RG, Dupuis J, Osborne M, et al. (2002) A mutation in the LDL receptor-related protein 5 gene results in the autosomal dominant high-bone-mass trait. Am J Hum Genet 70: 11–19.
14. Johnson ML, Gong G, Kimberling W, Recker SM, Kimmel DB, et al. (1997) Linkage of a gene causing high bone mass to human chromosome 11 (11q12-13). Am J Hum Genet 60: 1326–1332.
15. Sawakami K, Robling AG, Ai M, Pitner ND, Liu D, et al. (2006) The Wnt co-receptor LRP5 is essential for skeletal mechanotransduction but not for the anabolic bone response to parathyroid hormone treatment. J Biol Chem 281: 23698–23711.
16. Saxon LK, Jackson BF, Sugiyama T, Lanyon LE, Price JS (2011) Analysis of multiple bone responses to graded strains above functional levels, and to disuse, in mice in vivo show that the human Lrp5 G171V High Bone Mass mutation increases the osteogenic response to loading but that lack of Lrp5 activity reduces it. Bone 49: 184–193.
17. Zaman G, Suswillo RF, Cheng MZ, Tavares IA, Lanyon LE (1997) Early responses to dynamic strain change and prostaglandins in bone-derived cells in culture. J Bone Miner Res 12: 769–777.
18. Yadav VK, Ryu JH, Suda N, Tanaka KF, Gingrich JA, et al. (2008) Lrp5 controls bone formation by inhibiting serotonin synthesis in the duodenum. Cell 135: 825–837.
19. Rawlinson SC, el Haj AJ, Minter SL, Tavares IA, Bennett A, et al. (1991) Loading-related increases in prostaglandin production in cores of adult canine cancellous bone in vitro: a role for prostacyclin in adaptive bone remodeling? J Bone Miner Res 6: 1345–1351.
20. Rawlinson SC, McKay IJ, Ghuman M, Wellmann C, Ryan P, et al. (2009) Adult rat bones maintain distinct regionalized expression of markers associated with their development. PLoS One 4: e8358.
21. Koshihara Y, Hirano M, Kawamura M, Oda H, Higaki S (1991) Mineralization ability of cultured human osteoblast-like periosteal cells does not decline with aging. J Gerontol 46: B201–206.
22. Fedarko NS, Vetter UK, Weinstein S, Robey PG (1992) Age-related changes in hyaluronan, proteoglycan, collagen, and osteonectin synthesis by human bone cells. J Cell Physiol 151: 215–227.
23. Fedarko NS, D'Avis P, Frazier CR, Burrill MJ, Fergusson V, et al. (1995) Cell proliferation of human fibroblasts and osteoblasts in osteogenesis imperfecta: influence of age. J Bone Miner Res 10: 1705–1712.
24. Battmann A, Jundt G, Schulz A (1997) Endosteal human bone cells (EBC) show age-related activity in vitro. Exp Clin Endocrinol Diabetes 105: 98–102.
25. Kassem M, Ankersen L, Eriksen EF, Clark BF, Rattan SI (1997) Demonstration of cellular aging and senescence in serially passaged long-term cultures of human trabecular osteoblasts. Osteoporos Int 7: 514–524.
26. Yudoh K, Matsuno H, Nakazawa F, Katayama R, Kimura T (2001) Reconstituting telomerase activity using the telomerase catalytic subunit prevents the telomere shorting and replicative senescence in human osteoblasts. J Bone Miner Res 16: 1453–1464.
27. Bergman RJ, Gazit D, Kahn AJ, Gruber H, McDougall S, et al. (1996) Age-related changes in osteogenic stem cells in mice. J Bone Miner Res 11: 568–577.
28. Stenderup K, Justesen J, Clausen C, Kassem M (2003) Aging is associated with decreased maximal life span and accelerated senescence of bone marrow stromal cells. Bone 33: 919–926.
29. Jiang D, Fei RG, Pendergrass WR, Wolf NS (1992) An age-related reduction in the replicative capacity of two murine hematopoietic stroma cell types. Exp Hematol 20: 1216–1222.
30. Zha L, Hou N, Wang J, Yang G, Gao Y, et al. (2008) Collagen1[alpha]1 promoter drives the expression of Cre recombinase in osteoblasts of transgenic mice. Journal of Genetics and Genomics 35: 525–530.
31. Kalajzic I, Kalajzic Z, Kaliterna M, Gronowicz G, Clark SH, et al. (2002) Use of type I collagen green fluorescent protein transgenes to identify subpopulations of cells at different stages of the osteoblast lineage. J Bone Miner Res 17: 15–25.
32. Armstrong VJ, Muzylak M, Sunters A, Zaman G, Saxon LK, et al. (2007) Wnt/beta-catenin signaling is a component of osteoblastic bone cell early responses to load-bearing and requires estrogen receptor alpha. J Biol Chem 282: 20715–20727.
33. Sunters A, Armstrong VJ, Zaman G, Kypta RM, Kawano Y, et al. (2010) Mechano-transduction in osteoblastic cells involves strain-regulated estrogen receptor alpha-mediated control of insulin-like growth factor (IGF) I receptor sensitivity to Ambient IGF, leading to phosphatidylinositol 3-kinase/AKT-dependent Wnt/LRP5 receptor-independent activation of beta-catenin signaling. J Biol Chem 285: 8743–8758.
34. Shen L, Zhou S, Glowacki J (2009) Effects of age and gender on WNT gene expression in human bone marrow stromal cells. J Cell Biochem 106: 337–343.
35. Dwyer MA, Joseph JD, Wade HE, Eaton ML, Kunder RS, et al. (2010) WNT11 expression is induced by estrogen-related receptor alpha and beta-catenin and acts in an autocrine manner to increase cancer cell migration. Cancer Res 70: 9298–9308.
36. Almeida M, Han L, Bellido T, Manolagas SC, Kousteni S (2005) Wnt proteins prevent apoptosis of both uncommitted osteoblast progenitors and differentiated osteoblasts by beta-catenin-dependent and -independent signaling cascades involving Src/ERK and phosphatidylinositol 3-kinase/AKT. J Biol Chem 280: 41342–41351.
37. Tobimatsu T, Kaji H, Sowa H, Naito J, Canaff L, et al. (2006) Parathyroid hormone increases beta-catenin levels through Smad3 in mouse osteoblastic cells. Endocrinology 147: 2583–2590.
38. Boutahar N, Guignandon A, Vico L, Lafage-Proust MH (2004) Mechanical strain on osteoblasts activates autophosphorylation of focal adhesion kinase and proline-rich tyrosine kinase 2 tyrosine sites involved in ERK activation. J Biol Chem 279: 30588–30599.
39. Cheng M, Zaman G, Rawlinson SC, Mohan S, Baylink DJ, et al. (1999) Mechanical strain stimulates ROS cell proliferation through IGF-II and estrogen through IGF-I. J Bone Miner Res 14: 1742–1750.
40. Damien E, Price JS, Lanyon LE (2000) Mechanical strain stimulates osteoblast proliferation through the estrogen receptor in males as well as females. J Bone Miner Res 15: 2169–2177.
41. Fermor B, Gundle R, Evans M, Emerton M, Pocock A, et al. (1998) Primary human osteoblast proliferation and prostaglandin E2 release in response to mechanical strain in vitro. Bone 22: 637–643.
42. Kaspar D, Seidl W, Neidlinger-Wilke C, Ignatius A, Claes L (2000) Dynamic cell stretching increases human osteoblast proliferation and CICP synthesis but decreases osteocalcin synthesis and alkaline phosphatase activity. J Biomech 33: 45–51.
43. Neidlinger-Wilke C, Wilke HJ, Claes L (1994) Cyclic stretching of human osteoblasts affects proliferation and metabolism: a new experimental method and its application. J Orthop Res 12: 70–78.
44. Weyts FA, Bosmans B, Niesing R, van Leeuwen JP, Weinans H (2003) Mechanical control of human osteoblast apoptosis and proliferation in relation to differentiation. Calcif Tissue Int 72: 505–512.
45. Zhuang H, Wang W, Tahernia AD, Levitz CL, Luchetti WT, et al. (1996) Mechanical strain-induced proliferation of osteoblastic cells parallels increased TGF-beta 1 mRNA. Biochem Biophys Res Commun 229: 449–453.
46. Brighton CT, Fisher JR Jr., Levine SE, Corsetti JR, Reilly T, et al. (1996) The biochemical pathway mediating the proliferative response of bone cells to a mechanical stimulus. J Bone Joint Surg Am 78: 1337–1347.

47. Lee KC, Jessop H, Suswillo R, Zaman G, Lanyon LE (2004) The adaptive response of bone to mechanical loading in female transgenic mice is deficient in the absence of oestrogen receptor-alpha and -beta. J Endocrinol 182: 193–201.
48. Case N, Ma M, Sen B, Xie Z, Gross TS, et al. (2008) Beta-catenin levels influence rapid mechanical responses in osteoblasts. J Biol Chem 283: 29196–29205.
49. Kamel MA, Picconi JL, Lara-Castillo N, Johnson ML (2010) Activation of beta-catenin signaling in MLO-Y4 osteocytic cells versus 2T3 osteoblastic cells by fluid flow shear stress and PGE2: Implications for the study of mechanosensation in bone. Bone 47: 872–881.
50. Cullen D, Akhter M, Johnson M, Morgan S, Recker R (2004) Ulna loading response altered by the HBM mutation. J Bone Miner Res 19;Suppl.1): S396 p.
51. Akhter MP, Wells DJ, Short SJ, Cullen DM, Johnson ML, et al. (2004) Bone biomechanical properties in LRP5 mutant mice. Bone 35: 162–169.
52. Giladi M, Milgrom C, Simkin A, Danon Y (1991) Stress fractures. Identifiable risk factors. Am J Sports Med 19: 647–652.
53. Klein-Nulend J, van der Plas A, Semeins CM, Ajubi NE, Frangos JA, et al. (1995) Sensitivity of osteocytes to biomechanical stress in vitro. FASEB J 9: 441–445.

Cortical Bone Mechanical Properties Are Altered in an Animal Model of Progressive Chronic Kidney Disease

Christopher L. Newman[1], Sharon M. Moe[2,3], Neal X. Chen[2], Max A. Hammond[4], Joseph M. Wallace[4,5], Jeffry S. Nyman[6,7], Matthew R. Allen[1]*

1 Department of Anatomy and Cell Biology, Indiana University School of Medicine, Indianapolis, Indiana, United States of America, **2** Division of Nephrology, Department of Medicine, Indiana University School of Medicine, Indianapolis, Indiana, United States of America, **3** Roudebush VA Medical Center, Indianapolis, Indiana, United States of America, **4** Weldon School of Biomedical Engineering, Purdue University, West Lafayette, Indiana, United States of America, **5** Department of Biomedical Engineering, Indiana University—Purdue University, Indianapolis, Indiana, United States of America, **6** Department of Orthopaedic Surgery and Rehabilitation and Vanderbilt Center for Bone Biology, Vanderbilt University Medical Center, Nashville, Tennessee, United States of America, **7** Department of Veterans Affairs, Tennessee Valley Healthcare System, Nashville, Tennessee, United States of America

Abstract

Chronic kidney disease (CKD), which leads tocortical bone loss and increasedporosity,increases therisk of fracture. Animal models have confirmed that these changes compromise whole bone mechanical properties. Estimates from whole bone testing suggest that material properties are negatively affected, though tissue-level assessmentshavenot been conducted. Therefore, the goal of the present study was to examine changes in cortical bone at different length scales using a rat model with theprogressive development of CKD. At 30 weeks of age (~75% reduction in kidney function), skeletally mature male Cy/+ rats were compared to their normal littermates. Cortical bone material propertieswere assessed with reference point indentation (RPI), atomic force microscopy (AFM), Raman spectroscopy,and high performance liquid chromatography (HPLC). Bones from animals with CKD had higher (+18%) indentation distance increase and first cycle energy dissipation (+ 8%) as measured by RPI.AFM indentation revealed a broader distribution of elastic modulus values in CKD animals witha greater proportion of both higher and lower modulus values compared to normal controls. Yet, tissue composition, collagen morphology, and collagen cross-linking fail to account for these differences. Though the specific skeletal tissue alterations responsible for these mechanical differences remain unclear, these results indicate that cortical bone material properties are altered in these animals and may contribute to the increased fracture risk associated with CKD.

Editor: Damian Christopher Genetos, University of California Davis, United States of America

Funding: National Institutes of Health grants AR58005 (SM) and DL100093 (CN); Indiana Clinical Translational Science Institute grant TR000162 (CN). The funders had no role in study design, data collection and analysis, decision to publish, or preparation of the manuscript.

Competing Interests: The authors have declared that no competing interests exist.

* E-mail: matallen@iupui.edu

Introduction

Chronic kidney disease—mineral and bone disorder (CKD-MBD) is characterized by hyperphosphatemia, secondary hyperparathyroidism, and an increased risk offractures[1–3].Unlike osteoporosis, CKD-MBD appears to have a preferential impact on cortical bone, leading to reduced bone mass and increased porosity [4–6].These effects likely underlie the increased fracture risk observed in patients with CKD[7–9].

Whole bone (structural)mechanical properties are dependent upon a number of variables [10–11]. While bone mass is a major determinant, both the distribution of bone and its material properties (inherent physical and chemical properties) also play crucial roles. Most biomechanical studies in rodent models of CKD have focused on structural mechanical properties, employing three-point bending or dynamic mechanical analysis (DMA) [12–18]. These studies indicate that the bending and viscoelastic properties of bone are compromised in animals with CKD. Specifically, DMA indicates that diseased animals have lower storage modulus (a measure of stiffness) and tan delta (a measure of energy dissipation) [14–15], while three point bending studies indicate that ultimate load, stiffness, and energy to failure are lower in CKD animals [12].

While there is an increasing awareness of the importance of bone quality in CKD [19], few studies have explicitly examined material properties in animal models[14–15,20]. Material properties can be estimated from whole bone mechanical tests using standardengineering equations that account for whole bone structure and geometry.Because these estimates assume that skeletal tissue is homogeneous, isotropic, and linearly elastic, direct measures ofmaterial properties in bone would provide additionalinsight into how the disease is affecting fracture resistance. Therefore, the goal of the present study was to examine material-level changes in cortical bone at several length scales using a rat model with the progressive development of CKD. Specifically, we hypothesized that CKD adversely impacts cortical bone material properties as determined by material-level mechanical testing and assessments of bone composition and collagen morphology.

Materials And Methods

Animal Model

The current study utilized a slowly progressive animal model of CKD, the Cy/+ rat. Cy/+ ratsare characterized by autosomal dominant polycystic kidney disease [21]. These animals have a mutation (R823W) in *Anks6*, a gene that codes for the protein SamCystin. Currently, the function of this protein is unknown, and the specific role of this mutation in the development of polycystic kidney disease is unclear. Aside from its expression in the kidney, however, little is known about its role in the cell [22].Unlike most other PKD-related proteins, though, SamCystin does not localize to the primary cilia of kidney cells [23]. While there is no known human disease associated with this gene, thespontaneous onset of disease provides a helpful phenotypic model of human CKD [21].Unlike the more common surgical models[24], Cy/+ rats display a gradual onset of disease.And unlike most genetic models[25-26], they exhibit a slow enough progression that bone disease does not begin to occur until after skeletal maturity.

Skeletal tissuefrom animals in a previous study wasutilized [12]. All animals were fed a casein diet (Purina AIN-76A; 0.7% Pi) to increase phosphorus availability in order to produce a more consistent kidney disease phenotype.Fresh frozen tibiaefrom 30-week-old male Cy/+ ratsand their age-matched non-affected littermates were assessed mechanically, compositionally, and morphologically at several length scales.Fresh frozen femora were used for collagen cross-linking analyses. Blood was collected at the end of the experiment for biochemical analyses (previously reported in [12]).All procedures were conducted under the approval of Indiana University School of Medicine Institutional Animal Care and Use Committeeprotocol # 10479.

Reference Point Indentation

Tibiae were thawed to room temperature and soaked overnight in phosphate-buffered saline. The anteromedial surface of the proximal diaphysis of the tibia was assessed using reference point indentation (RPI) (Biodent Hfc, Active Life Scientific, Santa Barbara, CA). The reference probe, which housed a BP2 test probe, waslowered vertically, normal to the surface, until itrested on the surface of the bone.In order to stabilize the unit, a reference force of ~13 N was applied before each measurement was initiated.Each test included a series of 10 cycles at 2 Hz to a force of 10 N. Bones were maintained in a hydrated state throughout the test. Five locations per sample, each ~2 mm apart, were indented. Raw data from the RPI analysis software (version 2.0) were imported into a customized MATLAB code (Mathworks) designed to provide cycle-by-cycle data for each test [27], from which first cycle unloading slope, indentation distance increase, first cycle energy dissipation, creep indentation distance, first cycle indentation distance, total indentation distance, and total energy dissipation were calculated for each test. All five tests from each animal were averaged to produce a single value for each variable.

Tissue Composition

Raman spectroscopy was performed using a LabRAM HR 800 Raman Spectrometer (HORIBA JobinYvon, Edison, NJ) connected to a BX41 microscope (Olympus, Tokyo, Japan). A 660 nm laser was focused on the bone surface using a 50X objective to a spot size of ~10 μm. Five locations were imaged ~1 mm apart on the anteromedialmid-diaphysiswith five 20 second acquisitions at each location as previously published [28]. A five point linear baseline correction was applied in LabSpec 5 (HORIBA JobinYvon). Using OriginPro 8.6 (OriginLab, Northampton, MA), a single Gaussian peak was fit to the $PO_4^{3-}\nu1$ peak, and the areas under the $PO_4^{3-}\nu1$, $CO_3^{2-}\nu1$, and Amide I peaks were calculated at each location. Type B carbonate substitution was found by the band area ratio of $CO_3^{2-}\nu1/PO_4^{3-}\nu1$. The degree of matrix mineralization was determined by the band area ratios of $PO_4^{3-}\nu1$/Amide I. Mineral maturity (crystallinity) was determined by the inverse of the full width at half maximum (FWHM) of the $PO_4^{3-}\nu1$ peak.

AFM Indentation

The anteromedial portion of the mid-diaphysis used above was polished with a 3 μm polycrystalline water-based diamond suspension in order to create a flat region for testing. Nanoindentation was performed using a BioScope Catalyst atomic force microscope (Bruker, Santa Barbara, CA), operating in peak force tapping mode using previously published methods [29]. Indentations were performed using a polycrystalline diamond probe (NaDia ND-DYC series; Advanced Diamond Technologies, Inc.) with a measured spring constant of 29.25 N/m. Four locations per sample were indented and, at each location (20 μm×20 μm grid), 49 indentationswere performed. Samples were loaded to 200 nN with force-separation curves acquired from each indentation. Within each location, indentations were spaced about 2 μm apart in order to avoid interactions from neighboring indentations. In total, 196 indentations were performed for each sample. The indentation elastic modulus was calculated from 5% to 95% of the withdrawal curve using the classic Hertz model of contact between a rigid sphere and an elastic half space because the indentation depth is much smaller than the radius of curvature of the probe [29]. The indentation elastic modulus was determined from the following equation: E = 3F(1-v^2)/(4r^(1/2) δ^(3/2)) where E is the indentation elastic modulus, F is the indentation force, v is the Poisson's ratio of the sample (assumed to be 0.35), r is the tip radius (nominal radius of 50 nm, with the same probe used for all samples), and δ is the indentation depth. All of the individual indentations were averaged to produce a single value for each animal, though individual tests were used for distribution comparisons among the groups.

Collagen Morphology

Following AFMindentation, the polished surface was partially decalcified by soaking the bones in 0.5 M EDTA for 25 minutes followed by five minutes of sonication in a water bath. This process was repeated five times for each sample. For imaging, RTESPA probes were used (Bruker; radius nominally 8 nm, spring constant = 40 N/m). The scan size was set at 3.5 μm with 512×512 pixels and a scan rate of 0.5 lines/s. For measurements of collagen morphology, four locations were imaged per sample, and 10 to 15 fibrils were measured at each location. 40 to 50 fibrils per sample were averaged to produce a single value for each animal, though the individual tests were used for distribution comparisons. Using SPIP 5.1.10 (Image Metrology, Hrsholm, Denmark),D-periodic spacing was calculated using2D Fast Fourier Transformations (2D FFTs) as previously described [28].

Collagen Cross-Linking

Segments of bone (~3 mm in length) from the proximal femoral diaphysis were fully demineralized in 20% EDTA (0.68 M, pH 7.4). Approximately 10 mg of demineralized bonewerehydrolyzedin6 N HCl (~10 μL per 1 mg) at 110°C for 20 to 24 hours. After evaporating the acidusing a SpeedVAC centrifuge with coldtrap, each hydrolysate was resuspended in ultrapure water, split into two equal portions, and dried. Half the residue was resuspended in ultrapure water with an internal standard

(5×10^{-6} g/L pyridoxine). The solution was filtered and diluted with 0.05% heptafluorobutyric acid in 10% acetonitrile, and 50 μL of each hydrolysate were assayed by a high performance liquid chromatography (HPLC) system (Beckman-Coulter System Gold 168) with a silica-based column (Waters Spherisorb). Standards with varying concentrations of pyridinoline (Pyd) (Quidel),deoxypyridinoline (Dpd) (Quidel),pentosidine(PE) (International Maillard Reaction Society), and a constant amount of pyridoxinewere also assayed. Using a Waters 2475 fluorescence detector (excitation/emission of295/400 nm for Pyd and Dpd and 328/378 nm for PE), chromatograms were recorded to determine the amount of each crosslink. These amounts were then normalized by collagen content, which was determined from the other half of each hydrolysate by another HPLC assay [30]. Briefly, withα-amino-butyric acid (α-ABA) included as an internal standard, the amino acids were subjected to derivatization withphenyl isothiocyanate (PITC). Along with standards of varying concentrations of hydroxyproline (Sigma) and proline (Sigma)and a constant amount of α-ABA, the derivatized samples were resuspendedin a buffer solution of 5% acetonitrile in 5 mM disodium phosphate. Upon injecting 50 μLof this sample, chromatograms were generated with a UV detector (Beckman-Coulter System Gold 168). The calculated mass of hydroxyproline was then multiplied by 7.5 (assuming 13–14% of type I collagen by mass) and divided by the molecular weight of collagen (30,000 Da) [31], thereby giving crosslink concentration as mol/mol of collagen.

Statistical Analysis

All analyses were performed using SPSS software. Comparisons between groups were made with Student's t-tests (assumptions validated by Shapiro-Wilk and Levene tests). When non-normal distributions or unequal variances were present, comparisons were made using Wilcoxon ranked-sum tests and unequal variance t-tests, respectively. Distributions included all measures from each individual, and comparisons were made using Kolmogorov-Smirnov tests. *A priori* α-levels were set at 0.05 to determine significance.

Results

Animal Model

Details about the phenotype of these animals have been previous published [12]. Briefly, measures of kidney function, including BUN (+116%) and the albumin-to-creatinine ratio (+ 301%), weresignificantly higher in Cy/+ animals compared to the normal controls. Similar to what is observed in humans with CKD, there were no differences between groups for phosphorus or calcium levels, but both serum PTH (+240%) and FGF23 (+195%) weredrastically higher(**FIGURE 1**).Cy/+ animals had higher numbers of osteoclasts and higher levels of bone remodeling. Using three-point bending, they exhibited lower ultimate load (−28%), stiffness(−17%), and energy to fracture (−46%). Estimates of material properties indicate that they had lower ultimate stress (−20%) and toughness (−47%) (**FIGURE 2**)[12].

Reference Point Indentation

Indentation distance increase (IDI)provides an assessment of the change in depth between the first cycle and the final cycle. Cy/+ animals had significantly higher IDI (+18%), indicating that the tissue ismore prone to damage under the same applied load (**FIGURE 3**). The amount of energy dissipated during the first cycle was also significantlyhigher in animals with CKD (+8%). While the first cycle creep indentation distance (+18%) was higher in Cy/+ animals, there was no difference in microstructural stiffness (first cycle unloading slope)between the two groups.No differences were noted in first cycle indentation distance, total indentation distance, or total energy dissipation (**Table 1**).

AFM-based indentation

There was no difference in the indentation elastic modulus between the groups (**FIGURE 4a**). However, when all indentations within each groupwere considered as a population, the distribution of elastic modulus values did differ between the two groups. Animals with CKD had a greater proportion of both high and low values of elastic modulus than their normal counterparts (**FIGURE 4b**).

Tissue Composition

Raman spectroscopy revealed no differences between animals with CKD and their normal counterparts with regard to overall compositionof the mineral and organic matrices (**Table 2**). Specifically, there were no differences between the groups in the phosphate-to-amide I ratio (the mineral-to-matrix ratio), mineral crystallinity, or the carbonate-to-phosphate ratio (a reflection of type B carbonate substitution).

Collagen Morphology and Cross-Linking

There were no mean differences in D-periodicity between the two groups (**Table 2**). There were also no differences in the distribution of D-periodicity when all fibrils were considered. In addition, both enzymatic and non-enzymatic cross-linksas assessed by HPLC were similar between groups (**Table 2**).

Discussion

The mechanical integrity of skeletal tissue is determined by the amount of tissue present, its distribution, and its quality. Compromises in any of these factors can lead to an increased fracture risk. The notable loss of cortical bone mass associated with CKD is assumed to be primarily responsible for the increased fracture risk seen in patients [5]. The current study advances our understanding of bone fragility in CKD by showing that microscale and nanoscale mechanical properties are alteredindependently of changes in bone mass and porosity.

Our lab has previously documented reductions in both structural and estimated materialproperties in Cy/+ rats, animals with progressive CKD [12,32]. But, whole bone testing only provides indirect estimates of material properties, which is why wedirectly assessedmicroscale mechanical propertiesusing reference point indentation (RPI).RPI data from the present study indicate that animals with CKD had higher IDI, higher first cycle creep indentation distance, and first cycle energy dissipation. Taken together, these results indicatethat the tissue in animals with CKD is less resistant to indentation and more prone to damage. Indentation distance increase was nearly 20% higher in CKD animals compared to their normal counterparts. Similar differences in IDI have been previously reported in diabetic rats[33]. These data have two important implications. First, they show that CKD negatively affects skeletal tissue independently of bone mass, which means that estimates of bone massalone likely underestimate the overall mechanical effects of CKD.These differences in bone quality may explain the conflicting data available on BMD and fracture risk in CKD patients[6,34–40]. Second, our data provide a basis for considering *in vivo* applications of RPI in the clinical setting of CKD. RPI has been used to successfully differentiate patients with and without hip fractures[41] as well as those with and without atypical femoral fractures [42]. A related

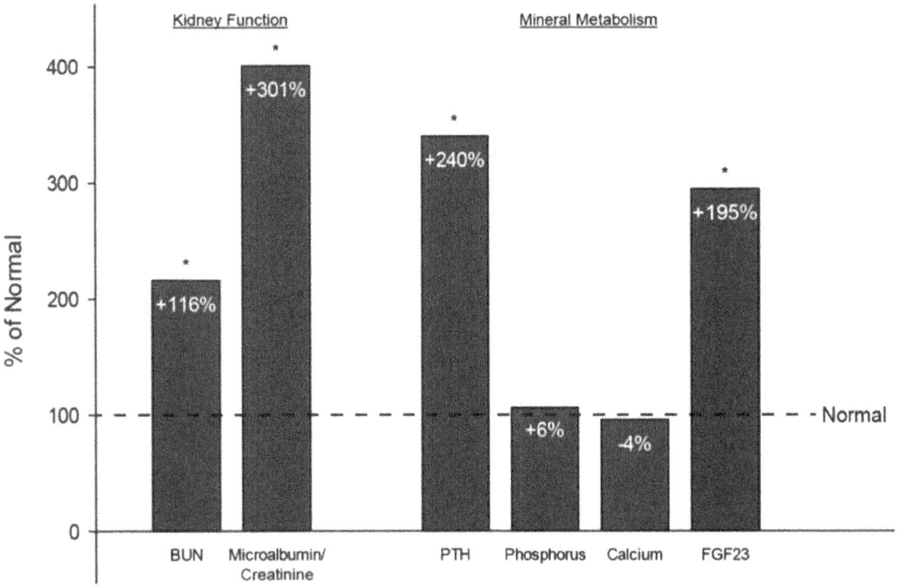

Figure 1. Biochemical assessment of kidney function and mineral metabolism. These previously published data (Allen *et al.*, 2013) show abnormalities in kidney function and mineral metabolism resulting from hyperparathyroidism in the animals utilized in the current work. Data are presented as a percentage of non-affected normal animals with (*) representing statistical significance.

indentation device has also been shown to discriminate patients with diabetes from their normal counterparts[43]. Assessment of tissue-level mechanical properties, combined with standard imaging modalities to measure bone mass, cortical geometry (especially porosity), and trabecular architecture, may prove to be an ideal combination by which to assess the overall mechanical integrity of bones in patients with CKD.

The current study also employed a hierarchical approach by examining nanoscale mechanical properties with atomic force microscopy. AFM indentation provides a direct assessment of the nanoscale stiffness produced by the collagen and mineral composite. Consistent with measurements of microscale stiffness (first cycle unloading slope), these results show that the average indentation elastic modulus was not significantly different between the two groups.Yet, the distribution of elastic modulus values was different. Animals with CKD displayed a greater degree of heterogeneity in nanoscale elasticity. Because increased material heterogeneity is often considered advantageous [44], these results may reflect an adaptive response to declining integrity at larger length scales. Alternatively, extreme variations in nanoscale properties maylead to localized stress concentrations that result in damage accumulation from lower forces[45]. Although heterogeneity is likely necessary for normal mechanical integrity, extreme heterogeneity may be problematic from a mechanical

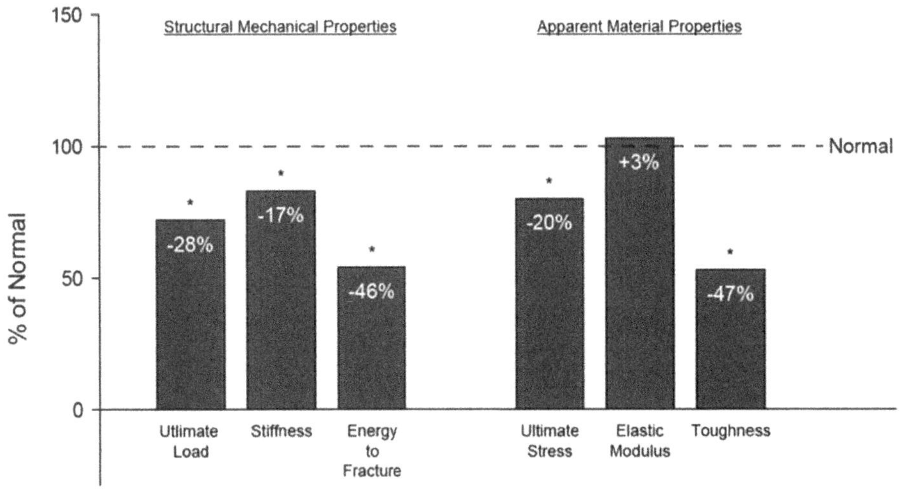

Figure 2. Structural mechanical properties and estimated material properties. These previously published data (Allen *et al.*, 2013) show compromised whole bone mechanical properties from femoral 3-point bending and apparent material-level mechanical properties derived from standard beam bending equations in the animals utilized in the current work. Data are presented as a percentage of non-affected normal animals with (*) representing statistical significance.

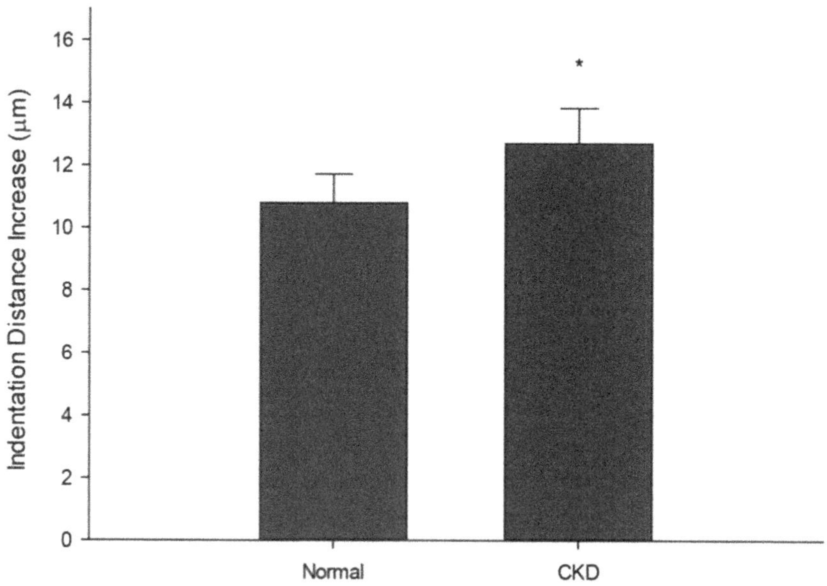

Figure 3. Microindentation reveals that CKD skeletal tissue is less able to resist damage. Using reference point indentation (RPI), the indentation distance increase (IDI) was found to be significantly higher in CKD animals compared to normal. These data indicate that the mechanical integrity of the bone is less able to resist microscale damage formation and propagation. Data are presented as mean and standard deviation. *p< 0.05 versus normal controls.

standpoint [46]. Future studies should attempt to better understand the role of material heterogeneity in CKD in order to specifythe contributionofmicroscale and nanoscalepropertiesto whole bone mechanical properties.

While whole bone, microscale, and nanoscale mechanical differences are present in animals with CKD, tissue composition, collagen morphology, and collagen cross-linking fail to account for the differences. These data conflict with studiesshowing higher mineral-to-matrix ratios, lower mineral crystallinity, increased advanced glycationendproducts (AGEs), and decreased gene expression of lysyl oxidase in alternative models of CKD [14–15,47]. One potential explanation for these disparate results is that these previous studies utilized younger animals that developed advanced CKD during skeletal growth. Teasing apart the interaction between growth and disease is difficult, which is why the present study employed the use of a model in which kidney disease occurs after skeletal maturity.

Previous studies have demonstrated that non-enzymatic cross-links (pentosidine, specifically) are increased in the circulation of patients with CKD[48–51]. These findings coincide with the accumulation of AGEs in soft tissues detected by fluorescence methods[52]. Because high levels in the circulation are associated with the deposition of AGEs in other tissues, this may be true of skeletal tissue as well. To date, this has only been confirmed in one small clinical study in patients on dialysis [53]. Currently, there are few data in animal models, and clinical trials examining predialysis patients are lacking. Using a low turnover 5/6 nephrectomy model, two studies have reported increased pentosidineusing

Table 1. Mechanical properties from microindentation and nanoindentation.

RPI	**Normal (n = 6)**	**Cy/+ (n = 6)**	**p-values**
First Cycle Indentation Distance (µm)	83.38±3.15	88.24±5.45	*0.088
First cycle Energy Dissipation (µJ)	275.53±14.00	297.94±19.35	***0.044**
First Cycle Unloading Slope (N/µm)	0.47±0.02	0.45±0.03	*0.113
First Cycle Creep Indentation Distance (µm)	6.08±0.43	7.17±0.95	***0.028**
Indentation Distance Increase (µm)	10.81±0.92	12.71±1.13	***0.009**
Total Indentation Distance (µm)	89.39±2.73	95.21±5.13	#0.080
Total Energy Dissipation (µJ)	663.06±43.53	712.30±89.19	*0.252
AFM	**Normal (n = 5)**	**Cy/+ (n = 4)**	**p-values**
Indentation Elastic Modulus (MPa)	962.99 345.98	996.73 588.99	0.920

Values are presented as mean ± standard deviation.
*equal variance t-test.
#Wilcoxon ranked-sum test.
p-values less than 0.05 are in bold.

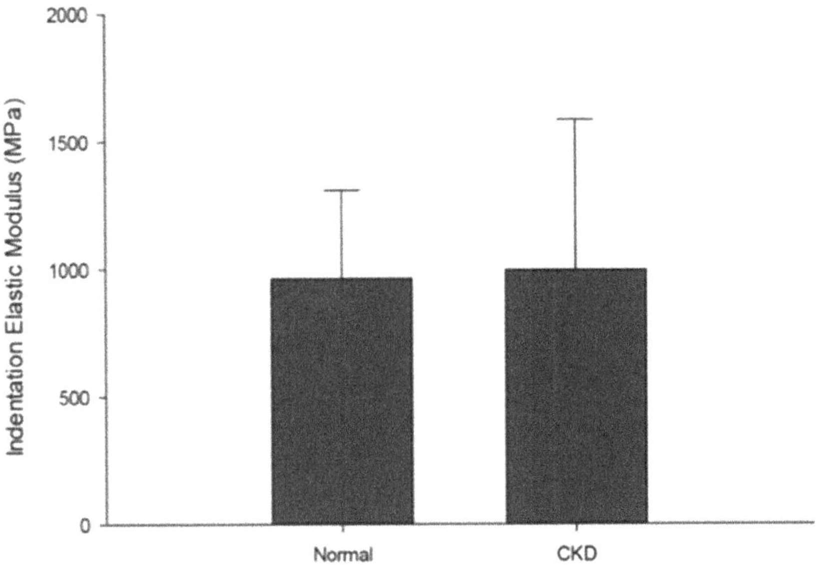

Figure 4b

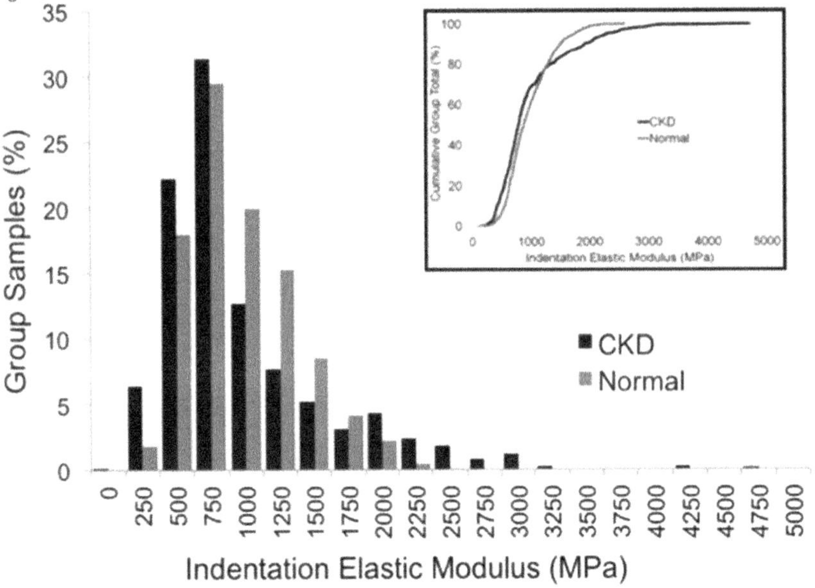

Figure 4. Nanoindenation reveals that CKD skeletal tissue has increased heterogeneity in the elastic modulus compared to normal bone. There was no significant difference in the average elastic modulus (A), but the distribution of elastic modulus values was significantly broader (B), with a greater proportion of both high and low values in CKD relative to normal ($p<0.0001$).

Raman spectroscopy[14–15]. While Raman spectroscopy has been utilized to detect AGEs in ocular tissue[54], its ability to detect changes in bone is unknown as HPLC is the standard method used to measure AGEs in skeletal tissue[53,55–58]. Here, having employed HPLC, thehypothesized increases in AGE content were not observed. While increases may occur with more advanced disease in theseanimals, the relationship between circulating pentosidineand its accumulation in bone collagen in CKDremains unresolved.

At present, clinical data on bone quality in CKD are minimal. Aside from the aforementioned dialysis study [53], CKD patients with high bone turnover had reduced stiffness and a decreased mineral-to-matrix ratio as assessed on iliac crest biopsies [59]. As these data are from cancellous bone, though, direct comparison with the current work on cortical bone is difficult. Connecting these dots by examining cortical bone properties in patients (which is possible with iliac crest biopsies) and cancellous properties in rats will be an essential step in moving forward.

Limitations to the current study should also be recognized. First, because tissue from a previous study was used, the sample sizes used here were small. Hence, any applications to other animal models or patients should occur with a measure of caution. Second, the mechanical assessments were localized to the periosteal surface, which may not be fully representative of the entire cortex. As such, the assessed parameters may differ at other cortical sites. Finally, this study assessed material properties in 30-week-old animals. As the disease progresses, differences in composition and morphologymay arise.Nevertheless, the advan-

Table 2. Tissue composition and collagen morphology.

Raman	Normal (n = 6)	Cy/+ (n = 6)	p-values
Crystallinity (1/FWHM PO_4^{3-}v1)	0.054±0.001	0.055±0.001	*0.4421
Carbonate Substitution (CO_3^{2-}v1/PO_4^{3-}v1)	0.618±0.037	0.608±0.019	#0.5375
Relative Mineralization (PO_4^{3-}v1/Amide I)	2.539±0.253	2.699±0.317	*0.9372
AFM	**Normal (n = 6)**	**Cy/+ (n = 5)**	**p-values**
D-Periodicity (nm)	65.641±0.646	65.864±0.838	*0.631
HPLC	**Normal (n = 8)**	**Cy/+ (n = 6)**	**p-values**
Pyridinoline per Collagen (mol/mol)	0.60±0.17	0.54±0.10	**0.252
Deoxypyridinoline per Collagen (mol/mol)	0.37±0.07	0.37±0.04	**0.974
Pentosidine per Collagen (mol/mol)	878± 153	921±148	*0.523

Values are presented as mean ± standard deviation.
*equal variances t-test.
**unequal variances t-test.
#Wilcoxon ranked-sum test.

tage of using 30-week-old animals is that these animals are skeletally mature but do not yet exhibit the rampant increase in cortical porosity present at 35 weeks [32].

In conclusion, these data show that both microscale and nanoscale cortical bone material properties are altered in an animal model of CKD. The specific skeletal tissue alterations responsible for these mechanical differences remain unclear. Nevertheless, in addition to bone loss and cortical porosity, defects in material-level mechanical properties may also contribute to the increased fracture risk associated with CKD.

Acknowledgments

We would like to thank Mr. Drew Brown for his assistance with analysis and tissue harvesting. We would also like to acknowledge the late Dr. Vincent H. Gattone II, who was instrumental in developing this animal model.

Author Contributions

Conceived and designed the experiments: CLN SMM JMW MRA. Performed the experiments: CLN NXC MAH JMW JSN. Analyzed the data: CLN MAH JMW JSN. Contributed to the writing of the manuscript: CLN SMM JMW JSN MRA.

References

1. Levey AS, Eckardt KU, Tsukamoto Y, Levin A, Coresh J, et al. (2005). Definition and classification of chronic kidney disease: a position statement from Kidney Disease Improving Global Outcomes (KDIGO). Kidney Int 67:2089–2100.
2. Levin A, Bakris GL, Molitch M, Smulders M, Tian J, et al. (2007) Prevalence of abnormal serum vitamin D, PTH, calcium, and phosphorus in patients with chronic kidney disease: results of the study to evaluate early kidney disease. Kidney Int 71:31–38.
3. KDIGO Working Group (2009) KDIGO clinical practice guideline for the diagnosis, evaluation, prevention, and treatment of Chronic Kidney Disease-Mineral and Bone Disorder (CKD-MBD). Kidney Int 76: S1–S130.
4. Cejka D, Patsch JM, Weber M, Diarra D, Riegersperger M, et al. (2011) Bone microarchitecture in hemodialysis patients assessed by HR-pQCT. Clin J Am Soc Nephrol 6:2264–71.
5. Nickolas TL, Stein E, Cohen A, Thomas V, Staron RB, et al. (2010) Bone mass and microarchitecture in CKD patients with fracture. J Am Soc Nephrol 21:1371–1380.
6. Nickolas TL, Cremers S, Zhang A, Thomas V, Stein E, et al. (2011) Discriminants of prevalent fractures in chronic kidney disease. J Am Soc Nephrol 22:1560–1572.
7. Fried LF, Biggs ML, Shlipak MG, Seliger S, Kestenbaum B, et al. (2007) Association of kidney function with incident hip fracture in older adults. J Am Soc Nephrol 18:282–286.
8. Nickolas TL, McMahon DJ, Shane E (2006) Relationship between moderate to severe kidney disease and hip fracture in the United States. J Am Soc Nephrol 17:3223–3232.
9. Nitsch D, Mylne A, Roderick PJ, Smeeth, Hubbard R, et al. (2009) Chronic kidney disease and hip-fracture-related mortality in older people in the UK. Nephrol Dial Transplant 24:1539–1544.
10. Cole JH, van der Muelen MCH (2011) Whole bone mechanics and bone quality. ClinOrthopRelat Res 469:2139–2149.
11. Seeman E, Delmas PD (2006) Bone quality: the material and structural basis of bone strength and fragility. N Engl J Med 354:2250–2261.
12. Allen MR, Chen NX, Gattone II VH, Chen X, Carr AJ, et al. (2013) Skeletal effects of zoledronic acid in an animal model of chronic kidney disease. OsteoporosInt 24:1471–1481.
13. Iwamoto J, Seki A, Sato Y, Matsumoto H (2012) Vitamin K2 improves renal function and increases femoral bone strength in rats with renal insufficiency. Calcif Tissue Int 90:50–59.
14. Iwasaki Y, Kazama JJ, Yamato H, Fukagawa M (2011) Changes in chemical composition of cortical bone associated with bone fragility in rat model with chronic kidney disease. Bone 48:1260–1267.
15. Iwasaki Y, Kazama JJ, Yamato H, Shimoda H, Fukagawa M (2013) Accumulated uremic toxins attenuate bone mechanical properties in rats with chronic kidney disease. Bone 57:477–483.
16. Jokihaara J, Porsti I, Pajamaki I, Vuohelainen T, Jolma P, et al. (2006) Paracalcitol [19-nor-1,25-(OH)2D2] in the treatment of experimental renal bone disease. J Bone Miner Res 21:745–751.
17. Moe SM, Radcliffe JS, White KE, Gattone VH II, Seifert MF, et al. (2011) The pathophysiology of early-stage chronic kidney disease–mineral bone disorder (CKD-MBD) and response to phosphate binders in the rat. J Bone Miner Res 26:2672–2681.
18. Sabbagh Y, Graciolli FG, O'Brien S, Tang W, dos Reis LM, et al. (2012) Repression of osteocyte Wnt/β-catenin signaling is an early event in the progression of renal osteodystrophy. J Bone Miner Res, 27:1757–1772.
19. Malluche HH, Porter DS, Pienkowski D (2013) Evaluating bone quality in patients with chronic kidney disease. Nat Rev Nephrol 9:671–680.
20. Kadokawa S, Matsumoto T, Naito H, Tanaka M (2011) Assessment of trabecular bone architecture and intrinsic properties of cortical bone tissue in a mouse model of chronic kidney disease. J Hard Tissue Biol 20: 79–86.
21. Moe SM, Chen NX, Seifert MF, Sinders RM, Duan D, et al. (2009) A rat model of chronic kidney disease-mineral bone disorder. Kidney Int 75:176–184.
22. Nagao S, Kugita M, Yoshihara D, Yamaguchi T (2012) Animal models for human polycystic kidney disease. Exp Anim Tokyo 61:477–488.
23. Stagner EE, Bouvrette DJ, Cheng J, Bryda EC (2009) The polycystic kidney disease-related proteins Bicc1 and SamCystin interact. BiochemBioph Res Co 383:16–21.
24. Shobeiri N, Adams MA, Holden RM (2010) Vascular calcification in animal models of CKD: a review. Am J Nephrol 31:471–481.
25. Gattone VH II, Tourkow BA, Trambaugh CM, Yu AC, Whelan S, et al. (2004)Development of multiorgan pathology in the *wpk* rat model of polycystic kidney disease. Anat Rec 277A:384–395.

26. Nagao S, Morita M, Kugita M, Yoshihara D, Yamaguchi T, et al. (2010) Polycystic kidney disease in Han:SPRD Cy rats is associated with elevated expression and mislocalizationof SamCystin. Am J Physiol Renal Physiol 299:F1078–F1086.
27. Aref M, Gallant MA, Organ JM, Wallace JM, Newman CL, et al. (2013) *In vivo* reference point indentation reveals positive effects of raloxifene on mechanical properties following 6 months of treatment in skeletally mature beagle dogs. Bone 56:449–53.
28. Hammond MA, Gallant MA, Burr DB, Wallace JM (2014) Nanoscale changes in collagen are reflected in physical and mechanical properties of bone at the microscale indiabetic rats. Bone 60:26–32.
29. Wallace JM (2012) Applications of atomic force microscopy for the assessment of nanoscale morphological and mechanical properties of bone. Bone 50:420–427.
30. Buckley A, Hill KE, Davidson JM (1988) Collagen metabolism. In:Colowick SP, Kaplan NO, Di SabatoG, editors. Methods in Enzymology: Immunochemical Techniques, Part M: Chemotaxis and inflammation. London: Academic Press. pp. 674–693.
31. Saito M, Marumo K, Fujii K, Ishioka N (1997) Single-column high-performance liquid chromatographic-fluorescence detection of immature, mature, and senescent cross-links of collagen. Anal Biochem 253:26–32
32. Moe SM, Chen NX, Newman CL, Gattone VH II, Organ JM, et al. (2014) A comparison of calcium to zoledronic acid for improvement of cortical bone in an animal model of CKD. J Bone Miner Res 29:902–910.
33. Gallant MA, Brown DM, Organ JM, Allen MR, Burr DB (2013) Reference-point indentation correlates with bone toughness assessed using whole-bone traditional mechanical testing. Bone 53:301–305.
34. Iimori S, Mori Y, Akita W, Kuyama T, Takada S, et al. (2012) Diagnostic usefulness of bone mineral density and biochemical markers of bone turnover in predicting fracture in CKD stage 5D patients—a single-center cohort study. Nephrol Dial Transplant 27:345–351.
35. Jamal SA, Hayden JA, Beyene J (2007) Low bone mineral density and fractures in long-term hemodialysis patients: a meta-analysis. Am J Kidney Dis 49:674–681.
36. Jamal SA, Cheung AM, West SL, Lok C (2012) Bone mineral density by DXA and HR pQCT can discriminate fracture status in men and women with stages 3 to 5 chronic kidney disease. OsteoporosInt 23:2805–2813.
37. Jassal SK, von Muhlen D, Barrett-Connor E (2007) Measures of renal function, BMD, bone loss, and osteoporotic fracture in older adults: the Rancho Bernardo study. J Bone Miner Res 22:203–210.
38. Klawansky S, Komaroff E, Cavanaugh PFJr, Mitchell DY, Gordon MJ, et al. (2003) Relationship between age, renal function and bone mineral density in the US population. OsteoporosInt 14:570–576.
39. Piraino B, Chen T, Cooperstein L, Segre G, Puschett J (1988) Fractures and vertebral bone mineral density in patients with renal osteodystrophy. ClinNephrol 30:57–62.
40. Yamaguchi T, Kanno E, TsubotaJ, Shiomi T, Nakai M, et al. (1996) Retrospective study on the usefulness of radius and lumbar bone density in the separation of hemodialysis patients with fractures from those without fractures. Bone 19:549–555.
41. Diez-Perez A, Güerri R, Nogues X, Caceres E, Pena MJ, et al. (2010)Micro-Microindentationfor in vivo measurement of bone tissue mechanical properties in humans. J Bone Miner Res 25:1877–1885.
42. Güerri-Fernández RC, Nogués X, Quesada Gómez JM, Torres Del Pliego E, Puig L, et al. (2013)Microindentation for in vivo measurement of bone tissue material properties in atypical femoral fracture patients and controls. J Bone Miner Res 28:162–168.
43. Farr JN, Drake MT, Amin S, Melton LJ III, McCready LK, et al. (2014) *In Vivo* assessment of bone quality in postmenopausal women with type 2 diabetes. J Bone Miner Res 29:787–795.
44. Tai K, Dao M, Suresh S, Palazoglu A, Ortiz C (2007) Nanoscale heterogeneity promotes energy dissipation in bone. Nat Mater 6:454–462.
45. Phelps JB, Hubbard GB, Wang X, Agrawal CM (2000) Microstructural heterogeneity and the fracture toughness of bone. J Biomed Mater Res 51:735–741.
46. Currey J (2005) Structural heterogeneity in bone: good or bad? J MusculoskeletNeuronal Interact 5:317.
47. Aoki C, Uto K, Honda K, Kato Y, Oda H(2013) Advanced glycation end products suppress lysyl oxidase and induce bone collagen degradation in a rat model of renal osteodystrophy. Lab Invest 93:1170–1183.
48. Galli F (2007) Protein damage and inflammation in uraemia and dialysis patients. Nephrol Dial Transplant 22 (Suppl 5):v20–36.
49. Miyata T, Ueda Y, Shinzato T, Iida Y, Tanaka S, et al. (1996) Accumulation of albumin-linked and free-form pentosidine in the circulation of uremic patients with end-stage renal failure: renal implications in the pathophysiology of pentosidine. J Am Soc Nephrol 7:1198–1206.
50. Sakata N, Noma A, Yamamoto Y, Okamoto K, Meng J, et al. (2003) Modification of elastin by pentosidine is associated with the calcification of aortic media in patients with end-stage renal disease. Nephrol Dial Transplant 18:1601–1609.
51. Zoccali C, Mallamaci F, Asahia K, Benedetto FA, Tripepi G, et al. (2001) Pentosidine, carotid atherosclerosis and alterations in left ventricular geometry in hemodialysis patients. J Nephrol 14:293–298.
52. Arsov S, Graaff R, van Oeveren W, Stegmayr B, Sikole A, et al. (2014) Advanced glycation end-products and skin autofluorescence in end-stage renal disease: a review. ClinChem Lab Med 52:11–20.
53. Mitome J, Yamamato H, Saito M, Yokoyama K, Marumo K, et al. (2011)Nonenzymaticcross-linking pentosidine increase in bone collagen and are associated with disorders of bone mineralization in dialysis patients. Calcif Tissue Int 88:521–529.
54. Glenn JV, Beattie JR, Barrett L, Frizzell N, Thorpe SR, et al. (2007) Confocal Raman microscopy can quantify advanced glycation end product (AGE) modifications in Bruch's membrane leading to accurate, nondestructive prediction of ocular aging. FASEB J 21:3542–52.
55. Nyman JS, Roy A, Acuna RL, Gayle HJ, Reyes MJ, et al. (2006). Age-related effect on the concentration of collagen crosslinks in human osteonal and interstitial bone tissue. Bone 39:1210–1217.
56. Odetti P, Rossi S, Monacelli F, Poggi A, Cirnigliaro M, et al. (2005) Advanced glycationend products and bone loss during aging. Ann NY AcadSci 1043:710–717.
57. Saito M, Fujii K, Mori Y, Marumo K (2006) Role of enzymatic and glycation induced cross-links as a determinant of bone quality in spontaneously diabetic WBN/Kob rats. Osteoporosis Int 17: 1514–1523.
58. Silva MJ, Brodt MD, Lynch MA, McKenzie JA, Tanouye KM, et al. (2009) Type 1 diabetes in young rats leads to progressive trabecular bone loss, cessation of cortical bone growth, and diminished whole bone strength and fatigue life. J Bone Miner Res 24: 1618–1627.
59. Malluche HH, Porter DS, Monier-Faugere M, Mawad H, Pienkowski D (2012)Differences in bone quality in low- and high-turnover renal osteodystrophy. J Am Soc Nephrol 23:525–532.

12

Disease Progression and Phasic Changes in Gene Expression in a Mouse Model of Osteoarthritis

Richard F. Loeser[1]*, Amy L. Olex[2], Margaret A. McNulty[3], Cathy S. Carlson[3], Michael Callahan[4], Cristin Ferguson[4], Jacquelyn S. Fetrow[2,5]

1 Department of Internal Medicine, Section of Molecular Medicine, Wake Forest University School of Medicine, Winston-Salem, North Carolina, United States of America, **2** Department of Computer Science, Wake Forest University, Winston-Salem, North Carolina, United States of America, **3** Department of Veterinary Population Medicine, College of Veterinary Medicine, University of Minnesota, St. Paul, Minneapolis, United States of America, **4** Department of Orthopedic Surgery, Wake Forest University School of Medicine, Winston-Salem, North Carolina, United States of America, **5** Department of Physics, Wake Forest University, Winston-Salem, North Carolina, United States of America

Abstract

Osteoarthritis (OA) is the most common form of arthritis and has multiple risk factors including joint injury. The purpose of this study was to characterize the histologic development of OA in a mouse model where OA is induced by destabilization of the medial meniscus (DMM model) and to identify genes regulated during different stages of the disease, using RNA isolated from the joint "organ" and analyzed using microarrays. Histologic changes seen in OA, including articular cartilage lesions and osteophytes, were present in the medial tibial plateaus of the DMM knees beginning at the earliest (2 week) time point and became progressively more severe by 16 weeks. 427 probe sets (371 genes) from the microarrays passed consistency and significance filters. There was an initial up-regulation at 2 and 4 weeks of genes involved in morphogenesis, differentiation, and development, including growth factor and matrix genes, as well as transcription factors including Atf2, Creb3l1, and Erg. Most genes were off or down-regulated at 8 weeks with the most highly down-regulated genes involved in cell division and the cytoskeleton. Gene expression increased at 16 weeks, in particular extracellular matrix genes including Prelp, Col3a1 and fibromodulin. Immunostaining revealed the presence of these three proteins in cartilage and soft tissues including ligaments as well as in the fibrocartilage covering osteophytes. The results support a phasic development of OA with early matrix remodeling and transcriptional activity followed by a more quiescent period that is not maintained. This implies that the response to an OA intervention will depend on the timing of the intervention. The quiescent period at 8 weeks may be due to the maturation of the osteophytes which are thought to temporarily stabilize the joint.

Editor: Francois Rannou, Cochin Hospital (AP-HP), and the University Paris Descarte, France

Funding: Supported by an Innovative Research Award from the Arthritis Foundation, The Wake Forest University Translational Science Institute, NIH Musculoskeletal Training Grant (T32 AR050938) and NIH Orthopaedics and Skeletal Biology Training Grant (T32 AR052272). The funders had no role in study design, data collection and analysis, decision to publish, or preparation of the manuscript.

Competing Interests: The authors have declared that no competing interests exist.

* E-mail: rloeser@wakehealth.edu

Introduction

Osteoarthritis (OA) affects over 27 million people in the United States and is similarly prevalent across the globe, making it the most common cause of chronic disability in adults [1,2]. There are a number of well established risk factors for OA that include age, obesity, prior joint injury, genetics, joint anatomy, and occupational history related to joint use [3]. Current treatments for OA are limited and no treatment has been conclusively shown to alter disease progression. A better understanding of the biological factors which drive disease progression, particularly early-stage disease, is needed in order to develop more targeted therapies to stop or slow progression.

Studies of human OA are limited by its multifactorial nature, the lack of tissue that can be obtained at various stages of the disease and difficulties in defining disease onset. Basic mechanistic studies often are performed with tissue obtained at the time of joint replacement, which represents end-stage disease. These studies have focused largely on changes present in the articular cartilage; however, OA is a condition that affects the joint as an organ including not only the cartilage but also subchondral bone, synovium, ligaments and, in the knee, the meniscus (reviewed in [4]).

Various animal models of OA have been developed in order to study the disease process under more controlled conditions where disease onset and stages of progression can be better defined and evaluated. A commonly used model in mice is the destabilized medial meniscus (DMM) model where OA is surgically induced by transection of the medial meniscotibial ligament. In this model, OA results from altered joint biomechanics and the pathologic changes of cartilage destruction, subchondral bone thickening, and osteophyte formation are similar to the changes seen in human OA [5]. We recently used this model to compare the changes in OA severity and gene expression in young and older adult mice at a single time point of 8 weeks after DMM surgery [6]. The severity of OA changes in the joint of the older adult mice (12 months old at the time of surgery) was about twice that of the younger adult mice (12 weeks old at surgery) and significant differences were noted in the genes that were up and down-regulated at that time point.

The present study was designed as a time-course experiment to evaluate changes in gene expression during the development of OA and to compare these changes to the histologic progression of the disease. The recently reported comparison of gene expression at the 8 week time point in young adult and older adult mice [6] was a sub-study of the present work, but because of the lack of sufficient numbers of older animals the time course study only includes the young adult mice. Similar to the previous report, the histological assessment and the gene microarray analysis were designed in a manner which considered OA as a disease of the joint as an organ and, thus, were not limited to a single tissue within the joint. The general hypothesis was that different stages of the disease process would be characterized by unique gene expression signatures. Knowledge of the biological processes regulated by these genes could provide new information about the OA disease process. The results demonstrated progressive histological changes of OA beginning within two weeks of DMM surgery and progressing over the 16 week time course. These were accompanied by phasic changes in gene expression, with the peak number of up-regulated genes found at 4 weeks after induction of OA, a significant decline in expression at 8 weeks, and an increase again at 16 weeks with different clusters of genes being more prominent at each time point.

Materials and Methods

Animals and surgical induction of OA

Male C57BL/6 mice (n = 129) were purchased from Charles River Inc. and were 12 weeks of age at the time of DMM surgery or sham surgery performed as a control. Animal use was carried out in strict accordance with the recommendations in the Guide for the Care and Use of Laboratory Animals of the National Institutes of Health. The protocol was approved by the Wake Forest School of Medicine Animal Care and Use Committee (protocol #A09-622). All surgery was performed under isoflurane anesthesia, and all efforts were made to minimize suffering. Butorphanol (2.5mg/kg) was administered in the event of pain.

Details of animal housing and induction of OA have been recently published [6]. Mice were operated on in waves and at the time of surgery were randomly assigned to a surgical group and termination time point so that the date when the surgery was performed would not influence the results. For the present study, a group of 9 mice was used for collection of RNA at time 0 (before surgery) when the animals were 12 weeks old. For the other time points, 6 DMM and 6 sham controls were sacrificed at 2, 4, 8, and 16 weeks after surgery for histological analysis and 9 DMM and 9 sham controls were sacrificed at each time point for RNA isolation. As noted above, the histological sections and RNA used for the 8 week time point were from the same samples as those previously reported [6] but here were reanalyzed as part of the time course study.

Histological analysis

Hind limbs from both the operated side and the contralateral side of each animal were dissected and processed for histological analysis. The details of fixation, processing, and sectioning, as well as the histological analysis, were as recently published [6,7]. In brief, hematoxylin and eosin and safranin-O mid-coronal sections of each stifle joint were obtained and representative sections from each joint graded by an evaluator (MAM) blinded to group assignment. The evaluation included the Articular Cartilage Structure (ACS) score (0–12), Safranin-O (Saf-O) staining score (0–12), articular cartilage thickness and area,% chondrocyte cell death, subchondral bone area and thickness, and osteophyte total area. Because the most severe changes were consistently found on the tibial side of the joints, the analysis was focused on the tibial plateaus. Synovitis is only apparent in severe disease in this model and given the lack of sufficient numbers of severe samples there was no attempt to score synovial changes.

Immunohistochemistry was performed on sections from 3 DMM and 4 sham control mice at the 16-week time point in order to examine tissue distribution of type III collagen, fibromodulin and proline-arginine-rich end leucine-rich repeat protein (Prelp). Antigen retrieval and blocking steps were as recently described [6]. Primary antibodies were acquired from Abcam Inc (Cambridge, MA) and included rabbit polyclonal antibodies to Collagen III (ab7778), Prelp (ab103868), and fibromodulin (ab81443). Secondary antibodies and detection were as described [6]. Immunostained sections were graded for cell and matrix staining using a scale of no immunopositivity (−) to marked immunopositivity (++++).

RNA preparation and microarray analysis

Knee joint tissue from the medial joint compartment was obtained from the time 0 group and the operated hind limbs from the other time points and processed for RNA isolation as described [6]. The tissue included tibial plateau and femoral condyle articular cartilage, subchondral bone with any osteophytes, meniscus, and the joint capsule with synovium. The tissue was treated with RNAlater® (Invitrogen) prior to freezing and storage at −80°C. RNA was extracted by homogenization using the Precellys 24 tissue homogenizer (Bertin Technologies purchased from MO BIO) as described [6] and the amount and quality of the RNA was determined using an Agilent 2100 Bioanalyzer.

RNA was pooled prior to microarray analysis such that 3 randomly selected samples from each surgical group and time point were pooled to create a each biological replicate. Because 9 mice were used for each experimental group, a total of three biological replicates per group were analyzed using the Affymetrix Mouse Genome 430 2.0 oligonucleotide arrays as described [6]. One replicate pool, which was from week two DMM mice, did not meet the RNA integrity level needed for microarray analysis; thus, this pool was not analyzed further, leaving two pools for the week two DMM mice.

Normalization and processing of microarray data

Microarrays were imaged and the resulting data normalized using systematic variation normalization (SVN) as previously described [6,8]. Reported data included the $\log_2$ of the signal intensity and the Affymetrix detection p-value for each probe set. Because some genes had more than one probe set, we provide results for both numbers of genes and probe sets when the numbers differed. The complete dataset has been provided to the Gene Expression Omnibus (GEO) repository (accession number GSE41342). Relative gene expression in the samples collected from the sham-operated control animals was calculated to identify those genes that changed as the animals aged over the 16 week time course independent of DMM-induced OA. For this analysis, sham gene expression was calculated as the signal log ratio (SLR) of the average time 0 intensity (baseline un-operated controls) to each sham replicate pool for each time point. The average of the time 0 intensity was used to ensure a consistent baseline, and each biological replicate of the sham arrays was analyzed individually to allow biological consistency to be measured in the analysis. The SLR is the $\log_2$ of the fold change and so an SLR of 0.5 = 1.4-fold. After SLR calculations, each probe set had 12 associated SLR values (3 for each time point—2, 4, 8 and 16 weeks), which together are referred to as the "sham time course".

Relative gene expression changes for the DMM time course were calculated to identify those genes that changed over time due to the DMM-induced changes in the joints. For this analysis, the sham results were used as a time-matched control (sham 2 weeks used as control for DMM 2 weeks etc.). Sham replicate signal intensities for each time point were averaged to ensure a consistent baseline for each replicate. DMM gene expression was then calculated as the time-matched signal log ratio of the average sham intensity to each DMM replicate for each time point, where each DMM replicate was analyzed individually. After SLR calculations, each probe set had 11 associated SLR values (2 for the 2 week time point, and 3 each for 4, 8 and 16 weeks), which are referred to as the "DMM time course".

Filtering and clustering of microarray data

Relative gene expression for the sham time course and DMM time course was filtered for differentially expressed genes with consistent expression changes over time as previously described [9] with a few alterations. Briefly, both data sets were filtered in a step-wise fashion as illustrated in **Figure 1**. Replicate time courses were filtered individually in the first two steps to identify those transcripts that were significantly detected on the chip over background (detection p-value $<=0.06$ for all time points and control), and for those that were differentially expressed in at least one time point (SLR ≥ 0.5 or ≤ -0.5 which converts to ≥ 1.4-fold and ≤ -1.4-fold). These data sets were intersected to identify those probe sets that passed the first two filtering steps independently in all replicates. Finally, transcripts were filtered for consistency of expression pattern (Pearson's correlation; PCC) and magnitude (Euclidean distance; ED) over time. An all-by-all comparison was done for each replicate time course profile resulting in 3 PCC and 3 ED scores for each probe set. Requiring all 6 scores to pass selected criteria was found to be too strict (data not shown). Therefore, only 2 of the 3 PCC and ED scores were required to pass selected cutoffs: PCC $>=0.70$ (a standard statistical threshold for positive correlation) and ED $<=0.60$ or $<=0.81$ for the DMM and sham time courses, respectively (the median ED score for each data set). Additionally, due to the missing 2-week DMM data for one of the replicates, all PCC and ED comparisons with this time course were done using only the 4-, 8- and 16-week time points. Probe sets passing all filtering criteria were considered to have been consistently and significantly expressed.

Filtered DMM time course gene expression data were clustered using the updated consensus clustering option provided by version 3 of SC^{2}ATmd [10]—sham time course data was not clustered in this work. The option to perform consensus clustering using a threshold to identify genes that cluster together less than 100% of the time was added to SC^{2}ATmd's functionality since its original release. This was implemented by converting the consensus matrix to an adjacency matrix and then using MATLAB's depth first search algorithm to identify consensus clusters. A figure of merit (FOM) analysis was run to determine the optimal number of clusters present in each replicate data set and to identify which clustering algorithm formed the most homogeneous clusters with respect to Euclidean distance [9,11]. As determined by the FOM analysis, consensus clustering was run using 10 starting clusters with k-means as the clustering algorithm and Euclidean distance as the distance metric. Each replicate data set was clustered 10 times, and a consensus over all 30 runs was calculated. Performing more than 10 iterations on each replicate did not significantly improve cluster homogeneity (data not shown). Probe sets clustering together 83% of the time were identified as a consensus cluster.

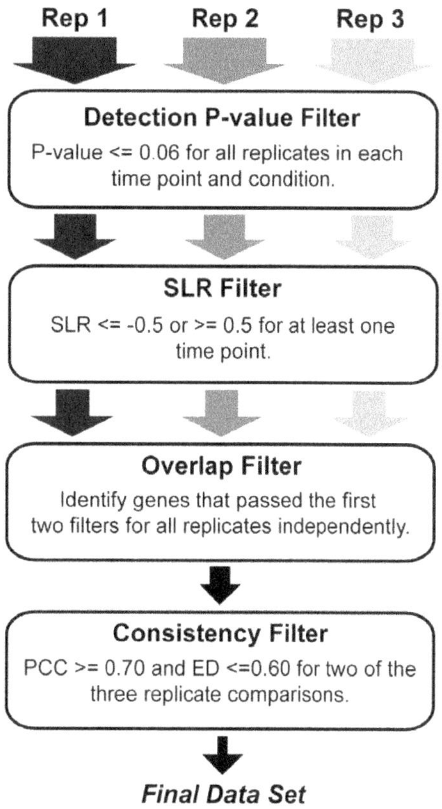

Figure 1. Flow chart of filtering process. After data normalization, SLR values were calculated as described in the methods, and replicate pools were randomly paired to obtain 3 complete time courses—referred to as Rep 1, Rep 2 and Rep 3. The first 2 filtering steps were done for each replicate independently, and identified probe sets that were significantly detected on the chip (detection p-value filter; all p-values $<=0.06$) as well as significantly differentially expressed (SLR filter; SLR was $<=-0.5$ or $>=0.5$ for any one time point). The overlap filter intersected all three filtered lists to identify the set of probe sets that passed the first 2 filtering steps independently in all replicates. Finally, probe sets were filtered for consistency in pattern (PCC score) and magnitude (ED score) of expression over time across all replicate time courses (consistency filter), where 2 of the 3 PCC scores had to be $>=0.70$, and 2 of the 3 ED scores had to be $<=0.60$. Those probe sets passing all filtering criteria were considered consistently and significantly differentially expressed across the time course in all 3 biological replicates, and were used for further analysis. Results of this process on each of the data sets described in the text can be found in Tables S1 and S2.

Increasing or decreasing this threshold resulted in small clusters with many singletons or large clusters that were uninformative, respectively; thus, the 83% threshold was chosen as an acceptable balance between these two extremes

Annotation analysis

Annotation enrichment analysis was performed using the Database for Annotation, Visualization, Integration and Discovery (DAVID) [12,13]. The Functional Annotation Clustering tool provided by DAVID was run using the Affymetrix Mouse 430 2.0 chip as background, with all other options left at their default settings. Annotations of clusters were considered significant if the Enrichment Score was greater than or equal to 1.3 (equivalent to a p-value $<=0.05$).

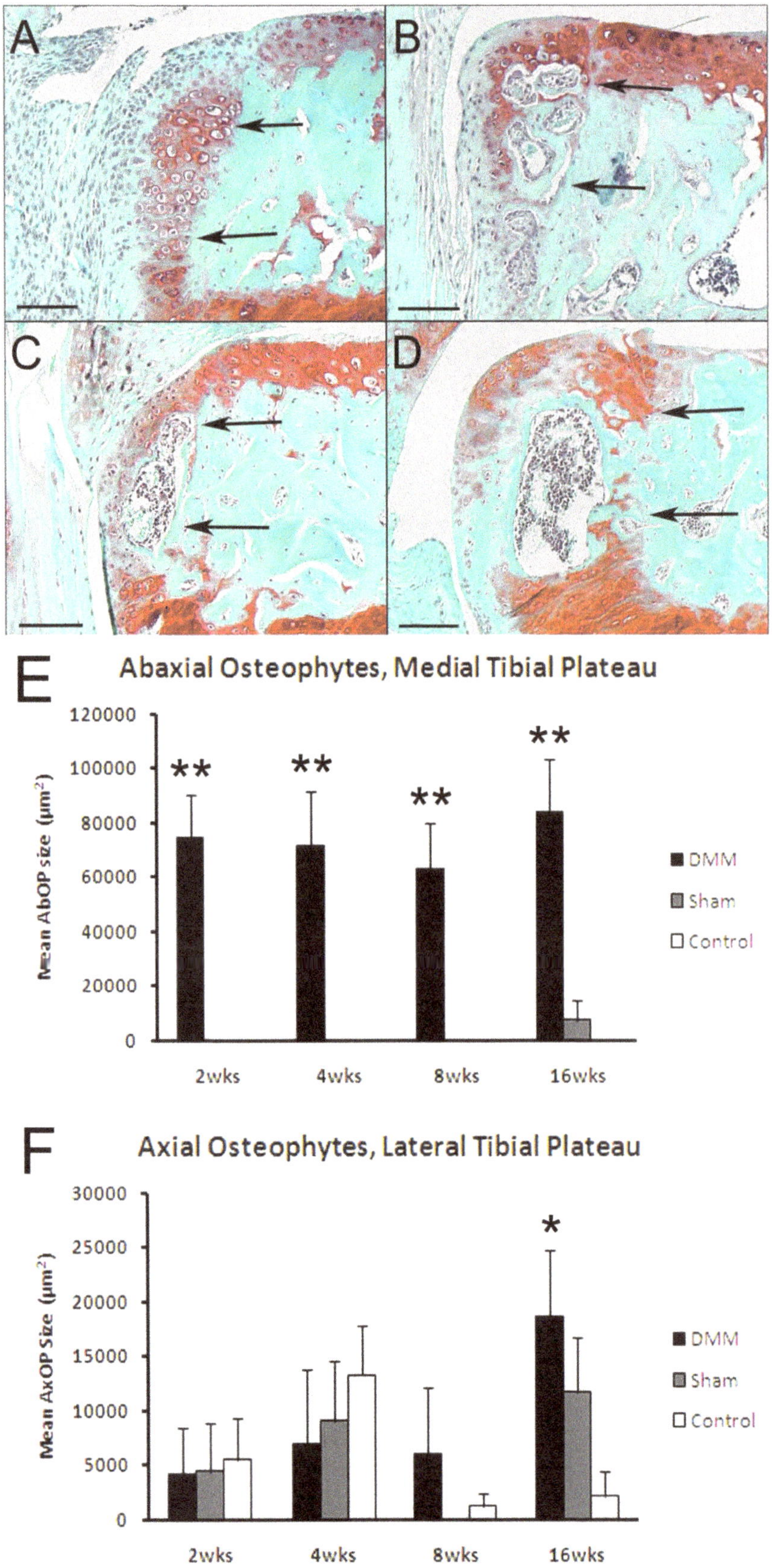

Figure 2. Histology results demonstrating osteophyte formation over the time course. Sections from DMM joints obtained 2 weeks (A), 4 weeks (B), 8 weeks (C), and 16 weeks (D) after DMM surgery were stained with safranin-O. Bar = 100 μm. Arrows point to the original medial abaxial joint margin and abaxial osteophytes that formed at this site. These start as chondrophytes at 2 weeks (A) and progressively mature.

Histomorphometric measures included the size of the abaxial osteophytes on the medial plateau (E) and axial osteophytes on the lateral plateau (F) for the DMM, sham, and contralateral control groups as indicated. $^{**}p<0.0001$ vs sham and control; $^{*}p=0.02$ vs sham and control by ANOVA.

Real-time PCR

Real-time PCR was performed using samples of RNA from the same pools used for the microarrays as previously described [6] using the SYBR®Green-based method with optimized primer sets obtained in the RT2 qPCR Primer Assays (SABiosciences/Qiagen) and with TATA box-binding protein (TBP) used to normalize relative expression.

Statistical analysis

Analysis of the microarray data is presented above. The histological data and the real time PCR data were found to be normally distributed. Histological data from both the lateral and medial tibial plateaus was evaluated using ANOVAs (intra-animal comparisons) and repeated measures analyses (inter-animal comparisons) using SPSS version 17.0 (IBM Corp, Somers, NY). The real time PCR results at each individual time point for sham controls and DMM animals were analyzed using t tests with StatView 5.0 software (SAS, Cary, NC).

Results

Histologic progression of joint tissue changes induced by DMM surgery

The sham operated joints and the contralateral control (non-operated joints from sham and DMM animals) demonstrated minimal to no pathological changes over the 16 week time course. Among the earliest changes observed in the DMM joints at 2 weeks after surgery were abaxial osteophytes in the medial tibial plateau. Osteophytes were primarily cartilaginous at 2 weeks, were ossified at 4 weeks, and were composed of trabecular bone that contained marrow spaces occupied by hematopoietic tissue at 8 and 16 weeks (**Figure 2A, B, C, D**). Interestingly, the cross-sectional area of the osteophytes did not change significantly from 2–16 weeks (**Figure 2E**). Much smaller and more variable axial osteophytes were noted on the lateral tibial plateaus but, unlike the medial abaxial osteophytes, their size was not significantly different among the three groups until 16 weeks after surgery, when they were significantly larger in the DMM relative to the sham and contralateral control joints (**Figure 2F**).

There were mild articular cartilage lesions noted at 2 weeks in the medial tibial plateaus of the DMM joints, resulting in an increase in the articular cartilage structure score and an increase in the Saf-O scores relative to sham and contralateral control joints at this time point (**Figure 3**). The articular cartilage structure scores increased progressively over the 16 weeks in the DMM joints while the Saf-O scores remained more stable over time. At 16 weeks, there was a mild increase in the articular cartilage structure score at the lateral tibial plateau in the DMM joints but the mean score was less than half of that seen in the medial tibial plateau (**Figure 3G**). No significant differences were seen among the groups or time points for Saf-O scores in the lateral tibial plateaus (data not shown). In addition, there were no significant differences in articular cartilage thickness over the course of the study in any of the groups (data not shown).

Chondrocyte death in the medial tibial plateau articular cartilage was significantly increased at 4 weeks in the DMM and sham joints relative to the non-operated controls, and increased further in the DMM joints at 8 and 16 weeks (**Figure 4A**). Dead chondrocytes also were apparent in the lateral tibial plateaus at week 16 but the area occupied by dead chondrocytes was less than half that in the medial tibial plateau, nor was there a difference in this parameter among the surgical groups at any time point (**Figure 4B**). We have recently published evidence for chondrocyte death in the DMM model at 8 weeks after surgery including findings of positive TUNEL staining consistent with apoptosis [14]; thus, the mechanism of cell death was not pursued in the present study.

The subchondral bone was thicker in the medial tibial plateau than the lateral tibial plateau in all three groups and at all time points (**Table 1**). At all time points, the subchondral bone thickness and area were larger in the medial tibial plateau of the DMM group than in the other two groups, although this difference was only significant at the 4-week time point. In all groups, there was a gradual increase in subchondral bone thickness and area over the 16 weeks of the study.

Changes in gene expression over time in the sham control joints

To detect changes in gene expression occurring over the 16 week time period of the study that could be due to aging of the animals, we analyzed the gene expression results in the sham joints relative to the time 0 baseline. Filtering of the data revealed 347 genes (406 probe sets) significantly and consistently regulated over time in the sham joints. A complete list of these genes is provided in File S1. The 2-week time point had the largest number of up-regulated genes and this was followed by a progressive decrease in expression of the majority of genes over the 16 week time course (**Figure 5A and 5B**). The set of 347 genes was analyzed by DAVID's Functional Annotation Clustering tool [12], which identified 36 groups of significantly over-represented annotations with enrichment scores ≥ 1.3 (File S1). Most of the annotations were related to signal peptide, extracellular matrix, development, differentiation and morphogenesis, consistent with a maturation process occurring over the 16 week time course.

A small subset of 25 genes remained up-regulated over the time course (File S1). Functional Annotation Clustering was performed on this subset of genes, and only one group of significantly over-represented annotations was identified. This group of terms included plasma membrane, glycoprotein, immune response, and cell surface linked signal transduction terms.

Gene expression in DMM joints relative to sham controls

The time course results for changes in expression in the DMM joints relative to time-matched sham joints revealed 371 genes (427 probe sets) that were significantly and consistently regulated over the three biological replicates (File S2). Examination of a heat map of these genes as well as the SLR distributions (**Figure 6A and 6B**) reveals a phasic pattern. The majority of genes were up-regulated at 2 and 4 weeks followed by reduced expression or down-regulation at 8 weeks and then some increase in expression at 16 weeks although not to the level of weeks 2 and 4.

These results were much different from the time course results noted in the sham joints, consistent with changes in gene expression due to induction of OA by the DMM surgery. An overlap analysis revealed 94 genes (97 probe sets) that were in common in the DMM/sham and sham/baseline control datasets (**Figure 7A** and File S3). Many of these were extracellular matrix genes including Prelp, fibromodulin, several collagens (Types IV, V, XII, XVI, and XXII), and biglycan. A heat map revealed that

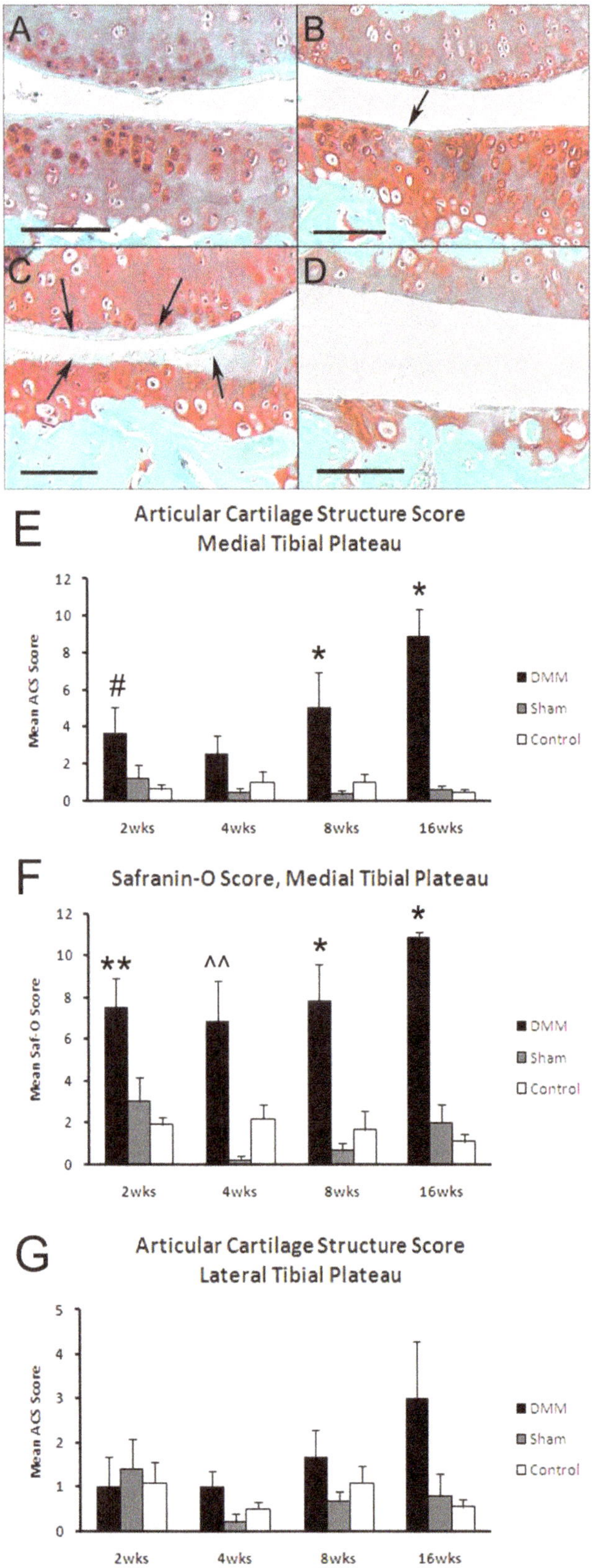

Figure 3. Histology results demonstrating articular cartilage lesions over the time course. Sections from DMM joints obtained 2 weeks (A), 4 weeks (B), 8 weeks (C), and 16 weeks (D) after DMM surgery were stained with safranin-O. Bar = 100 μm. Arrows indicate an early cartilage lesion in the medial tibial plateau at 4 weeks (B) and a more severe lesion at 8 weeks (C) on the medial tibial plateau (lower tissue in image) and the femoral condyle (upper tissue in image). Note advanced articular cartilage loss at 16 weeks. Articular cartilage structure scores (E) and safranin-O scores (F) for the medial tibial plateaus and articular cartilage structure scores for the lateral tibial plateau (G) are shown for the DMM, sham, and contralateral control groups as indicated. *p<0.05 vs sham and control; ^p = 0.01 vs sham; **p<0.01 vs control; #p<0.05 vs control by ANOVA.

almost all of these genes displayed very different expression profiles. Most were down-regulated over time in the sham controls but up-regulated in the DMM joints, particularly at 2 and 4 weeks (**Figure 7B**). Of the 94 genes in common between the DMM and sham joints, almost all were up-regulated in the DMM joint, with the exception of three: H2afz (predicted gene 6722///H2A histone family, member Z), Alms1(Alstrom syndrome 1), and Adhfe1(iron-containing alcohol dehydrogenase), which were down-regulated in the DMM joints. These genes do not have any known role in joint development or in OA.

The 94 genes in common between DMM/sham and sham/baseline were analyzed by DAVID. This returned 10 significant annotation groups (File S3) that included terms such as extracellular matrix, cell adhesion, collagen, skeletal development, EGF-like domains, fibronectin, leucine rich repeats, and endoplasmic reticulum.

Consensus clustering of the genes regulated during the development of OA in the DMM joints

Consensus clustering of genes with altered expression after DMM surgery identified 27 clusters with 2 or more probe sets and 38 genes (39 probe sets) that were classified as outliers (singletons). The complete list of the genes found in each cluster and the DAVID analysis for the clusters are found in File S2. Heat maps of the largest 16 clusters are shown in **Figure 8** and reveal striking differences in the temporal patterns of gene expression over the 16 week time course. The significant annotations for these clusters from DAVID analysis are shown in **Table 2**.

Only clusters 5, 7, 10 and 12 exhibited significant down-regulation at specific time points. Cluster 5 contained genes down-regulated at week 4; cluster 10, genes down-regulated at weeks 4 and 8; and clusters 7 and 12, genes down-regulated at week 8. Cluster 5 genes were not associated with any significantly over-represented annotations, but this cluster of 27 genes (32 probe sets) included Cytl1 (cytokine-like 1), which has been shown to be expressed during chondrogenesis and to promote chondrocyte differentiation through stimulation of Sox9 transcriptional activity [15]. Cluster 10, also down-regulated at week 4, with continuing down-regulation in week 8, contained 11 genes. No functions were significantly over-represented in this cluster and none of these genes were associated with osteoarthritis in the literature. Cluster 10 contained a phosphatase, several kinases and four genes whose function involves nucleotide binding. Clusters 7 and 12, both down-regulated at week 8, consisted of 19 and 11 genes (21 and 11 probe sets), respectively. Significantly over-represented annotations identified by DAVID in cluster 7 included mitotic cell cycle, cell cycle process, cell division, and cytoskeleton. S100b, which had been used in the past as a marker for chondrogenesis [16] was in this cluster. Over-represented annotations in cluster 12 all involved carbohydrate metabolism.

Significant up-regulation of gene expression at 16 weeks was seen in clusters 15 and 16, both of which also exhibited high up-regulation at week 4. Cluster 15 consisted of 7 probe sets covering three genes; Prelp, Col3a1 (collagen, type III, alpha 1), and Fmod (fibromodulin). Prelp and fibromodulin were also present in the

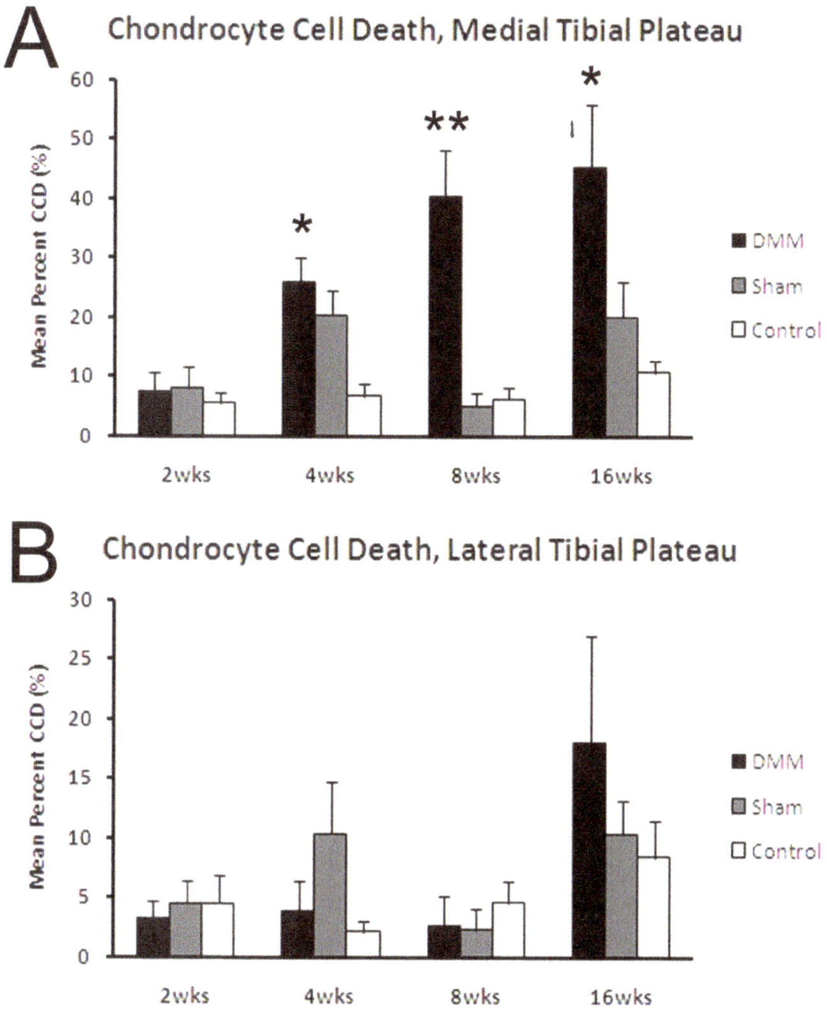

Figure 4. Histologic analysis of chondrocyte death over the time course. Dead chondrocytes were counted on H&E sections from the medial tibial plateau (A) and lateral tibial plateau (B) from DMM, sham, and contralateral control joints at the various time points after surgery. *$p<0.05$ vs sham and control joints; **$p<0.001$ vs sham and control joints by ANOVA.

DMM/sham-Sham/baseline overlap gene list reported above, where they were found to be highly down-regulated at 16 weeks in the sham joints; however, these genes were highly up-regulated in the DMM joints. Cluster 16 was comprised of four probe sets, representing 3 genes: Col14a1 (collagen, type XIV, alpha 1), Bgn (biglycan), and Fbln7 (fibulin 7), all associated with the extracellular matrix. Col14a1 was identified in a microarray analysis of human tissue [17]; while Bgn was previously associated with chondrogenesis and extracellular matrix turnover in osteoarthritis [18].

Genes in clusters 3 and 11 displayed temporal profiles of up-regulation only at 4 weeks, with little significant change in expression from control at any other time point. Cluster 3 contained 45 genes (48 probe sets), with significant annotations that included regulation of transcription, DNA binding, regulation of RNA metabolic process, zinc ion binding, and transcription. Potential genes of interest were NFκB activating protein, Atf2 and Erg. Cluster 11 was composed of 11 genes, which exhibited no significantly over-represented functions. One of the genes in this cluster was Asb13, an ankyrin repeat and SOCS box-containing protein.

Clusters 1, 2, 4, 9, and 14 contained genes that exhibit strong up-regulation at 4 weeks, with less up-regulation at 2 weeks. Cluster 1 contained 48 genes (54 probe sets) representing genes whose significant annotations include embryonic organ morphogenesis, positive regulation of cell differentiation and developmental process. This cluster included several genes thought to be involved in joint biology and/or OA including syndecan 4, Bmp-1, and Timp-2. Cluster 2 contained 39 genes (52 probe sets) for genes also up-regulated at 2 and 4 weeks. The cluster included over-represented annotations for collagen, signal peptide, extracellular region, extracellular matrix, cell adhesion and glycosaminoglycan binding. Genes of potential interest in this cluster included collagen genes such as Col5a1 and Col16a1, growth factor-related genes such as Igf1 and Egfr, MMP-14, and biglycan. (Note, biglycan is represented by three probe sets on this mouse chip, two of which are found in cluster 16 and 1 in cluster 2). Clusters 4, 9, and 14 contained 33, 16 and 8 genes (33, 18, and 8 probe sets), respectively. DAVID did not identify any function annotations over-represented any of these clusters. Cluster 4 genes included two glutathione peroxidases, Gpx7 and Gpx8, perhaps suggesting some redox-related event.

Table 1. Histomorphometric measures of subchondral bone area and thickness in DMM and sham control joints.

	Time	Treatment Group	Medial Tibial Plateau	ANOVA	Lateral Tibial Plateau	ANOVA
SCB Area	2 week	DMM	85777 (±12232)	NS	42703 (±5768)	NS
SCB Area	2 week	Sham	66140 (±8668)	NS	46342 (±6410)	NS
SCB Area	2 week	Control	70557 (±5895)	NS	48279 (±4694)	NS
SCB Area	4 week	DMM	116943 (±18235)	p = 0.011	67074 (±5367)	NS
SCB Area	4 week	Sham	71067 (±11028)	p = 0.011	57426 (±8690)	NS
SCB Area	4 week	Control	71758 (±5284)	p = 0.011	55541 (±5293)	NS
SCB Area	8 week	DMM	147622 (±13141)	NS	50446 (±8643)	NS
SCB Area	8 week	Sham	122046 (±19956)	NS	68432 (±11352)	NS
SCB Area	8 week	Control	103391 (±9112)	NS	62735 (±5925)	NS
SCB Area	16 week	DMM	144786 (±21706)	NS	75524 (±16120)	NS
SCB Area	16 week	Sham	124481 (±23749)	NS	62240 (±10563)	NS
SCB Area	16 week	Control	116784 (±15843)	NS	66090 (±7798)	NS
SCB Thickness	2 week	DMM	74.1 (±9.4)	NS	40.5 (±4.6)	NS
SCB Thickness	2 week	Sham	58.7 (±6.2)	NS	45.7 (±5.7)	NS
SCB Thickness	2 week	Control	63.3 (±5.3)	NS	45.5 (±4.1)	NS
SCB Thickness	4 week	DMM	99.2 (±13.4)	p = 0.011	56.3 (±4.0)	NS
SCB Thickness	4 week	Sham	64.2 (±9.8)	p = 0.011	51.9 (±7.8)	NS
SCB Thickness	4 week	Control	63.5 (±4.3)	p = 0.011	49.8 (±4.1)	NS
SCB Thickness	8 week	DMM	120.8 (±9.9)	NS	48.4 (±5.1)	NS
SCB Thickness	8 week	Sham	99.4 (±11.3)	NS	69.0 (±11.7)	NS
SCB Thickness	8 week	Control	90.8 (±7.2)	NS	57.0 (±4.7)	NS
SCB Thickness	16 week	DMM	111.9 (±20.4)	NS	66.2 (±9.8)	NS
SCB Thickness	16 week	Sham	106.8 (±15.7)	NS	60.1 (±7.9)	NS
SCB Thickness	16 week	Control	101.2 (±12.6)	NS	60.1 (±6.2)	NS

Subchondral bone (SCB) area (μm^2) and thickness (μm) were measured as detailed in the Materials and Methods. The p values are the ANOVA values between the treatment groups within each time point and the significance noted was between the DMM vs sham and contralateral controls. For each group and each time point sections from an n of 6 animals were measured.

Clusters 6, 8, and 13 also displayed the most up-regulation at week 4, but to a lesser extent than clusters 1, 2, 4, 9, and 14. Cluster 6 included 23 genes (24 probe sets) whose DAVID-identified over-represented annotations included signal peptide, glycoprotein, cell adhesion, serine/threonine kinase signaling pathway, skeletal system development and growth factor activity. Genes of particular interest included TGFβ2 and TGFβ3, latent TGFβ binding protein and Ddr2. Cluster 8 contained 19 genes for which the significant gene annotations included cell adhesion and contained COMP and Mmp13 which are thought to be important markers of the OA process. Cluster 13 included 9 genes for which there were no significantly over-represented functions. One of these, Enpp3, a pyrophosphatase, has been previously associated with osteoarthritis [19].

Overall, the analysis of gene clusters based on the metrics of both shape and magnitude of the time profile provided insight into the temporal process of osteoarthritis development. Only a few genes were down-regulated as part of this process, and those were down-regulated mainly at 4 and/or 8 weeks. Many more genes were up-regulated and most of the up-regulated genes displayed up-regulation at 4 weeks, with lesser up-regulation at 2 and 16 weeks. The phasic process was clearly visualized in these clusters, with the gene expression at 8 weeks being significantly different from gene expression at the other time points. This difference was consistent across all replicates.

Tissue distribution of type III collagen, fibromodulin, and Prelp

Based on the results of the consensus clustering, we choose to immunostain for type III collagen, fibromodulin, and Prelp, in order to determine which tissues might be providing the signals noted by gene expression at week 16. A total of 3 DMM and 4 sham control mice were studied and representative images are shown in **Figure 9** The tissue distribution of immunopositivity was similar between the two surgical groups; however, certain tissue types (e.g. fibrocartilage) were more prevalent in the DMM mice. Type III collagen immunopositivity was present in a pericellular distribution in articular cartilage and the meniscus and was located more diffusely in ligaments, the joint capsule, and the synovium as well as in the fibrocartilage located over osteophytes (**Table 3**). It was also present in the vascular endothelium. Fibromodulin immunopositivity was present in low numbers of articular chondrocytes, minimally in meniscus, and variably in synovium. Immunopositivity was more intense and involved more chondrocytes in fibrocartilage, notably over osteophytes, than in articular cartilage. Some bone marrow cells, including megakaryocytes also were positive. Immunopositivity for Prelp was present in ligaments (particularly at the site of ligamentous attachments to bone), periosteum, and fibrous connective tissue. Most chondrocytes were negative; however the

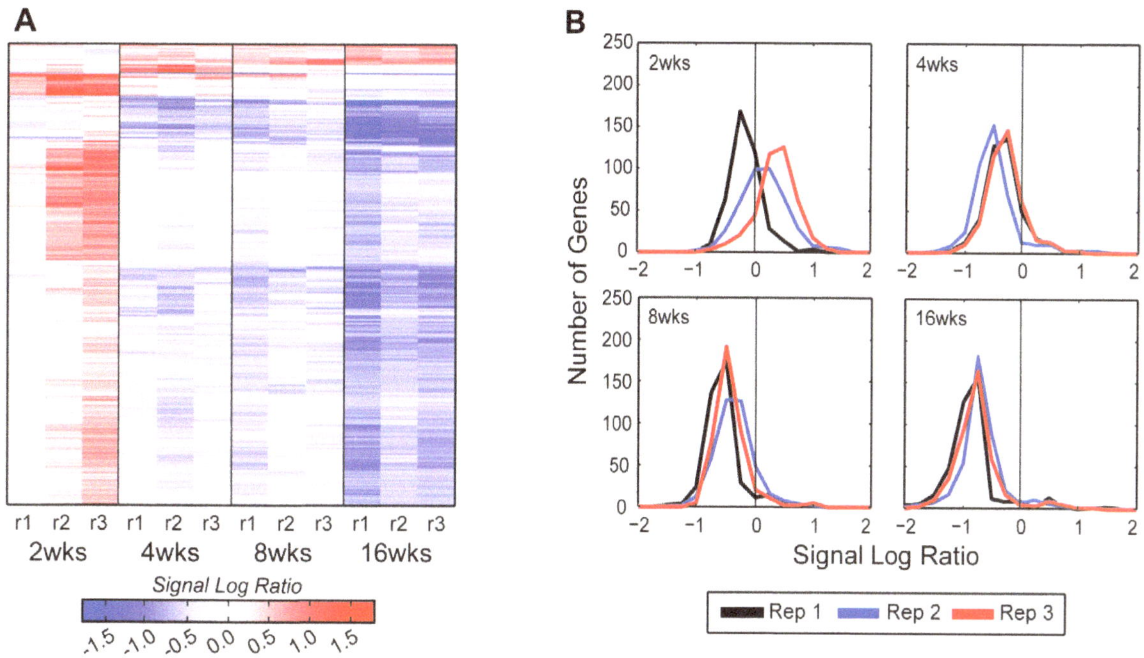

Figure 5. Global view of the differentially expressed genes in the sham time course. A) A heat map illustrates that the majority of differentially expressed genes (406 probe sets for 347 genes), in the sham time course are down-regulated, with few being up-regulated over time. Heat map rows represent genes, and columns represent replicates of each time points. Red indicates up-regulation, blue down-regulation and white indicates no change in gene expression from the respective control (see Methods). B) Gene expression distributions of the sham time course exhibit a uni-modal distribution throughout the experiment; however, the distributions center becomes shifted toward the negative side of zero at 4 weeks, indicating a global down-regulation of these genes over time due to aging. An SLR of zero is marked by a vertical line on the graph, and replicate time courses are colored as follows: replicate 1 = black, replicate 2 = blue, replicate 3 = red.

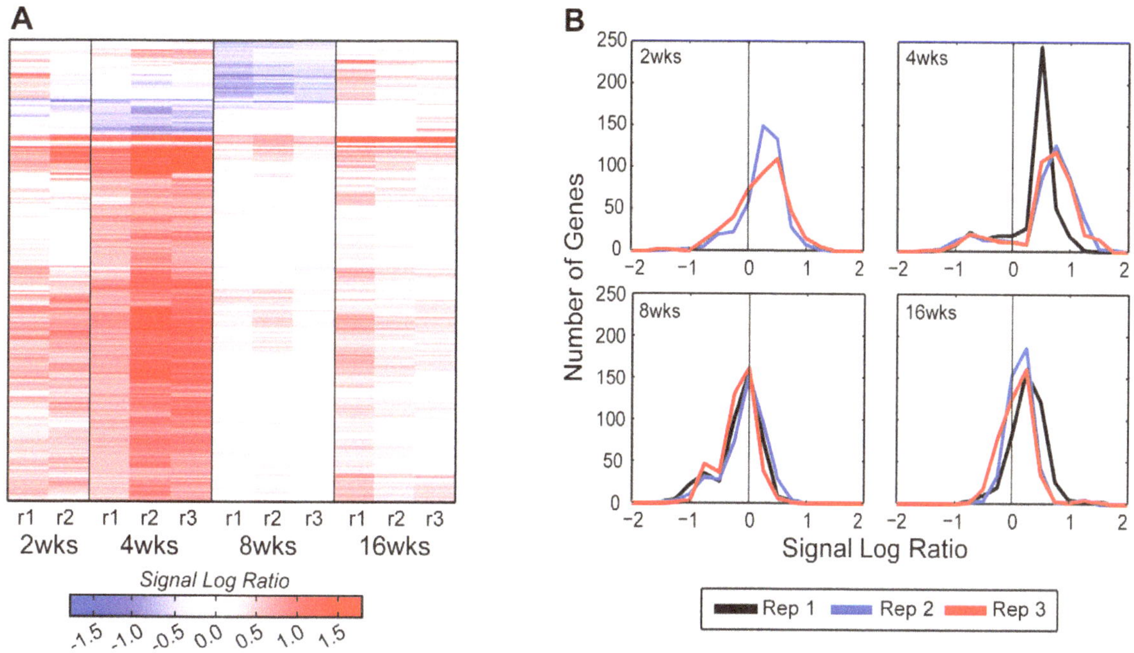

Figure 6. Global view of the differentially expressed genes in the DMM time course. A) The heat map illustrates that the majority of differentially expressed genes (427 probe sets for 371 genes) were up-regulated throughout the DMM time course, except for a small group of genes, which were down-regulated 4 and 8 weeks after surgery (see Figure 5A legend for heat map formatting details). B) The DMM time course exhibits a bi-modal distribution at 4 and 8 weeks after surgery, with the majority of genes being up-regulated at 4 weeks and not different from control at 8 weeks (see Figure 5B legend for formatting details).

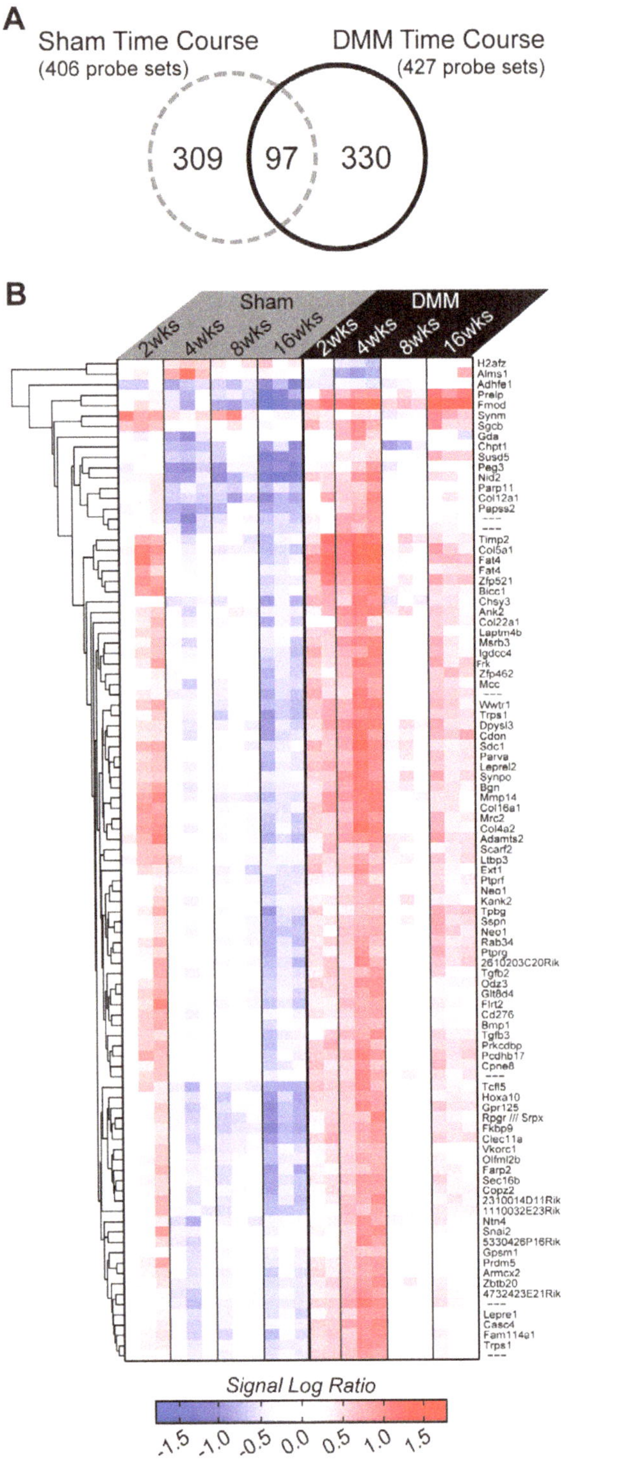

Figure 7. The group of genes differentially expressed in both sham and DMM data sets. Intersection of the 406 differentially expressed sham time course probe sets and the 427 DMM time course probe sets revealed 97 probe sets (94 genes) found in both data sets. A) A Venn diagram illustrates the number of probe sets in each data set as well as the overlap, and indicates that the majority of genes with OA induced expression changes are not altered in sham joints. B) A heat map of gene expression changes for the 97 intersecting probe sets was created using hierarchical agglomerative clustering and Euclidean distance, with sham expression on the left and DMM expression on the right. The heat map is formatted as in Figures 5A and 6A with the addition of the hierarchical dendrogram on the left and the gene names on the right.

matrix of degenerative cartilage and fibrocartilage was strongly immunopositive.

Real-time PCR results for selected genes

We selected a set of 16 genes to evaluate using RT-PCR based on genes tested in our previous study [6] where we had compared RT-PCR results at the 8 week time point in young and older adult mice. The average fold change in the DMM relative to sham controls for this gene set was highest at 4 weeks and lowest at 8 weeks (**Table 4**) which was consistent with the overall pattern of the 371 genes found to be significantly regulated in DMM vs sham joints on the microarrays (**Figure 6**). Genes with significant upregulation at 4 weeks included aggrecan, asporin, Ccl21, Cxcr7, Dkk3, Htra1, Igf-1, periostin, and Sfrp2. Looking across the time course, none of the genes examined were significantly up- or down-regulated in DMM relative to sham joints at all 4 time points; however, Ccl21, Cxcr7, Igf-1, and Sfrp2 were up-regulated at 3 of 4 time points. The two Wnt pathway regulators that were examined, Dkk3 and Sfrp2, were both significantly up-regulated at the early time points as was Col3a1. Unlike Dkk3 and Sfrp2, Col3a1 was also highly expressed at 16 weeks, consistent with the microarray results. Although type X collagen has been used as a marker of chondrocyte hypertrophy, which is thought to contribute to the development of OA, we actually observed a decrease in its expression at two weeks and no significant increase at the later time points. MMP-13 was increased at 2, 4, and 16 weeks in DMM relative to joints, as was noted on the microarrays, but due to variability among the 3 pools it did not reach statistical significance.

Discussion

Both the histologic and gene expression analysis support a phasic process for the development of OA in this model. The early phases at 2 and 4 weeks after DMM surgery were the most active in terms of gene expression at a time when the earliest cartilage lesions in the medial tibial plateau were very mild but abaxial chondrophytes had already formed. The chondrophytes matured to osteophytes as the articular cartilage lesions became more severe but, interestingly, this was accompanied by a significant decline in overall gene expression at the 8 week time point. In addition to the differences in overall gene expression, the findings from cluster analysis showed that each time point studied had a unique gene signature that also supports a phasic process.

Perhaps most striking was the decline in gene expression at 8 weeks after surgery. There was a significant down-regulation of genes regulating cell proliferation while matrix remodeling genes that were up-regulated at 2 and 4 weeks were mostly off, suggesting that a quiescent phase had been reached. However, at 16 weeks this pattern had changed and was accompanied by significant cartilage loss in the medial tibial plateau while cartilage damage and chondrocyte death was beginning to be evident in the lateral tibial plateau along with the appearance of lateral axial osteophytes. Because RNA for the gene arrays was only isolated from the medial side of the joint, the changes in gene expression observed at 16 weeks were not due to the disease progressing laterally but rather reflect more advanced disease medially. The lack of time points between 4 and 8 weeks and 8 and 16 weeks prevents any conclusions about the length of the quiescent phase.

The significant expression of Prelp, Col3a1, and fibromodulin at 16 weeks suggests that a matrix repair or a "wound healing response" was active. At 16 weeks, the articular cartilage from the DMM group had severe lesions in the medial tibial plateau with some loss of cartilage. This suggested that the signal at 16 weeks

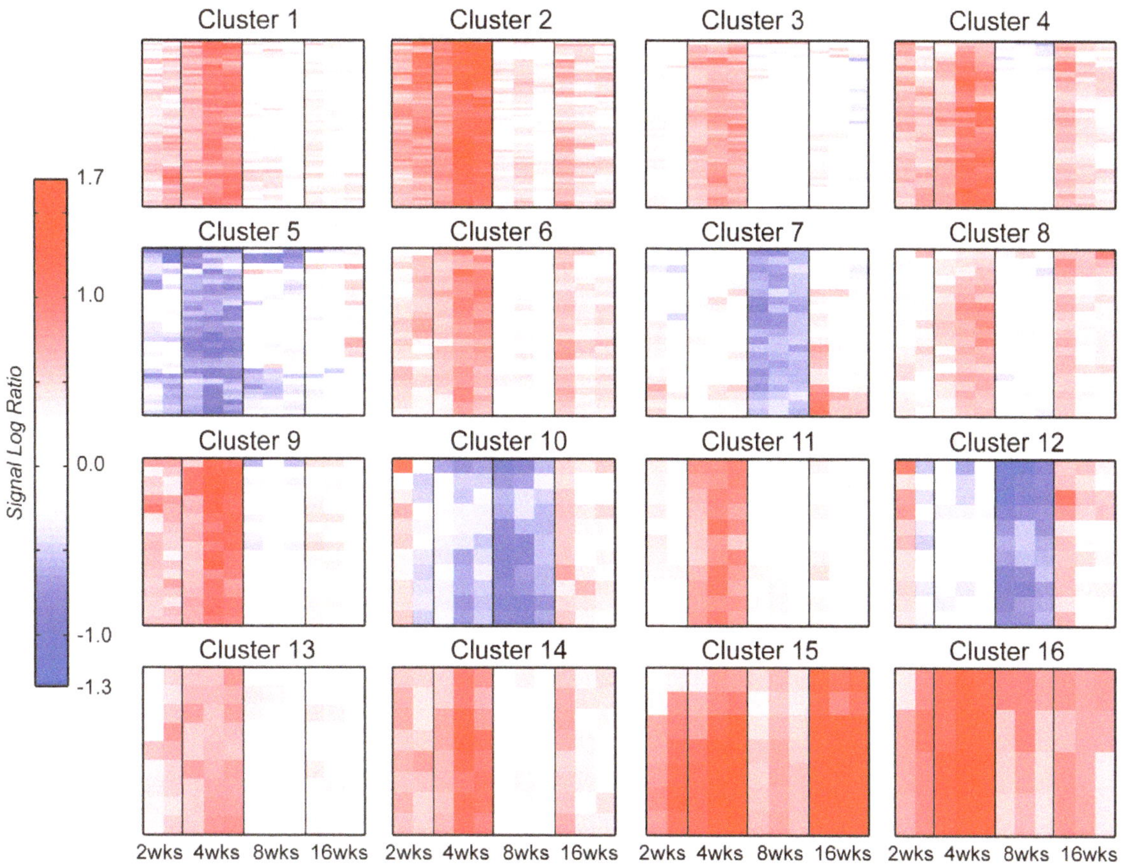

Figure 8. Heat maps of the largest 16 consensus clusters in the DMM time course. Rows represent genes and columns are time point replicates in the following order: 2 weeks rep2, rep3; 4-, 8- and 16 weeks rep1, rep2, rep3. Red indicates up-regulation, blue down-regulation and white indicates no change in expression from the sham time-matched control. All heat maps in this figure are colored on the same scale for easy comparison with maximum up-regulation at 1.7 SLR and maximum down-regulation at −1.3 SLR. A variety of expression patterns are present with most including significant up-regulation at 4 weeks. Only four clusters contain down-regulated genes (clusters 5, 7, 10 and 12), and cluster 15 is the only one with significant up-regulation 16 weeks after surgery.

for these genes may have come from either early changes on the femoral side, since some femoral tissue was included for RNA extraction, or more likely, from other joint structures such as the meniscus, synovium, ligaments and subchondral bone. Immunostaining revealed that ligaments and the fibrocartilage found over osteophytes were common locations for all three proteins. These results are consistent with previous studies that examined the location and function of these proteins. Prelp is thought to play a role in matrix organization through interactions with collagen, as does the small leucine-rich proteoglycan fibromodulin [20,21]. Deletion of fibromodulin in mice leads to OA, possibly via weakened ligaments and tendons [22]. However, a recent study that revealed a role for complement activation in OA demonstrated increased levels of fibromodulin in OA synovial fluid and found that fibromodulin could promote the activation of complement [23]. Overexpression of Prelp has been shown to disrupt normal collagen fiber formation in skin [24] and, in contrast to fibromodulin, it is an inhibitor of complement activation [25]. Thus, too little or too much fibromodulin and Prelp could contribute to OA.

Increased expression of type III collagen has been previously noted in human OA cartilage [26,27] and it has been found in normal cartilage in fibrils containing type II collagen [28]. We noted a pericellular location for type III collagen in articular cartilage and the meniscus. It is not known what role type III collagen could have in the OA joint. In the set of 371 genes that were differentially expressed in DMM vs sham joints, we observed increased expression, at one or more time points, in a large number of collagen genes that are likely part of an attempted repair response. These included the alpha 1 chain of types III, V, XII, XIV, XVI, and XXII collagen and the alpha 2 chain of type IV collagen, along with the collagen processing genes, procollagen c-endopeptidase enhancer protein and procollagen-lysine, 2-oxoglutarate 5-dioxygenase 1.

The phasic changes in gene expression noted in the DMM knees were not the result of aging of the animals over the 16 week time course. Changes in gene expression were noted when we compared the 12 week old animals at baseline (un-operated) and the sham controls over the 16 week time course but these differed significantly from the changes in gene expression noted in the DMM relative to sham joints. This was seen in the overlap analysis where the changes over time in expression in the DMM joints were most often in the opposite direction to changes over time in the sham joints. This was most evident for Prelp and fibromodulin which were significantly down-regulated at week 16 in the sham controls but increased in the DMM joints. Interestingly, immunopositivity for both of these proteins was notably stronger and more extensive in fibrocartilage over osteophytes than in

Table 2. Significant DAVID annotations for the top 16 Gene Clusters.

Cluster	Significant DAVID Annotations
1	Embryonic organ morphogenesis, inner ear morphogenesis, embryonic organ development, positive regulation of cell differentiation, positive regulation of developmental process, regulation of cell proliferation
2	Collagen, signal peptide, disulfide bond, glycoprotein, extracellular region, extracellular matrix, cell adhesion, glycosaminoglycan binding
3	Regulation of transcription, DNA binding, regulation of RNA metabolic process, Zinc finger C2H2-like, transition metal ion binding
4	None significant
5	None significant
6	Signal, signal peptide, glycoprotein, glycosylation site:N-linked, disulfide bond, cell adhesion, phosphorus, metabolic process, transmembrane receptor protein serine/threonine kinase signaling pathway, skeletal system development/morphogenesis, enzyme linked receptor protein signaling pathway, protein amino acid phosphorylation, growth factor, growth factor activity, regulation of cell proliferation
7	Mitotic cell cycle, cell cycle phase/process, nuclear/cell division, organelle fission, cytoskeletal protein binding, intracellular non-membrane-bounded organelle,
8	Cell adhesion, biological adhesion
9	None significant
10	None significant
11	None significant
12	Carbohydrate metabolism, glucose/hexose/monosaccharide metabolic process
13	None significant
14	None significant
15	Extracellular matrix, secreted, disulfide bond, signal peptide, glycoprotein
16	Extracellular matrix, secreted, disulfide bond, signal peptide, glycosylation site:N-linked, glycoprotein

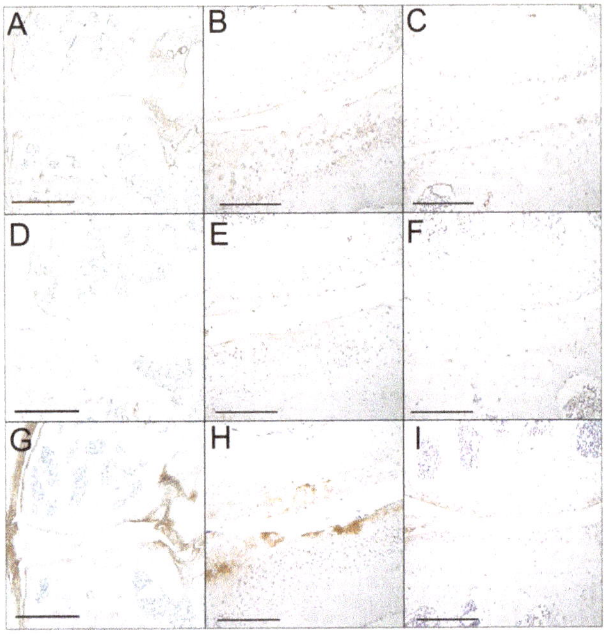

Figure 9. Immunolocalization of type III collagen, fibromodulin, and Prelp. Sections from mice in the 16 week-old sham and DMM groups were immunostained as detailed in the Methods using antibodies to type III collagen (A,B,C), fibromodulin (D,E,F) and Prelp (G,H,I). A, D, and G are 4x views of sham control joints to demonstrate overall tissue distribution. B, E, and H are 20x views of DMM joints and C, F, and I are 20x views of sham control joints. Bar =1 mm for 4X, 200um for 20X.

articular or meniscal cartilage. In addition, immunopositivity for Prelp was increased in degenerative cartilage matrix compared with normal cartilage. In the sham time course analysis, most genes exhibited an up-regulation of expression at 2 weeks followed by a progressive decline out to 16 weeks, compared to time zero. Many of these genes were involved in morphogenesis and development, suggesting the animals were more actively growing at the start of the study and then growth likely slowed. Importantly, the progressive increase in subchondral bone area and thickness were the only histologic measures that changed with time in all groups (control, sham and DMM).

We have recently reported a comparison of the 8 week time point results included in the present study with results from the same time point in animals that were 12 months-old at the time of DMM surgery [6]. The histologic OA severity in the older mice was about twice that of the younger mice and significantly more genes were up-regulated in the older mice. The 8 week comparisons suggest that the older mice develop OA more rapidly after DMM surgery than the younger mice, a result which could have contributed to the differences in gene expression at 8 weeks. A major difference between the young and older mice was in the expression of muscle related genes which were up-regulated in the older mice and either down-regulated or unchanged in the younger mice. Consistent with greater importance of the muscle-related genes in the older mice, we did not find significant annotations for muscle in the time course study using young mice. It would be of interest to do a time course study in the 12 month-old mice to determine if a phasic progression is also found. We did compare the DMM vs sham gene expression from the 8 week time point in the 12 month old mice to the other time points in the younger mice and found the most genes in common at 16 weeks (158 genes) suggesting more rapid progression in the older mice (data not shown).

Table 3. Immunostaining results for Prelp, Type III collagen, and Fibromodulin.

Tissue	Prelp	Type III collagen	Fibromodulin
Ligaments	+++/++++	+	+/−
Periosteum	+++	+	+/−
Fibrous connective tissue	++	+	−
Articular cartilage chondrocytes	−	−	+/−
Articular cartilage matrix	+/−	++ (mainly pericellular matrix)	−
Meniscus chondrocytes	+/−	+	+/−
Meniscus matrix	+/− −	++ (mainly pericellular matrix)	+
Bone	−	−	−
Bone marrow	−	−	++
Growth plate chondrocytes	+/−	−	−
Growth plate matrix	+/−	+/−	+
Fibrocartilage	++	++ (mainly pericellular matrix of chondrocytes)	++
Skeletal muscle	−	+ (perimysium only)	+/−
Synovium	−	+++	+/++
Degenerate/fibrillated cartilage	++/+++	++	++
Vascular endothelium	−	++++ (also vessel wall)	−

Prelp = proline-arginine-rich end leucine-rich repeat protein. Sections from 3 DMM and 4 sham control animals at 16 weeks after surgery were graded on a scale from no immunopositivity (−) to marked immunopositivity (++++). The results presented are the consensus grades from all animals evaluated. The degenerate/fibrillated cartilage was only present in the DMM animals.

A phasic progression of OA was suggested by a previous study in humans where radiographic progression was related to changes in serial measures of serum COMP, as an OA biomarker [29]. Interestingly, we found that COMP, along with MMP-13, clustered with genes that were up-regulated during times of increased activity at 2, 4, and 16 weeks and were down-regulated at 8 weeks when activity was lowest. One potential explanation for a phasic process would be the maturation of osteophytes which have been proposed to stabilize the joint mechanics [30]. Our observation that chondrophytes had already formed by 2 weeks after surgery to destabilize the meniscus is consistent with the hypothesis that joint destabilization stimulates their formation.

Table 4. Real time PCR results for selected genes showing fold change in DMM joints relative to sham controls.

Time point	2 weeks		4 weeks		8 weeks		16 weeks	
Gene name	fold change	p value	fold change	p value	fold change	p value	fold change	p value
Adamts5	0.37	NS	0.26	NS	0.86	NS	0.96	NS
Aggrecan	2.53	NS	5.90	0.006	1.06	NS	2.00	NS
Asporin	1.45	NS	2.50	0.04	1.60	0.05	2.00	NS
Ccl21	1.48	NS	2.41	0.001	2.27	0.003	1.57	0.05
Ccr7	0.48	0.006	1.00	NS	1.83	0.05	1.00	NS
Cxcr7	2.43	NS	2.77	0.03	1.51	0.02	2.99	0.03
Col3	2.24	0.05	4.28	NS	1.93	NS	3.34	0.004
Col10	0.48	0.02	0.25	NS	1.75	NS	1.17	NS
Dkk 3	4.27	0.01	2.50	0.02	1.77	NS	2.50	NS
Htra1	1.39	NS	4.09	0.01	1.81	0.008	3.00	NS
Igf-1	1.88	NS	3.50	0.0004	3.00	0.002	3.00	0.008
IL33	1.50	NS	1.50	NS	1.61	0.05	1.88	NS
Mmp3	3.68	0.03	10.57	NS	2.32	0.007	2.22	NS
Mmp13	1.48	NS	2.00	NS	1.08	NS	1.46	NS
Periostin	4.48	NS	3.38	0.009	1.44	NS	1.75	NS
Sfrp2	2.92	0.01	2.81	0.002	1.56	0.01	1.29	NS
Average fold change	2.07		3.11		1.71		2.01	

Increased expression of Bmp-1, TGFβ2 and TGFβ3 at the early time points is also consistent with their presumed role in stimulating osteophyte formation [31]. The stabilization, however, appeared to be transient because cartilage loss was marked at 16 weeks and gene expression was increased relative to 8 weeks.

There are important limitations to the present study. Because RNA was not isolated from individual tissues it is not possible to determine which specific tissue (cartilage, bone, meniscus, ligament, synovium) contributed to the changes in gene expression. Also, if a gene is expressed in a single tissue, pooling of tissues will reduce the signal to a lower level than what would have been observed in the individual tissue. That is the likely explanation for the overall lower levels of gene expression observed in the present study when compared to work using a single tissue. Based on the immunostaining for type III collagen, fibromodulin, and Prelp, as well as immunostaining for IL-33, periostin, and CCL21 reported in our previous study [6], it appears that multiple joint tissues can be responsible for changes in gene expression consistent with the joint operating as an organ rather than as individual tissues. Therapeutic interventions for OA which target key processes occurring in multiple joint tissues rather than a single tissue should be more effective than those targeting a single tissue. Another limitation is that the DMM model may or may not reflect human OA disease pathogenesis. Certainly the histologic features in cartilage and bone are similar, but in human OA there may be more disease activity in the synovium than in the DMM model. Finally, we studied gene expression, and not protein production, and these do not always correlate. Immunohistochemical studies to assess changes at the protein level are not sensitive enough to detect differences noted at the level of gene expression, unless either the differences in expression are marked, or the protein being examined is only detected in diseased tissue and not in normal tissue.

Further studies will be needed to determine the importance of these findings for human OA. An important implication of the results is that the degree of response to an intervention given during a phasic process will depend on the timing of the intervention. Pre-clinical studies using animal models most often start the intervention at the same time or just after the start of the OA process while in human trials participants are likely to be at various stages of the disease process when the intervention is initiated. Finding markers of various disease stages in OA could be used to direct targeted therapy to the proper phase of the disease when the target is most active.

Supporting Information

Table S1 Filtering results for the sham time course.

Table S2 Filtering results for the DMM time course.

File S1 Excel file of 406 Sham filtered probe sets and DAVID results. Results are presented as signal log ratio (SLR) which is the $\log_2$ of the fold change and so an SLR of 0.5 = 1.4-fold. A positive number would be up-regulation and negative number down-regulation.

File S2 Excel file of 427 DMM filtered probe sets and DAVID results. Results are presented as signal log ratio as described for supplemental file 1.

File S3 Excel file of 97 common probe sets and DAVID results.

Acknowledgments

We thank Mary Zhao for technical assistance and the microarray core facility of the Comprehensive Cancer Center of Wake Forest University for performing the microarrays. We also thank Paula Overn in the Comparative Pathology Shared Resource of the Masonic Cancer Center, University of Minnesota, for developing the immunostaining protocols and preparing the immunohistochemistry sections.

Author Contributions

Conceived and designed the experiments: RFL ALO MAM CSC MC CF JSF. Performed the experiments: RFL ALO MAM CSC MC. Analyzed the data: RFL ALO MAM CSC JSF. Contributed reagents/materials/analysis tools: ALO JSF. Wrote the paper: RFL ALO MAM CSC MC CF JSF.

References

1. Lawrence RC, Felson DT, Helmick CG, Arnold LM, Choi H, et al. (2008) Estimates of the prevalence of arthritis and other rheumatic conditions in the United States: Part II. Arthritis Rheum 58: 26–35.
2. (2010) Prevalence of doctor-diagnosed arthritis and arthritis-attributable activity limitation --- United States, 2007–2009. MMWR Morb Mortal Wkly Rep 59: 1261–1265.
3. Blagojevic M, Jinks C, Jeffery A, Jordan KP (2010) Risk factors for onset of osteoarthritis of the knee in older adults: a systematic review and meta-analysis. Osteoarthritis Cartilage 18: 24–33.
4. Loeser RF, Goldring SR, Scanzello CR, Goldring MB (2012) Osteoarthritis: A disease of the joint as an organ. Arthritis Rheum 64: 1697–1707.
5. Glasson SS, Blanchet TJ, Morris EA (2007) The surgical destabilization of the medial meniscus (DMM) model of osteoarthritis in the 129/SvEv mouse. Osteoarthritis Cartilage 15: 1061–1069.
6. Loeser RF, Olex A, McNulty MA, Carlson CS, Callahan M, et al. (2012) Microarray analysis reveals age-related differences in gene expression during the development of osteoarthritis in mice. Arthritis Rheum 64: 705–717.
7. McNulty MA, Loeser RF, Davey C, Callahan MF, Ferguson CM, Carlson CS (2011) A comprehensive histological assessment of osteoarthritis lesions in mice. Cartilage 2: 354–363.
8. Chou JW, Paules RS, Bushel PR (2005) Systematic variation normalization in microarray data to get gene expression comparison unbiased. J Bioinform Comput Biol 3: 225–241.
9. Olex AL, Hiltbold EM, Leng X, Fetrow JS (2010) Dynamics of dendritic cell maturation are identified through a novel filtering strategy applied to biological time-course microarray replicates. BMC Immunol 11: 41.
10. Olex AL, Fetrow JS (2011) SC(2)ATmd: a tool for integration of the figure of merit with cluster analysis for gene expression data. Bioinformatics 27: 1330–1331.
11. Yeung KY, Haynor DR, Ruzzo WL (2001) Validating clustering for gene expression data. Bioinformatics 17: 309–318.
12. Huang DW, Sherman BT, Lempicki RA (2009) Systematic and integrative analysis of large gene lists using DAVID bioinformatics resources. Nat Protoc 4: 44–57.
13. Huang DW, Sherman BT, Lempicki RA (2009) Bioinformatics enrichment tools: paths toward the comprehensive functional analysis of large gene lists. Nucleic Acids Res 37: 1–13.
14. McNulty MA, Loeser RF, Davey C, Callahan MF, Ferguson CM, et al. (2012) Histopathology of naturally occurring and surgically induced osteoarthritis in mice. Osteoarthritis Cartilage 20: 949–956.
15. Kim JS, Ryoo ZY, Chun JS (2007) Cytokine-like 1 (Cytl1) regulates the chondrogenesis of mesenchymal cells. J Biol Chem 282: 29359–29367.
16. Wolff DA, Stevenson S, Goldberg VM (1992) S-100 protein immunostaining identifies cells expressing a chondrocytic phenotype during articular cartilage repair. J Orthop Res 10: 49–57.
17. Karlsson C, Dehne T, Lindahl A, Brittberg M, Pruss A, et al. (2010) Genome-wide expression profiling reveals new candidate genes associated with osteoarthritis. Osteoarthritis Cartilage 18: 581–592.
18. Embree MC, Kilts TM, Ono M, Inkson CA, Syed-Picard F, et al. (2010) Biglycan and fibromodulin have essential roles in regulating chondrogenesis and extracellular matrix turnover in temporomandibular joint osteoarthritis. Am J Pathol 176: 812–826.

19. Johnson K, Hashimoto S, Lotz M, Pritzker K, Goding J, et al. (2001) Up-regulated expression of the phosphodiesterase nucleotide pyrophosphatase family member PC-1 is a marker and pathogenic factor for knee meniscal cartilage matrix calcification. Arthritis Rheum 44: 1071–1081.
20. Bengtsson E, Neame PJ, Heinegard D, Sommarin Y (1995) The primary structure of a basic leucine-rich repeat protein, PRELP, found in connective tissues. J Biol Chem 270: 25639–25644.
21. Neame PJ, Tapp H, Azizan A (1999) Noncollagenous, nonproteoglycan macromolecules of cartilage. Cell Mol Life Sci 55: 1327–1340.
22. Jepsen KJ, Wu F, Peragallo JH, Paul J, Roberts L, et al. (2002) A syndrome of joint laxity and impaired tendon integrity in lumican- and fibromodulin-deficient mice. J Biol Chem 277: 35532–35540.
23. Wang Q, Rozelle AL, Lepus CM, Scanzello CR, Song JJ, et al. (2011) Identification of a central role for complement in osteoarthritis. Nat Med 17: 1674–1679.
24. Grover J, Lee ER, Mounkes LC, Stewart CL, Roughley PJ (2007) The consequence of PRELP overexpression on skin. Matrix Biol 26: 140–143.
25. Happonen KE, Furst CM, Saxne T, Heinegard D, Blom AM (2012) PRELP protein inhibits the formation of the complement membrane attack complex. J Biol Chem 287: 8092–8100.
26. Aigner T, Bertling W, Stoss H, Weseloh G, von der Mark K (1993) Independent expression of fibril-forming collagens I, II, and III in chondrocytes of human osteoarthritic cartilage. J Clin Invest 91: 829–837.
27. Fukui N, Ikeda Y, Ohnuki T, Tanaka N, Hikita A, et al. (2008) Regional differences in chondrocyte metabolism in osteoarthritis: A detailed analysis by laser capture microdissection. Arthritis Rheum 58: 154–163.
28. Young RD, Lawrence PA, Duance VC, Aigner T, Monaghan P (2000) Immunolocalization of collagen types II and III in single fibrils of human articular cartilage. J Histochem Cytochem 48: 423–432.
29. Sharif M, Kirwan JR, Elson CJ, Granell R, Clarke S (2004) Suggestion of nonlinear or phasic progression of knee osteoarthritis based on measurements of serum cartilage oligomeric matrix protein levels over five years. Arthritis Rheum 50: 2479–2488.
30. Pottenger LA, Phillips FM, Draganich LF (1990) The effect of marginal osteophytes on reduction of varus-valgus instability in osteoarthritic knees. Arthritis Rheum 33: 853–858.
31. Scharstuhl A, Glansbeek HL, Van Beuningen HM, Vitters EL, Van Der Kraan PM, et al. (2002) Inhibition of endogenous tgf-Beta during experimental osteoarthritis prevents osteophyte formation and impairs cartilage repair. J Immunol 169: 507–514.

13

Chondrocyte Deformations as a Function of Tibiofemoral Joint Loading Predicted by a Generalized High-Throughput Pipeline of Multi-Scale Simulations

Scott C. Sibole, Ahmet Erdemir*

Computational Biomodeling (CoBi) Core and Department of Biomedical Engineering Lerner Research Institute, Cleveland Clinic, Cleveland, Ohio, United States of America

Abstract

Cells of the musculoskeletal system are known to respond to mechanical loading and chondrocytes within the cartilage are not an exception. However, understanding how joint level loads relate to cell level deformations, e.g. in the cartilage, is not a straightforward task. In this study, a multi-scale analysis pipeline was implemented to post-process the results of a macro-scale finite element (FE) tibiofemoral joint model to provide joint mechanics based displacement boundary conditions to micro-scale cellular FE models of the cartilage, for the purpose of characterizing chondrocyte deformations in relation to tibiofemoral joint loading. It was possible to identify the load distribution within the knee among its tissue structures and ultimately within the cartilage among its extracellular matrix, pericellular environment and resident chondrocytes. Various cellular deformation metrics (aspect ratio change, volumetric strain, cellular effective strain and maximum shear strain) were calculated. To illustrate further utility of this multi-scale modeling pipeline, two micro-scale cartilage constructs were considered: an idealized single cell at the centroid of a $100\times100\times100$ μm block commonly used in past research studies, and an anatomically based (11 cell model of the same volume) representation of the middle zone of tibiofemoral cartilage. In both cases, chondrocytes experienced amplified deformations compared to those at the macro-scale, predicted by simulating one body weight compressive loading on the tibiofemoral joint. In the 11 cell case, all cells experienced less deformation than the single cell case, and also exhibited a larger variance in deformation compared to other cells residing in the same block. The coupling method proved to be highly scalable due to micro-scale model independence that allowed for exploitation of distributed memory computing architecture. The method's generalized nature also allows for substitution of any macro-scale and/or micro-scale model providing application for other multi-scale continuum mechanics problems.

Editor: Hani A. Awad, Cleveland Clinic, United States of America

Funding: Th[illegible] supported by the grant R01EB009643 provided by the National Institute of Biomedical Imaging and Bioengineering, National Institutes of Health (http://www.nibib.nih.gov/). The funders had no role in study design, data collection and analysis, decision to publish, or preparation of the manuscript.

Competing Interests: The authors have read the journal's policy and have the following conflicts: Ahmet Erdemir owns and operates innodof, LLC, a consulting company for modeling and simulation. Scott Sibole has declared that no competing interests exist. This does not alter the authors' adherence to all the PLoS ONE policies on sharing data and materials.

* E-mail: erdemira@ccf.org

Introduction

The phenomenon of cell behavior being directed by mechanical stimuli, referred to as mechanotransduction or mechanoregulation, as well as cell damage resulting from mechanical disruption, have been a topic of research in medicine and biology for several decades [1–3]. Often, research has been conducted at the spatial scale of the cell and its immediate extracellular environment. While cellular activity at the micro-scale alters the mechanical environment, loading transferred from higher spatial scales also plays a role [4]. For this reason, the search for a better understanding of multi-scale spatial interactions has become an increasingly desirable objective, in order to establish the causal mechanical relationships between the loading of joints, tissues, and cells.

In the field of biomechanics, a strong motivation to better understand the mechanics of articular cartilage exists [5]. This is due to the high prevalence of pathologies such as osteoarthritis (OA), which affects approximately 27 million adults in the United States [6] and can drastically reduce quality of life. The progression of OA exhibits changes in tissue structure [7–9], as well as changes in cellular (chondrocyte) distribution and behavior [10–14]. While these changes occur at the tissue or cellular scales, a general consensus exists that the loading of the joints likely plays a role in their onset. Even in the absence of pathology, cartilage may experience changes simply as a result of aging. As with OA, these changes occur at the tissue [15,16] and cellular scale [17,18]. In addition, modifications of joint-scale mechanics also occur with aging [19–21]. Clearly, cartilage mechanics is a multi-scale paradigm and a means to investigate the interplay between scales is crucial to extending the understanding of the *in vivo* function of this biological material.

While pathology and aging impact cartilage mechanics at multiple scales, before addressing such complexities, understanding the normal joint, tissue, and cellular mechanical behavior is necessary. Experimental acquisition of mechanical data, while attainable in animal studies [22], becomes more difficult as the spatial scale decreases. If one attempts to gather data at different spatial scales simultaneously under lifelike loading scenarios, e.g. synchronous measurement of joint level kinematics and/or kinetics and cell deformation, the present technology is inadequate. Computational modeling techniques provide an avenue to obtain additional insights about mechanics at various spatial scales. Further, passing information between models at different spatial scales allows for investigation of load transfer mechanisms.

Extensive research utilizing computational modeling, particularly finite element analysis (FEA), has been conducted at each of these individual spatial scales. At the tissue and cellular scale, complex constitutive models have been applied to simplified geometric and loading cases [23]. In contrast, at the joint scale, simpler material models were typically employed, allowing representation of complex geometry and physiological loading conditions to be considered [24]. Ultimately, relating models at both scales will provide insights about the mechanics a chondrocyte experiences *in vivo*.

An array of approaches can be taken to understand the mechanical coupling between joint function and chondrocyte response. Explicitly modeling the micro-scale components in the macro-scale model constitutes the method with the least abstraction. This approach is often used in the modeling of cancellous bone [25], but requires a tremendous finite element count for even small volumes. For the dimensions and added complexities of a joint, the computational cost is too excessive given current technology.

Computational homogenization, in which the material behavior at the macro-scale at each non-linear solution step is a result of the solution of a micro-scale model at every integration point in the macro-scale mesh, provides another avenue for relating spatial scales [26]. While still very computationally expensive, solutions can be obtained with this method [27], but for advanced problems, require access to large shared-memory architectures which are less common than distributed-memory platforms. It should also be noted that robust simulations using this method may not be possible since the failure of a single micro-scale model to converge, if not contained, results in the failure of the entire macro-scale solution.

Finally, a simple post-processing method can be employed. This involves first obtaining a solution of the macro-scale model, possibly using FEA. The deformation experienced by each finite element in this model can then be used to generate boundary conditions for an array of micro-scale models, which are then solved to determine the micro-scale response. While this provides a weaker coupling between scales than the previously described methods, and therefore must satisfy multiple assumptions about consistency between scales, it provides a unique advantage in that all models are independent or autonomous. This allows for exploitation of distributed-memory architectures which can provide tremendous computing power, since there is no need to communicate information between micro-scale models. Further, this approach is more robust in that, failure of a micro-scale model does not result in failure of the entire process. While the macro-scale mechanics are not a direct function of micro-scale response (as in computational homogenization), a post-processing pipeline would provide a cost-effective platform for descriptive analysis of cell deformations under different joint loading.

The post-processing approach, to relate joint mechanics to cell mechanics, was used to achieve the three-fold objective in this study: i) to establish a pipeline to post-process macro-scale finite element analysis results to estimate micro-scale cell deformations for desired macro-scale regions at a desired time point of macro-scale loading, ii) to illustrate the pipeline's utility through estimation of cell deformations in middle-zone cartilage for compressive loading of the tibiofemoral joint, and iii) to explore the differences in the results of multi-scale modeling of state-of-the-art and anatomically-based assumptions of cell distribution in a micro-scale volume.

Methods

The autonomous approach implemented in this study, involved a series of stages beginning with the FEA of a single macro-scale model at the joint scale, calculation of deformation gradients at element centroids, using these deformation gradients to prescribe boundary conditions for micro-scale models for each macro-scale element of interest, and finally, solving and post-processing many micro-scale models in parallel (Figure 1).

Macro-scale Model

A free and open access finite element representation of the tibiofemoral joint with modified material properties and boundary conditions (Open Knee version 1.0.0) was used to obtain a macro-scale solution [28]. The tibia, femur, medial collateral ligament (MCL), lateral collateral ligament (LCL), anterior cruciate ligament (ACL), posterior cruciate ligament (PCL), medial and lateral menisci, and femoral and tibial cartilage were represented (Figure 2A). All soft tissue structures were discretized with 56433 linear hexahedral (8 node) finite elements (Figure 3) and assigned hyperelastic material properties valid for finite strain, based on literature values (Table 1), while the bones were discretized with 25220 quadrilateral shell elements with a thickness of 1 mm and assumed to be rigid.

An uncoupled isotropic Mooney-Rivlin constitutive model was used to define articular cartilage [29]. Model parameters were assigned to agree with literature values for instantaneous (fast-loading) elastic modulus (10 MPa) [30] and to simulate nearly incompressible (Poisson's ratio of 0.48) behavior (Table 1). Ligaments [31–33] and menisci [34–36] were modeled as transversely isotropic with a Mooney-Rivlin ground substance and a piecewise non-linear fiber term [37] (Table 1).

Frictionless contact was defined between all soft tissue structures which may interface. The tibia was fixed in space for the entire solution time, while the femur was prescribed a distal (compressive) displacement of 2 mm linearly ramped from $time = 0 - 1s$ with flexion fixed. Displacement, rather than force, was prescribed as this was a better numerically conditioned problem. All other femoral degrees of freedom were free, allowing the femoral trajectory to be decided by the combined effects of soft tissue structures. Implicit dynamic analysis was conducted using FEBio version 1.4 [38]. A dynamic model was used to exploit the lumped mass matrix to condition the stiffness matrix at each non-linear time step and aid in model convergence. The deformed nodal positions were the outputs of the macro-scale model to be processed for multi-scale coupling.

Joint-scale to Cell-scale Mechanical Coupling

Mechanical coupling between spatial scales was achieved by passing deformation gradients occurring at the macro-scale to the micro-scale. The deformation gradient is a second-order tensor that maps a position vector from the undeformed state, X, to a deformed state, x. The undeformed and deformed nodal positions from the macro-scale model were used to calculate the deformation gradients occurring at element centroids for user-specified element sets at user-specified simulation times. For the current study, the results reported were for the tibial and femoral cartilage at a simulation time of $0.395s$. At this converged time point in the simulation, a compressive force of approximately $1\times$ specimen body weight ($780N$) occurred. The last converged time step in the macro-scale model was $0.4685s$, at which a compressive force of $1310N$ occurred. This solution set therefore allows for the potential consideration of up to nearly $1.7\times$ specimen body weight.

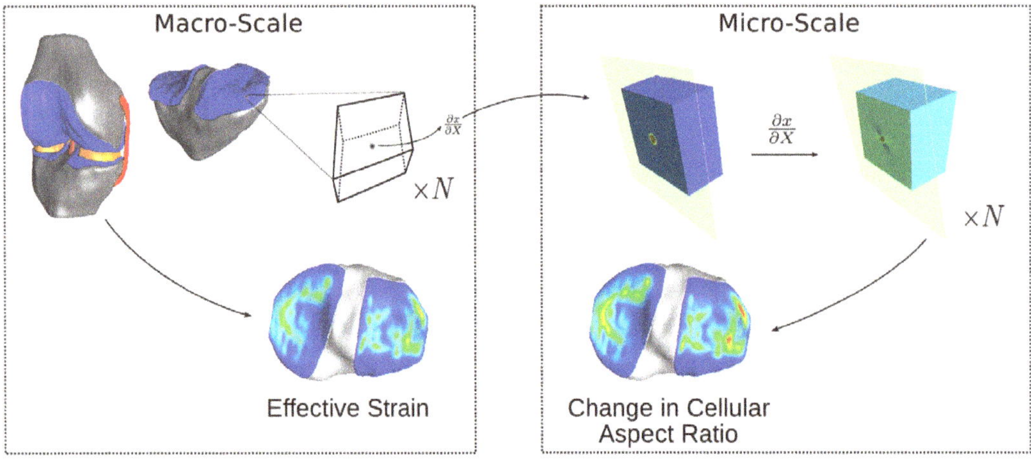

Figure 1. The autonomous approach to couple joint, tissue, and cell scales is shown above. Left: The method began with the FEA of a macro-scale model for a kinetic/kinematic scenario. Deformation gradients at the centroids of finite elements in tissue regions of interest were calculated from element nodal positions. Right: Displacement boundary conditions were prescribed to surface nodes of independent micro-scale models corresponding to the deformation gradient of each finite element experiencing deformation in tissue regions considered. Results of micro-scale FEA solutions were post-processed to calculate deformation metrics of interest.

Calculating the deformation gradient from the deformed nodal positions made use of the isoparametric formulation technique often employed in FEA. Briefly, this formulation maps an element in the global space to an element of idealized geometry where calculations can be performed in a simplified manner. To calculate the deformation gradient at the element centroids the following equations were evaluated.

$$\frac{\partial X_i}{\partial \xi_j} = \sum_{a=1}^{8} (\mathbf{X_a})_i \frac{\partial N_a}{\partial \xi_j} \tag{1}$$

$$\frac{\partial N_a}{\partial X_i} = \sum_{j=1}^{3} \left(\left[\frac{\partial X}{\partial \xi} \right]_{ij}^{-T} \frac{\partial N_a}{\partial \xi_j} \right) \tag{2}$$

$$F_{ij} = \sum_{a=1}^{8} (\mathbf{x_a})_i \frac{\partial N_a}{\partial X_j} \tag{3}$$

where, $\xi = [0,0,0]$ was the centroid position vector in the idealized geometry space, $\mathbf{X_a}$ were the undeformed nodal position vectors, N_a

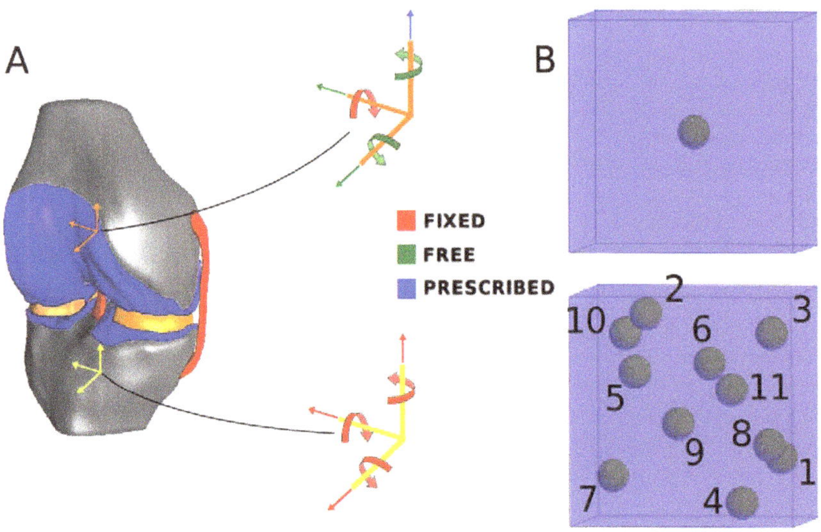

Figure 2. Macro and micro-scale models used in study. A. A model of the tibiofemoral joint was employed at the macro-scale. Boundary conditions were prescribed for the bones, modeled as rigid bodies, to approximate compressive loading of the joint. The tibia was fixed in space. Femoral compression was prescribed at fixed flexion with other degrees of freedom unconstrained. **B.** The single (top) and 11 cell (bottom) models. The single cell model was the popular scenario considered in previous studies [39], while the 11 cell model better represented the cell densities observed *in situ* for the middle layer of articular cartilage in the knee [40].

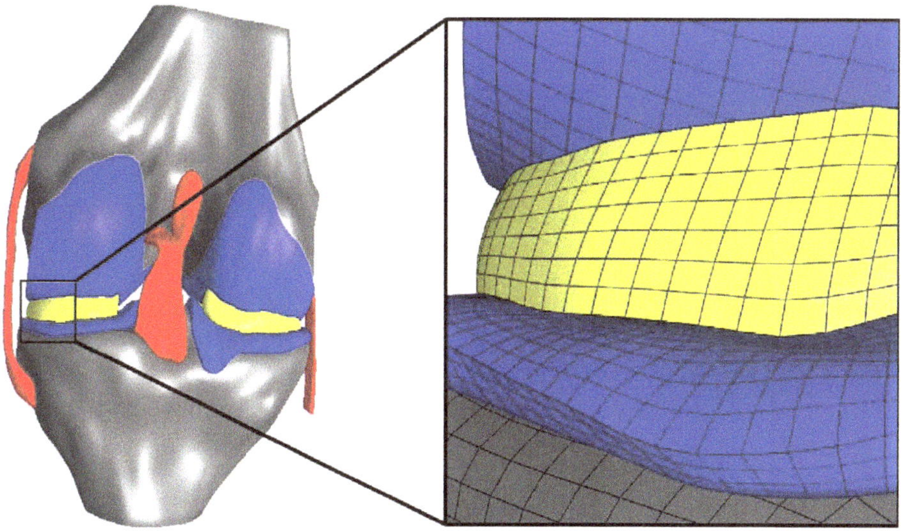

Figure 3. A finite element model of the tibiofemoral joint with representation of ACL, PCL, MCL, LCL, tibial and femoral cartilage, lateral and medial menisci, femur, and tibia. Soft tissue structures were discretized with 56433 linear hexahedral finite elements with an average edge length of approximately 1mm. The bones were discretized with 25220 quadrilateral shell elements with an assigned thickness of 1 mm. An enlarged model region is shown on the right to illustrate the mesh resolution. The femoral and tibial cartilage each had 3 hexahedral elements through their thickness.

were the trilinear nodal shape functions, $\mathbf{x_a}$ were the deformed nodal position vectors, X was the position vector of the element in the global space corresponding to the point in the idealized space, ξ, and F_{ij} was the deformation gradient. The deformation gradients calculated from Equation 3 were used to prescribe boundary conditions for each micro-scale model.

Micro-scale Models

Micro-scale model input decks for elements that experienced deformation (characterized by having a deformation gradient that varied from the identity tensor by greater than ± 0.01 in any component) were generated. A total of 7882 elements in the tibial and femoral cartilage were above this threshold and warranted model generation. Two micro-scale cases were considered: a single cell and an 11 cell configuration (Figure 2B). In the single cell case, a spherical cell (of radius 5 μm) surrounded by a pericellular matrix (PCM) (of thickness 2.5 μm) located at the centroid of a $100 \times 100 \times 100$ μm block of extracellular matrix (ECM), similar to previous studies [39], was considered. For the 11 cell case, cells and PCMs of the same dimension as the single cell configuration were randomly positioned in the ECM block, with the constraint that all chondrons (chondrocyte + PCM) were separated by at least 2.5 μm (equivalent to pericellular matrix thickness) and were at least 1.25 μm from the outer boundary. Eleven cells corresponded to the mean number of cells that occur in a block of middle layer tibiofemoral articular cartilage of this size [40]. Materials were defined with an uncoupled Mooney-Rivlin constitutive model with values from [41] adjusted to approximately satisfy mechanical consistency across spatial scales (Table 2). This was achieved by assigning the ECM, which comprises 99.5% and 94.2% of the construct volume for the single and 11 cell cases, respectively, identical properties to that of the cartilage in the macro-scale model. Previous studies have reported the PCM may have a strain amplification/attenuation effect on the cell due to the stiffness mismatch between ECM, PCM, and cell [42–44]. Therefore, the cell and PCM properties were scaled to maintain the same ratios as values reported in [41].

The nodes on the six faces of the ECM block were prescribed displacement boundary conditions, u_i, derived from the application of the macro-scale element deformation gradients, F, to their undeformed position vectors, X (Equation 4).

Table 1. Material parameters for articular cartilage [30], ligaments [31–33], and meniscus [34–46].

	ρ	c_1	c_2	c_3	c_4	c_5	K	λ^*
Cartilage	**1.5e3**	**1.6892**	**0**	**-**	**-**	**-**	**83.3333**	**-**
ACL	**1.5e3**	**1.95**	**0**	**0.0139**	**116.22**	**535.039**	**73.2**	**1.046**
PCL	**1.5e3**	**3.25**	**0**	**0.1196**	**87.178**	**431.063**	**122**	**1.035**
MCL	**1.5e3**	**1.44**	**0**	**0.57**	**48**	**467.1**	**397**	**1.063**
LCL	**1.5e3**	**1.44**	**0**	**0.57**	**48**	**467.1**	**397**	**1.063**
Meniscus	**1.5e3**	**4.6115**	**0**	**0.12**	**150**	**400**	**227.5**	**1.02**

Units: $\rho = \frac{kg}{m^3}$; $c_1, c_2, c_3, c_5, K = MPa$; $c_4, \lambda^* = unitless$.

Table 2. Material parameters for micro-scale model [41].

	c_1	c_2	K
ECM	1.6892	0	83.3333
PCM	0.6838	0	1.0570
Cell	0.0405	0	1.9980

Units: $c_1, c_2, K = MPa$.

$$u_i = \sum_{j=1}^{3} (F_{ij}X_j) - X_i \tag{4}$$

Micro-scale models were solved using implicit static analysis in FEBio version 1.4. For verification, a mesh convergence study was conducted for the single cell geometry subjected to −30% nominal strain in the z-dimension with free lateral (x- and y-dimensions) expansion boundary conditions (in other words, unconfined uniaxial loading). The maximum effective strain and maximum shear strain that occurred in the model changed by 3.6% and 1.9%, respectively, when the mesh was increased from 15168 to 25889 linear hexahedral elements. Therefore, the 25889 element model (Figure 4) was assumed to be mesh-converged. The 77880 hexahedral element model of the 11 cell geometry was assumed to be mesh-converged because the cells and PCMs had the same mesh densities as the converged single cell case, 9 elements across the cell diameter and 2 elements through the PCM thickness, and the ECM had higher density.

Micro-scale Model Deformation Analysis

To quantify the deformation of cells in the micro-scale models, the volume-averaged effective (von Mises) strain, effective stress, and maximum shear strain, as well as, the initial and deformed aspect ratios were calculated for the cell, by operations on the stress and strain tensors generated by the model simulations for each element. Cell level deformation metrics required volume-averaging across the cell. Undeformed (V_e^0) and deformed (V_e) element volumes within the cells were used for volume-averaging. The undeformed element volumes were determined from nodal positions read from the micro-scale mesh definition file. Likewise, the deformed nodal positions, the result of the undeformed nodal positions plus the nodal displacement vector, were used to calculate the deformed element volumes. The mesh definition file also contained element sets, which were used to define micro-scale sub-regions e.g. the cell(s). The volume of each element, e, in the mesh was calculated with Equation 5,

$$V_e = v_e det(J_e) \tag{5}$$

where, J_e were the Jacobian matrices evaluated at each element centroid (the determinants of which were the volume ratios) and v_e were the isoparametric element volumes. For the hexahedral case, the isoparametric element was defined as a $2 \times 2 \times 2$ cube (with the same units as the model units), thus v_e was always $8\,\text{mm}^3$. The Jacobian matrix maps the isoparametric space ξ to the global or model space, X. Element volume was calculated in this manner for both the deformed cases as well as the undeformed case.

Change in cell volume. Volumetric strain for each cell was calculated by Equation 6.

$$\epsilon_v = \frac{\sum_e V_e}{\sum_e V_e^0} - 1 \tag{6}$$

where, V_e^0 was the undeformed volume of element e in the cell.

Change in cellular aspect ratio. The shape(s) of the cell(s) was calculated by assembling the moment of inertia tensor for the finite elements contained in the cellular subsets. With the assumption of unit density, the moment of inertia tensor, **I**, was calculated with Equation 7,

$$\mathbf{I} = \sum_e V_e \begin{vmatrix} (y_e^2 + z_e^2) & -x_e y_e & -x_e z_e \\ -y_e x_e & (x_e^2 + z_e^2) & -y_e z_e \\ -z_e x_e & -z_e y_e & (x_e^2 + y_e^2) \end{vmatrix} \tag{7}$$

where, e was each finite element belonging to a cell set, V_e was the element volume, and x_e, y_e, and z_e were the components of the element centroid position vector.

The eigenvalues, λ_i in descending order, of this tensor correspond to the principal moments of inertia which can be related to the length of the axes of the ellipsoid of best fit for the object's shape, L_i, via Equation 8 [45].

$$L_i = \frac{1}{\sqrt{\lambda_i}} \tag{8}$$

Three aspect ratios were measured: $\kappa_{31} = \frac{L_3}{L_1}$, $\kappa_{32} = \frac{L_3}{L_2}$, and $\kappa_{21} = \frac{L_2}{L_1}$, the major-minor, major-middle, and middle-minor axes ratios, respectively. The change in cellular aspect ratio was then taken as the difference between the undeformed and deformed aspect ratios.

Stress and strain metrics. The effective stress and strain were positive definite scalar values calculated from the Cauchy stress and Green-Lagrange strain tensors via Equation 9,

$$\psi = \sqrt{\frac{1}{2}\left[(\lambda_1 - \lambda_2)^2 + (\lambda_2 - \lambda_3)^2 + (\lambda_3 - \lambda_1)^2\right]} \tag{9}$$

where, λ_i are the eigenvalues of the stress or strain tensor in descending order. These eigenvalues correspond to the principal stresses or strains.

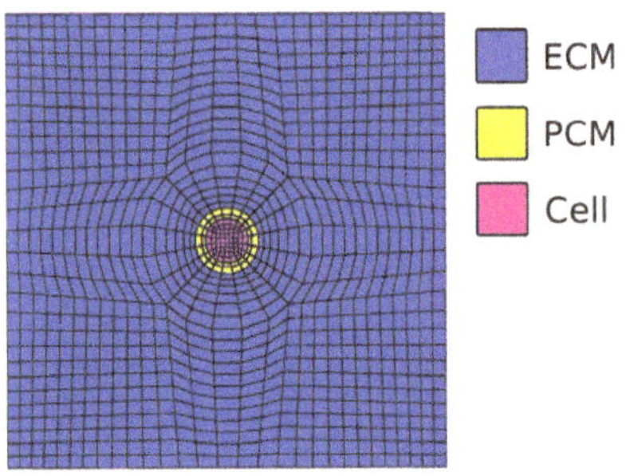

Figure 4. A cross-section of the 25889 finite element mesh of the single cell micro-scale case, which was determined to be mesh-converged. The extracellular matrix (ECM), pericellular matrix (PCM), and chondrocyte (Cell) were discretized with linear hexahedral elements. The chondrocyte had 9 elements across its diameter and the pericellular matrix had 2 elements through its thickness. For the eleven cell case, the chondrocyte and pericellular matrix had the same mesh densities.

Likewise, maximum shear strain, calculated by Equation 10, was also positive definite, and scalar.

$$\psi = max\{ |\lambda_2 - \lambda_3| \quad |\lambda_3 - \lambda_1| \quad |\lambda_1 - \lambda_2| \} \tag{10}$$

Since these metrics were positive definite scalars, volume-averaging was valid for a set of finite elements. This was performed for the cell(s), PCM, and ECM as follows:

$$\bar{\psi} = \frac{\sum_e V_e \psi_e}{\sum_e V_e} \tag{11}$$

where, V_e and ψ_e were the deformed volume and stress or strain metrics for each finite element contained in the respective set.

Parallelization

Since all micro-scale models were independent; generation, solution, and analysis of them could be performed easily on a distributed memory computational platform. All micro-scale computational work for this study was performed on Ohio Supercomputer Center's Glenn Cluster (http://www.osc.edu), which provides up to 9572 compute cores, ranging in frequencies of 2.4–2.6 GHz, offering a peak performance of more than 75 teraflops. A collection of Python and shell scripts were used to generate, solve with FEBio, and analyze a unique micro-scale model for each finite element experiencing deformation in the middle layer of tibial and femoral cartilage. 7882 model generation, solution, and analysis processes were divided between 101 compute threads, with 78 process sets carried out in serial on 100 threads and 82 on the 101st thread. The pipeline completed in a wall-clock time of approximately 2 hours for the single cell case and 19 hours for the 11 cell case. These corresponded to CPU times of approximately 8.4 and 72.3 days, respectively; demonstrating the importance of parallelization.

Results

The FEA solution of the tibiofemoral joint model under 1× body weight compression (780*N*), resulted in strain distributions with concentrations under the menisci-cartilage interfaces for both tibial and femoral cartilage (Figure 5A). The cell(s) in both the single cell and 11 cell models experienced amplified deformation when compared to the macro-scale finite element deformation which drove the mechanics at the micro-scale model exterior. This was expected due to the large mismatch in micro-scale component material properties, i.e. cells being softer than their surrounding medium, resulting in inhomogeneous deformation occurring in the interior. Although the magnitudes were different, the regional distribution of deformation was similar to that which occurred at the macro-scale (Figure 5B and 5C).

The change in cellular aspect ratio, $\Delta\kappa_{31}$, was linearly proportional to the macro-scale effective strain for both the single cell and 11 cell cases, with the 11 cell case consistently lower for all cells than the single cell case (Figure 6). In both configurations, the data spread increased as the corresponding macro-scale deformation increased, with the effect magnified in the 11 cell case. This behavior can be quantified by considering the sum of squares of residuals (SSR) attained for the linear fits. A greater SSR value indicates a larger spread (Table 3).

Regardless of the presentation of the results in the form of linear relationships between macro-scale and micro-scale, the micro-scale solutions had an inhomogeneous strain distribution internally. This was of particular interest when comparing single and 11 cell configurations, where cellular proximity altered distribution in the 11 cell models (Figure 7). A more detailed look to cell deformation metrics for this specific case of macroscopic deformation also illustrated that magnitudes of individual cell deformations may differ, potentially based on their location (Table 4). As described in the methods, deformation metrics were also obtained for the ECM and PCM. These results, although not presented, may have utility when investigating matrix damage mechanisms.

Discussion

The method employed in this study was a preliminary step toward the realization of relating joint level mechanics to the mechanics of the cellular environment. While a similar method has been employed for simplified tissue geometries at a small subset of spatial coordinates [46], to the best of the authors' knowledge, this was the first study which investigated large tissue regions, and considered anatomically-based geometry (both at macro- and micro-scales). This provided coarse insight into how cells may be deforming *in situ*.

Some notable observations were made in comparison of single and 11 cell micro-scale models. In both cases, the deformations determined at the macro-scale, when applied to the micro-scale, resulted in amplified deformations of the cell(s). This behavior was expected, because the chondrocytes were much softer than the surrounding ECM. However, every cell in the 11 cell model experienced smaller deformations for a given macro-scale deformation than the single cell model did. If one considers a simple 1D analogy of springs in series to model the ECM-chondron composites, the addition of more soft springs, as is the case in the 11 cell model, would result in less displacement occurring in each of the soft springs when displacement is prescribed at the series ends. Extending this to 3D supports the model results. This strain-shielding trend in the 11 cell models may suggest that the single cell case provides an upper bound for the observed macro-micro deformation amplification. Cells within the 11 cell models also experienced different deformation from one another. Although the cell positions were assigned randomly for this model without input from histological observation other than cell count, it is conceivable that, in reality, cells within the middle layer of cartilage do not experience the same mechanics, and the resolution of this variance may be at the order of several microns. The proximity of chondrocytes to each other may have dictated their mechanics. While an analysis was not specifically conducted to explore the relationship between cell-to-cell distance and intercellular mechanical interaction; this study, through macro-to-micro response metrics (Figure 6), supported by a comparison of single and 11 cell model results for a specific macroscopic deformation (Figure 7 and Table 4), indicates that such an influence may exist. This is certainly an important issue to address in the future where evaluation of single cell mechanics within a large group may be a necessity.

In spite of using simplified geometries (at the micro-scale) and constitutive models (i.e. non-linear, isotropic elastic rather than anisotropic, poroelastic), this study presented opportunities to make several observations from a mechano-biological perspective. Elongation of cells of 10% has been shown to induce catabolic processes in SW1353 chondrocyte-like cells, while 5% was not shown to have an effect [47]. These elongations correspond to aspect ratio changes (major-minor) of approximately 0.154 and 0.024 respectively. Given the low femoral compressive force of 1 ×

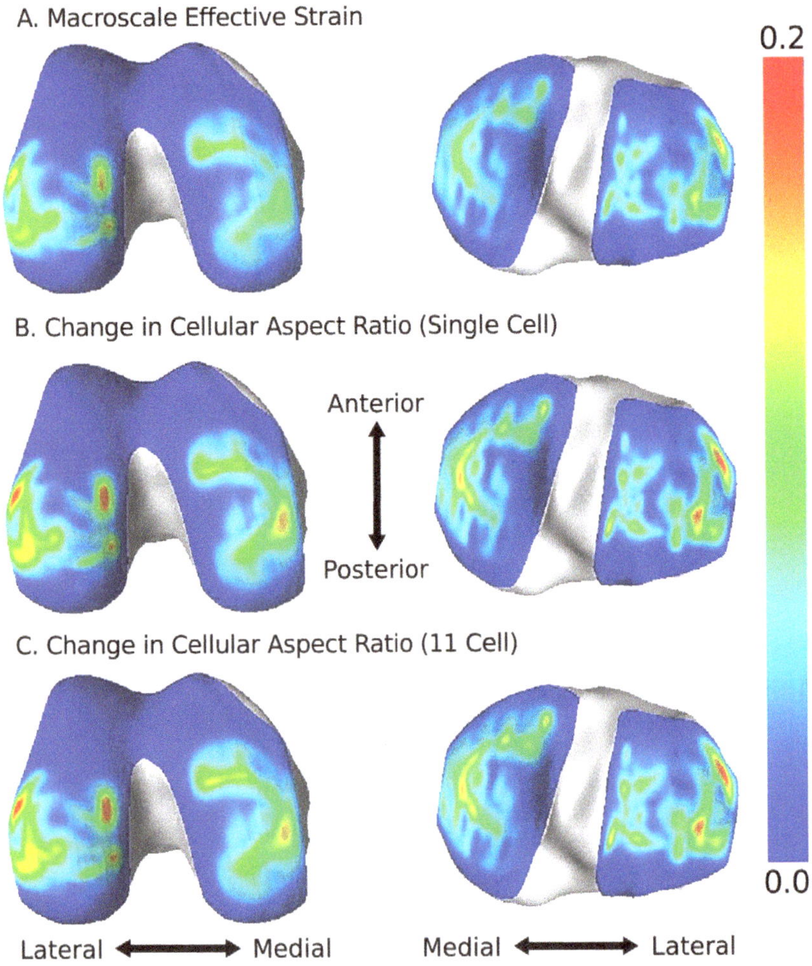

Figure 5. Fringe plots showing macro-scale and micro-scale deformation metric regional distributions in the middle layer of cartilage of the femur (left) and tibia (right). A. The effective strain which occurred at the macro-scale. **B**. The change in cellular aspect ratio (major-minor) calculated for the single cell model. **C**. The maximum change in cellular aspect ratio (major-minor) experienced by a cell in the 11 cell model.

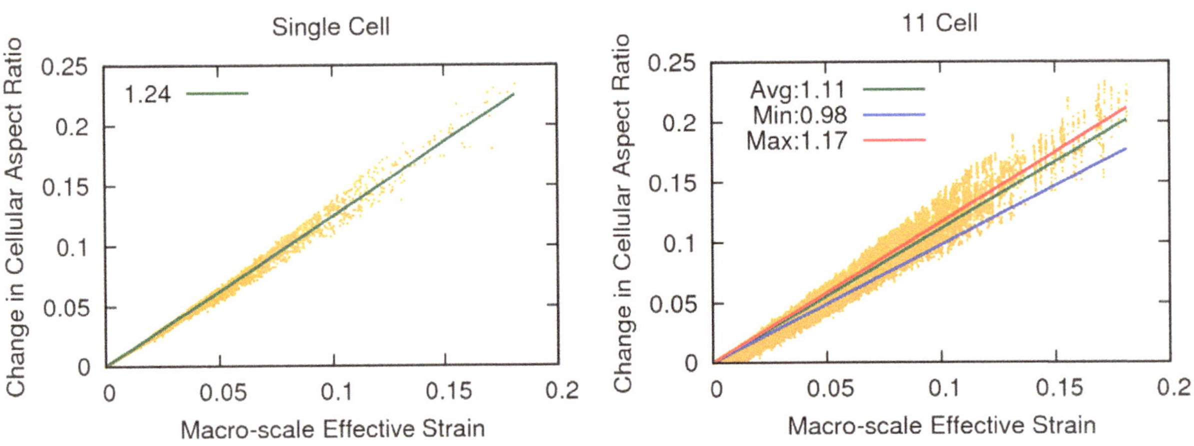

Figure 6. The change in cellular aspect ratio measured in each micro-scale model for the single cell (left) and 11 cell (right) cases was plotted as a function of macro-scale effective strain occurring at the corresponding finite element. The solid lines were linear least-squares regressions performed with the requirement that the lines passed through the origin. The slopes of each of these lines were provided in the legend. In the 11 cell case, the line labeled "Max" considered only data from the cell which experienced the greatest change in aspect ratio. Likewise, the line labeled "Min" was the cell which experienced the least change in aspect ratio, and the "Avg" was the average of the linear regressions for all 11 cells. These slopes indicated the distribution of the 11 cell change in aspect ratios was skewed left.

Table 3. Linear regression slopes and sum of squared residuals of single and 11 cell cases for change in cellular aspect ratio vs macro-scale effective strain.

	Single Cell	11 Cell Average	11 Cell Minimum	11 Cell Maximum
Slope	1.2429	1.1119	0.9765	1.1652
SSR	0.0513	0.1718	0.0949	0.1986

body weight prescribed in this study, in comparison to, the 3 × body weight or greater joint distal forces typically observed during walking [48], one would not expect cellular deformations to occur which may induce catabolic processes, yet changes in aspect ratios greater than 0.154 were observed. This indicated a limitation in the modeling at the macro-scale, micro-scale, or likely both, potentially related to the suitability of macro- and/or micro-scale material representations.

Modeling the material behavior of the macro-scale cartilage as too soft would be an obvious source of over-prediction of deformation. If this is the case in this study, the predicted macro-scale cartilage deformations, which would be necessary to equilibrate the desired level of joint loading, would be larger than expected. This will in turn result in higher chondrocyte deformations. Likewise, adjusting the PCM and cell stiffnesses will also have strong influence on the cellular deformation. The material properties assigned to the ECM, PCM, and cell were taken from a numerical study that optimized the PCM modulus to agree with experimental observation. The optimized PCM modulus found in this study resulted in a 2.11 ratio (cell/ECM) of effective strain, which varied from the experimentally observed ratio by 0.5% [41]. For the current study, the optimized material properties reported by [41] were scaled while maintaining the same ratios, and the case of multiple cells was considered. To assess potential sources of error due to this scaling, a simple sensitivity study was conducted in which the eleven cell model was subjected to a nominal compressive strain of 10% with volume-preserving lateral expansion for substantially different ECM properties: 1) $c_1 = 0.0268$ MPa, $K = 0.25$ MPa [41], 2) $c_1 = 1.6892$ MPa, $K = 83.3333$ MPa [reported study], 3) $c_1 = 16.8919$ MPa, $K = 833.3333$ MPa [reported study × 10]) while maintaining equivalent stiffness ratios between components. Additionally, a case in which the PCM stiffness reported in Table 2 was reduced by a factor of 10, 4) $c_1 = 0.0684$ MPa, $K = 0.1057$ MPa, while the other components were unchanged, was considered. The quartile analysis of the ratios of the average effective strain occurring in the ECM vs that occurring in each cell for these four cases are presented in Figure 8. The scaling of the material properties from those reported in [41] to those used in this study resulted in small changes in cellular deformation, indicating the scaling approach did not necessarily influence the amplification of macro-scale strains on the cells. Likewise, scaling the material properties by an additional factor of 10, resulted in little change. In contrast, reducing the PCM stiffness by tenfold resulted in a decrease in cellular effective strain, in agreement with the trends observed in [41].

For informative results, computational models should ideally employ anatomical geometry, realistic constitutive representations, and physiological joint loading. In addition, simulation results should be confirmed by comparisons against experimental studies. This study provided an adequate representation of anatomy at both joint and cell levels. The use of constitutive models that capture the anisotropic, lamellar, and poroelastic behavior of cartilage at the macro-scale would likely alter the strain distribution and magnitude within the tissue. While these complicated material models have commonly been employed at the micro-scale [23], their advent was quite recent at the joint scale. These state-of-the-art joint models incur high computational cost, and are currently only capable of simulating loads smaller than those observed *in vivo* [49], and also lower than forces

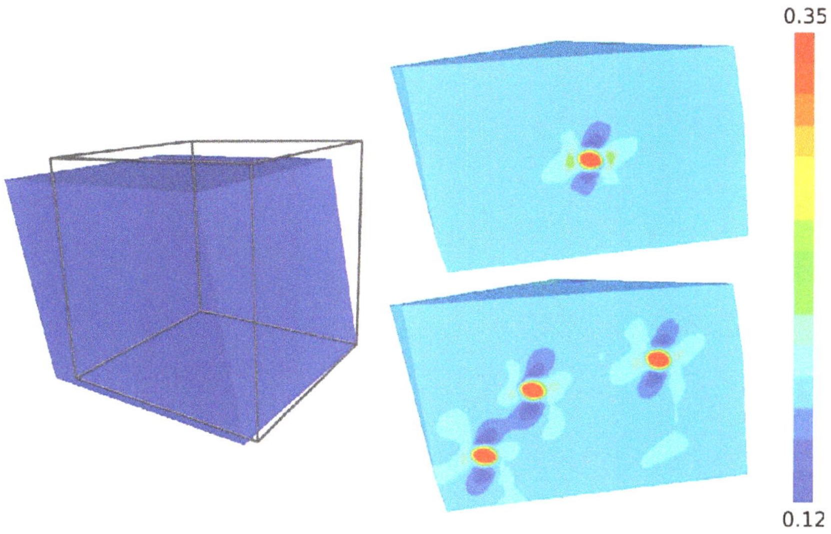

Figure 7. An example of the internal effective strain distributions observed in a single (top right) and 11 cell (bottom right) micro-scale solution for the same deformation gradient passed from the macro-scale (left). A macro-scale finite element experienced a combined loading deformation gradient which resulted in a shape change from the gray cube to the blue hexahedron shown on the left. The single and 11 cell models were deformed in the same way with the resulting effective strain distributions in a cross-section of the model shown on the right. While the cells experienced qualitatively similar strains in both cases, the strain in the ECM around the cells in the 11 cell model differed from the single cell in regions of close cellular proximity. See Table 4 for cell-specific quantitative results.

Table 4. Chondrocyte deformation metric set for a single and eleven cell model with boundary conditions prescribed via a specific deformation gradient passed from the macro-scale.

Cell ID	Δ Aspect Ratio	Volumetric Strain	Effective Strain	Maximum Shear Strain	Effective Stress
Single	0.226	−0.130	0.341	0.197	1.028
Cell 1	0.215	−0.108	0.334	0.193	0.301
Cell 2	0.200	−0.100	0.314	0.181	0.270
Cell 3	0.202	−0.100	0.317	0.183	0.272
Cell 4	0.196	−0.096	0.309	0.178	0.276
Cell 5	0.224	−0.113	0.345	0.199	0.311
Cell 6	0.220	−0.111	0.339	0.196	0.306
Cell 7	0.218	−0.110	0.336	0.193	0.302
Cell 8	0.216	−0.109	0.334	0.193	0.300
Cell 9	0.220	−0.111	0.338	0.195	0.304
Cell 10	0.212	−0.107	0.329	0.190	0.293
Cell 11	0.216	−0.109	0.334	0.193	0.301
Mean ± SD	0.213±0.009	−0.107±0.006	0.330±0.011	0.190±0.007	0.294±0.015

See Figure 7 for visualization and Figure 2B for the location of individual cells within the eleven cell model.

employed in this study. In addition to material assumptions, the loading conditions utilized in this study, while large in magnitudes, were not necessarily physiological, i.e. representative of gait. Joint scale models driven by physiological dynamics exist, but these must employ simplified material models, like those used in this study, and revert to explicit time integration for speed and robustness [50]. The highly non-linear behavior of cartilage, when modeled accurately, may be better suited for implicit time integration and the non-linear solution convergence checks it bestows. Currently, even at the single spatial scale of joints,

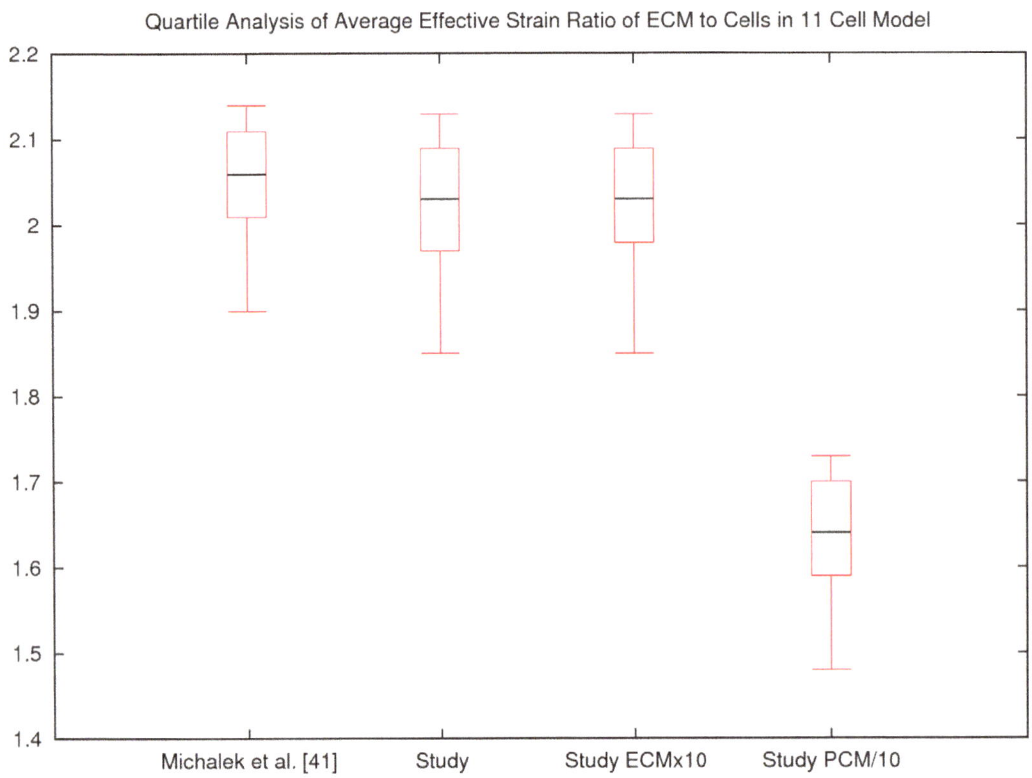

Figure 8. The quartile analyses of the ratios of average cellular effective strain to extracellular matrix (ECM) effective strain for the four cases considered in the material sensitivity study of the 11 cell model are shown above. In agreement with [41], scaling of material properties while maintaining ratio (Study and Study ×10) does not strongly impact chondrocyte deformation, but modifying the stiffness ratio between micro-scale components, i.e. by decreasing pericellular matrix stiffness by tenfold (Study PCM/10), does.

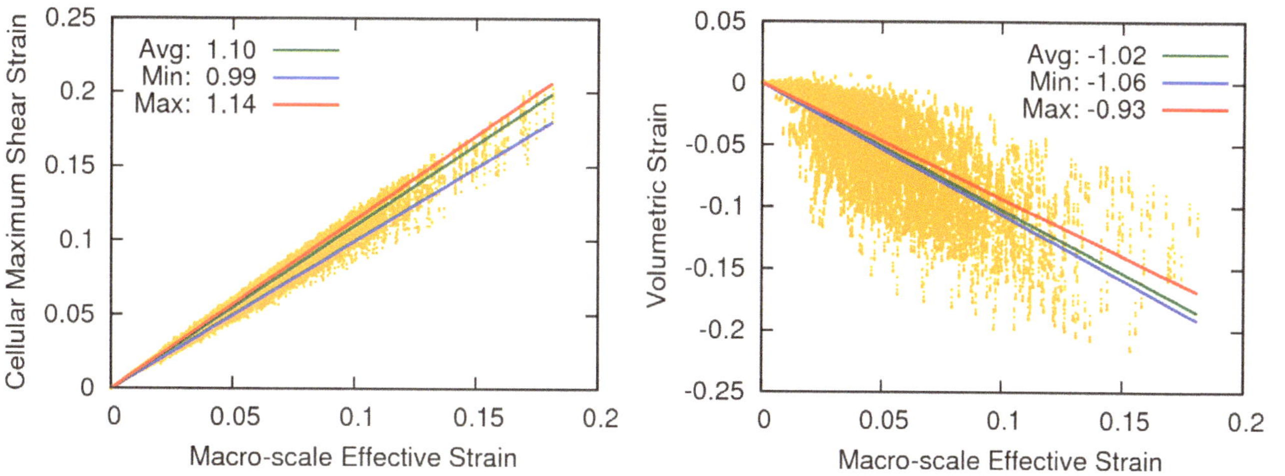

Figure 9. The volume-averaged maximum shear strain (left) and volumetric strain (right) for the 11 cell model plotted against the macro-scale effective strain. Deformation metrics such as those shown here, may have additional implications to understand cellular damage mechanisms as well as the onset of mechano-biological function, which change in aspect ratio may not provide. For example, pure cell dilation will result in a volumetric strain, but not a change in aspect ratio. The large bandwidth of the volumetric strain also suggests that a direct linear relationship between the macro- and micro-scales may not be acceptable for all characterizations of deformation.

modeling and simulation studies employing both physiologically accurate constitutive behavior and lifelike loading do not seem to be available.

As in any modeling study, verification and validation are necessary. The micro-scale models were verified through a mesh convergence study, but were not validated against an experimental study. In contrast, a mesh convergence study was not performed on the macro-scale model. However, a previous study found tibial and femoral cartilage modeled with elastic material properties converged with an approximate linear hexahedral element edge length of 2 mm [51]. Therefore, the cartilage mesh used in this study, with an approximate element edge length of 1 mm, was assumed sufficient for elastic analysis. Adequate validation of biological structures at any scale; joint, tissue, or cellular, presents substantial challenges. In addition, the further complication of multi-scale coupling exacerbates the difficulty. The macro-scale model was weakly validated through assessing its ability to reproduce experimentally-observed joint kinematics [52], but this level of validation was not ultimately sufficient to the aspects of this study which were dependent on the strain distribution within the tissue rather than joint kinematics. Contact pressure, which can better reflect the internal strain state, is an obtainable measure [53], but in addition to added experimental difficulty, the introduction of measurement devices may modify the mechanics of the joint. Predictions of large chondrocyte deformations under one body weight suggests that further validation of the multi-scale modeling strategy may be necessary. While a direct validation to confirm chondrocyte deformations in the human knee, under physiological loading, may not be possible; recent animal studies may provide possible avenues to establish confidence in the multi-scale modeling approach presented in this study. For example, a recent application of multi-photon confocal microscopy quantified chondrocyte deformation *in situ* while an intact joint of a mouse was subjected to physiological muscle loading [22].

Change in aspect ratio has often been employed as the metric to evaluate deformation in experimentation [45]. Nonetheless, other variables of interest, such as those related to shear and volumetric strains, may have significant value to understand cellular damage mechanisms as well as thresholds of mechano-biological function. This modeling pipeline has the capacity to summarize such variables, as illustrated by Figure 9, showing cellular volumetric strain and maximum shear strain exhibited by cells of the eleven cell model.

This study also provided a large database of input-output relationships between macro-scale and micro-scale mechanics. The slopes obtained from linear regression analysis of this data provide a direct proportionality constant to relate mechanics obtained at the macro-scale to the deformation the chondrocytes may experience, with the uncertainty in that relationship quantifiable by the residuals of the fit. In addition, this database contained loading states which were a direct result of joint mechanics. While a similar database may be obtained with either idealized interval stepping through a series of deformation gradients or through the solution of a stochastic set of deformation gradient applied boundary conditions, the former may not capture all loading states which may possibly occur, while the latter may introduce states which may not occur *in situ*. This database was specific to the joint-level case of vertical compression of 1 × body weight. It could be repeated for another joint scenario i.e. stair-climbing, to obtain another activity-specific database. The collection of these databases can provide a widely applicable surrogate model, i.e. analogous to approaches used in coupling of movement and tissue deformation simulations [54], to efficiently relate macro-micro scale mechanics without the need to perform micro-scale analyses.

The pipeline developed was proven to be highly scalable allowing for reasonably fast solution of the multi-scale problem. Since iterative multi-scale communications were not required during the processing and analysis stages of the many micro-scale simulations, the network overhead only involved movement of files to and from each parallel node at the beginning and end of the generation, solution, and analysis process. It was therefore, fair to hypothesize that this method, although tested on 101 parallel threads, should scale well to thousands of threads. This scalability will prove invaluable when more complex micro-scale models or a larger array of macro-scale elements are considered.

Only passing the deformation gradient at the macro-scale finite element centroids potentially introduced error. A hexahedral finite element can deform such that the deformation gradient is non-uniform across its volume. Depending on the mode of loading, this variation could be high, and sampling only at the macro-scale

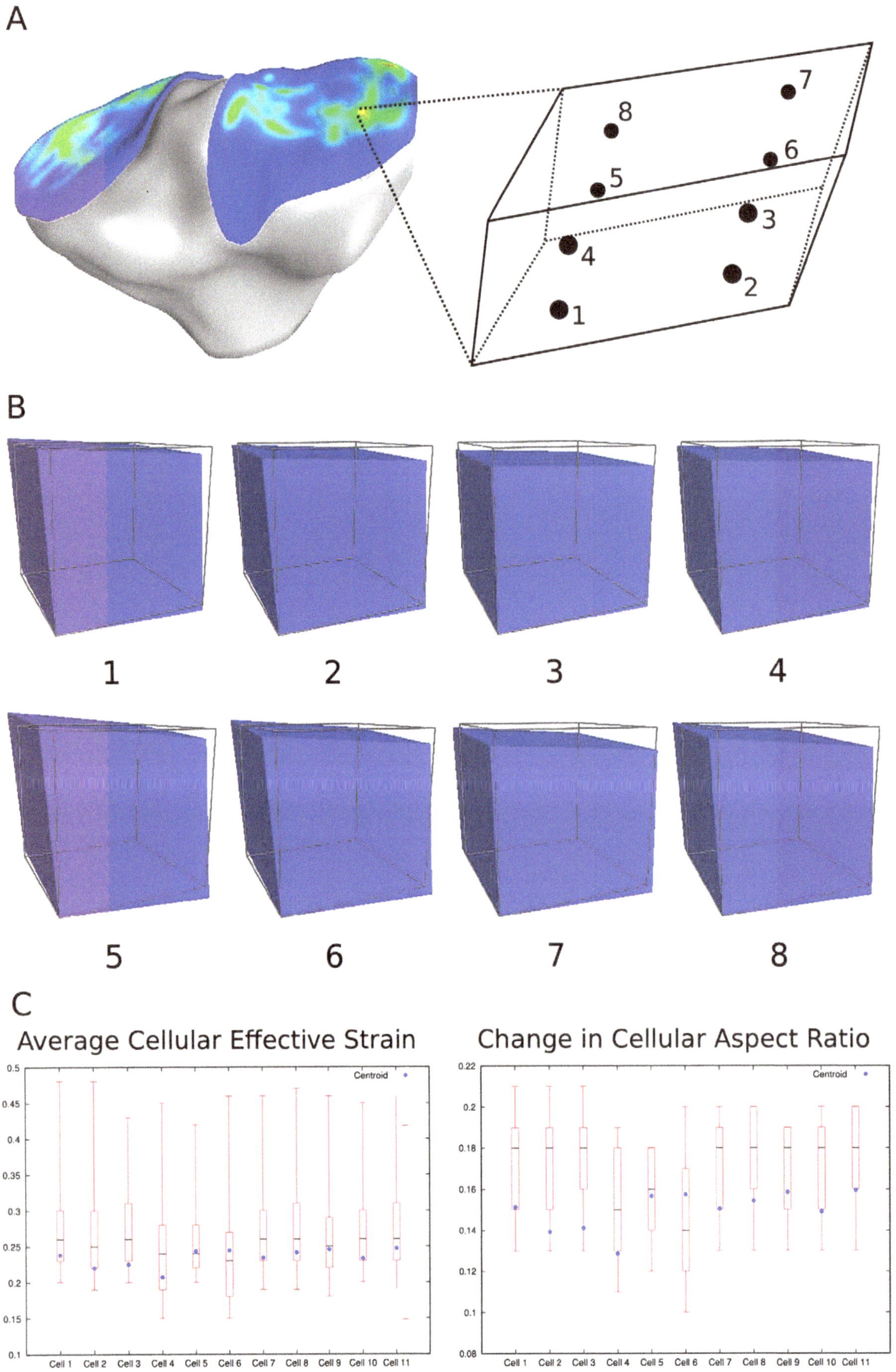
A
8
7
6
5
3
4
2
1
B
1
2
3
4
5
6
7
8
C
Average Cellular Effective Strain
Centroid
0.5
0.45
0.4
0.35
0.3
0.25
0.2
0.15
0.1
Cell 1 Cell 2 Cell 3 Cell 4 Cell 5 Cell 6 Cell 7 Cell 8 Cell 9 Cell 10 Cell 11
Change in Cellular Aspect Ratio
Centroid
0.22
0.2
0.18
0.16
0.14
0.12
0.1
0.08
Cell 1 Cell 2 Cell 3 Cell 4 Cell 5 Cell 6 Cell 7 Cell 8 Cell 9 Cell 10 Cell 11

Figure 10. To investigate the potential error due to sampling of the deformation gradient at element centroids, 11 cell micro-scale models were solved for the eight Gaussian integration points of the macro-scale element determined to have the highest variation in deformation gradient. A. Deformation gradients were calculated at the eight integration points of macro-scale element ID 20585. **B.** The micro-scale model boundary conditions, assigned for each integration point and identified in the image sequence, resulted in a range of deformations. **C.** The variation in deformation gradient associated with integration point sampling resulted in a variation in cellular deformation metrics. The quartile analysis of the resulting volume-averaged cellular effective strain and change in cellular aspect ratio is shown above with the value determined from the analysis performed at the macro-scale element centroid overlaid.

element centroids may alias the deformation occurring on the continuum discretized by the finite elements. To assess this sampling error, the deformation gradients were calculated at each of the 8 Gaussian integration points in the macro-scale finite elements. Deformation gradient variation on each element was then characterized by taking the difference of every unique combination of the 8 deformation gradient tensors, summing the absolute value of the components of the tensor resulting from each difference to get a scalar residual value, and then taking the highest of these 8 scalar residuals and using that as a metric to describe the deformation gradient variation on the particular element. The deformation gradients calculated at the element with the highest variation metric, element ID 20585 with a residual of 0.317, (Figure 10A) were used to assign boundary conditions to eight different eleven cell micro-scale models (Figure 10B). The deformation modes ranged from compression dominated, e.g. integration point 3, to shear dominated e.g. integration point 5. The cellular deformation metrics were calculated from the results of these 8 models for each chondrocyte and a quartile analysis for each cell was performed (Figure 10C). The range in the resulting cellular deformation metrics is high, e.g. 30% in effective strain. While this is the worst case element, it certainly illustrates the sensitivity to spatial sampling. To reduce this error, one can either increase the spatial sampling resolution, e.g. sample at integration points rather than centroids, or refine the macro-scale mesh. Both cases can easily be implemented in this approach, with the acceptance of added computational cost.

Prescribing boundary conditions based on the deformation gradient modeled the finite strain as a first order Taylor series. For problems that experience a highly non-uniform deformation gradient, this may not be an adequate approximation. Including an additional term in the series would capture the gradient of the deformation gradient, and therefore, include information about how the deformation gradient varies spatially [26]. From a temporal perspective, the macro-scale deformation information was only passed to the micro-scale at a single instant in time. The time history of the macro-scale element deformation prior to this instant was not communicated. While this is not relevant in an elastic analysis, including this information will be necessary when considering rate-dependent phenomena such as poro- or visco-elasticity.

The mechanical consistency across spatial scales was satisfied in a weak sense through the use of the same constitutive models at the macro and micro-scales. The PCM(s) and cell(s), although much softer were negligible in volume compared to the ECM. The error associated with this assumption would not be present when using a computational homogenization approach in which the macro-scale material behavior resulted from the micro-scale constitutive models(s). However, the computational scalability advantage provided by the employed method was considered to outweigh the weaknesses in mechanical consistency satisfaction. With advances in shared-memory platform technology, the computational homogenization approach can be revisited in the future.

Due to the infancy of the presented research, a vast array of extensions can be made to the approach in the future. Considering more complex material behaviors at the macro and micro-scales should not only improve the predictivity of the modeling pipeline, but will also permit more accurate investigation of mechano-biological processes. Regarding predictivity, the crude linear relationship, presented in this study for elastic deformations of chondrocytes and joint loading, may take more complicated forms with more accurate constitutive modeling. Extension to a poroelastic model will supply a fluid flux vector field providing insights into bulk fluid flow for transport of nutrients, wastes, and signaling agents. It has been shown that chondrocytes respond to fluid shear stress at the cellular membrane [55], but not to the hydrostatic pressure acting normal to it [56,57]. The fluid flux vector field returned by a poroelastic model will allow for quantitative measures of these transverse and perpendicular quantities. Likewise, the incorporation of fibrous structures into the material models of the micro-scale constituents will also have mechano-biological implications. Such additions will provide a coarse means to model, for example, cytoskeleton fibril interaction with integrin binding sites [4] and stretch-induced ion channel activation [56,57]. An additional coupling to mechano-biological models may also be possible, providing a link between daily activity and phenomena such as matrix remodeling, cell migration, and apoptosis [58]. Ultimately, this will aid in the understanding of the pathological and/or age-related evolution of cartilage anatomy, physiology, and mechanics.

Acknowledgments

Computational resources were provided by Ohio Supercomputer Center (http://www.osc.edu). Open source, freely available software: FEBio, PostView (http://mrl.sci.utah.edu/software), Python (http://www.python.org), and Gnuplot (http://www.gnuplot.info); and models: Open Knee (https://simtk.org/home/openknee) were extensively employed. A download package incorporating the macro- and micro-scale mesh definitions and scripts for model generation, solution, and post-processing of results, is freely accessible in the 'Downloads' section of the project web site https://simtk.org/home/j2c.

Author Contributions

Conceived and designed the experiments: AE SCS. Performed the experiments: SCS. Analyzed the data: SCS AE. Contributed reagents/materials/analysis tools: SCS AE. Wrote the paper: SCS AE. Developed models: SCS AE. Ran simulations: SCS. Interpreted results: SCS AE.

References

1. Wang JHC, Thampatty BP (2006) An introductory review of cell mechanobiology. Biomechanics and Modeling in Mechanobiology 5: 1–16.
2. Schwartz MA (2010) Integrins and extracellular matrix in mechanotransduction. Cold Spring Harbor Perspectives in Biology 2: a005066.
3. Kolahi KS, Mofrad MRK (2010) Mechanotransduction: a major regulator of homeostasis and development. Wiley Interdisciplinary Reviews Systems Biology and Medicine 2: 625–639.
4. Chen CS, Ingber DE (1999) Tensegrity and mechanoregulation: from skeleton to cytoskeleton. Osteoarthritis and Cartilage/OARS, Osteoarthritis Research Society 7: 81–94.
5. Herzog W, Federico S (2006) Considerations on joint and articular cartilage mechanics. Biomechanics and Modeling in Mechanobiology 5: 64–81.

6. Lawrence RC, Felson DT, Helmick CG, Arnold LM, Choi H, et al. (2008) Estimates of the prevalence of arthritis and other rheumatic conditions in the united states. part II. Arthritis and Rheumatism 58: 26–35.
7. Pritzker K, Gay S, Jimenez S, Ostergaard K, Pelletier J, et al. (2006) Osteoarthritis cartilage histopathology: grading and staging. Osteoarthritis and Cartilage 14: 13–29.
8. Alexopoulos LG, Haider MA, Vail TP, Guilak F (2003) Alterations in the mechanical properties of the human chondrocyte pericellular matrix with osteoarthritis. Journal of Biomechanical Engineering 125: 323–333.
9. Heinegrd D, Saxne T (2011) The role of the cartilage matrix in osteoarthritis. Nature Reviews Rheumatology 7: 50–56.
10. Ryu J, Treadwell BV, Mankin HJ (1984) Biochemical and metabolic abnormalities in normal and osteoarthritic human articular cartilage. Arthritis and Rheumatism 27: 49–57.
11. Kim HA, Lee YJ, Seong SC, Choe KW, Song YW (2000) Apoptotic chondrocyte death in human osteoarthritis. The Journal of Rheumatology 27: 455–462.
12. Meachim G, Collins DH (1962) Cell counts of normal and osteoarthritic articular cartilage in relation to the uptake of sulphate (35SO4) in vitro. Annals of the Rheumatic Diseases 21: 45–50.
13. Yutani Y, Yamano Y (1996) The distribution of differentiated phenotypes of chondrocytes in osteoarthritic knee. Osaka City Medical Journal 42: 37–44.
14. Donkelaar CC, Wilson W (2011) Mechanics of chondrocyte hypertrophy. Biomechanics and Modeling in Mechanobiology: In Press.
15. Hudelmaier M, Glaser C, Hohe J, Englmeier KH, Reiser M, et al. (2001) Age-related changes in the morphology and deformational behavior of knee joint cartilage. Arthritis and Rheumatism 44: 2556–2561.
16. Charlebois M, McKee MD, Buschmann MD (2004) Nonlinear tensile properties of bovine articular cartilage and their variation with age and depth. Journal of Biomechanical Engineering 126: 129–137.
17. Temple MM, Bae WC, Chen MQ, Lotz M, Amiel D, et al. (2007) Age- and site-associated biomechanical weakening of human articular cartilage of the femoral condyle. Osteoarthritis and Cartilage/OARS, Osteoarthritis Research Society 15: 1042–1052.
18. Hsieh C, Lin Y, Lin S, Tsai-Wu J, Herbert Wu CH, et al. (2008) Surface ultrastructure and mechanical property of human chondrocyte revealed by atomic force microscopy. Osteoarthritis and Cartilage/OARS, Osteoarthritis Research Society 16: 480–488.
19. Barela AMF, Duarte M (2008) Biomechanical characteristics of elderly individuals walking on land and in water. Journal of Electromyography and Kinesiology: Official Journal of the International Society of Electrophysiological Kinesiology 18: 446–454.
20. Messier SP (1994) Osteoarthritis of the knee and associated factors of age and obesity: effects on gait. Medicine and Science in Sports and Exercise 26: 1446–1452.
21. Karamanidis K, Arampatzis A (2009) Evidence of mechanical load redistribution at the knee joint in the elderly when ascending stairs and ramps. Annals of Biomedical Engineering 37: 467–476.
22. Abusara Z, Seerattan R, Leumann A, Thompson R, Herzog W (2010) A novel method for determining articular cartilage chondrocyte mechanics in vivo. Journal of Biomechanics 44: 930–934.
23. Wilson W, van Donkelaar CC, van Rietbergen R, Huiskes R (2005) The role of computational models in the search for the mechanical behavior and damage mechanisms of articular cartilage. Medical Engineering & Physics 27: 810–826.
24. Mackerle J (2006) Finite element modeling and simulations in orthopedics: a bibliography 1998 2005. Computer Methods in Biomechanics & Biomedical Engineering 9: 149–199.
25. Guilln T, Zhang Q, Tozzi G, Ohrndorf A, Christ H, et al. (2011) Compressive behaviour of bovine cancellous bone and bone analogous materials, microCT characterisation and FE analysis. Journal of the Mechanical Behavior of Biomedical Materials 4: 1452–1461.
26. Kouznetsova VG, Geers MG, Brekelmans WA (2004) Multi-scale second-order computational homogenization of multi-phase materials: a nested finite element solution strategy. Computer Methods in Applied Mechanics and Engineering 193: 5525–5550.
27. Breuls RGM, Sengers BG, Oomens CWJ, Bouten CVC, Baaijens FPT (2002) Predicting local cell deformations in engineered tissue constructs: a multilevel finite element approach. Journal of Biomechanical Engineering 124: 198–207.
28. Erdemir A, Sibole S (2010) Open Knee: A Three-Dimensional Finite Element Representation of the Knee Joint, User's Guide, Version 1.0.0.
29. Maas S, Rawlins D, Weiss J, Ateshian G (2010) FEBio Theory Manual. University of Utah.
30. Shepherd DE, Seedhom BB (1999) The 'instantaneous' compressive modulus of human articular cartilage in joints of the lower limb. Rheumatology (Oxford, England) 38: 124–132.
31. Butler DL, Sheh MY, Stouffer DC, Samaranayake VA, Levy MS (1990) Surface strain variation in human patellar tendon and knee cruciate ligaments. Journal of Biomechanical Engineering 112: 38–45.
32. Gardiner JC, Weiss JA (2003) Subject-specific finite element analysis of the human medial collateral ligament during valgus knee loading. Journal of Orthopaedic Research: Official Publication of the Orthopaedic Research Society 21: 1098–1106.
33. Peña E, Calvo B, Martínez MA, Doblaré M (2006) A three-dimensional finite element analysis of the combined behavior of ligaments and menisci in the healthy human knee joint. Journal of Biomechanics 39: 1686–1701.
34. Fithian DC, Kelly MA, Mow VC (1990) Material properties and structure-function relationships in the menisci. Clinical Orthopaedics and Related Research. pp 19–31.
35. Tissakht M, Ahmed AM (1995) Tensile stress-strain characteristics of the human meniscal material. Journal of Biomechanics 28: 411–422.
36. Yao J, Snibbe J, Maloney M, Lerner AL (2006) Stresses and strains in the medial meniscus of an ACL deficient knee under anterior loading: a finite element analysis with image-based experimental validation. Journal of Biomechanical Engineering 128: 135–141.
37. Weiss JA, Maker BN, Govindjee S (1996) Finite element implementation of incompressible, transversely isotropic hyperelasticity. Computer Methods in Applied Mechanics and Engineering 135: 107–128.
38. Maas S, Ellis BJ, Rawlins DS, Weiss JA (2009) A comparison of FEBio, ABAQUS, and NIKE3D results for a suite of verification problems. SCI Technical Report.
39. Guilak F, Mow VC (2000) The mechanical environment of the chondrocyte: a biphasic finite element model of cell-matrix interactions in articular cartilage. Journal of Biomechanics 33: 1663–1673.
40. Hunziker EB, Quinn TM, Huselmann H (2002) Quantitative structural organization of normal adult human articular cartilage. Osteoarthritis and Cartilage/OARS, Osteoarthritis Research Society 10: 564–572.
41. Michalek AJ, Iatridis JC (2007) A numerical study to determine pericellular matrix modulus and evaluate its effects on the micromechanical environment of chondrocytes. Journal of Biomechanics 40: 1405–1409.
42. Guilak F, Alexopoulos LG, Haider MA, Ting-Beall HP, Setton LA (2005) Zonal uniformity in mechanical properties of the chondrocyte pericellular matrix: Micropipette aspiration of canine chondrons isolated by cartilage homogenization. Annals of Biomedical Engineering 33: 1312–1318.
43. Alexopoulos LG, Setton LA, Guilak F (2005) The biomechanical role of the chondrocyte pericellular matrix in articular cartilage. Acta Biomaterialia 1: 317–325.
44. Cao L, Guilak F, Setton LA (2009) Pericellular matrix mechanics in the anulus fibrosus predicted by a Three-Dimensional finite element model and in situ morphology. Cellular and Molecular Bioengineering 2: 306–319.
45. Peeters EAG, Bouten CVC, Oomens CWJ, Bader DL, Snoeckx LHEH, et al. (2004) Anisotropic, three-dimensional deformation of single attached cells under compression. Annals of Biomedical Engineering 32: 1443–1452.
46. Korhonen RK, Han S, Herzog W (2010) Osmotic loading of in situ chondrocytes in their native environment. Molecular & Cellular Biomechanics: MCB 7: 125–134.
47. Tetsunaga T, Nishida K, Furumatsu T, Naruse K, Hirohata S, et al. (2011) Regulation of mechanical stress-induced MMP-13 and ADAMTS-5 expression by RUNX-2 transcriptional factor in SW1353 chondrocyte-like cells. Osteoarthritis and Cartilage/OARS, Osteoarthritis Research Society 19: 222–232.
48. Worsley P, Stokes M, Taylor M (2011) Predicted knee kinematics and kinetics during functional activities using motion capture and musculoskeletal modelling in healthy older people. Gait & Posture 33: 268–273.
49. Kazemi M, Li LP, Savard P, Buschmann MD (2011) Creep behavior of the intact and meniscectomy knee joints. Journal of the Mechanical Behavior of Biomedical Materials 4: 1351–1358.
50. Yang NH, Nayeb-Hashemi H, Canavan PK, Vaziri A (2010) Effect of frontal plane tibiofemoral angle on the stress and strain at the knee cartilage during the stance phase of gait. Journal of Orthopaedic Research: Official Publication of the Orthopaedic Research Society 28: 1539–1547.
51. Donahue TLH, Hull ML, Rashid MM, Jacobs CR (2002) A finite element model of the human knee joint for the study of tibio-femoral contact. Journal of Biomechanical Engineering 124: 273–280.
52. Erdemir A, Sibole S (2011) Open knee: capacity to reproduce passive joint kinematics. In: 23rd Congress of the International Society of Biomechanics Brussels, Belgium.
53. Hofer JK, Gejo R, McGarry MH, Lee TQ (2011) Effects of kneeling on tibiofemoral contact pressure and area in posterior Cruciate-Retaining and posterior Cruciate-Sacrificing total knee arthroplasty. The Journal of Arthroplasty: In Press.
54. Halloran JP, Erdemir A, van den Bogert AJ (2009) Adaptive surrogate modeling for efficient coupling of musculoskeletal control and tissue deformation models. Journal of Biomechanical Engineering 131: 011014.
55. Wang P, Zhu F, Tong Z, Konstantopoulos K (2011) Response of chondrocytes to shear stress: antagonistic effects of the binding partners toll-like receptor 4 and caveolin-1. The FASEB Journal: Official Publication of the Federation of American Societies for Experimental Biology 25: 3401–3415.
56. Martinac B (2004) Mechanosensitive ion channels: molecules of mechanotransduction. Journal of Cell Science 117: 2449–2460.
57. Sokabe M, Sachs F, Jing ZQ (1991) Quantitative video microscopy of patch clamped membranes stress, strain, capacitance, and stretch channel activation. Biophysical Journal 59: 722–728.
58. Ramage L, Nuki G, Salter DM (2009) Signalling cascades in mechanotransduction: cell-matrix interactions and mechanical loading. Scandinavian Journal of Medicine & Science in Sports 19: 457–469.

14

The BMP Ligand Gdf6 Prevents Differentiation of Coronal Suture Mesenchyme in Early Cranial Development

Dawn E. Clendenning, Douglas P. Mortlock*

Department of Molecular Physiology and Biophysics, Center for Human Genetics Research, Vanderbilt University School of Medicine, Nashville, Tennessee, United States of America

Abstract

Growth Differentiation Factor-6 (*Gdf6*) is a member of the Bone Morphogenetic Protein (BMP) family of secreted signaling molecules. Previous studies have shown that *Gdf6* plays a role in formation of a diverse subset of skeletal joints. In mice, loss of *Gdf6* results in fusion of the coronal suture, the intramembranous joint that separates the frontal and parietal bones. Although the role of GDFs in the development of cartilaginous limb joints has been studied, limb joints are developmentally quite distinct from cranial sutures and how *Gdf6* controls suture formation has remained unclear. In this study we show that coronal suture fusion in the *Gdf6−/−* mouse is due to accelerated differentiation of suture mesenchyme, prior to the onset of calvarial ossification. *Gdf6* is expressed in the mouse frontal bone primordia from embryonic day (E) 10.5 through 12.5. In the *Gdf6−/−* embryo, the coronal suture fuses prematurely and concurrently with the initiation of osteogenesis in the cranial bones. Alkaline phosphatase (ALP) activity and *Runx2* expression assays both showed that the suture width is reduced in *Gdf6+/−* embryos and is completely absent in *Gdf6−/−* embryos by E12.5. ALP activity is also increased in the suture mesenchyme of *Gdf6+/−* embryos compared to wild-type. This suggests *Gdf6* delays differentiation of the mesenchyme occupying the suture, prior to the onset of ossification. Therefore, although BMPs are known to promote bone formation, *Gdf6* plays an inhibitory role to prevent the osteogenic differentiation of the coronal suture mesenchyme.

Editor: Cheng-Ting Chien, Academia Sinica, Taiwan

Funding: DPM was supported by United States National Institutes of Health (NIH) grant HD047880. DEC was supported by NIH Genetics Training Grant T32GM080178 and NIH Developmental Biology Training Grant T32HD07502. The funders had no role in study design, data collection and analysis, decision to publish, or preparation of the manuscript.

Competing Interests: The authors have declared that no competing interests exist.

* E-mail: mortlock@chgr.mc.vanderbilt.edu

Introduction

The mammalian cranial vault is composed of five main flat bones separated by joints known as the cranial sutures. These sutures are composed of fibrous connective tissue and act as the main sites for cranial growth during development. As the cranial vault expands, bone is deposited at the growing edges of the bone (the bone fronts), while the suture mesenchyme remains undifferentiated. Sutures provide flexible joints for passage through the birth canal, act as shock absorbers, prevent separation of the cranial bones, and accommodate room for the rapidly growing brain [1]. With the exception of the metopic suture, human sutures normally do not fuse until the third or fourth decade of life [2], when the undifferentiated mesenchyme of the suture space becomes obliterated by bone.

Craniosynostosis is defined as the premature fusion of one or more of the cranial sutures and occurs in approximately 1 in 2,500 live births [3]. When a suture fuses prematurely, cranial growth ceases perpendicular to the fused suture, producing a dysmorphic skull shape. In turn, when the calvarial vault cannot expand sufficiently to accommodate the rapidly growing brain, increased intracranial pressure can occur [4]. Coronal craniosynostosis can result from several potential mechanisms. For example, a failure to form the developmental boundary between the neural crest-derived frontal bone and the paraxial mesoderm-derived parietal bone can result in impaired suture formation. This failed mechanism is evident as a mixing of the frontal and parietal cell populations at sites of suture fusion in utero, as seen in the *Twist1* mutant mouse [5]. It is thought that *Twist1* functions with *Msx2* to control the localization of ephrin-A2 and ephrin-A4, which are known to play roles in boundary formation at the frontal/parietal junction by restricting cell migration [5]. Several additional mechanisms could also lead to fusion of a cranial suture. These include changes in proliferation, apoptosis, or the rate of differentiation in the suture mesenchyme or at the leading edges of the ossifying bone. For example, gain of function mutations in *Fibroblast growth factor receptors (FGFRs)* have been associated with craniosynostosis in humans. Studies in mice have shown that *Fgfr2* is expressed in proliferating osteoprogenitor cells surrounding the ossifying bones while *Fgfr1* is expressed more centrally in osteoid of the developing frontal and parietal bones. As differentiation progresses, *Fgfr2* is downregulated and *Fgfr1* is upregulated, suggesting that signaling through FGFR2 mainly plays a role in proliferation, while FGFR1 signaling regulates osteogenic differentiation. The contribution of FGFR3 is less clear though its expression overlaps with FGFR1 and −2 [6]. However, the P250R gain-of-function mutation in FGFR3 has been associated with coronal craniosynostosis, either isolated or as part of syndromes such as Muenke syndrome [7]. While defects in boundary formation between lineage compartments (e.g. neural crest and paraxial mesoderm) can explain some of the etiology of coronal craniosynostosis, it remains less clear how proposed changes in differentiation or maintenance can affect certain sutures while sparing others.

Growth Differentiation Factors (GDFs) 5, 6, and 7 are members of the Bone Morphogenetic Protein (BMP) family of secreted signaling molecules. The GDF subgroup (GDF5/6/7) is highly conserved in vertebrates and has been shown to play a critical role in limb joint formation and chondrogenesis [8]. *Gdf6* homozygous knockout mice display multiple joint defects, including fusions of tarsal and carpal bones, morphological abnormalities in the malleus, incus, and stapes bones of the middle ear, and hypoplasia of the thyroid cartilage. In addition to these defects, *Gdf6* knockout mice lack the coronal suture [9]. However, the detailed expression pattern of *Gdf6* in the developing skull and its relationship to the onset of cranial suture fusion in this mutant has not been shown. Another GDF family member, *Gdf5*, is mutated in the *brachypodism* mouse and normally stimulates cartilage development, growth, and maturation [8]. Therefore, *Gdf5* can be viewed as promoting aspects of endochondral bone growth. *Gdf5* and *Gdf6* share approximately 80% identity in the mature signaling region [10] and therefore it is likely the *Gdf5* and *Gdf6* operate by similar ligand-receptor interactions. Like *Gdf5*, *Gdf6* (a.k.a. CDMP2) can promote chondrogenic differentiation in vitro [11]. This makes the craniosynostosis phenotype in the *Gdf6*−/− mouse particularly interesting because unlike the long bones, the cranial bones form through intramembranous ossification without a cartilage intermediate. Therefore, the mechanism of *Gdf6* function in the coronal suture may be drastically different than its function in joints of the axial skeleton.

The aim of this study was to gain a more thorough developmental understanding of craniosynostosis in the *Gdf6*−/− mouse and the underlying cause of suture fusion. We found that the coronal suture is obliterated in *Gdf6*−/− embryos before the first evidence of cranial bone ossification is detectable at E14.5, with changes in early osteogenic markers detected prior to the onset of ossification. Our data suggests that *Gdf6* may self-regulate its expression in the developing frontal bone primordium. Additionally, fusion in the *Gdf6*−/− is not due to a failure to form the boundary properly between the frontal and parietal bones, or changes in cell survival or proliferation, but is likely due to a failure of the suture mesenchyme to remain in an undifferentiated state.

Results

Gdf6−/− Coronal Suture Fuses Early in Development

The entire coronal suture was absent in *Gdf6*−/− fetal mice (Fig. 1C, F), with complete penetrance (not shown). This defect was not observed in wild-type (Fig. 1A, D) and *Gdf6* heterozygote littermates (Fig. 1B, E) through embryonic development and weaning. To determine the time point during development at which the suture first became fused, *Gdf6*−/− embryos were collected at various stages and stained with alizarin red. At E14.0, ossification centers in either the frontal or parietal bone were not yet visible by alizarin red staining. By E14.5, frontal and parietal bones were first visible as two separate ossification centers (Fig. 1G, J; H, K). The nascent coronal suture was apparent in the wild-type embryo as the gap between the two bones. Yet in *Gdf6*−/− embryos, a single continuous ossification center was present (Fig. 1I, L). Analysis of multiple *Gdf6*−/− embryos at E13.5–14.5 failed to identify visibly separate sites of alizarin staining for frontal and parietal rudiments in any specimens (not shown). At E15.5, the frontal and parietal bones were fused into one continuous bone in the *Gdf6*−/− embryo (Fig. 1O), while the bones remained separated by the coronal suture in the wild-type and heterozygote (Fig. 1M, N) embryos. The coronal suture continued to fuse along its entire length as ossification progresses outward in the *Gdf6*−/− embryo, whereas the sagittal, lambdoid, and squamosal sutures (Fig. 1A–F) remained unaffected in *Gdf6*−/− mice throughout prenatal development. At the macroscopic level, the ossification centers and suture in *Gdf6*+/− appear to develop identically to wild-type embryos with regards to the onset of ossification and size of the bones (not shown). This data suggests that *Gdf6* plays a role in coronal suture formation at or prior to the onset of ossification.

Gdf6−/− has Normal Suture Boundary Formation

Coronal craniosynostosis can result from a failure to form a proper boundary between cells of the neural crest-derived frontal bone and the paraxial mesoderm-derived parietal bone. The formation of this boundary involves the cooperation of *Twist1* and *Msx2* to control of the expression domains of ephrin-A2, ephrin-A4, and EphA4 [5]. Ephrin signaling has been shown to inhibit cell mixing and provide guidance cues for migrating cell populations [12]. Failed boundary formation is evident as a mixing of the two cell lineages within the suture mesenchyme, as in the *Twist1* mutant mouse [5].

To determine whether a similar cell mixing was the cause of the craniosynostosis in the *Gdf6*−/− embryos, we visualized the suture boundary using the *Wnt1-Cre* and *R26R* transgenic lines, which together stably label derivates of the neural crest [13], including the frontal bone. At E16.5, coronal suture fusion was evident in whole-mount stained *Gdf6*−/− embryos (Fig. 2A,B). Transverse sections showed the presence of ossified bone across the boundary between the frontal and parietal bones in *Gdf6*−/− (Fig. 2D, arrow), while the suture remained open and undifferentiated in wild-type (Fig. 2C, arrow). Also of note was a general thinning of the bone in this region of the *Gdf6*−/− (Fig. 2D) along with the loss of the characteristic suture mesenchyme blastema, seen in wild-type embryos (Fig. 2C, arrow). In the regions of the frontal bone more distal to the suture, there was no thinning of the *Gdf6*−/− bone compared to wild-type (not shown).

In the *Gdf6*−/− embryo, ossified tissue disrupted the boundary between the frontal and parietal domains (as seen in Fig. 2D) making it difficult to determine if cells have crossed the normal boundary. Therefore embryos were examined at E14.5, when portions of the *Gdf6*−/− calvaria were not yet ossified through the suture. Coronal sections through the region of the presumptive coronal suture reveal that although the *Gdf6*−/− lacked an identifiable suture, the cellular boundary between the frontal and parietal bones remained distinct just like the wild-type suture (Fig. 2E,F). We could find no evidence of cell mixing between these tissue populations and there were no other obvious differences between wild-type and *Gdf6*+/− embryos with regards to the suture boundary (not shown). Furthermore, we observed a surprisingly uniform and continuous surface between the frontal and parietal bones of *Gdf6*−/−, where the suture should reside.

Gdf6−/− and *Gdf6*+/− Present with Pre-ossification Changes in the Suture

Transverse sections through the E12.5 wild-type suture were stained for alkaline phosphatase (ALP) activity, an early osteoblast marker, to highlight the frontal and parietal bone primordia with the presumptive coronal suture in between (Fig. 3A); ALP was weaker in the band of cells between the primordia, but was faintly visible across the suture region (Fig. 3A). In *Gdf6*+/− embryos, ALP activity extended through the presumptive suture region which was shorter as defined by the distance between the flanking bone primordia (Fig. 3B), revealing less undifferentiated suture

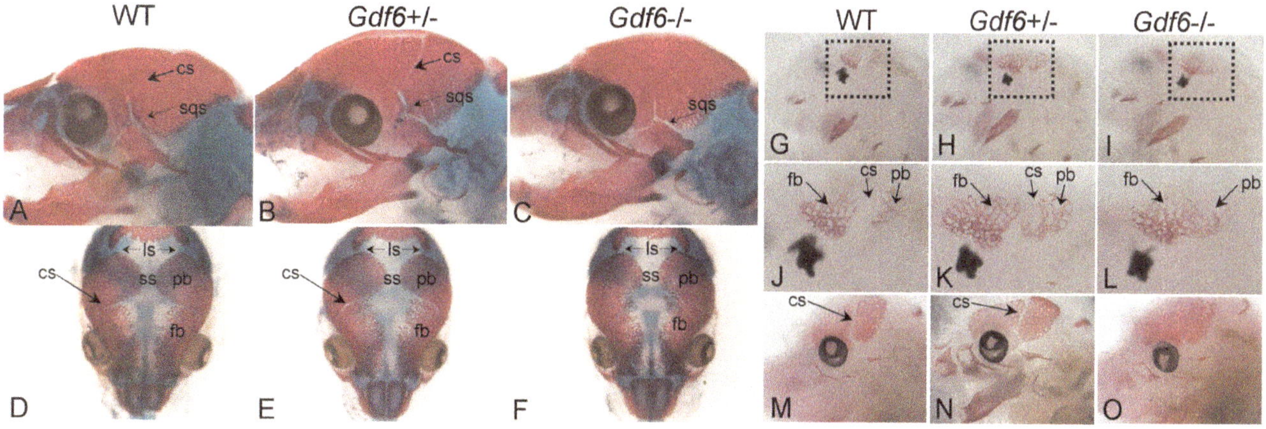

Figure 1. Analysis of coronal suture development in wild-type and *Gdf6−/−* embryos with alizarin red. The coronal suture separated the frontal and parietal bones in wild-type and heterozygote embryos (A, B), but was lacking in the *Gdf6−/−* embryos (C). At E14.5, the early coronal suture was a distinct gap between the frontal and parietal ossification centers (G, H, J, K). The coronal suture appeared fused in *Gdf6−/−* embryos at the onset of ossification (I, L). The frontal and parietal bones fused into one continuous bone in the *Gdf6−/−* at E15.5 (O). The sagittal, lambdoid (D–F), and squamosal (A–C) sutures remained unfused through weaning in both wild-type and *Gdf6−/−* animals. fb, frontal bone; pb, parietal bone, cs, coronal suture; ls, lambdoid suture; sqs, squamosal suture.

mesenchyme relative to the wild-type suture. Although *Gdf6+/−* mice develop normal sutures, ALP was also increased in the presumptive suture relative to wild-type. This points to a dosage effect, where loss of one copy of *Gdf6* does increase ALP activity in the suture, but this slightly increased differentiation does not reach the threshold required for fusion of the suture. In addition, the suture gap width was reduced in the *Gdf6+/−* compared to wild-type (Fig. 3B). In E12.5 *Gdf6−/−* embryos, the frontal primordium was clearly visible, but there was no clear region of concentrated ALP in the parietal primordium; rather, there was continuous, moderate ALP staining across the region of the presumptive suture and extending into the region where the parietal primordia has concentrated ALP activity in wild-type and *Gdf6+/−* embryos (Fig. 3C).

Differentiation of the suture mesenchyme was also examined by expression of *Runx2*, another marker for early bone differentiation. Like ALP, *Runx2* marked the presumptive frontal and parietal bones, with a gap of undifferentiated mesenchyme in between (Fig. 3D). Again, the distance between the frontal and parietal rudiments was reduced in the *Gdf6+/−* (Fig. 3E). In the *Gdf6−/−*, *Runx2* was expressed continuously through the suture region at E12.5 (Fig. 3F). These data suggest the presumptive suture region

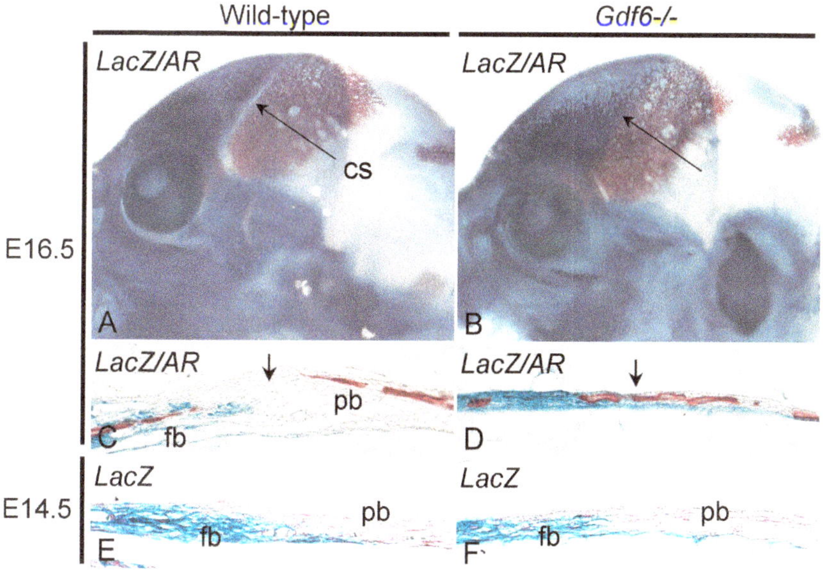

Figure 2. Analysis of boundary formation in *Gdf6−/−* embryos. E16.5 *Wnt1Cre+/−; R26R+/−; Gdf6+/+* (A) and *Wnt1Cre+/−; R26R+/−; Gdf6−/−* (B) embryos were stained with Xgal to label the frontal bone followed by alizarin red to highlight the parietal bone. Sections through the *lacZ*/alzarin red stained embryos show the boundary between the labeled frontal bone and unlabeled parietal bone at the site of the wild-type suture (C, arrow), with bone continuing through the suture boundary in the *Gdf6−/−* embryo (D, arrow). E14.5 *Wnt1Cre+/−; R26R+/−; Gdf6+/+* (E) and *Wnt1Cre+/−; R26R+/−; Gdf6−/−* (F) embryos were stained with Xgal and counterstained with nuclear fast red. In both the wild-type and *Gdf6−/−* coronal sutures, the boundary was distinct, with no evidence of cell mixing. AR, alizarin red; cs, coronal suture; fb, frontal bone; pb, parietal bone.

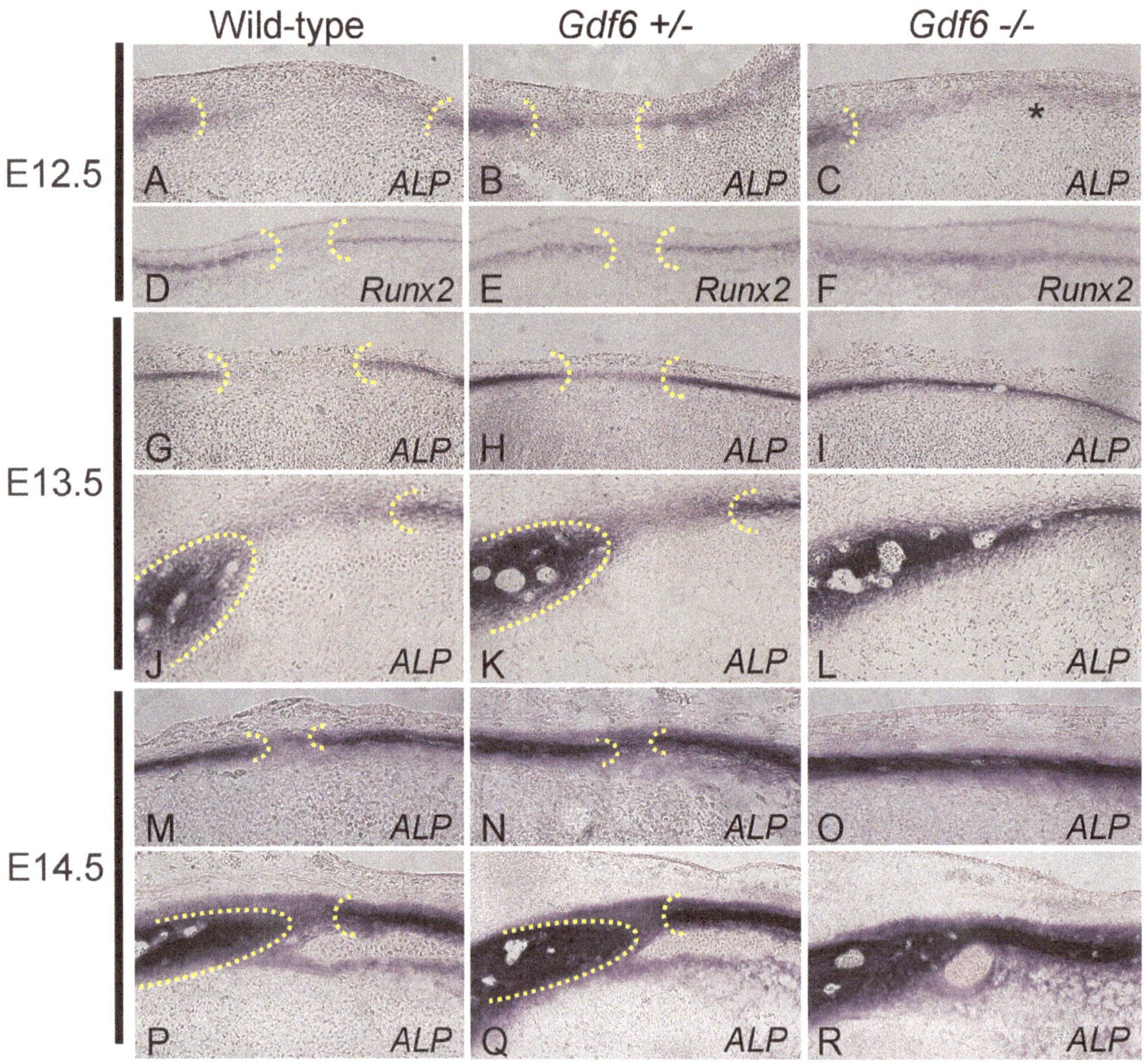

Figure 3. Alkaline-phosphatase (ALP) staining in the presumptive suture. Transverse sections through the E12.5 wild-type suture showed a gap in ALP activity between the frontal and parietal bones (A). The width of the gap was reduced in the *Gdf6*+/−, with an increase in ALP activity within the suture (B). In the *Gdf6*−/−, there is a continuous line of ALP activity through the region, with a reduction in ALP activity in the parietal portion of the fused bone (C). Similar changes in ALP staining were observed in the E13.5 and E14.5 rostral (G–I, M–O) and caudal (J–L, P–R) coronal sutures and through *in situ* hybridization for *Runx2* (D–F).

of *Gdf6*−/− embryos is prematurely differentiating by E12.5, as characterized by abnormally high ALP and *Runx2* expression. Interestingly, ALP activity is apparently delayed in the parietal rudiment of *Gdf6*−/− embryos although *Runx2* expression is not.

Increased ALP activity was confirmed at both caudal (closer to the eye) and rostral (newly formed) levels of the presumptive coronal suture at E13.5 and E14.5 (caudal, Fig. 3J–L, P–R and rostral, Fig. 3G–I, M–O). This suggests an increase in osteogenic differentiation of the cells in the developing suture of the *Gdf6*+/− and *Gdf6*−/− embryos, and also a dosage effect where *Gdf6*+/− has intermediately increased differentiation between wild-type and *Gdf6*−/− embryos.

A decrease in both the intensity (Fig. 3C,I) and span (not shown) of ALP activity in the parietal bone rudiment of *Gdf6*−/− embryos was noted, suggesting a decrease in the rate of differentiation in this structure. This was also observed in the alizarin red staining of E14.5 embryos, with a reduction of the size of the *Gdf6*−/− parietal bone ossification center compared to wild-type and *Gdf6*+/− (not shown). This could be a potential secondary effect of loss of the suture, or a direct effect of the loss of *Gdf6*.

Loss of Gdf6 does not Significantly Affect Proliferation in the Nascent Suture

In principle, suture fusion could result from changes in the number of cells in the suture or bone fronts proliferating or undergoing apoptosis, thereby increasing or decreasing the number of cells in the pre-osteogenic pool. Between E14.0 and E14.5, the frontal and parietal rudiments in the *Gdf6*−/− are clearly fused as shown by alizarin red staining into a single ossified element (Fig. 1I, L). Therefore the sutures of wild-type, *Gdf6*+/−, and *Gdf6*−/− littermates were examined for changes in proliferation or apoptosis at E12.5, concurrent with the earliest detectable changes in ALP staining (Fig. 3) but before the formation of osteoid. Adjacent sections were stained for ALP in order to help localize the suture (Fig. 4A–C). Immunohistochemistry for phospho-histone H3 (Fig. 4A'–C') showed no significant overall changes in the number of proliferating cells in heterozygous or homozygous mutants as compared to wild-type, nor when the suture mesenchyme, frontal bone, and parietal bone were analyzed separately (Fig. 4D,E). Proliferation assays at E13.5 also failed to detect significant differences across genotypes (Fig. S1) although some trends toward altered proliferation rates in mutant mice were suggested; although not significant statistically, these trends may be secondary to the increased rate of differentiation in the mutant sutures and thus, to changes in the pool of pre-osteogenic proliferating cells.

To assay apoptosis, we used cleaved-caspase 3 immunohistochemistry. Few to no apoptotic cells were detectable in the suture mesenchyme or bone front in pre-ossified calvaria (Fig. S1), consistent with previous reports that there are very few apoptotic cells in fetal mouse calvaria prior to E16.5 [14] and likewise, no significant difference between genotypes was found.

Gdf6 is Expressed in the Frontal Bone Primordia

The neural crest/paraxial mesoderm tissue boundary that determines the future site of the coronal suture is formed by E10.5 [13]. In order to pinpoint the pattern of *Gdf6* expression during cranial development and specifically in relation to coronal suture formation, we performed *in situ* hybridization on embryos at E9.5–E14.5. *Gdf6* mRNA was first detected in the developing cranial region in a triangular-shaped area just anterior to the eye at E10.5 (Fig. 5A–C, arrow). This corresponded closely with the neural crest-derived frontal bone rudiment, as labeled in *Wnt1-Cre; R26R* embryos (Fig. 5D, arrow). *Gdf6* was expressed in the frontal bone rudiment at E11.5 (Fig. 5H–J), as the rudiment begins to grow and expand. Transverse sections through the E10.5 frontal rudiment (depicted in Fig. 5E, dotted line) reveal that the site of expression anterior to the eye was localized to several layers of mesenchyme underlying the surface ectoderm (Fig. 5F,G). At E12.5, *Gdf6* continued to be exclusively expressed in the frontal bone rudiment (Fig. 5K–M, arrow), with no evidence of expression in the suture mesenchyme or parietal bone rudiment. By E14.5, when fusion of the ossification centers was first visible by alizarin red staining, *Gdf6* is no longer expressed in the suture region (Fig. S2).

Although no functional Gdf6 protein can be made from the *Gdf6* knockout allele, the mutant *Gdf6* transcript can be detected by our *in situ* RNA probe, which targets the 3′ UTR of *Gdf6*. *In situ* hybridization revealed that *Gdf6* transcripts were still present in *Gdf6−/−* embryos (Fig. 5C,J,M). Interestingly, the *Gdf6* transcript was more highly expressed in *Gdf6−/−* embryos than in either wild-type or *Gdf6+/−*, with staining in *Gdf6+/−* at intermediate levels (Fig. 5A–C, H–J). Increased staining was also observed for *Gdf6* in the branchial arches of *Gdf6−/−* embryos (Fig. 5, A–C, H–J asterix). These observations suggest that *Gdf6* expression may be self-regulated in these structures by a negative feedback loop. In cross-section, *Gdf6* expression was also observed in the orbital bone rudiment (Fig. 5L) of wild-type, *Gdf6+/−*, and *Gdf6−/−* embryos (not shown). *Gdf6* is also normally expressed in the dorsal retina where it functions in promoting eye development [15,16]. However, *Gdf6* transcript was observed in the dorsal retina wild-type and *Gdf6+/−* embryos (Fig. 5K,L), but was lost in *Gdf6−/−* embryos (Fig. 5M), suggesting that in the retina *Gdf6* autoregulates through a positive feedback loop, in contrast to the negative autoregulation in frontal bone and branchial arches.

Discussion

Here we present data indicating that *Gdf6* is genetically required for osteogenic differentiation in the developing coronal suture during its formation. *Gdf6* is absolutely required for formation of the suture, as in *Gdf6−/−* embryos there is an initial failure to establish a region of delayed differentiation between the frontal and parietal condensations. We observed that *Gdf6* mRNA is strongly downregulated in wild-type calvaria by E14.5. It remains unknown if *Gdf6* plays roles at later stages to maintain patency of

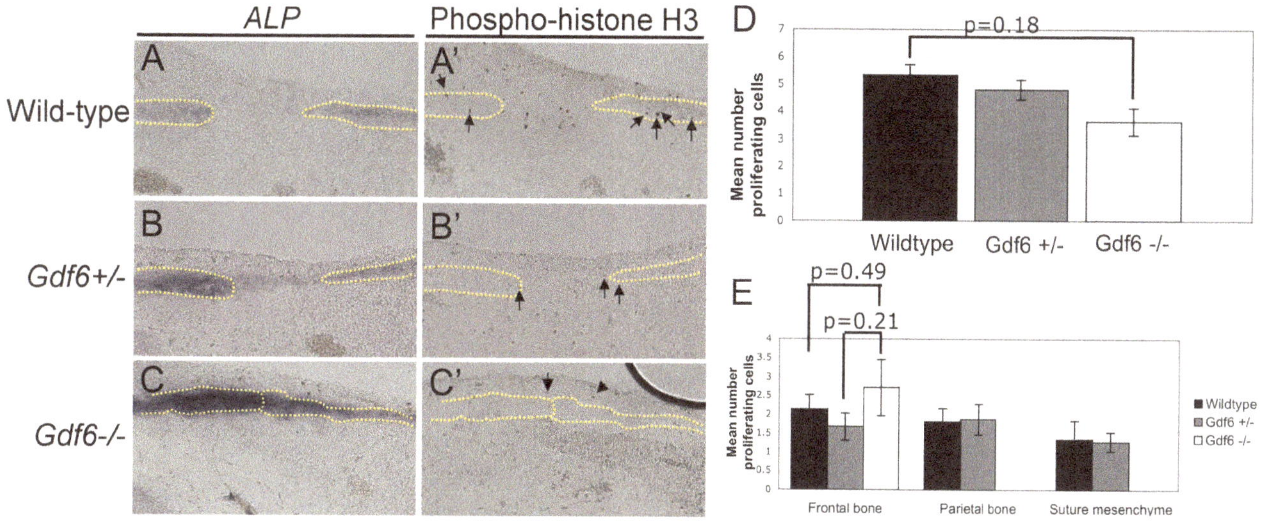

Figure 4. Analysis of cell proliferation in the E12.5 coronal suture. Adjacent sections stained for ALP activity, highlighting the location of the frontal and parietal bones (A–C dotted lines), and immunohistochemistry for phospho-histone H3 (A′–C′). Examples of positive cells are marked with arrows. (D) Quantification of the mean number of proliferating cells counted in the combined frontal/suture/parietal region. (E) Quantification of the mean number of proliferating cells counted in each region separately (the frontal bone, parietal bone, and suture mesenchyme) (x-axis). Since the suture mesenchyme cannot be distinguished from the parietal in Gdf6−/− embryos at this time, only data for the frontal rudiment is shown for this genotype. N = 3 embryos for each genotype with 5 sections per embryo quantified. Differences the number of proliferating cells per suture region were analyzed using a t-test.

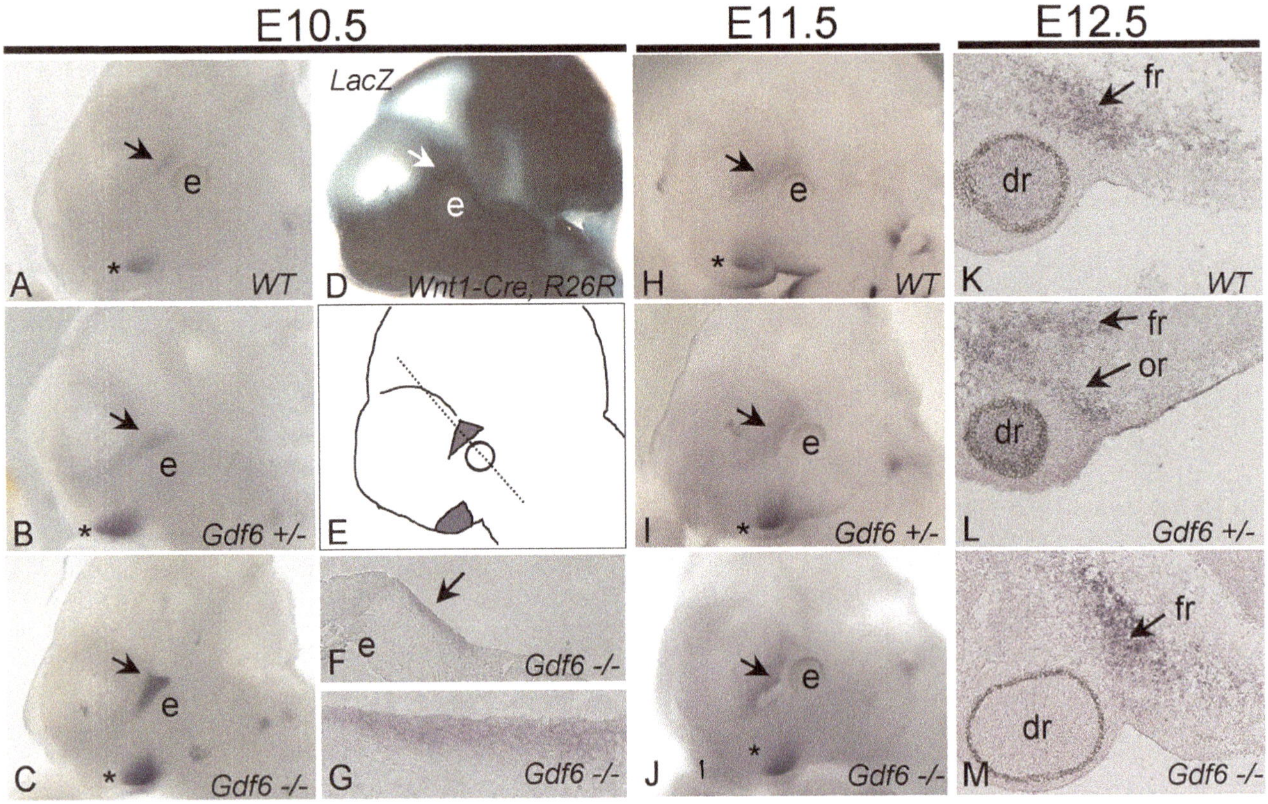

Figure 5. Expression of *Gdf6*. *In situ* hybridization for *Gdf6* at E10.5 (A–C, F,G), E11.5 (H–J), and E12.5 (K–M). *Gdf6* was expressed in the frontal bone primordia (arrow), which is labeled as neural crest-derived in the *Wnt1-Cre; R26R* transgenic embryos (D). *Gdf6* transcript was expressed more strongly in the *Gdf6*−/− embryo (C, J) than either the wild-type (A, H) or *Gdf6*+/− embryo (B, I), in both the frontal bone rudiment (arrow) and branchial arches (asterix). In transverse cross section through the eye and frontal bone primordia at E10.5 (dotted line, E), *Gdf6* was expressed in several layers of mesenchyme underlying the surface ectoderm (F, G). At E12.5, *Gdf6* continues to be expressed in the frontal bone rudiment, in addition to the dorsal retina (K–L) and orbital bone rudiment (L). Expression of *Gdf6* in the dorsal retina seen in the wild-type and *Gdf6*+/− (K,L) was absent in the *Gdf6*−/− (M). dr, dorsal retina; e, eye; fr, frontal rudiment; or, orbital bone rudiment.

the established suture; such a notion would be consistent with a report that *Gdf6* expression is detectable in calvarial sutures by E16.5 [9]. The question of whether *Gdf6* plays a role in suture maintenance will require examination of Gdf6 protein stability and localization, and/or conditional deletion of *Gdf6* at later stages.

Gdf6 Represses Osteogenic Differentiation but not Boundary Formation in the Coronal Suture

We found no evidence for disruption in the frontal/parietal cell boundary in *Gdf6*− /− mice. This is in contrast to the mechanism of suture fusion in the *Twist*+/−, and *Epha4*− /− mice where, before E14.5, osteogenic cells from the frontal bone abnormally cross into the suture mesenchyme [5]. In *Twist*+/− mice, ALP activity in the frontal/parietal rudiments is normal in appearance up to at least day E13.5 [5]. In contrast, ALP activity abnormalities are detectable by E12.5 in *Gdf6*− /− embryos, before ephrin ligands are expressed in the frontal/parietal region [5]. Therefore *Gdf6* is required for a mechanism of suture formation that is distinct from that controlled by the *Twist/Ephrin* pathway. *Twist* also regulates osteogenic condensation via interaction with *Msx2* [17]. Our data does not exclude *Gdf6/Twist* interactions during osteogenic differentiation, although a combined reduction of *Twist* and *Msx2* levels was shown to primarily affect differentiation of the frontal, but not the parietal bone, suggesting this is possible [17].

Effects of Gdf6 Signaling in the Developing Calvarium

Somewhat surprisingly, *Gdf6* mRNA was not detected in the suture mesenchyme itself but in the frontal bone primordia. This is in contrast to the sites of wrist and ankle joint fusion in *Gdf6*− /− embryos, where *Gdf6* is clearly expressed in the developing joint interzones [9]. However, several studies suggest that the action of GDFs in limb joint development is not explained by direct autocrine suppression of chondrogenesis; for example, both the direct application of GDF5 protein to developing limb cartilage and transgenic *Gdf5* overexpression are pro-chondrogenic [8,18], although in limb joints the pro-chondrogenic effects of GDFs are probably inhibited by Noggin [19]. *Gdf5/6/7* form a closely related subfamily of BMPs, sharing >80% identity in their mature C-terminal signaling domains [10]. The strong similarity of *Gdf5* and *Gdf6* suggest they share similar signaling properties. Genetic evidence from analysis of *Gdf5/Gdf6* compound mutant mice supports the idea that they have similar, partly redundant roles in skeletal development that are determined largely by site of expression rather than distinct signaling mechanisms [20]. A unifying theme of both limb joints and the frontal bone is that both are important paracrine signaling centers for adjacent targets (that is, cartilage in the limb and the suture mesenchyme in the cranium). We propose that *Gdf6* expression in the frontal bone primordium enables it to serve as a paracrine signaling center to affect cellular processes in the suture mesenchyme and the parietal rudiment. It is not yet clear if this occurs via direct signaling or through indirect effects transmitted by downstream effectors.

Interestingly, the onset of ALP activity is delayed in the parietal, but not frontal, primordia in *Gdf6−/−* embryos. Since *Gdf6* is expressed in the frontal but not parietal primordia, this suggests *Gdf6* signaling from the frontal primordium also acts in a paracrine manner to influence maturation of the parietal. In this view, Gdf6 actually stimulates osteogenic maturation of the parietal rudiment, although it is not clear if this affect is direct or indirect (for example, it could be a secondary effect mediated by Gdf6 regulating a separate factor in the suture mesenchyme). Therefore, data regarding Gdf6's possible roles in skeletal differentiation are important for interpretation of our results. Several reports indicate that like Gdf5, Gdf6 can stimulate chondrogenic differentiation in cell culture models [11]. Whether Gdf6 is pro- or anti-osteogenic is less clear. Some studies indicate that in vitro, Gdf6 can have pro-osteogenic effects on osteoblastic cells in similar manner to Gdf5, albeit its ability to induce osteoblast markers is much less than that of the "canonical" osteogenic BMPs such as BMP2 or BMP7 [21]. However, Gdf6 can inhibit ALP expression and mineralization in bone marrow-derived mesenchymal stem cells [22]. *In vitro* experiments must be interpreted with caution, due to potential differences in expression of BMP receptors and/or inhibitors across cell lines. In general, *in vitro* studies indicate that Gdf6 seems consistently capable of promoting differentiation of chondrogenic cells but relatively poor, or inhibitory, at promoting osteogenesis.

However, injection of GDF5 into perinatal mouse calvaria *in vivo* led to increased bone formation [23]. While this suggest GDFs can have stimulatory effects on calvarial osteogenic differentiation, the different timing and context of Gdf5 application may not lead to the same effects as Gdf6 in the prenatal calvaria and Gdf6 may have distinct signaling effects compared to Gdf5, despite similar receptor usage [24]. Other studies indicate that the effects of *Gdf6* on ALP induction are context dependent [25]. This effect might be mediated by receptor subunit combinations, interactions with inhibitors such as Noggin, or even heterodimerization with other BMP family members. Noggin is expressed in layers surrounding the developing frontal and parietal bones and can bind Gdf6 and inhibit its signaling ability [26]. Noggin can repress BMP signaling in the coronal suture [27], so it likely inhibits Gdf6-mediated signaling. However, Noggin is not required for suture formation, as *Noggin−/−* embryos do form coronal sutures (not shown). Therefore, Noggin is probably dispensable for the function of Gdf6 in suppressing suture differentiation. However, our data would not exclude the possibility that the reduction of ALP activity in the Gdf6−/− E12.5 parietal bone could be caused by increased Noggin activity, secondary to a reduction of Gdf6 that normally suppresses Noggin. Xenopus GDF6 can heterodimerize with other BMPs, such as BMP2, *in vivo* [26,28] and other BMP heterodimers can have distinct and potent effects as compared to homodimers [29]. Therefore it is possible that Gdf6/BMP heterodimers have unique signaling properties.

Alternatively, it is possible that the relative temporal development of the frontal and parietal rudiments is critical, and that the relative delay of the parietal ossification sequence leads indirectly to failure of suture establishment. However, the onset of *Runx2* transcription is not delayed in *Gdf6−/−* embryos, suggesting *Gdf6* is not required for temporal control of *Runx2* mRNA in calvarial rudiments. We postulate that the suture mesenchyme and the parietal rudiment may be differentially sensitive to *Gdf6* signaling.

Gdf6 Autoregulation and Interaction with other BMPs

We observed that *Gdf6* transcription is increased in frontal bone, but reduced in eyes, of *Gdf6−/−* embryos. This suggests differential, tissue-specific autoregulation of *Gdf6*. Interestingly, *Gdf5* represses its own transcription in limb joints [8]. We propose that *Gdf6* autoregulates itself in the frontal bone and that Gdf6/BMP signaling levels are fine-tuned during normal coronal suture development to coordinate proper differentiation and morphogenesis. Interestingly, *Bmp4* and *Gdf6* are coexpressed in both the dorsal retina and the frontal bone primordia [16]. Mutations in *Bmp4* and *Gdf6* independently disrupt eye development [15,30,31]. Although *Gdf6* is expressed in the frontal bone rudiment, there is no evidence for a frontal bone defect in *Gdf6−/−*. This is likely due to compensation by *Bmp4*. *Bmp4+/−; Gdf6−/−* mice at E18.5 do in fact have a frontal bone defect, with the persistence of large fontanelles that is not observed in either single heterozygotes (data not shown; manuscript in preparation). We speculate that these two BMP ligands cooperate to regulate suture and/or calvarial development.

Conclusions

In summary, we found that *Gdf6* is required to control an early stage of repressed osteogenic differentiation in the coronal suture. Not only does this suggest potential new mechanisms for this BMP family member in regulating bone growth, it nominates *GDF6* as a candidate gene harboring mutations in individuals with coronal craniosynostosis. *GDF6* mutations in humans have been associated with eye and postcranial skeletal abnormalities although these effects are characterized by incomplete penetrance and phenotypic heterogeneity [15,32]. Interestingly, genomic lesions close to the *GDF6* genomic region are associated with Nablus Mask-Like Facial Syndrome [33,34,35] which is a complex multigene deletion syndrome characterized by loss of a critical region just proximal to *GDF6*. In one of only two known patients where the genomic deletion included *GDF6*, coronal craniosynostosis was observed [33,34]. We propose that some individuals having coronal craniosynostosis with unknown etiology may harbor mutations in *GDF6*.

Materials and Methods

Mice, Crosses and Genotyping

The *Gdf6−/−* mouse [9] was a gift from Dr. David Kingsley and was backcrossed onto a C57BL/6J background for more than 10 generations. Since the loss of *Gdf6* is perinatal lethal on this background (not shown), all time points were collected prenatally. For fate mapping experiments, *Gdf6+/−* mice were crossed to *R26R+/−* [36] to produce *Gdf6+/−; R26R+/−* (double heterozygotes), which were then crossed to *Wnt1Cre+/−* [37]; *Gdf6+/−* mice. Embryonic age was determined through detection of the vaginal plug, with noon of that day observed as E0.5. DNA samples for genotyping were isolated using tail snips from postnatal mice and yolk sacs from embryos, and processed as previously described [38]. The *Gdf6* [9], *R26R* [36], and *Wnt1-Cre* [39] lines were genotyped by PCR analysis as previously described. The use of animals in this study was approved by the Vanderbilt University Institutional Animal Care and Use Committee as part of animal use protocol M/09/293, approved on 1/25/10 and 1/25/11.

Whole Mount Skeletal Preps

Mid-gestation mice from E14.5 to E18.5 were collected, organs removed and skinned. Each specimen was placed in a separate 50 ml conical tube and then soaked in 95% ethanol for 1 day. Specimens were agitated constantly on a shaker. Preps were then stained in alcian blue solution [20% glacial acetic acid, 0.015% alcian blue in 95% ethanol] for 14 days, destained in 95% ethanol for 1 day, then transferred into 1% KOH until cleared. Once cleared, the skeletal preps were placed in alizarin red staining solution [0.00125% alizarin red in 1% KOH] for 1 day. Skeletal preps were then transferred into graded changes of increasing glycerol for storage (15%, 30%, 50%, 70%, 90% glycerol made in 1× PBS, 100% glycerol).

Whole Mount and Slide *in situ* Hybridization

The *Gdf6* RNA probe was generated by cloning a PCR fragment using the primers 5′- AAGCATGGAAGGAGGAT-GAAAGGG- 3′ and 5′- CGACCTCCAGTAACTT-TAGTGTTGTCA -3′, targeting the *Gdf6* 3′ untranslated region, into the pGEM-Teasy vector (Promega). The *Runx2* RNA probe was made using the primers and protocol described previously [40]. Hybridization was performed over night at 63°C, with embryos incubated in 200 ng/ml (whole-mount) or 30 ng of probe per slide (sections). For sectioning, embryos were equilibrated in 30% sucrose and then embedded in Tissue-Tek O.C.T. compound (Sakura Finetek). Frozen sections were collected at 18 um. For each time-point, embryos were from the same litter and stained for an equal length of time.

Histology

Embryos were dissected in 1× PBS and fixed for 60 min at 4° in 10% neutral buffer formalin (Sigma), decapitated, bisected sagittally, the skin removed, and fixed for another 15 min. Embryos were prepared for X-Gal staining as previously described [38]. Whole-mount specimens were further stained with alizarin red overnight. Sectioned specimens were dehydrated through ethanol series and embedded in paraffin. 10 µM sections were collected and counterstained with nuclear fast red (Vector Laboratories).

For staining for ALP activity, frozen sections were collected at 18 um and stored at −80°C until ready for staining. Slides were brought to room temperature, then washed in acetone, TBST [Tris-buffered saline pH 8.0, 1% Tween-20], and NTMT [0.1 M NaCl, 0.1 M Tris-HCl pH 9.5, 50 mM MgCl2, 0.1% Tween-20] at 4°C, stained with nitro-blue tetrazolium chloride (NBT) and bromo-4-chloro-3′-indolyphosphate p-toluidine (BCIP) at room temperature, then counterstained with nuclear fast red.

Immunohistochemistry for Phospho-Histone-H3 (Ser10) and Cleaved Caspase-3 (Asp175) was carried out on cryosections. Slides were fixed in neutral buffer formalin, treated with 0.3% H_2O_2 to quench endogenous peroxidase activity, and blocked with 5% normal goat serum in PBS. Diluted primary antibody (Phospho-Histone-H3 1:200, Cleaved Caspase-3 1:12,800) was applied overnight at 4°C. Sections were developed using a biotinylated rabbit secondary antibody with ABC solution (Vector Laboratories) and DAB.

Supporting Information

Figure S1 Analysis of cell proliferation and apoptosis in the coronal suture. Adjacent sections stained for ALP activity, highlighting the location of the frontal and parietal bones (A–F dotted lines), and antibodies for phospho-histone H3 (A'–C') or cleaved caspase-3 (D'–F'). Positive cells are marked with arrows. (G) Quantification of the mean number of proliferating cells (y-axis) counted in the suture region (x-axis). (H) Quantification of the mean number of proliferating cells (y-axis) counted in each region of the suture; the frontal bone, parietal bone, and suture mesenchyme (x-axis). The mean number of proliferating cells in each region of the suture was not counted for *Gdf6*−/− embryos since there is no suture mesenchyme and the border between the frontal and parietal bones cannot be distinguished. N = 3 embryos for each genotype and antibody treatment with 5 sections per embryo quantified. Differences the number of proliferating cells per suture region were analyzed using a t-test.

Figure S2 *Gdf6* expression at E14.5. Gdf6 expression was downregulated in the frontal bone by E14.5 in wild-type (B), *Gdf6*+/− (D), and *Gdf6*−/− embryos (F). Adjacent sections were stained for ALP to highlight the locations of the frontal and parietal bones (E–G, dotted lines). Previously reported *Gdf6* expression in the middle ear bone joints was clearly visible in sections from the same series, acting as a positive control (G,H).

Acknowledgments

We gratefully thank Dr. Robert Maxson and Nancy Wu for experimental training and advice, and for many helpful discussions. We thank Dr. Michelle Southard-Smith, Carrie Weise, and Yue Hou for technical assistance. We thank Dr. David Kingsley for sharing the *Gdf6* knockout mouse. We thank Dr. Kelly Chandler for the generation of the *Gdf6 in situ* RNA probe. We thank Dr. Michelle Southard-Smith and Dr. Trish Labosky for sharing the *Wnt1-Cre* and *R26R* mouse lines. We thank Dr. Xiangli Yang, Dr. Steven Pregizer, and Eva Broeckelmann for critical comments on the manuscript and helpful discussions.

Author Contributions

Conceived and designed the experiments: DEC DPM. Performed the experiments: DEC. Analyzed the data: DEC DPM. Contributed reagents/materials/analysis tools: DEC DPM. Wrote the paper: DEC DPM.

References

1. Cohen MM Jr. (2005) Editorial: perspectives on craniosynostosis. Am J Med Genet A 136A: 313–326.
2. Furuya Y, Edwards MS, Alpers CE, Tress BM, Ousterhout DK, et al. (1984) Computerized tomography of cranial sutures. Part 1: Comparison of suture anatomy in children and adults. J Neurosurg 61: 53–58.
3. Wilkie AO (1997) Craniosynostosis: genes and mechanisms. Hum Mol Genet 6: 1647–1656.
4. Kabbani H, Raghuveer TS (2004) Craniosynostosis. Am Fam Physician 69: 2863–2870.
5. Merrill AE, Bochukova EG, Brugger SM, Ishii M, Pilz DT, et al. (2006) Cell mixing at a neural crest-mesoderm boundary and deficient ephrin-Eph signaling in the pathogenesis of craniosynostosis. Hum Mol Genet 15: 1319–1328.
6. Iseki S, Wilkie AO, Morriss-Kay GM (1999) Fgfr1 and Fgfr2 have distinct differentiation- and proliferation-related roles in the developing mouse skull vault. Development 126: 5611–5620.
7. Doherty ES, Lacbawan F, Hadley DW, Brewer C, Zalewski C, et al. (2007) Muenke syndrome (FGFR3-related craniosynostosis): expansion of the phenotype and review of the literature. Am J Med Genet A 143A: 3204–3215.
8. Storm EE, Kingsley DM (1999) GDF5 coordinates bone and joint formation during digit development. Dev Biol 209: 11–27.
9. Settle SH Jr., Rountree RB, Sinha A, Thacker A, Higgins K, et al. (2003) Multiple joint and skeletal patterning defects caused by single and double mutations in the mouse Gdf6 and Gdf5 genes. Dev Biol 254: 116–130.
10. Storm EE, Huynh TV, Copeland NG, Jenkins NA, Kingsley DM, et al. (1994) Limb alterations in brachypodism mice due to mutations in a new member of the TGF beta-superfamily. Nature 368: 639–643.

11. Nochi H, Sung JH, Lou J, Adkisson HD, Maloney WJ, et al. (2004) Adenovirus mediated BMP-13 gene transfer induces chondrogenic differentiation of murine mesenchymal progenitor cells. J Bone Miner Res 19: 111–122.
12. Poliakov A, Cotrina M, Wilkinson DG (2004) Diverse roles of eph receptors and ephrins in the regulation of cell migration and tissue assembly. Dev Cell 7: 465–480.
13. Jiang X, Iseki S, Maxson RE, Sucov HM, Morriss-Kay GM (2002) Tissue origins and interactions in the mammalian skull vault. Dev Biol 241: 106–116.
14. Rice DP, Kim HJ, Thesleff I (1999) Apoptosis in murine calvarial bone and suture development. Eur J Oral Sci 107: 265–275.
15. Asai-Coakwell M, French CR, Berry KM, Ye M, Koss R, et al. (2007) GDF6, a novel locus for a spectrum of ocular developmental anomalies. Am J Hum Genet 80: 306–315.
16. Mortlock DP, Guenther C, Kingsley DM (2003) A general approach for identifying distant regulatory elements applied to the Gdf6 gene. Genome Res 13: 2069–2081.
17. Ishii M, Merrill AE, Chan YS, Gitelman I, Rice DP, et al. (2003) Msx2 and Twist cooperatively control the development of the neural crest-derived skeletogenic mesenchyme of the murine skull vault. Development 130: 6131–6142.
18. Tsumaki N, Tanaka K, Arikawa-Hirasawa E, Nakase T, Kimura T, et al. (1999) Role of CDMP-1 in skeletal morphogenesis: promotion of mesenchymal cell recruitment and chondrocyte differentiation. J Cell Biol 144: 161–173.
19. Brunet LJ, McMahon JA, McMahon AP, Harland RM (1998) Noggin, cartilage morphogenesis, and joint formation in the mammalian skeleton. Science 280: 1455–1457.
20. Settle S, Marker P, Gurley K, Sinha A, Thacker A, et al. (2001) The BMP family member Gdf7 is required for seminal vesicle growth, branching morphogenesis, and cytodifferentiation. Dev Biol 234: 138–150.
21. Bobacz K, Ullrich R, Amoyo L, Erlacher L, Smolen JS, et al. (2006) Stimulatory effects of distinct members of the bone morphogenetic protein family on ligament fibroblasts. Ann Rheum Dis 65: 169–177.
22. Shen B, Bhargav D, Wei A, Williams LA, Tao H, et al. (2009) BMP-13 emerges as a potential inhibitor of bone formation. Int J Biol Sci 5: 192–200.
23. Yoshimoto T, Yamamoto M, Kadomatsu H, Sakoda K, Yonamine Y, et al. (2006) Recombinant human growth/differentiation factor-5 (rhGDF-5) induced bone formation in murine calvariae. J Periodontal Res 41: 140–147.
24. Mazerbourg S, Sangkuhl K, Luo CW, Sudo S, Klein C, et al. (2005) Identification of receptors and signaling pathways for orphan bone morphogenetic protein/growth differentiation factor ligands based on genomic analyses. J Biol Chem 280: 32122–32132.
25. Williams LA, Bhargav D, Diwan AD (2008) Unveiling the bmp13 enigma: redundant morphogen or crucial regulator? Int J Biol Sci 4: 318–329.
26. Chang C, Hemmati-Brivanlou A (1999) Xenopus GDF6, a new antagonist of noggin and a partner of BMPs. Development 126: 3347–3357.
27. Warren SM, Brunet LJ, Harland RM, Economides AN, Longaker MT (2003) The BMP antagonist noggin regulates cranial suture fusion. Nature 422: 625–629.
28. Lyons KM, Hogan BL, Robertson EJ (1995) Colocalization of BMP 7 and BMP 2 RNAs suggests that these factors cooperatively mediate tissue interactions during murine development. Mech Dev 50: 71–83.
29. Butler SJ, Dodd J (2003) A role for BMP heterodimers in roof plate-mediated repulsion of commissural axons. Neuron 38: 389–401.
30. den Hollander AI, Biyanwila J, Kovach P, Bardakjian T, Traboulsi EI, et al. Genetic defects of GDF6 in the zebrafish out of sight mutant and in human eye developmental anomalies. BMC Genet 11: 102.
31. Dunn NR, Winnier GE, Hargett LK, Schrick JJ, Fogo AB, et al. (1997) Haploinsufficient phenotypes in Bmp4 heterozygous null mice and modification by mutations in Gli3 and Alx4. Dev Biol 188: 235–247.
32. Tassabehji M, Fang ZM, Hilton EN, McGaughran J, Zhao Z, et al. (2008) Mutations in GDF6 are associated with vertebral segmentation defects in Klippel-Feil syndrome. Hum Mutat 29: 1017–1027.
33. Raas-Rothschild A, Dijkhuizen T, Sikkema-Raddatz B, Werner M, Dagan J, et al. (2009) The 8q22.1 microdeletion syndrome or Nablus mask-like facial syndrome: report on two patients and review of the literature. Eur J Med Genet 52: 140–144.
34. Salpietro CD, Briuglia S, Rigoli L, Merlino MV, Dallapiccola B (2003) Confirmation of Nablus mask-like facial syndrome. Am J Med Genet A 121A: 283–285.
35. Shieh JT, Aradhya S, Novelli A, Manning MA, Cherry AM, et al. (2006) Nablus mask-like facial syndrome is caused by a microdeletion of 8q detected by array-based comparative genomic hybridization. Am J Med Genet A 140: 1267–1273.
36. Soriano P (1999) Generalized lacZ expression with the ROSA26 Cre reporter strain. Nat Genet 21: 70–71.
37. Danielian PS, Muccino D, Rowitch DH, Michael SK, McMahon AP (1998) Modification of gene activity in mouse embryos in utero by a tamoxifen-inducible form of Cre recombinase. Curr Biol 8: 1323–1326.
38. Chandler KJ, Chandler RL, Broeckelmann EM, Hou Y, Southard-Smith EM, et al. (2007) Relevance of BAC transgene copy number in mice: transgene copy number variation across multiple transgenic lines and correlations with transgene integrity and expression. Mamm Genome 18: 693–708.
39. Chai Y, Jiang X, Ito Y, Bringas P Jr., Han J, et al. (2000) Fate of the mammalian cranial neural crest during tooth and mandibular morphogenesis. Development 127: 1671–1679.
40. Chandler RL, Chandler KJ, McFarland KA, Mortlock DP (2007) Bmp2 transcription in osteoblast progenitors is regulated by a distant 3′ enhancer located 156.3 kilobases from the promoter. Mol Cell Biol 27: 2934–2951.

15

Load Regulates Bone Formation and Sclerostin Expression through a TGFβ-Dependent Mechanism

Jacqueline Nguyen[1]ⁿ, Simon Y. Tang[2], Daniel Nguyen[2], Tamara Alliston[1,2,3,4,5]*

1 Graduate Program in Oral and Craniofacial Sciences, University of California San Francisco, San Francisco, California, United States of America, 2 Department of Orthopaedic Surgery, University of California San Francisco, San Francisco, California, United States of America, 3 Department of Bioengineering and Therapeutic Sciences, University of California San Francisco, San Francisco, California, United States of America, 4 Department of Otolaryngology Head and Neck Surgery, University of California San Francisco, San Francisco, California, United States of America, 5 Eli and Edythe Broad Center of Regeneration Medicine and Stem Cell Research, University of California San Francisco, San Francisco, California, United States of America

Abstract

Bone continually adapts to meet changing physical and biological demands. Osteoblasts, osteoclasts, and osteocytes cooperate to integrate these physical and biochemical cues to maintain bone homeostasis. Although TGFβ acts on all three of these cell types to maintain bone homeostasis, the extent to which it participates in the adaptation of bone to mechanical load is unknown. Here, we investigated the role of the TGFβ pathway in load-induced bone formation and the regulation of Sclerostin, a mechanosensitive antagonist of bone anabolism. We found that mechanical load rapidly represses the net activity of the TGFβ pathway in osteocytes, resulting in reduced phosphorylation and activity of key downstream effectors, Smad2 and Smad3. Loss of TGFβ sensitivity compromises the anabolic response of bone to mechanical load, demonstrating that the mechanosensitive regulation of TGFβ signaling is essential for load-induced bone formation. Furthermore, sensitivity to TGFβ is required for the mechanosensitive regulation of Sclerostin, which is induced by TGFβ in a Smad3-dependent manner. Together, our results show that physical cues maintain bone homeostasis through the TGFβ pathway to regulate Sclerostin expression and the deposition of new bone.

Editor: Lin Mei, Medical College of Georgia, United States of America

Funding: This work was funded by the National Institutes of Health F30DE022680, F32AR059497, and R01DE019284 grants. The funders had no role in study design, data collection and analysis, decision to publish, or preparation of the manuscript.

Competing Interests: The authors have declared that no competing interests exist.

* E-mail: tamara.alliston@ucsf.edu

These authors contributed equally to this work.

Introduction

Osteocytes coordinate the adaptation of bone to changing physical demands on the skeleton [1]. Upon sensing mechanical load through their canalicular processes, osteocytes initiate a series of biochemical signaling events that coordinate the activity of osteoblasts and osteoclasts to increase bone mass [2]. In this way, physical stimuli employ established biochemical pathways long known to participate in the maintenance of bone homeostasis, including parathyroid hormone (PTH) [3], insulin-like growth factor-I (IGF-1) [4], and prostaglandin signaling (PGE_2) [5]. Despite recent progress in deciphering the molecular mechanisms by which physical signals regulate bone homeostasis, many questions remain.

Sclerostin, a secreted protein expressed by osteocytes, responds to mechanical load and antagonizes bone formation [6]. Loss of function mutations in either the sclerostin-encoding gene, *SOST*, or in its regulatory sequence cause the human syndromes known as sclerosteosis and van Buchem disease, both of which are characterized by high bone mass [7]. Sclerostin acts by binding to the Wnt co-receptor Lrp5/6 on osteoblasts to inhibit Wnt-inducible osteogenesis [8]. Sclerostin plays a central role in the anabolic response of bone to mechanical loading. Applied mechanical loads repress Sclerostin mRNA and protein expression [6], thereby releasing the brakes on new bone synthesis. Conversely, Sclerostin-antagonizing antibodies prevent bone loss due to unloading of the bone [9]. Several pathways that control bone development and metabolism also regulate *SOST* expression. The BMP pathway induces *SOST* expression during bone development [10]. PTH, an essential regulator of mineral homeostasis, represses *SOST* expression [11]. This PTH-mediated repression of *SOST* requires MEF2 recruitment to a highly conserved regulatory region 35-kb downstream from the *SOST* gene [12]. The rapid increase in PGE_2 following mechanical load also contributes to the mechanosensitive repression of *SOST*, though the mechanism remains to be identified [13]. The master osteoblast transcription factor Runx2 binds and induces transcription from a more proximal element of the *SOST* promoter [14]. Although many pathways modulate *SOST* expression, these pathways do not fully explain the complexity of mechanotransduction in bone and the regulation of *SOST* expression.

TGFβ is a critical regulator of bone homeostasis. Through its effects on osteoblast and osteoclast migration, proliferation, differentiation and viability, TGFβ couples bone formation with bone resorption [15,16]. In this way, TGFβ maintains both bone mass and bone quality [17–18]. Activated TGFβ binds to its receptors, TβRI and TβRII, causing their heterotetramerization and transphosphorylation. Many intracellular proteins, including Smad2, Smad3 and other non-canonical effectors, are phosphorylated upon recruitment to the activated TβRI/TβRII complex [19]. Phosphorylated Smad3 translocates to the nucleus where it can activate or repress the activity of sequence-specific transcription factors, such as Runx2 [20]. Through crosstalk at each the ligand, receptor and effector levels, the TGFβ pathway integrates signals from multiple stimuli. For example, fluid flow induces TGFβ1 mRNA expression in SAOS-2 cells [21]. Cell-generated tension by myofibroblasts converts the TGFβ ligand from the latent to active form [22]. PTH receptors drive clustering and internalization of TβRI and TβRII, leading to desensitization of the pathway [23]. The nuclear localization of Smads is sensitive to other biochemical and physical cues, including Wnt signaling [24], cytoskeletal tension [25], and extracellular matrix stiffness [26]. However, the net effect of mechanical load on the overall activity of the TGFβ pathway remains unknown. Therefore, we hypothesize that the TGFβ pathway integrates signals provided by mechanical load to maintain bone homeostasis, in part by regulating the expression of Sclerostin.

Using a combination of genetically modified mouse models and *in vitro* approaches, we investigated the effect of mechanical load on TGFβ activity, the role of TGFβ in load-induced bone formation, and the regulatory relationship between TGFβ and Sclerostin. Taken together, our results suggest that TGFβ plays a critical role in the mechanosensitive regulation of Sclerostin and is required for the anabolic response of bone to mechanical load.

Materials and Methods

Mouse models

Treatments and protocols used for the animal studies were approved by the University of California, San Francisco Institution Animal Care and Use Committee (Protocol # AN082159-03A) and were designed to minimize discomfort to the animals. This study used 8–9 week-old male SBE-luciferase mice [27] or DNTβRII mice, which express a dominant negative version of TβRII under control of 1.8 kb of the osteocalcin promoter [28]. Wild type littermates were used as comparative controls.

In vivo mechanical loading of the tibiae

Axial compressive loads equivalent to 10 times the mouse's body weight were delivered by a Bose Electroforce ELF3200 desktop load frame (Bose, MN, USA) fitted with two custom-made hemi-spherical fixtures that gripped the mouse knee and ankle. Similar methods of *in vivo* loading have been shown to upregulate bone anabolism [29]. In our preliminary studies of *ex vivo* limb loading using in situ strain rosettes, these loading parameters produce maximum principal strains in the range of 1500–2500 με on the mid-diaphyseal surface of the tibiae. For each mouse, only the right hind limb was loaded, while the left hind limb was not loaded to serve as the contralateral control (nonloaded). Each round of loading consisted of 600 cycles of axial compression at 1 Hz administered under general injectable anesthesia. Mice were subjected to this loading regimen once daily for either 1 day (short-term) or once a day for 5 days (prolonged).

In vivo luciferase imaging

Five hours after a single bout of loading, the SBE-luc mice (n = 6) were anesthetized using isoflurane, injected with 150 mg D-luciferin (Xenogen) per kg body weight, and imaged using the IVIS-200 Bioluminescence system 10 minutes after injection (Caliper Bioscience, MA, USA) [22,30]. Photons emitted from living mice were acquired as photons per second per cm^2 per steradian (sr) by using LIVINGIMAGE software (Xenogen) and integrated over 20 min. For photon quantification, a region of interest was manually selected and kept constant within all experiments; the signal intensity was converted into photons/s/cm^2/sr. The resulting quantitative measures were segmented and contoured at the tibiae to determine the relative levels of Smad2/3 activity between the loaded and non-loaded limb.

Immunohistochemistry

The loaded and nonloaded tibiae from SBE-luciferase (n = 5), DNTβRII (n = 5), or WT mice (n = 5) were dissected and fixed in 2% paraformaldehyde for 24 h at 4°C. The bones were decalcified in 19% EDTA solution for 7–10 days and decalcification was confirmed with x-ray imaging. Bones were then infiltrated with a series of 10%, 20%, and 30% sucrose solutions [31]. After sucrose infiltration, each tibia was cut into three fragments, with the distal fragment being 8 mm long and the middle fragment being 6 mm long, to ensure that comparable sections of each region were analyzed for each bone. Each fragment was embedded in OCT for frozen sectioning (10 μm sections). The tissue sections were permeabilized with 0.3% Triton X-100, processed for antigen retrieval with Ficin (Invitrogen 00–3007), and blocked for intrinsic peroxidase activity with 3% hydrogen peroxide. For detection of luciferase, the sections were blocked with 1.5% normal goat serum (Vectastain) and incubated with anti-Luciferase primary antibodies (Abcam ab21176) at a dilution of 1:100. For detection of Sclerostin, the sections were blocked in 1.5% normal rabbit serum (Vectastain) and incubated with anti-Sclerostin primary antibodies (R&D Systems AF1589) at a dilution of 1:13 with 0.05% Tween-20. Normal rabbit IgG (Caltag Lab 10500) and normal goat IgG (Santa Cruz sc-2028) were used at the same concentrations as primary luciferase and Sclerostin antibodies, respectively, to control for the specificity of immunostaining. The binding of peroxidase-conjugated secondary antibodies was detected with a DAB kit (Vector Lab).

Three to five immunostained sections for each bone were analyzed quantitatively. A composite of 20X images was generated for each immunostained section, from which all DAB-stained (brown) and unstained lacunae were counted and recorded using ImageJ. The percent of osteocytes expressing luciferase or Sclerostin was determined by dividing the number of DAB-positive lacunae by the total number of lacunae for each section. The percent change in luciferase or Sclerostin expression due to load was determined by subtracting the averaged percentage of luciferase or Sclerostin expression in the nonloaded tibia from the loaded tibia as describe [6]. Since quantitative analyses consider the effect of loading only on the number of stained and unstained lacunae, not on the staining intensity, they likely underrepresent the effects of mechanical loading on Sclerostin and luciferase expression.

Micro-computed tomography

Five hours after the last session of *in vivo* loading of the DNTβRII mice and their WT littermates (n = 6), tibiae were dissected from euthanized mice, fixed in 4% paraformaldehyde in PBS, and serially dehydrated in graded ethanol. The bones were then scanned using micro-CT to determine the relative changes in bone geometry (VivaCT40, Scanco Medical AG). The micro-CT scanner was operated at the peak energy of 70 kVp, current of 114 μA, integration time of 381 ms, and a 10 μm voxel resolution. The scans were segmented using an attenuation constant of 200, and then the structural parameters of bone were evaluated. The proximal tibial trabecular bone was evaluated for changes in trabecular connectivity, trabecular thickness, and volume fraction. The cortical bone changes were evaluated at the tibio-fibular junction for cortical thickness, cross-sectional area, and moment of inertia.

Dynamic histomorphometry

Two intraperitoneal injections of calcein were administered at 0.02 mg/g body weight to DNTβRII mice and their WT littermates (n = 3) that underwent a prolonged 5-day loading regimen. The first injection was administered on the same day as the first loading bout, and the second injection was administered on the same day as the fifth and final loading bout (4 days apart). The mice were euthanized two days after the final loading bout and then the tibiae were collected and fixed in 4% paraformaldehyde in PBS, serially dehydrated in graded ethanol, and embedded in a plastic resin (TechnoVit 5, EMS, Pennsylvania). The embedded blocks were sectioned using a tungsten carbide blade and mounted on glass slides. The mineral apposition rate (MAR, mean inter-label thickness divided by the time between the two labeling periods) was computed at both the periosteal and the endosteal surfaces using ImageJ by evaluating fluorescent micrographs taken with a 20X optical objective. The Mineral Apposition Rate (MAR) was calculated in accordance with the ASBMR nomenclature [32].

Cell culture

UMR-106 cells (ATCC), a rat osteosarcoma cell line, and SAOS-2 cells (ATCC), a human osteosarcoma cell line, were used for the *in vitro* studies because they both express Sclerostin [12] [14]. UMR-106 cells were grown in DMEM 50% high glucose/50% F-12 media with 10% fetal bovine serum supplemented with 1% nonessential amino acids. SAOS-2 cells were grown in McCoy's 5A media with 15% fetal bovine serum. At 80% confluence, UMR-106 or SAOS-2 cells were treated with 5 ng/ml TGFβ1 (Peprotech, 100–36E) or 10 μM SB431542 (Sigma, S4317) for the indicated times. Cycloheximide (10 μg/ml, Sigma) or actinomycin D (1 μg/ml, Sigma) were added to cells 30 min prior to TGFβ treatment. For *Runx2* knockdown in SAOS-2 cells, cells were transiently transfected with 50 nM of human *Runx2* siRNA r(GGUUC AACGAUCUGAGAUU)d(TT) or AllStars negative control using Qiagen Hi-Perfect. For *Runx2* knockdown in UMR-106 cells, cells were transfected with 60 nM of rat *Runx2* siRNA (GACUCUAAACCUAGUUUGU[dt][dt]) and *Runx2* siRNA AS(ACAAACUAGGUUUAGAGUC[dt][dt]) (Sigma) or Sigma siRNA negative control (Sigma sic-001) using Qiagen Hi-Perfect. SAOS-2 cells were treated with TGFβ1 (5 ng/ml) for 24 h and cells were harvested 48h after transfection. UMR-106 cells were transfected for 72 h with repeated transfection every 24 h. At the last transfection, UMR-106 cells were treated with 5 ng/ml TGFβ1 and harvested 24 h later. All results shown are from UMR-106 cells, but they were repeated in SAOS-2 cells with similar but not identical conclusions.

RNA extraction and quantitative PCR

RNA was extracted from cells using the Qiagen RNeasy Mini Kit. cDNA was generated from up to 1 μg of RNA with the iScript cDNA Synthesis kit (Bio-Rad). Quantitative PCR was performed using iQ SYBR Green Supermix (Bio-Rad) with the following primers: rat *L19*-F (GCATATGGGCATAGGGAAGA); rat *L19*-R (CCATGAGAATCCGCTTGTTT); rat *SOST*-F (GCACCATGCAGCTCTCATTA); rat *SOST*-R (CATTCTTGAAGGCTTGCCAC); rat Runx2-F (ACCCAGGCGTATTTCAGATG); rat Runx2-R (AGTGAGGGATGAAATGCCTG); human *L19*-F (GGGATTTGCATTCAGAGATCAG); human *L19*-R (GGAAGGGCATCTCGTAAG); human *SOST*-F (GGACTCCAGTGCCTTTTGAA); human *SOST*-R (CTGAATTCTGGAAGTGACCTTG); human *Runx2*-F (CCCCACGACAACCGCACCAT); human *Runx2*-R (CACTCCGGCCCACAAATC).

Western Analysis

For Western analysis of cortical bone protein, both tibiae were collected 3–5 h after one application of unilateral load (n = 4). Bones were trimmed to remove the distal and proximal epiphyses and flushed with PBS to remove bone marrow. The remaining cortical bone was homogenized with a rotor-stator homogenizer (Omni) in radioimmunoprecipitation assay (RIPA) buffer (10 mM Tris-HCl pH 8, 140 mM NaCl, 1 mM EDTA, 0.5 mM EGTA, 1% Triton X-100, 0.1% Sodium deoxycholate, 0.1% SDS) supplemented with 5 mM Na_3VO_4, 10 mM $NaPP_i$, 100 mM NaF, 500 μM PMSF, and 5 mg/ml eComplete Mini protease inhibitor tablet (Roche) [33]. Western analyses was also used to examinee lysates from SAOS-2 or UMR-106 cells collected after the indicated treatments. Cells were lysed using RIPA buffer on ice. Equal concentrations of the clarified protein from bone or cell lysate were resolved on a 10% SDS-PAGE gel and transferred to a nitrocellulose membrane. Subsequently, the membrane was blocked with 5% milk and the proteins were detected using primary antibodies against pSmad3 (gift from Dr. E. Leof), Smad3 (abcam ab28379), Sclerostin (Santa Cruz, S-19) and β-actin (Abcam, ab8226) and secondary antibodies tagged with an infrared fluorophore. Blots were imaged using a Licor infrared imaging system and are representative of at least 3 experiments.

Statistical Analyses

Statistics were performed using GraphPad Prism 5. T-tests were used to compare the differences between groups of normally distributed data. The Mann-Whitney nonparametric tests were used for non-normally distributed data. Significance of comparisons is defined by p-values equal to or less than 0.05.

Results

Load represses TGFβ signaling through Smad2/3

We used the murine one-limb loading model [29] to evaluate the role of TGFβ in load-induced bone formation. Mechanical stimulation was applied to one tibia of anesthetized SBE-Luc transgenic mice, which express luciferase under control of a Smad2/3-responsive synthetic promoter [30] [34]. By assessing the functional outcome of Smad2/3 activity, this approach evaluates the net effect of mechanical load on canonical TGFβ signaling – whether those effects occur at the ligand, receptor, or effector levels. Five hours after loading, *in vivo* bioluminescent imaging revealed that Smad2/3 reporter activity was consistently reduced in the loaded limb relative to the nonloaded limb of the same mouse (Figure 1A). Loading significantly repressed TGFβ-mediated Smad2/3 reporter activity by an average of 40% (Figure 1B). Immunolocalization of luciferase expression confirms that the load-mediated repression of Smad2/3 activity occurs in osteocytes within the cortical bone. In addition to generalized reduction in luciferase staining of cortical bone (Figure 1C), the number of luciferase positive osteocyte lacunae was significantly reduced in response to mechanical loading (Figure 1D). To further examine the mechanism by which load represses Smad2/3-mediated transactivation, we compared the effect of *in vivo* mechanical loading to the effect of *in vitro* TGFβ stimulation or inhibition on Smad3 phosphorylation. The level of phosphorylated Smad3 in the loaded cortical bone was consistently reduced relative to that in the nonloaded bone of the same animal (Figure 1E, lower panel). The magnitude of this load-dependent

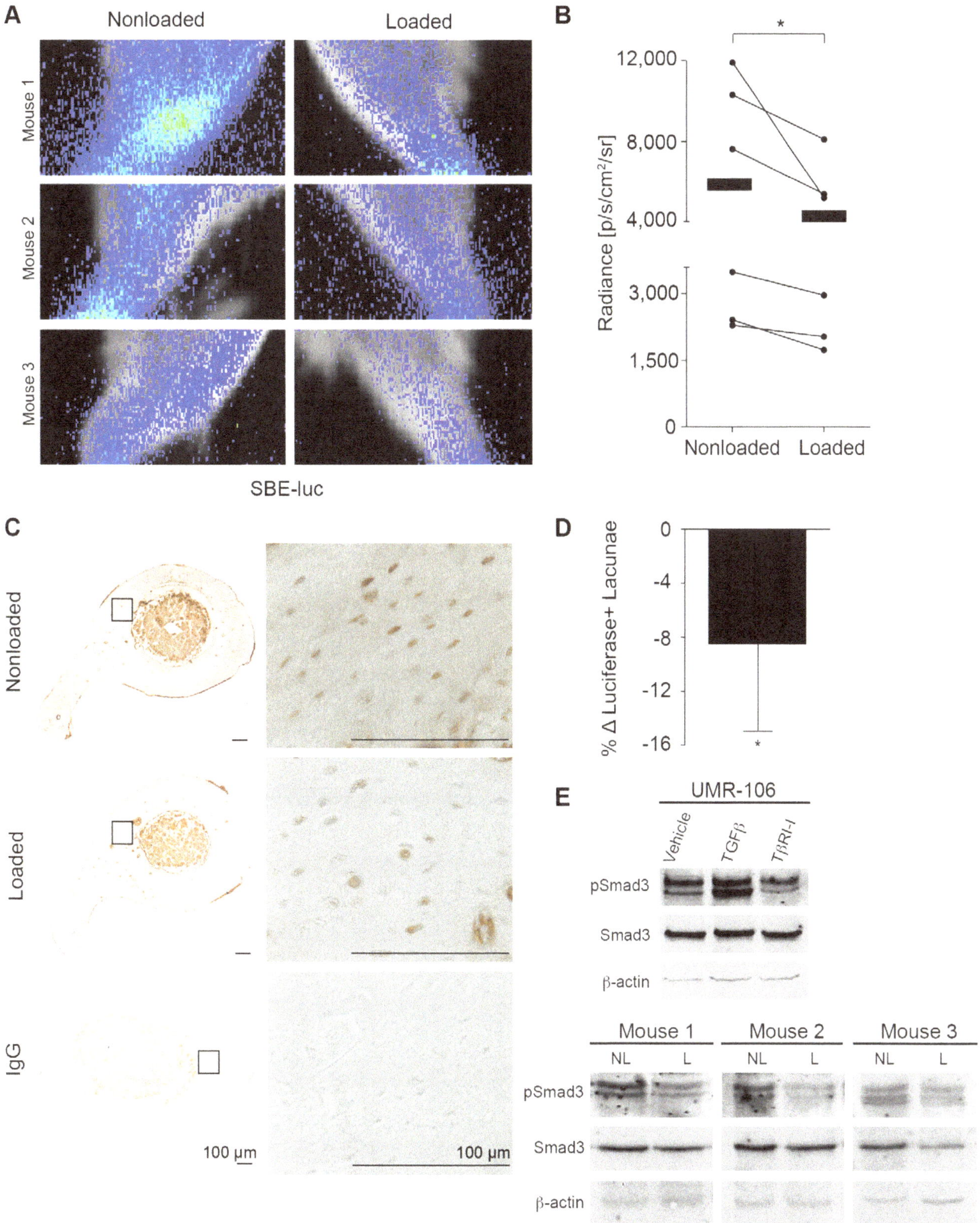

Figure 1. Mechanical load represses transactivation by Smad2/3 in tibial osteocytes. Images of luciferase activity in three individual SBE-luciferase mice 5h after *in vivo* loading reveals less Smad2/3-mediated transactivation in the loaded tibiae compared to nonloaded tibiae. Bioluminescence imaging and quantitation (A, B) show consistent reductions in luminescence in the loaded tibiae as opposed to the nonloaded tibiae. Radiance measurements from the nonloaded and loaded limb of the same animal are denoted by a line connecting the dots; black bars indicate the average radiance from nonloaded and loaded tibiae of 6 mice. Immunostaining for luciferase (C) in sections of tibial cortical bone and quantitation of luciferase-expressing osteocytes (D) reveal a decrease in luciferase-positive osteocytes in the loaded tibiae compared to the nonloaded control. UMR-106 whole cell lysates (E, upper panel) and tibial cortical bone lysates (E, lower panel) were evaluated for the level of

phosphorylated Smad3, total Smad3, and β-actin by Western analysis. UMR-106 cells were harvested 2 h after treatment with vehicle (DMSO), TGFβ1 (5 ng/ml), or an inhibitor of the TGFβ type 1 receptor, Alk5 (TβRI-I, SB431542). Tibiae were harvested 3h after loading (n = 4 mice). Loaded tibiae (L) were compared to the nonloaded tibiae (NL) from the same mouse. (* $p<0.05$).

effect is comparable to that achieved in UMR-106 cells treated with an inhibitor of the TGFβ type I receptor (Figure 1E, upper panel). Therefore, the phosphorylation and activity of the key TGFβ effector, Smad3, is rapidly and significantly reduced in osteocytes following mechanical loading of the limb.

The anabolic response of bone to mechanical load requires TGFβ signaling

We next examined whether the mechanosensitive regulation of TGFβ is necessary for load-induced bone formation. Mechanical load was applied to one limb of DNTβRII mice that have impaired TGFβ signaling due to expression of a dominant negative TGFβ type II receptor under control of the osteocalcin promoter [28]. In wild-type littermates, 5 days of mechanical loading stimulates a 19% increase in trabecular bone volume fraction (BV/TV) relative to the nonloaded limb (Table 1), similar to other studies [35,36]. However, mechanical stimulation in DNTβRII mice only increases bone formation by 9%. Mechanical load also failed to stimulate the same magnitude of increase in DNTβRII trabecular connectivity (Tb. Conn), cortical thickness (Cort. Th.), and moment of inertia (MOI) compared to wild-type animals (Figure 2A, Table 1). Impaired TGFβ signaling in DNTβRII mice compromises load-induced bone formation at both the periosteal and endosteal surfaces, as determined by the reduced fluorochrome intensity in the loaded DNTβRII bone compared to the loaded WT bone (Figure 2B). Despite a slightly increased basal mineral apposition rate (MAR) in DNTβRII mice, relative to WT, mechanical load was unable to further stimulate a significant increase in the DNTβRII MAR. In contrast, mechanical load stimulated large (>40%) and significant increases in WT MAR relative to the nonloaded WT limb (Figure 2C). These results demonstrate that the anabolic effect of mechanical load on bone formation requires an active TβRII-dependent signaling pathway.

TGFβ sensitivity is required for regulation of Sclerostin by mechanical load

Since the repression of *SOST*/Sclerostin by mechanical load is a key event in bone anabolism [6,37], we sought to determine if *SOST* regulation requires an intact TGFβ signaling pathway. We evaluated the effect of mechanical load on Sclerostin expression in DNTβRII mice. Following 5 days of loading, Sclerostin expression in wild-type cortical bone is reduced (Figure 3A). Specifically, the percentage of Sclerostin positive lacunae decreases by 9% following mechanical loading of the tibia (Figure 3B). However, in DNTβRII bone, the application of mechanical load produced no distinguishable difference in Sclerostin expression between the loaded and control limbs (Figures 3A, 3B), suggesting that the load-mediated regulation of Sclerostin requires sensitivity to TGFβ.

TGFβ signaling through Smad3 induces SOST expression

To examine mechanisms by which TGFβ sensitivity is required to regulate *SOST*, we first evaluated the effect of TGFβ on *SOST* mRNA levels in UMR-106 osteosarcoma cells. TGFβ rapidly induces *SOST* mRNA expression, with maximal induction following 8 h of treatment (Figure 4A). Conversely, *SOST* mRNA expression is repressed by a specific inhibitor of the TGFβ type I

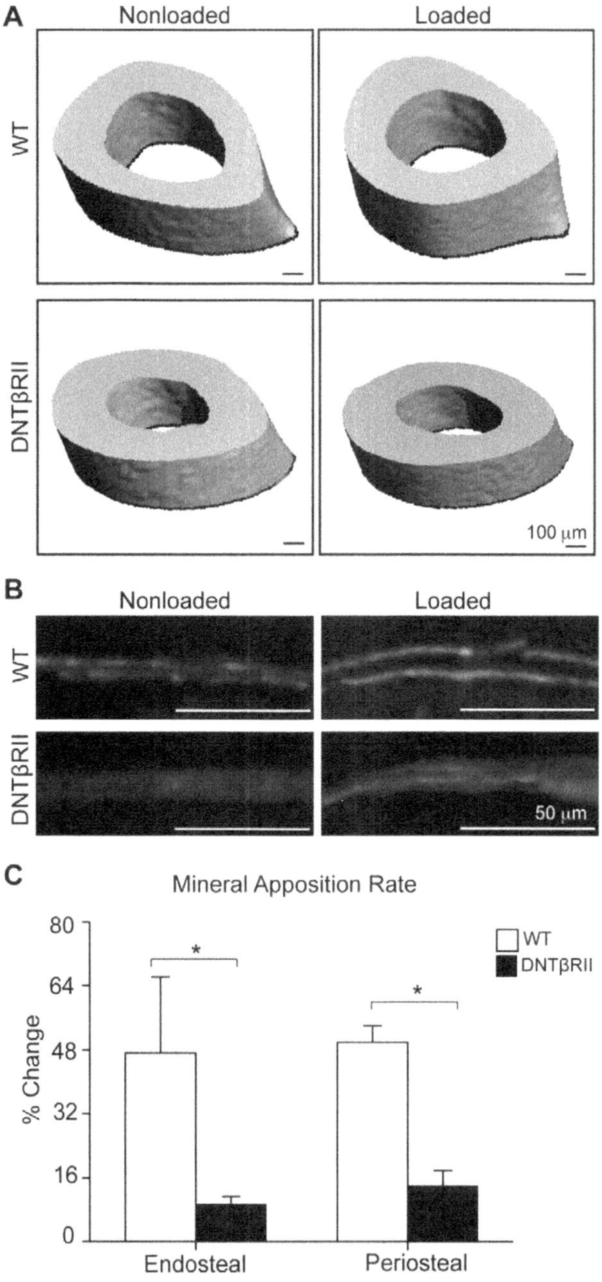

Figure 2. TGFβ signaling is required for load-induced bone formation. Micro-computed tomography images of loaded and nonloaded WT and DNTβRII tibiae (A) show that loading increases cortical bone thickness of WT bone more than DNTβRII bone. The overall fluorochrome intake was reduced in the DNTβRII mice despite a slightly increased basal mineral apposition rate in DNTβRII mice relative to WT (B). Results of dynamic bone histomorphometry are consistent with micro-CT, showing that the relative load-mediated increase in bone mineral apposition rate is significantly lower in DNTβRII tibiae than in WT (C) (* $p<0.05$).

Table 1. Quantitative measures of micro-computed tomography analyses.

Parameters	WT			DNTβRII		
	Nonloaded	*Loaded*	*% Change*	*Nonloaded*	*Loaded*	*% Change*
BV/TV	0.180+/−0.082	0.215+/−0.13*	19.4+/−5.5%	0.280+/−0.062	0.303+/−0.091*	**8.92+/−6.6%**
Tb. Conn. [1/mm³]	30.5+/−5.5	33.3+/−6.7*	9.20+/−7.3%	36.8+/−6.5	37.8+/−8.7	**2.90+/−3.1%**
Cort. Th. [mm]	0.218+/−0.11	0.249+/−0.096*	14.0+/−4.6%	0.265+/−0.13	0.287+/−0.15*	**8.30+/−3.4%**
MOI [1/mm⁴]	0.0530+/−0.022	0.0640+/−0.024*	12.0+/−4.3%	0.0665+/−0.014	0.0731+/−0.019*	**9.00+/−3.2%**

Values represent means and standard deviations for n = 5 mice. An asterisk (*) represents significant differences between loaded and nonloaded bones ($p<0.05$). Bolded values indicate parameters that differ significantly between WT and DNTβRII mice ($p<0.05$).

receptor (TβRI, Alk5) inhibitor SB431542 (Figures 4A). Consequently, TGFβ rapidly induces *SOST* expression *in vitro*.

Since mechanical load represses TGFβ signaling through Smad2/3 in osteocytes (Figure 1), as well as *SOST* expression [6], we hypothesized that TGFβ induction of *SOST* is Smad2/3-dependent. Even without exogenous TGFβ, cotransfected Smad3 was sufficient to activate a promoter-reporter construct that expresses luciferase under control of the human *SOST* promoter and 3 copies of a previously identified *SOST*-regulatory enhancer sequence (ECR5) (Figure 4B). Cotransfected Smad3 further enhanced the TGFβ-inducibility of this construct.

TGFβ/Smad3 induction of SOST is indirect and insensitive to Runx2

Though Smad3 increases *SOST*-reporter activity, these effects are indirect. As expected, incubation of UMR-106 cells with actinomycin D, an inhibitor of transcription, blocks TGFβ-inducible *SOST* mRNA expression (Figure 4C). However, TGFβ-inducible *SOST* mRNA expression is also completely abrogated in the presence of cycloheximide, an inhibitor of translation, even at the earliest 2 h time point (Figure 4C). These data suggest that TGFβ-inducible *SOST* expression occurs through an indirect Smad3-mediated pathway.

TGFβ and Smad3 regulate the expression and activity of the osteoblast transcription factor Runx2 [20]. Since *SOST* is a Runx2-target gene [14], we sought to determine if Runx2 was required for

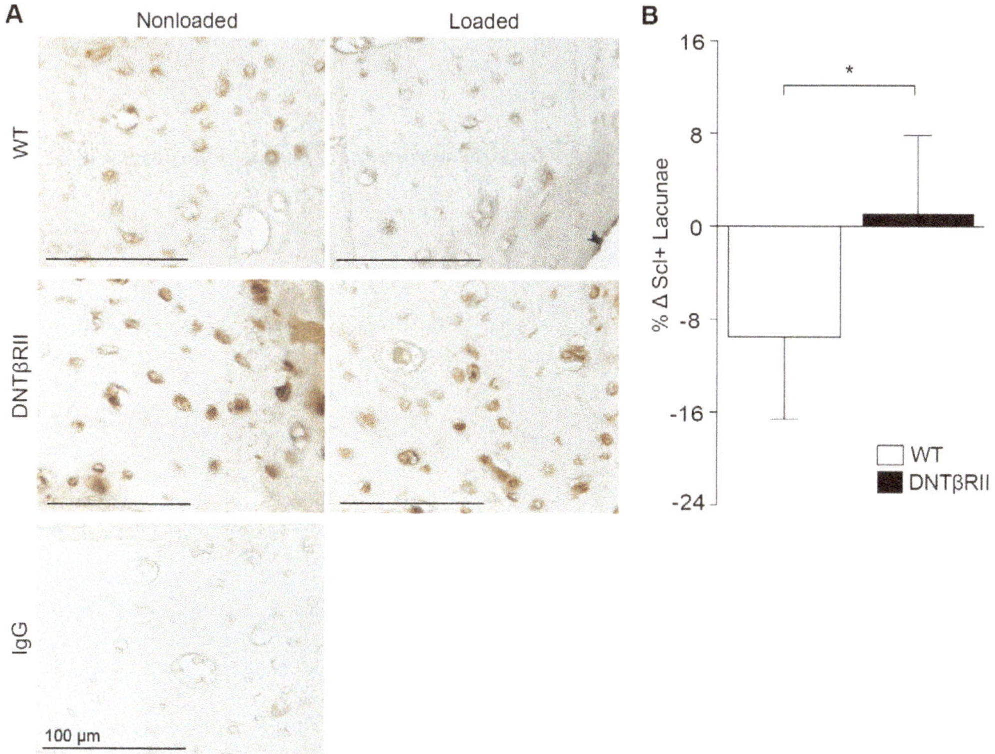

Figure 3. Load-sensitive Sclerostin regulation requires TGFβ signaling. Immunohistochemistry shows reduced Sclerostin expression between the loaded and nonloaded tibiae of WT mice, but no difference in Sclerostin expression in tibiae of DNTβRII mice (A). Control IgG used in the primary step of immunohistochemistry verifies the specificity of the SOST staining. Quantitation of Sclerostin-positive osteocytes in the tibiae confirm an 8% reduction in Sclerostin expression in loaded WT, but not in DNTβRII tibiae (B). (* $p<0.05$).

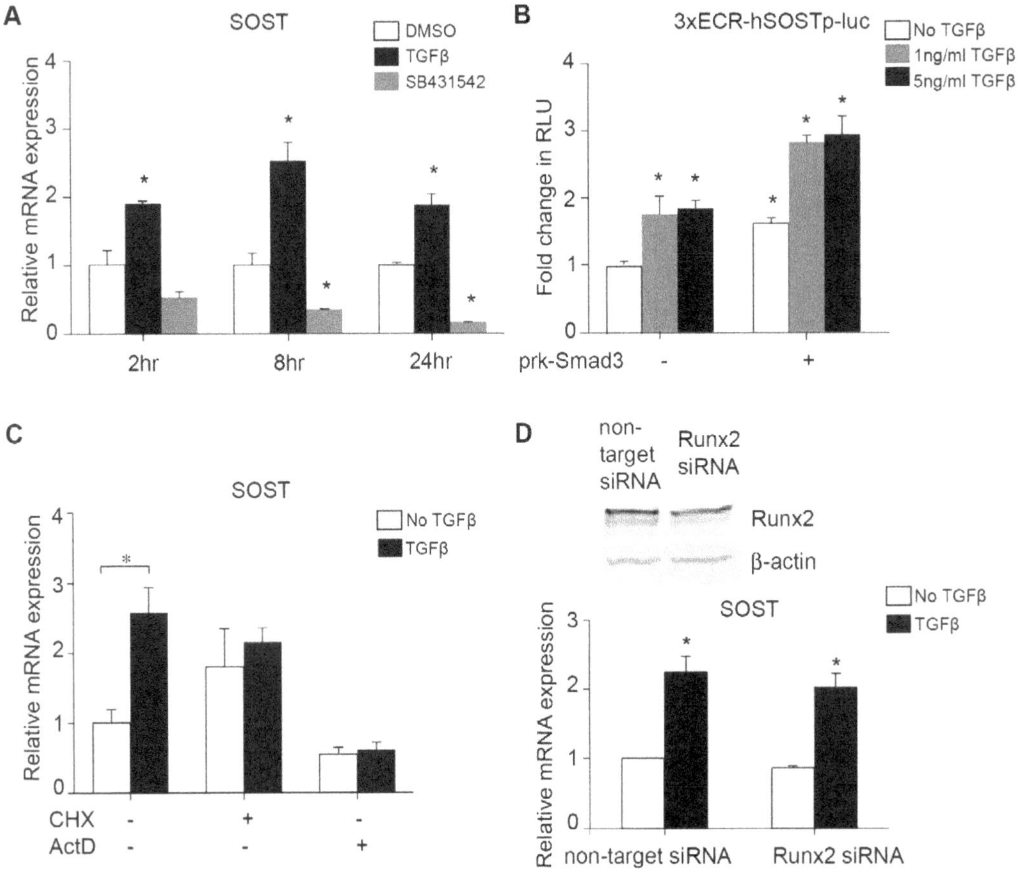

Figure 4. TGFβ induces *SOST* expression through Smad3. Treating UMR-106 cells with TGFβ1 (5 ng/ml) for 2, 8, or 24 h results in an increase in *SOST* mRNA, while inhibiting TGFβ signaling with SB431542 results in a decrease in *SOST* expression (A). Smad3 overexpression with pRK5-Smad3 induces the *SOST* promoter-reporter construct, 3XECR-hSOSTpLuc, in a TGFβ dose-dependent manner within 24 h of TGFβ treatment (B). Blocking translation with cycloheximide (CHX) or transcription with actinomycin-D (ActD) for 2 h prevents TGFβ (5 ng/ml) induction of *SOST* expression (C). siRNA mediated knockdown of *Runx2* did not prevent TGFβ (5 ng/ml) induction of *SOST* expression (D). (For panel C, * represents $p<0.05$ computed by comparing samples with added TGFβ to samples without added TGFβ in each treatment group; for all other panels, * $p<0.05$ computed by comparing samples to untreated cells).

the indirect TGFβ/Smad3-dependent regulation of *SOST* expression. *Runx2*-targetting siRNA yielded a 35–80% decrease in *Runx2* mRNA levels in UMR-106 and SAOS cells (not shown), with a corresponding reduction in Runx2 protein expression (Figure 4D). This treatment was sufficient to reduce the expression of Runx2-inducible RANKL by 35% (not shown). However, even with reduced levels of *Runx2*, the TGFβ-mediated induction of *SOST* mRNA was intact (Figure 4D), demonstrating that TGFβ-mediated induction of *SOST* is insensitive to the level of Runx2 activity. Together these findings show that TGFβ regulates SOST mRNA expression indirectly through a Smad3-dependent, Runx2-insensitive mechanism.

Discussion

Here, we report that mechanical load represses TGFβ activity, which is required for load-induced bone formation and the regulation of Sclerostin, an inhibitor of bone anabolism (Figure 5). Loading of mice tibiae rapidly inhibits phosphorylation of Smad3, a TGFβ effector, and consequently represses Smad3 activity in osteocytes. TGFβ signals through Smad3 to indirectly stimulate *SOST* mRNA expression. Furthermore, intact TGFβ signaling is required for load to repress Sclerostin expression and induce bone formation. Taken together, our results demonstrate that TGFβ plays a critical role in the mechanosensitive regulation of Sclerostin and is required for the anabolic response of bone to mechanical load.

Several lines of evidence implicate TGFβ as a regulator of bone homeostasis. Many mouse models with mutations in components of the TGFβ pathway have altered bone mass and bone matrix material properties, resulting from disruption of the tightly controlled balance between osteoblast and osteoclast activity. For example, reducing TGFβ signaling in mice by expression of a dominant negative TβRII allele in the osteoblast lineage increased bone mass by indirect reduction in osteoclast activity [28]. In addition, mice deficient in Smad3 have lower bone mass but an increased bone matrix elastic modulus indicating the importance of TGFβ in the maintenance of bone mass and bone quality [38]. Furthermore, inhibiting TGFβ signaling with a chemical inhibitor of TβRI affects postnatal bone formation and bone quality [30]. Stimuli that shift bone metabolism, including mechanical load, exert their effects by acting on pathways that normally maintain homeostasis. The extent to which TGFβ mediates the anabolic effect of mechanical load on bone has not previously been shown. Here, we show that disrupting TGFβ sensitivity in osteoblasts prevents mechanical

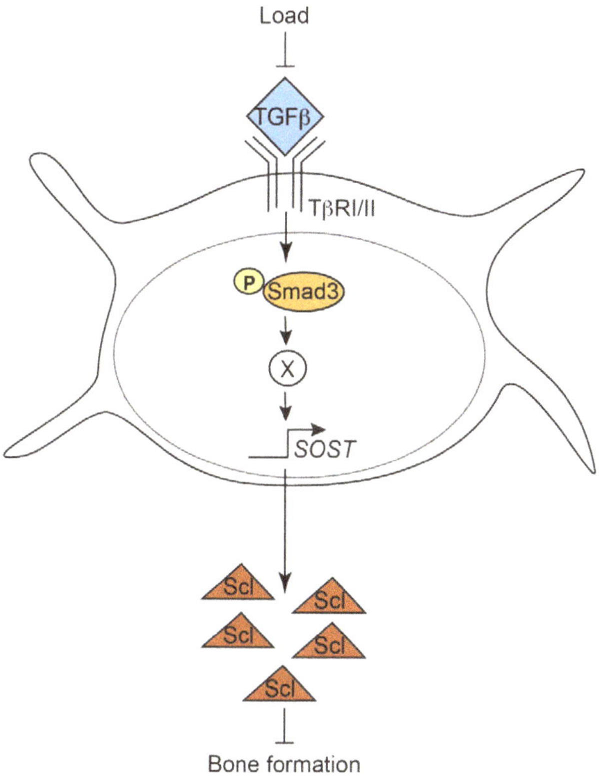

Figure 5. The role of TGFβ signaling in load-induced bone formation. Load represses TGFβ signaling through Smad2/3 in osteocytes, which is required for the activation of SOST expression through an indirect, Runx2-independent mechanism. Loss of function mutations in the TGFβ type II receptor impair load-mediated repression of SOST and new bone formation.

load from inducing bone formation. This suggests that mice with mutations in the TGFβ pathway uncouple the normal regulation of bone mass from stimuli such as mechanical load; likely contributing to the high or low bone mass phenotypes observed in a several mouse models and human diseases in which TGFβ signaling is deregulated.

Mechanical load regulates TGFβ signaling at multiple levels. Cell-generated tensile stress induces the activation of the latent TGFβ ligand by myocytes [22]. *In vitro* fluid flow stimulates the expression of TGFβ1 mRNA in osteoblast cells [21]. Also, loading of the rat ulna induces TGFβ1 mRNA expression in the periosteal bone within 4h [39]. Still unclear, however, is the net functional effect of these mechanosensitive changes at multiple hierarchical levels of the TGFβ pathway. Unexpectedly, our results show that mechanical load rapidly inhibits Smad3 phosphorylation and, thus, represses the activity of key TGFβ effectors, Smad2 and Smad3, in osteocytes. Therefore, mechanical stimulation regulates the TGFβ pathway at the transcriptional level, as described above, as well as through post-transcriptional regulation of Smad2/3 activity.

TGFβ can be added to the list of pathways found to be mechanosensitive in bone that also regulate Sclerostin. PGE_2 regulates both osteoblast and osteoclast activities and is produced within 5 mins of mechanical stimulation [40]. Once mechanically stimulated, PGE_2 signals through the EP4 receptor to repress *SOST* transcription in osteoblast cells [41]. Several lines of evidence implicate PTH in load regulation of SOST activity. First, PTH levels are elevated in serum during high impact exercises such as running [3]. Second, *SOST* overexpression desensitizes mice to PTH-induced bone formation, suggesting that *SOST* acts as a downstream target of PTH [42–43]. Third, PTH represses *SOST* expression by inhibiting MEF2 transcriptional activity at the *SOST* enhancer [12] [11]. Some gaps in the connection between load, PGE_2 and PTH, and *SOST* remains to be filled.

Here we find that load fails to repress Sclerostin expression by osteocytes or new bone formation in the tibia of DNTβRII mice. Along with the mechanosensitive regulation of Smad2/3 function in osteocytes, these findings establish a clear link between mechanical load, TGFβ signaling, *SOST* levels, and new bone formation. It is important to note that modest bone formation was detected in the loaded tibia of DNTβRII mice (3–9%). Clearly, multiple other pathways in addition to TGFβ cooperate to regulate bone anabolism following mechanical load. Since the PTH and TGFβ pathways induce desensitization of one another via receptor internalization [23], some of the PTH-dependent effects may occur through TGFβ-dependent mechanisms. *SOST* may be a target of crosstalk between the PTH and TGFβ pathways. For example, the *SOST* regulatory transcription factor, MEF2, is repressed by PTH in osteoblasts [12] as well as by TGFβ/Smad3 in myocytes [44]. Furthermore, MEF2 is required for the activation of *SOST* transcription by TGFβ in osteogenic cells [45]. Thus, MEF2 may be a common target of both PTH and TGFβ and a point of convergence in their regulation of *SOST* and load-induced bone formation. Although mechanical load represses Smad2/3 activity in osteocytes, it remains possible that load regulation of *SOST* through TGFβ occurs indirectly through the effects of TGFβ on osteoblasts since DNTβRII is not expressed exclusively in osteocytes but also in osteoblasts. Further studies using osteocyte-specific mutations would clarify the precise role of TGFβ in each cell type in the response to load.

In conclusion, we find that load represses Smad3 activity in osteocytes and signals through the TGFβ pathway to maintain bone homeostasis. TGFβ indirectly induces *SOST* expression, which is mediated by Smad3. Although Runx2 was previously shown to regulate *SOST* expression [14], the TGFβ and Smad3-dependent induction of *SOST* is insensitive to the level of Runx2 activity. Finally, our data reveal a novel mechanism in load regulation of bone formation, which could provide insights for treating bone diseases such as osteoporosis.

Acknowledgments

The authors gratefully acknowledge Dr. Andrea Alford for the bone protein extraction protocol, Dr. Yan-Yiu Yu for technical help and scientific discussion, and Dr. Gabriella Loots for the SOST promoter-reporter construct. In addition, we gratefully acknowledge Ellora Berthet for expert technical assistance.

Author Contributions

Conceived and designed the experiments: JN SYT DN TA. Performed the experiments: JN SYT DN. Analyzed the data: JN SYT DN TA. Contributed reagents/materials/analysis tools: TA. Wrote the paper: JN SYT DN TA.

References

1. Bonewald LF (2011) The amazing osteocyte. J Bone Miner Res 26: 229–238. doi:10.1002/jbmr.320.
2. Duncan R, Turner C (1995) Mechanotransduction and the Functional-Response of Bone to Mechanical Strain. Calcified Tissue Int 57: 344–358.
3. Salvesen H, Johansson AG, Foxdal P, Wide L, Piehl-Aulin K, et al. (1994) Intact serum parathyroid hormone levels increase during running exercise in well-trained men. Calcified Tissue Int 54: 256–261.
4. Reijnders CMA, Bravenboer N, Tromp AM, Blankenstein MA, Lips P (2007) Effect of mechanical loading on insulin-like growth factor-I gene expression in rat tibia. J Endocrinol 192: 131–140.
5. Price JS, Sugiyama T, Galea GL, Meakin LB, Sunters A, et al. (2011) Role of Endocrine and Paracrine Factors in the Adaptation of Bone to Mechanical Loading. Curr Osteoporos Rep 9: 76–82.
6. Robling AG, Niziolek PJ, Baldridge LA, Condon KW, Allen MR, et al. (2007) Mechanical Stimulation of Bone in Vivo Reduces Osteocyte Expression of Sost/Sclerostin. J Biol Chem 283: 5866–5875.
7. Moester MJC, Papapoulos SE, Lowik CWGM, van Bezooijen RL (2010) Sclerostin: current knowledge and future perspectives. Calcified Tissue Int 87: 99–107.
8. Li X, Zhang Y, Kang H, Liu W, Liu P, et al. (2005) Sclerostin binds to LRP5/6 and antagonizes canonical Wnt signaling. J Biol Chem 280: 19883–19887.
9. Tian X, Jee WSS, Li X, Paszty C, Ke HZ (2011) Sclerostin antibody increases bone mass by stimulating bone formation and inhibiting bone resorption in a hindlimb-immobilization rat model. Bone 48: 197–201.
10. Kamiya N, Ye L, Kobayashi T, Mochida Y, Yamauchi M, et al. (2008) BMP signaling negatively regulates bone mass through sclerostin by inhibiting the canonical Wnt pathway. Development 135: 3801–3811.
11. Keller H, Kneissel M (2005) SOST is a target gene for PTH in bone. Bone 37: 148–158.
12. Leupin O, Kramer I, Collette NM, Loots GG, Natt F, et al. (2007) Control of the SOST bone enhancer by PTH using MEF2 transcription factors. J Bone Miner Res 22: 1957–1967.
13. Kitase Y, Barragan L, Qing H, Kondoh S, Jiang JX, et al. (2010) Mechanical induction of PGE2 in osteocytes blocks glucocorticoid-induced apoptosis through both the β-catenin and PKA pathways. J Bone Miner Res 25: 2657–2668.
14. Sevetson B, Taylor S, Pan Y (2004) Cbfa1/RUNX2 directs specific expression of the sclerosteosis gene (SOST). J Biol Chem 279: 13849–13858.
15. Janssens K, Dijke ten P, Janssens S, Van Hul W (2005) Transforming growth factor-β1 to the bone. Endocr Rev 26: 743–774.
16. Fox SW, Lovibond AC (2005) Current insights into the role of transforming growth factor-β in bone resorption. Mol Cell Endocrinol 243: 19–26.
17. Geiser AG, Zeng QQ, Sato M, Helvering LM, Hirano T, et al. (1998) Decreased bone mass and bone elasticity in mice lacking the transforming growth factor-beta1 gene. Bone 23: 87–93.
18. Dabovic B, Levasseur R, Zambuto L, Chen Y, Karsenty G, et al. (2005) Osteopetrosis-like phenotype in latent TGF-β binding protein 3 deficient mice. Bone 37: 25–31.
19. Rahimi RA, Leof EB (2007) TGF-β signaling: A tale of two responses. J Cell Biochem 102: 593–608.
20. Alliston T, Choy L, Ducy P, Karsenty G, Derynck R (2001) TGF-beta-induced repression of CBFA1 by Smad3 decreases cbfa1 and osteocalcin expression and inhibits osteoblast differentiation. EMBO J 20: 2254–2272.
21. Sakai K, Mohtai M, Iwamoto Y (1998) Fluid shear stress increases transforming growth factor beta 1 expression in human osteoblast-like cells: modulation by cation channel blockades. Calcified Tissue Int 63: 515–520.
22. Wipff P-J, Rifkin DB, Meister J-J, Hinz B (2007) Myofibroblast contraction activates latent TGF-beta1 from the extracellular matrix. J Cell Biol 179: 1311–1323.
23. Qiu T, Wu X, Zhang F, Clemens TL, Wan M, et al. (2010) TGF-β type II receptor phosphorylates PTH receptor to integrate bone remodelling signalling. Nat Cell Biol 12: 224–234.
24. Jian H, Shen X, Liu I, Semenov M, He X, et al. (2006) Smad3-dependent nuclear translocation of beta-catenin is required for TGF-beta1-induced proliferation of bone marrow-derived adult human mesenchymal stem cells. Gene Dev 20: 666–674.
25. Wang Y-K, Yu X, Cohen DM, Wozniak MA, Yang MT, et al. (2012) Bone Morphogenetic Protein-2-Induced Signaling and Osteogenesis Is Regulated by Cell Shape, RhoA/ROCK, and Cytoskeletal Tension. Stem Cells Dev 21: 1176–1186.
26. Allen JL, Cooke ME, Alliston T (2012) ECM stiffness primes the TGF pathway to promote chondrocyte differentiation. Mol Biol Cell 23: 3731–3742.
27. Lin AH, Luo J, Mondshein LH, Dijke ten P, Vivien D, et al. (2005) Global analysis of Smad2/3-dependent TGF-beta signaling in living mice reveals prominent tissue-specific responses to injury. J Immunol 175: 547–554.
28. Filvaroff E, Erlebacher A, Ye J, Gitelman SE, Lotz J, et al. (1999) Inhibition of TGF-beta receptor signaling in osteoblasts leads to decreased bone remodeling and increased trabecular bone mass. Development 126: 4267–4279.
29. Fritton JC, Myers ER, Wright TM, van der Meulen MCH (2005) Loading induces site-specific increases in mineral content assessed by microcomputed tomography of the mouse tibia. Bone 36: 1030–1038.
30. Mohammad KS, Chen CG, Balooch G, Stebbins E, McKenna CR, et al. (2009) Pharmacologic inhibition of the TGF-beta type I receptor kinase has anabolic and anti-catabolic effects on bone. PLoS One 4: e5275.
31. Whitlon DS, Szakaly R, Greiner MA (2001) Cryoembedding and sectioning of cochleas for immunocytochemistry and in situ hybridization. Brain Res Protoc 6: 159–166.
32. Parfitt AM, Drezner MK, Glorieux FH, Kanis JA, Malluche H, et al. (1987) Bone histomorphometry: standardization of nomenclature, symbols, and units. Report of the ASBMR Histomorphometry Nomenclature Committee. J Bone Miner Res 2: 595–610.
33. Alford AI, Reddy AB, Goldstein SA, Murthy P, Tayim R, et al. (2012) Two Molecular Weight Species of Thrombospondin-2 Are Present in Bone and Differentially Modulated in Fractured and Nonfractured Tibiae in a Murine Model of Bone Healing. Calcif Tissue Int 90: 420–428.
34. Zawel L, Dai JL, Buckhaults P, Zhou S, Kinzler KW, et al. (1998) Human Smad3 and Smad4 are sequence-specific transcription activators. Mol Cell 1: 611–617.
35. van der Meulen MCH, Morgan TG, Yang X, Baldini TH, Myers ER, et al. (2006) Cancellous bone adaptation to in vivo loading in a rabbit model. Bone 38: 871–877.
36. van der Meulen MCH, Yang X, Morgan TG, Bostrom MPG (2009) The effects of loading on cancellous bone in the rabbit. Clin Orthop Relat Res 467: 2000–2006.
37. Li X, Ominsky MS, Niu Q-T, Sun N, Daugherty B, et al. (2008) Targeted Deletion of the Sclerostin Gene in Mice Results in Increased Bone Formation and Bone Strength. J Bone Miner Res 23: 860–869.
38. Balooch G, Balooch M, Nalla RK, Schilling S, Filvaroff EH, et al. (2005) TGF-beta regulates the mechanical properties and composition of bone matrix. Proc Natl Acad Sci USA 102: 18813–18818.
39. Raab-Cullen DM, Thiede MA, Petersen DN, Kimmel DB, Recker RR (1994) Mechanical loading stimulates rapid changes in periosteal gene expression. Calcified Tissue Int 55: 473–478.
40. Ajubi NE, Klein-Nulend J, Nijweide PJ, Vrijheid-Lammers T, Alblas MJ, et al. (1996) Pulsating fluid flow increases prostaglandin production by cultured chicken osteocytes–a cytoskeleton-dependent process. Biochem Biophys Res Commun 225: 62–68.
41. Galea GL, Sunters A, Meakin LB, Zaman G, Sugiyama T, et al. (2011) Sost down-regulation by mechanical strain in human osteoblastic cells involves PGE2 signaling via EP4. FEBS Letters 585: 2450–2454.
42. Kramer I, Loots GG, Studer A, Keller H, Kneissel M (2010) Parathyroid Hormone (PTH)-Induced Bone Gain Is Blunted in SOST Overexpressing and Deficient Mice. J Bone Miner Res 25: 178–189.
43. Rhee Y, Allen MR, Condon K, Lezcano V, Ronda AC, et al. (2011) PTH Receptor Signaling in Osteocytes Governs Periosteal Bone Formation and Intracortical Remodeling. J Bone Miner Res 26: 1035–1046.
44. Liu D, Kang JS, Derynck R (2004) TGF-β-activated Smad3 represses MEF2-dependent transcription in myogenic differentiation. EMBO J 23: 1557–1566.
45. Loots GG, Keller H, Leupin O, Murugesh D, Collette NM, et al. (2011) TGF-β regulates sclerostin expression via the ECR5 enhancer. Bone 50: 663–669.

Mechanical Loading in Osteocytes Induces Formation of a Src/Pyk2/MBD2 Complex That Suppresses Anabolic Gene Expression

Julia M. Hum[1], Richard N. Day[1], Joseph P. Bidwell[2], Yingxiao Wang[3], Fredrick M. Pavalko[1]*

1 Department of Cellular and Integrative Physiology, Indiana University School of Medicine, Indianapolis, Indiana, United States of America, 2 Department of Anatomy and Cell Biology, Indiana University School of Medicine, Indianapolis, Indiana, United States of America, 3 School of Engineering, University of California San Diego, San Diego, California, United States of America

Abstract

Mechanical stimulation of the skeleton promotes bone gain and suppresses bone loss, ultimately resulting in improved bone strength and fracture resistance. The molecular mechanisms directing anabolic and/or anti-catabolic actions on the skeleton during loading are not fully understood. Identifying molecular mechanisms of mechanotransduction (MTD) signaling cascades could identify new therapeutic targets. Most research into MTD mechanisms is typically focused on understanding the signaling pathways that stimulate new bone formation in response to load. However, we investigated the structural, signaling and transcriptional molecules that suppress the stimulatory effects of loading. The high bone mass phenotype of mice with global deletion of either Pyk2 or Src suggests a role for these tyrosine kinases in repression of bone formation. We used fluid shear stress as a MTD stimulus to identify a novel Pyk2/Src-mediated MTD pathway that represses mechanically-induced bone formation. Our results suggest Pyk2 and Src function as molecular switches that inhibit MTD in our mechanically stimulated osteocyte culture experiments. Once activated by oscillatory fluid shear stress (OFSS), Pyk2 and Src translocate to and accumulate in the nucleus, where they associate with a protein involved in DNA methylation and the interpretation of DNA methylation patterns –methyl-CpG-binding domain protein 2 (MBD2). OFSS-induced Cox-2 and osteopontin expression was enhanced in Pyk2 KO osteoblasts, while inhibition of Src enhanced osteocalcin expression in response to OFSS. We found that Src kinase activity increased in the nucleus of osteocytes in response to OFSS and an interaction activated between Src (Y418) and Pyk2 (Y402) increased in response to OFSS. Thus, as a mechanism to prevent an over-reaction to physical stimulation, mechanical loading may induce the formation of a Src/Pyk2/MBD2 complex in the nucleus that functions to suppress anabolic gene expression.

Editor: Nic D. Leipzig, The University of Akron, United States of America

Funding: Grant support was provided by NIH 5R01AR052682 (https://public.era.nih.gov). The funder had no role in study design, data collection and analysis, decision to publish, or preparation of the manuscript.

Competing Interests: The authors have declared that no competing interests exist.

* E-mail: fpavalko@iupui.edu

Introduction

Pyk2 plays an important role in bone remodeling. [1–5]. Pyk2 null mice exhibit increased bone mass. [1,6]. Reports differ on the explanation of the osteopetrotic phenotype of the Pyk2 knockout mouse. Once group reports the phenotype results from defective osteoclast function implicating Pyk2's role in osteclast driven bone resporption, while another group contends increased osteoblast differentiation contributes to the osteopetrosis [7,8]. Pyk2's more well-known family member, FAK, serves as an important positive regulator of mechanical stimuli in osteoblasts [9]. Pyk2's role in mediating the response of bone cells to mechanotransduction is unknown, but is suggested to be different than FAK's [10]. Additionally, Src phosphorylates both FAK and Pyk2, while FAK and Pyk2 also associate and phosphorylate Src [11–14].

Similar to Pyk2, global disruption of Src, non-receptor tyrosine kinase, resulted in a mouse with a high bone mass phenotype, demonstrating the importance of Src in osteoblastogenesis. The function of both osteoclasts and osteoblasts is altered in Src−/− mice [15–17]. Osteoclast numbers are increased at the bone surface, but lack a ruffled border and are inactive [18–20]. Accelerated osteoblastogenesis was observed in the Src-null mice, suggesting Src activity plays a suppressive role in osteoblast differentiation [16]. These findings led to studies focused on producing a Src inhibitor to treat osteoporosis [21–24].

If both Pyk2 and Src function to balance bone mass by suppressing anabolic bone genes, it is also likely to affect the response of bone to mechanical loading. In the healthy mammalian skeleton, this process is mediated by osteocytes and osteoblasts that coordinate an appropriate response to mechanical loading resulting in localized net bone gain or loss depending on the type of load experienced at specific sites [25–27]. Osteocytes and osteoblasts sense and react to mechanical loads generated by the fluid flow through the canalicular system within bone [28–30]. *In vitro*, osteoblasts and osteocytes respond to mechanical load simulated via the application of oscillatory fluid shear stress (OFSS). Fluid shear stress causes distortions of the membranes of osteoblasts and osteocytes resulting in the enhanced expression of genes associated with osteoblast activity, up regulating cell proliferation and increasing the release of paracrine factors required for bones to elicit an anabolic response [31–33]. Both Pyk2 and Src increase their activation in response to OFSS [34–36].

We tested the hypothesis that Pyk2 and Src suppress anabolic targets of OFSS-induced MTD in osteoblasts and osteocytes. In this study we sought to determine Pyk2 and Src's localization, effect on anabolic protein expression and gene transcription, and association with other signaling molecules under static and OFSS conditions.

Methods

Cell Culture Conditions

MC3T3 osteoblasts were obtained from ATCC, mouse calvarial osteoblasts (MCOB) were derived from WT neonatal mouse pups, as previously described [37], and Pyk2−/− osteoblasts were derived from Pyk2−/− mice as previously described [10]. Osteoblasts were cultured in minimal essential media alpha (MEM-α, Gibco, Life Technologies, Carlsbad, CA) containing 10% fetal calf serum (FCS) and 1% penicillin/streptomycin (Gibco, Life Technologies, Grand Island, NY). MLO-Y4 osteocytes were obtained from Dr. Linda Bonewald, UMKC and were cultured on collagen-coated plates (rat tail collagen type I, BD Biosciences, San Jose, CA) in MEM-α (Gibco, Life Technologies, Carlsbad, CA) supplemented with 5% FCS, 5% fetal bovine serum (FBS) and 1% penicillin/streptomycin (Gibco, Life Technologies, Grand Island, NY). Cells were maintained in 5% CO_2 at 37°C during experiments and imaging.

Fluid Flow Conditions

Two methods were used to induce fluid shear stress over the surface of cells. An oscillatory pump connected to parallel plate flow chambers via hard–walled tubing was used to induce a shear rate of 10 dynes/cm^2 across the surface of cells plated on glass slides. Additionally, a reservoir was created for the movement of fluid and 5% CO_2 exchange using hard-walled tubing attached to the outlet of the parallel plate. Static controls were incubated in the same volume of media. Prior to exposure to fluid flow, cells were serum starved (MEM-α, 0.5% FCS) overnight to reduce basal metabolic activity of cells prior to exposure to OFSS. During fluid flow experiments the parallel plate flow chambers and attached hard-walled tubing were placed in an incubator set to 37°C and 5% CO_2.

Similarly, an orbital shaking platform was used to induce fluid flow over the surface of MC3T3 osteoblasts and MLO-Y4 osteocytes. Cells plated in 6 well culture dishes were placed on an orbital shaking platform within a tissue culture incubator set to 37°C and 5% CO_2. Prior to experimentation, cells were grown overnight in low-serum α-MEM media supplemented with 0.5% FCS and antibiotics. Cells were subjected to fluid flow generated by 1 mL of media on an orbital platform shaker rotating at a speed of ~200 rpm (2 Hz) producing a estimated shear rate of ~10–25 dynes/cm^2 while inside a tissue culture incubator [10,38–40].

Src Inhibitor

MC3T3 osteoblasts and MLO-Y4 osteocytes were treated with Src Inhibitor 1 (Santa Cruz Biotechnology, Santa Cruz, CA) (10 μM) for 1 hour before experiments were conducted. Control samples were treated with DMSO.

Western Blotting Analysis

Cells exposed to static or flow conditions were harvested directly into SDS sample buffer and protein concentrations were determined using amino black method [41]. Equal amounts of protein were loaded onto SDS-PAGE gels for separation and transferred to nitrocellulose. The subsequent primary and secondary antibodies were used: phospho-Src (Y418) (Cell Signaling, Boston, MA), total Src (Cell Signaling, Boston, MA), γ-tubulin (Sigma-Aldrich, St. Louis, MO), lamin B (Santa Cruz, Santa Cruz, CA), HRP conjugated goat anti-rabbit and HRP conjugated goat anti-mouse (Jackson Immunoresearch, West Grove, PA). The secondary antibody signals were detected using a Luminescent Image Analyzer LAS-3000 system (Fujifilm Life Science, Stamford, CT). Densitometry was quantified using Image J software (NIH).

RNA Extraction, cDNA Synthesis and Quantitative Real-time PCR (qRT-PCR) Analysis

RNA was harvested from cultured MC3T3 osteoblasts and MLO-Y4 osteocytes in Trizol (Invitrogen, Carlsbad, CA). RNA was extracted with chloroform and precipitated with isopropanol. M-MLV reverse transcriptase (Promega, Madison, WI) was used to perform first strand cDNA synthesis. GAPDH (Mm99999915_g1), osteopontin (Mm00436767_m1), and RPLP2 (Mm03059047_gH) real-time PCR primers were obtained (Applied Biosystems, Grand Island, NY). Custom designed primer/probes were prepared for osteocalcin. (forward) 5(-CTGA-CAAAGCCTTCATGTCCAA-)3 (probe) 5(-AGGAGGGCAA-TAAGGTAGT-)3 and (reverse) 5(-GGTAGCGCCG-GAGTCTGTT-)3. TaqMan Universal PCR Master Mix (Applied Biosystems, Grand Island, NY) was used for amplification in a Mastercycler ep realplex^2 real-time PCR system (Eppendorf, Westbury, NY). The reaction conditions were as follows: 2 minutes at 50°C; 10 minutes at 95°C; 40 cycles of 15 seconds at 95°C and 1 minute at 60°C. The ΔΔCT method was used to evaluate gene expression between samples. RPLP2 and GAPDH were used as loading control genes.

Immunofluorescence

Images for all experiments were captured using a Nikon inverted immunofluorescence microscope equipped with a CCD camera. MLO-Y4 osteocytes cells were plated onto coverslips and placed into 6 well culture dishes. Cells were serum starved for 24 hrs (0.5% FCS), subjected to static conditions and fixed immediately or fixed after 20 minutes of OFSS (via orbital shaking platform) with 4% paraformaldehyde solution and permeablilized with 0.2% triton after rinsing with Tris-buffered saline (TBS). Coverslips were treated with normal donkey serum for 30 minutes at 37°C to block non-specific antibody binding. The following primary and secondary antibodies were used: Src and Src Y418 (Cell Signaling, Boston, MA) followed by FITC-conjugated donkey anti-rabbit (Jackson Immunoresearch, West Grove, PA). Texas-Red, phalloidin, and DAPI (Molecular Probes, Eugene, OR) were used for visualizing F-actin and the nucleus, respectively.

Osteoblasts were plated on glass coverslips, ~2.0×10^5 cells per slide (~1.1×10^5 cells/cm^2), following 24 hrs of serum starvation (0.5% FCS), cells subjected to static culture conditions were fixed immediately (static) or fixed after OFSS (30 minutes, 1 hour, or 1 hour plus 1 hour) (via oscillatory pump) with 4% paraformaldehyde solution and processed for immunofluorescence by permeabilization with 0.2% triton followed by rinsing in Tris-buffered saline (TBS). Slides were then treated with 1% BSA solution in TBS for 30 minutes at 37°C to block non-specific antibody binding. The following primary and secondary antibodies were used: Pyk2 (BD Biosciences, San Jose, CA), DAPI (Molecular Probes, Eugene, OR), and FITC-conjugated donkey anti-rabbit (Jackson Immunoresearch, West Grove, PA).

DNA Plasmids

The Src biosensor and Src mutant biosensor were generously obtained from Dr. Yingxiao Wang [42].

FRET Microscopy

One day prior to imaging, MLO-Y4 cells were electroporated (150 V, 9 ms) with either the Src biosensor or the Src mutant biosensor (10 µg). Cells were plated into 35 mm glass bottom dishes (MatTech, Ashland, MA) and maintained in phenol-free, MEM-α media supplemented with 0.5% FCS and antibiotics. The following day, FRET microscopy was performed using an ISS ALBA FastFLIM system (ISS Inc., Champagne, IL) coupled to an Olympus IX71 microscope equipped with a 60 X/1.2 NA water-immersion objective lens. A 5 mW 448 nm diode laser was modulated by the FastFLIM module of the ALBA system at a fundamental frequency of 20 MHz with up to six sinusoidal harmonics. The modulated 5 mW 448 nm laser was used to excite the donor fluorophore of either the Src biosensor or Src mutant biosensor. The frequency domain FLIM method was used to obtain fluorescent lifetime(s) based on changes in the phase and amplitude of the emission signal compared to the excitation source. The phasor plots, lifetime maps and intensity images were analyzed using ISS VistaVision software (ISS Inc., Champagne, IL). Lifetime maps were generated using a two-component fit for the calculation of the donor lifetime. The phasor plots are used to display the modulation and phase characteristics of the emission signal for every pixel in an image, providing a quantitative determination of the biosensor probe fluorescence lifetime [43,44]. Lifetime data from MLO-Y4 cells were extracted from three different regions of interest (ROI): plasma membrane, cytoplasm and nucleus. To ensure lifetime measurements were taken at the appropriate position Bodipy C12 (Invitrogen Corp., Grand Island, NY) (0.01 mg/ml) was used to identify the position of the plasma membrane from the cytosol, as well as mark the outline of the nucleus.

Nuclear Fractionation

Cells subjected to either static or OFSS treatment in 6 well dishes were washed with phosphate buffered saline, harvested in ice-cold hypotonic buffer (10 mM HEPES, 10 mM KCL, 1.5 mM $MgCl_2$, 1 mM DTT and protease inhibitors), passed through a 22-gauge needle five times and were centrifuged for 10 minutes at 13,000 rpm. The cytosolic fraction was saved while the nuclear fraction pellet was resuspended in buffer C (10 mM HEPES, 0.42 M NaCl, 25% Glycerol, 1.5 mM $MgCl_2$, 0.5 mD EDTA, ddH_2O and protease inhibitors) placed on ice and vortexed for 15 seconds every 10 minutes for an hour to swell nuclear proteins out the nuclei. Finally the samples were centrifuged at 4°C for 15 minutes at 14,000 rpm. The clear supernatant was collected and prepared for western blot analysis.

Immunoprecipitation

For detecting protein-protein interactions *in vivo* co-immunoprecipitation was performed in MC3T3 osteoblasts and MLO-Y4 osteocytes. Immunoprecipitation was performed using Src protein, Src (Y416), MBD2, normal rabbit serum, or normal mouse serum. Immunoprecipitation buffer contained 1% Triton-X-100, 145 mM NaCl, 10 mM Tric-Cl, pH 7.4, 5 mM EDTA, 2 mM EGTA, and 1 mM PMSF. Immune complexes were captured using Protein A sepharose beads (Sigma-Aldrich, Saint Louis, MO) conjugated to either goat-anti rabbit or goat-anti mouse antibody (Jackson Immunoresearch Laboratories, West Grove, PA).

Statistical Analysis

Statistical significance was assessed by either a two-tailed t-test or a two-way analysis of variance (ANOVA) with a p-value of $p < 0.05$ or less interpreted as statistically significant.

Results

To examine the role of Pyk2 in fluid shear stress-induced expression of anabolic targets of OFSS wild-type osteoblasts and Pyk2−/− osteoblasts were subjected to either static culture or 1 hour of OFSS. OFSS induced a significant 1.8 fold increase in Cox-2 expression in wild-type osteoblasts (Figure 1A). However, in the absence of Pyk2 (Pyk2 KO osteoblasts), Cox-2 expression was significantly elevated compared to wild-type osteoblasts both in static culture and following exposure to OFSS (Figure 1A). OFSS did not alter Pyk2 protein expression in either the wild-type osteoblasts or Pyk2 KO osteoblasts (Figure 1A). To determine if Pyk2 plays a role in regulating other anabolic genes in response to OFSS, relative expression of osteopontin (OPN) mRNA was examined in Pyk2 KO osteoblasts. Under static conditions, Pyk2 KO osteoblasts expressed significantly higher levels of OPN mRNA (Figure 1B). When wild-type osteoblasts and Pyk2 KO osteoblasts were exposed to either static or OFSS conditions using either the OFSS pump or orbital shaking platform, Pyk2 KO osteoblasts expressed enhanced levels of OPN mRNA compared to wild-type osteoblasts in response to OFSS (Figure 1B).

Although Src KO osteoblasts were not available, we evaluated the role of Src in expression of osteogenic genes in MC3T3 osteoblasts and MLO-Y4 osteocytes following treatment with a pharmacologic inhibitor of Src activity (Src inhibitor-1, SI1). We first confirmed that SI1 effectively inhibited Src activity by showing that SI1 inhibited fluid flow-induced Akt phosphorylation (Figure 2A). Osteocalcin expression was significantly increased in both MC3T3 osteoblasts and MLO-Y4 osteocytes treated with SI1 under static culture. (Figure 2B). Most importantly, OFSS further enhanced the expression of osteocalcin in both MC3T3 osteoblasts and MLO-Y4 osteocytes treated with SI1 compared to static controls treated with carrier (DMSO) only (2.7 and 3.4 fold change, respectively; Figure 2C). Knocking down Src protein expression via siRNA was attempted, but consistent knockdown of was unsuccessful.

Pyk2 and Src Accumulate in Perinuclear and Nuclear Regions in Response to OFSS

The localization pattern of both Pyk2 and Src in response to OFSS was analyzed using immunofluorescence microscopy. The cellular distribution of Pyk2 in osteoblasts was observed under static and OFSS (30 minutes, 1 hour, or 1 hour+1 hour of rest) conditions. Static osteoblasts displayed a relatively even distribution of Pyk2 throughout the cells, with a subtle concentration of Pyk2 in the perinuclear/nuclear region (Figure 3A). We found that Pyk2 preferentially accumulated in the nuclei following exposure to 30 minutes of OFSS. After exposure to one hour of OFSS, the accumulation of Pyk2 in the nucleus was less robust than at the 30 minute OFSS time point (Figure 3A). In response to 1 hour of OFSS and 1 hour of rest, Pyk2's absence in the nucleus was even further enhanced compared to static. Comparable results were observed in MLO-Y4 osteocytes (not shown). These results suggest that Pyk2 is capable of shuttling between the cytoplasm and the nucleus in response to OFSS.

We next examined changes in the distribution of Src in response to OFSS. Immunofluorescence microscopy indicated a shift in the distribution of both total Src and activated Src (as assessed by phosphorylation at tyrosine residue Y416) following as little as

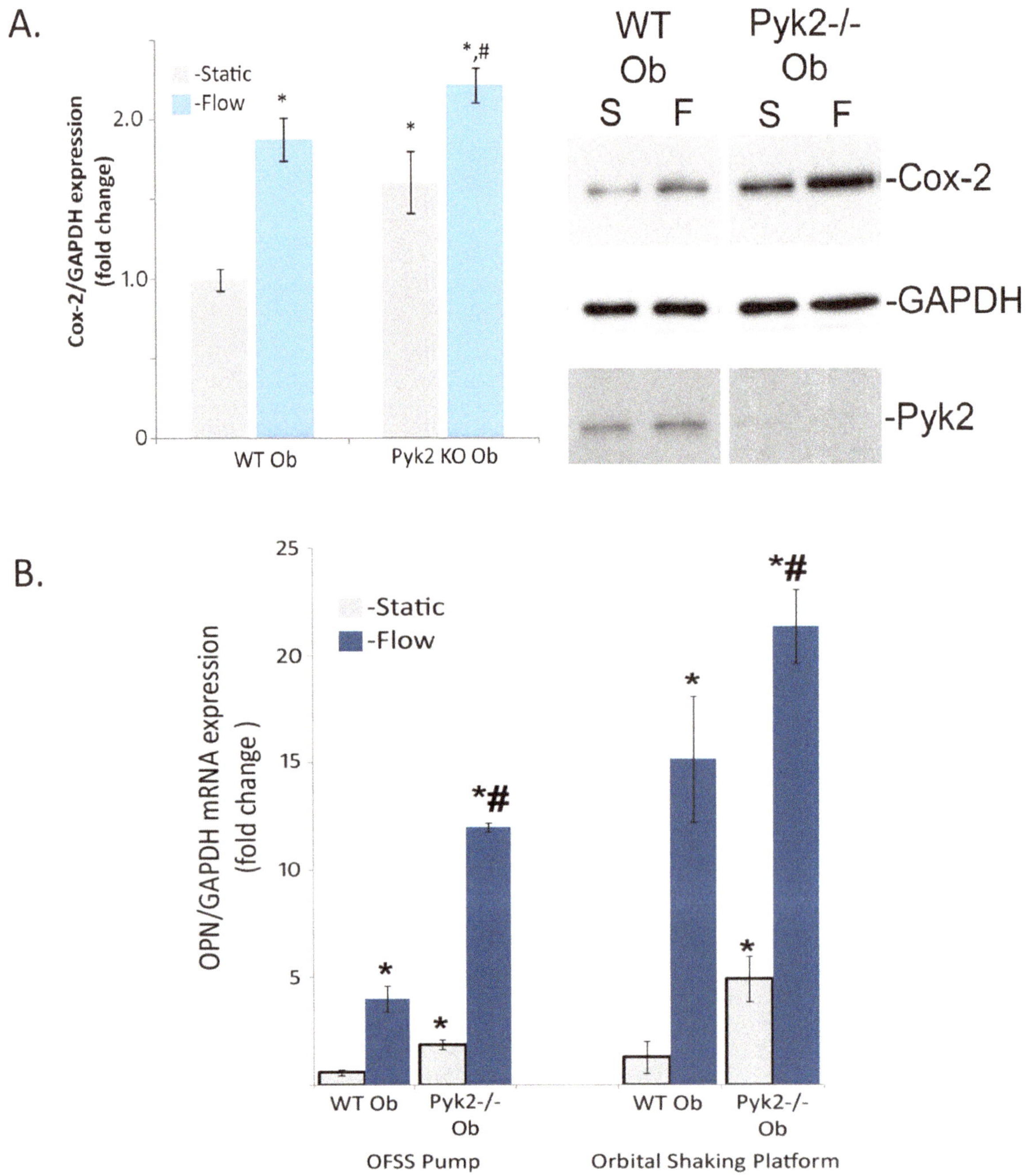

Figure 1. Anabolic protein and gene expression is effected in Pyk2−/− osteoblasts under static and OFSS conditions. (A) Wild-type osteoblasts and Pyk2−/− osteoblasts were exposed to either static of one hour of OFSS. Representative of immunoblots for Cox-2, GAPDH, and Pyk2 show a OFSS-induced increase in Cox-2 protein expression. OFSS does not cause a change in the loading control, GAPDH. Graph represents the densitometry units of Cox-2, normalized to GAPDH. In wild-type osteoblasts, OFSS results in a 1.8 fold change in Cox-2 protein expression. Pyk2−/− osteoblasts have an elevated protein expression of Cox-2 under static conditions, and after OFSS the level of Cox-2 protein expression is highest compared to all other groups (static control, wild-type osteoblasts static control, and wild-type osteoblasts OFSS). Error bars represent standard error. *$p<0.05$ vs wild-type static control, #$p<0.05$ vs. wild-type osteoblasts. $N=3$ in three separate trials. (B) Wild-type osteoblasts and Pyk2−/− osteoblasts were exposed to either static or 1 hour of OFSS conditions, using either an OFSS pump or orbital shaking platform. Static Pyk2−/− osteoblasts expressed significantly higher levels of osteopontin compared to static wild-type osteoblasts. In response to OFSS, using either method, the absence of Pyk2 further enhances the OFSS-induced osteopontin expression increase. Error bars represent standard error. *$p<0.05$ vs. wild-type static control, #$p<0.05$ vs wild-type osteoblasts. $N=3$ in three separate trials.

20 minutes of exposure to OFSS in MLO-Y4 osteocytes. Using an antibody that recognizes only activated Src phosphorylated at tyrosine 416 (Y416) we found that activated Src accumulated in the perinuclear/nuclear area of MLO-Y4 osteocytes after exposure to OFSS (Figure 3B). Total Src protein also increased modestly in the perinuclear/nuclear regions after OFSS, but was not as pronounced as that of the activated (Y416) Src (Figure 3B). These results suggest that Src activation (as measured by

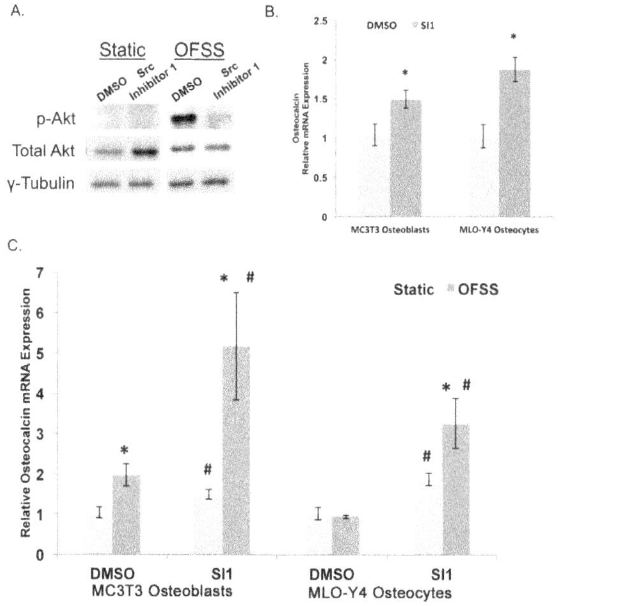

Figure 2. Src kinase represses osteocalcin in static and OFSS conditions. (A) Treating MC3T3 osteoblasts and MLO-Y4 osteocytes with Src Inhibitor 1 (SI1) (10 μM) for 1 hour inhibits Src kinase activity. Western blot analysis of phosphorylated-Akt (Ser308), Total Akt, and γ-tubulin under static and OFSS conditions (1 hour). (B) One hour of SI1 treatment significantly increases the expression of osteocalcin in MC3T3 osteoblasts and MLO-Y4 osteocytes (*$p<0.05$). (C) OFSS (1 hour) further enhanced the expression of osteocalcin in both MC3T3 osteoblasts and MLO-Y4 osteocytes compared to static controls treated with carrier (DMSO) ($p<0.05$). *Represents a statically significant increase compared to wild-type static control ($p<0.05$). #Represents a statically significant difference between treatment groups (#$p<0.05$) Error bars represent standard error. An $n\geq3$ were used in all experiments and each experiment was repeated at least three times.

phosphorylation at Y416) may be required for Src to accumulate in the nucleus of the cell. We saw no evidence that Src was shuttling back out of the nucleus during the time course of these experiments.

Nuclear Src Activity Increases in Response to OFSS

To examine the observation of increased perinuclear/nuclear Src accumulation in response to OFSS we used live cell imaging to monitor changes in Src activity in response to OFSS. To directly examine changes in the sub-cellular distribution of Src tyrosine kinase activity in MLO-Y4 osteocytes in response to OFSS we utilized a Src biosensor to measure Src activity by FRET microscopy. The changing FRET signal from the Src biosensor probe was detected using fluorescent lifetime imaging microscopy (FLIM), which measures the shortened donor lifetime that results from FRET. This approach allows us to map with pixel level resolution the sub-cellular locations of changing Src protein activity. The Src biosensor used here is in a closed conformation under conditions of low endogenous Src activity, resulting in high FRET efficiency and a shortened donor lifetime. Upon phosphorylation of the substrate peptide, a sequence derived from p130cas, by endogenous Src, the substrate binds to the phosphopeptide-binding pocket of the SH2 domain, resulting in a more open conformation and diminished FRET leading to an increased donor lifetime. Thus, an increase in Src biosensor lifetime indicates an increase in Src kinase activity.

The phasor plot analysis comparing the total population of Src biosensor in MLO-Y4 cells prior to or following exposure to OFSS clearly showed a shift towards longer lifetimes of the Src biosensor, indicating a global increase in Src activity throughout MLO-Y4 cells in response to OFSS (Figure 4A). Following exposure to 5 minutes of OFSS, lifetimes of the Src biosensor donor fluorophore were determined for three distinct sub-cellular compartments (regions of interest, ROI) – the membrane, cytoplasm and nucleus - at 10, 15 and 20 minutes post-OFSS using FLIM analysis. Prior to OFSS, Src activity in the nucleus was significantly lower than at either the membrane or in the cytoplasm (Figure 4B). Most importantly, a significant increase in nuclear Src activity was seen at each time point following OFSS and increased steadily during the 20 min post-OFSS period (Figure 4C). Lifetime maps of the nucleus under static and post-OFSS conditions illustrate the increase in Src activity in response to OFSS (Figure 4D). In contrast, Src activity at the membrane and in the cytoplasm peaked at 10 and 15 minutes post-OFSS, respectively, and then decreased at 20 minutes post-OFSS (Figure 4B). Prior to OFSS, the average lifetime of the Src biosensor in the nucleus was 1.69±0.01 nanoseconds. At 10, 15 and 20 minutes post-OFSS nuclear Src biosensor lifetimes significantly increased compared to static (1.80±0.01, 1.90±0.02, and 1.95±0.02 nanoseconds, respectively) (Figure 4B).

In sharp contrast, there was no change in the fluorescent lifetime of a mutant Src biosensor (Y662F Y664F) following 5 minutes of OFSS (Figure S1). The mutation of the tyrosine residues in the p130cas substrate blocks Src tyrosine kinase activation of the biosensor, and also changes its conformation, resulting in higher basal lifetimes compared to the Src biosensor.

Src Activation Increases in the Nucleus in Response to OFSS

To validate the observation of increased Src activity in the nucleus of MLO-Y4 cells in response to OFSS; nuclear fractionation followed by Western blot analysis was performed. MLO-Y4 osteocytes were exposed to either static conditions (control) or 5 minutes of OFSS. The control cells or OFSS cells were collected 10 minutes-post-OSS. Src activation, as measured by phosphorylation at Y416, was performed by Western blot. In response to 5 minutes of OFSS activated Src in the nucleus was increased at 10 minutes post-OFSS compared to static conditions (Figure 5).

Pyk2 and MBD2 Complex under Basal Conditions and Increase their Association in Response to OFSS

To examine the functional significance of Pyk2 translocation to the nucleus in response to OFSS we evaluated Pyk2's association with MBD2. In muscle cells the interaction of FAK, a closely related family member to Pyk2, and MBD2 in the nucleus has been observed during differentiation, leading to the disruption of the repression complex and increased expression of myogenin [45]. Therefore, we performed a co-immunoprecipitation assay to examine the possibility that OFSS was inducing the formation of a Pyk2-MBD2 complex. Antibodies to either Pyk2 or MBD2 were used to detect co-immunoprecipitated proteins by reciprocal western blot analysis. In osteocyte lysates from cells maintained in static culture, endogenous Pyk2 formed a complex with MBD2 (Figure 6A). A complex of Pyk2/MBD2 was detected using antibodies to either Pyk2 or MBD2. Next, we compared the association of Pyk2/MBD2 under static and OFSS conditions using antibodies that are specific for the activated form of Pyk2 (Y402). Under static culture conditions no association between

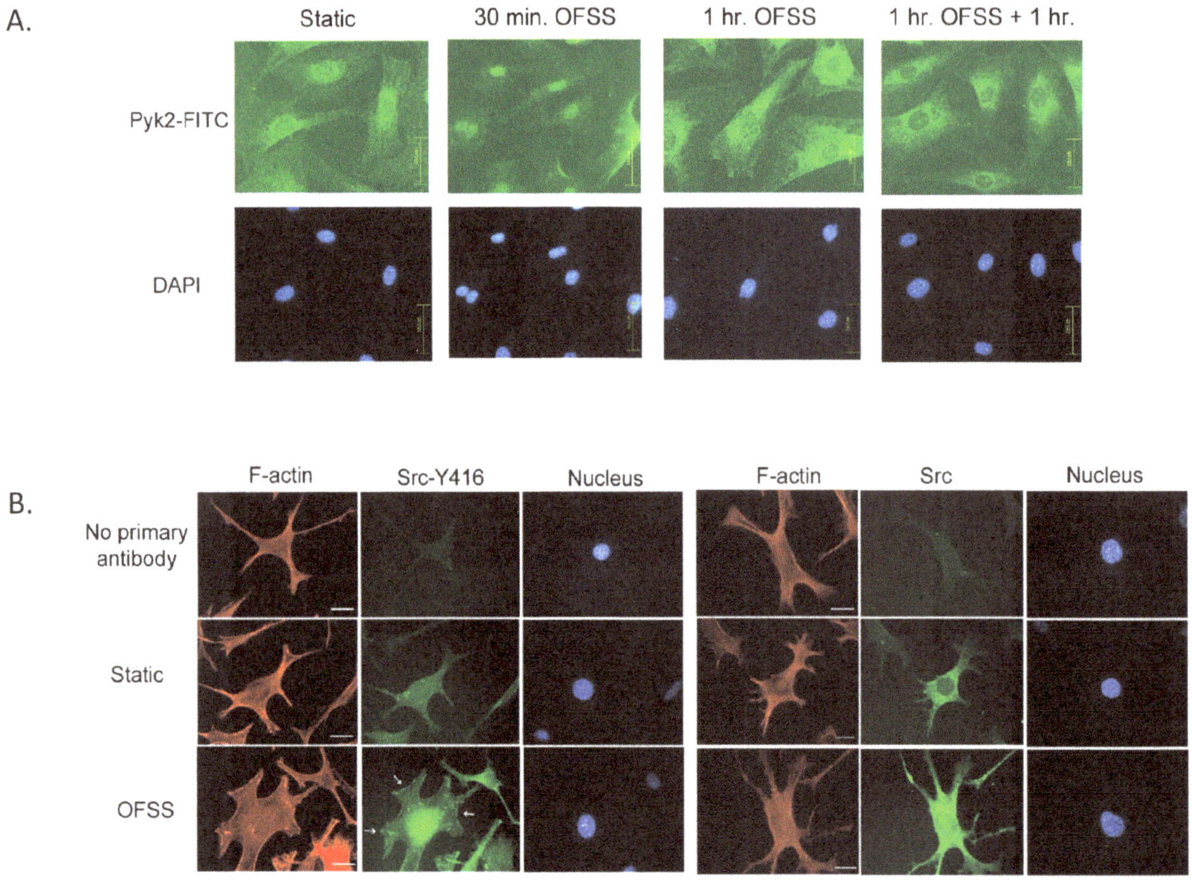

Figure 3. Pyk2 and Src accumulate in perinuclear and nuclear regions in response to OFSS. (A) Immunofluorescence microscopy of osteoblast's subjected to either static culture conditions or OFSS (30 minutes, 1 hour, or 1 hour+1 hour of rest). Slides were fixed immediately and processed for immunofluorescence using antibodies against Pyk2, followed by FITC-conjugated secondary antibodies. The nucleus was visualized using DAPI. Scale bars = 100 μm (B) OFSS induces accumulation of Src at perinuclear/nuclear regions in MLO-Y4 osteocytes. Immunofluorescence microscopy of MLO-Y4 osteocytes subjected to static culture conditions or OFSS for 20 minutes. Slides were fixed immediately and processed for immunofluorescence using antibodies against activated Src (Y416 followed by FITC-conjugated secondary antibodies). F-actin was visualized using Texas-Red Phalloidin and the nucleus was visualized using DAPI. White arrows indicate focal adhesions. Scale bars = 25 μm (B) Immunofluorescence microscopy of MLO-Y4 osteocytes subjected to static culture conditions or OFSS for 20 minutes. Slides were fixed immediately and processed for immunofluorescence using antibodies against total Src followed by FITC-conjugated secondary antibodies. F-actin was visualized using Texas-Red Phalloidin and the nucleus was visualized using DAPI. Scale bars = 25 μm.

MBD2 and Pyk2 was detected. However, in response to 20 minutes of OFSS, MBD2 was detected in the Pyk2 IP complex suggesting that MBD2 may interact with activated Pyk2 that is phosphorylated at tyrosine 402 (Figure 6B) in response to OFSS. Interestingly, OFSS also induced an association between Pyk2 (Y402) and Src (Y418) suggesting the formation of a Pyk2-Src-MBD2 complex in the nucleus (Figure 6B).

Discussion

We suggest that Pyk2 and Src may serve as an "off switch" to suppress the anabolic response of bone subjected to mechanical load. We have previously proposed the mechanosomes model to describe how mechanical stimuli sensed at the plasma membrane, results in changes of gene transcription [46–48]. A mechanosome consists of an adhesion-associated protein and a nucleocytoplasmic shuttling transcription factor. There are two forms of mechanosomes, a "GO" mechanosome and a "STOP" mechanosome. A "GO" mechanosome functions to promote the anabolic response of bone to mechanical loading, while a "STOP" mechanosome functions to suppress the anabolic response of bone to loading. Our findings suggest Pyk2 and Src have the capacity to function as a "STOP" mechanosome. Once activated by mechanical stimulation, Pyk2 and Src change their pattern of localization and serve as a nuclear mechanism to prevent an over-reaction to physical stimulation.

The aim of this study was to better understand the signaling mechanisms that osteoblasts and osteocytes use to suppress the anabolic response of bone to mechanical loading. Src and Pyk2 were examined due to their shared knockout phenotype, increased bone mass. In the absence of Pyk2, Cox-2 and osteopontin expression are modestly increased. OFSS further enhanced Cox-2 and osteopontin expression in Pyk2 null osteoblasts. Therefore, Pyk2 functions to suppress the expression of the anabolic bone gene osteopontin, as well as the expression of Cox-2 protein under static and OFSS conditions. Immunofluorescence microscopy was performed to evaluate if OFSS induced changes in the subcellular localization of Pyk2. Osteoblasts under static conditions displayed a relatively even distribution of Pyk2 throughout the cytoplasm, with a subtle concentration of Pyk2 in the perinuclear/nuclear region (Figure 3A). Evidence that Pyk2 was capable of shuttling into and out of the nucleus in response to OFSS was seen by an

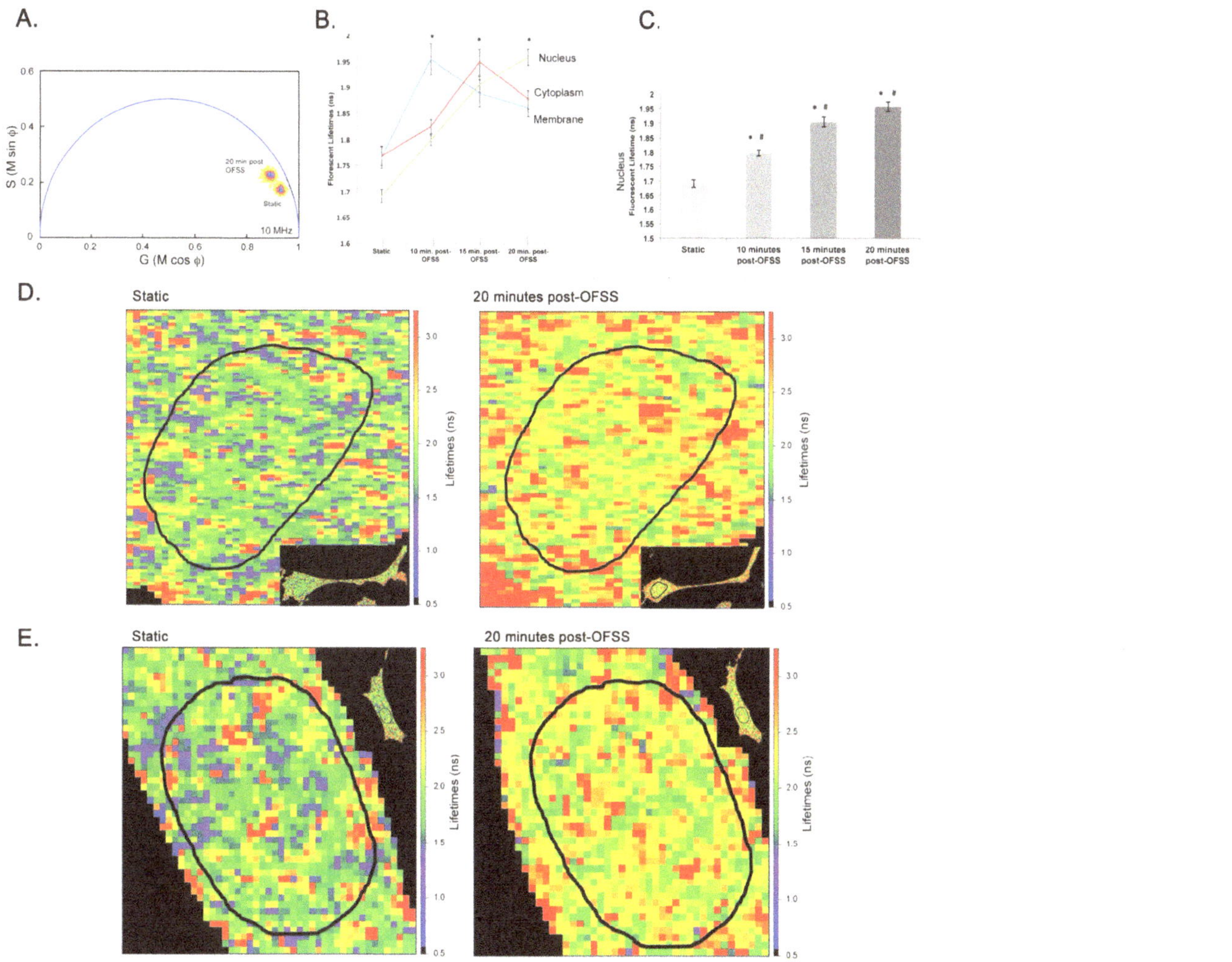

Figure 4. OFSS causes an increase in nuclear Src activity. (A) Composite phasor plot analysis of static Src biosensor lifetime and 20 minutes post-OFSS Src biosensor lifetime. (B) Graph represents n = 3 in which the average lifetime of each ROI (30) at each time point analyzed. Error bars represent standard error. (C) Graph of nuclear Src lifetimes. *Represents a statically significant increase compared to static control (*$p<0.001$). #Represents a statically significant difference between other OFSS time points examined (#$p<0.05$) Error bars represent standard error. (D, E) Lifetime maps of the same MLO-Y4 osteocyte under static, 10 minutes, 15 minutes or 20 minutes post-OFSS.

initial accumulation of Pyk2 in the nucleus (after 30 minutes of OFSS) followed by an absence in the nucleus (following 1 hour of OFSS and 1 hour of rest). An OFSS-induced nucleocytoplasmic shuttling mechanism for Pyk2 has yet to be described, but other studies in fibroblasts have observed Pyk2's nucleocytoplasmic shuttling behavior in response to membrane depolarization [49,50]. Nucleocytoplasmic shuttling of Pyk2 is possible through the nuclear localization sequence (NLS) and the nuclear export sequence (NES) that are both located in the FERM domain [51–53]. The changes observed in Cox-2 expression and osteopontin transcription might be mediated by an OFSS-induced association of Pyk2 and MBD2. In MLO-Y4 osteocytes a basal interaction between Pyk2 and MBD2 was observed. When examining the activated form of Pyk2 (Y402), an increase in its association with MDB2 occurs in response to 20 minutes of OFSS. While not a transcription factor, MBD2 is a member of the methyl CpG-binding protein family and functions to repress transcription [54–56]. Specifically, MBD2 and methyl CpG binding protein 2 (MeCP2) bind heterochromatin through their interaction with methylated DNA at CpG islands. The complex then translates the DNA methylation signal into transcriptional repression by recruiting histone deacetylases and other silencing complexes to sustain a heterochromatic state [57,58]. In muscle cells an interaction between FAK and MBD2 in the nucleus has been observed during differentiation, leading to the disruption of the repression complex and increased expression of myogenin [45]. Similarly, in response to membrane depolarization Pyk2 binds MBD2 in the nucleus of nerve cells, but the functional outcome of this observation has yet to be explained [49]. These findings suggest the possibility that MBD2 might be a component of a mechanosome containing Pyk2 and/or Src kinase.

A second aspect of this study was to investigate a potential role for Src tyrosine kinase in transcriptional regulation of anabolic gene expression in MC3T3 osteoblasts and MLO-Y4 osteocytes, principally in response to OFSS. Expression of osteocalcin, a marker of bone formation *in vivo*, was increased when Src activity was inhibited in MC3T3 osteoblasts and MLO-Y4 osteocytes. Furthermore, we show for the first time that the increase in osteocalcin expression normally induced by OFSS was further enhanced in MC3T3 osteoblasts and MLO-Y4 osteocytes when Src activity was inhibited by treatment with SI1 (compared to control cells in which Src activity was not inhibited). Thus, our

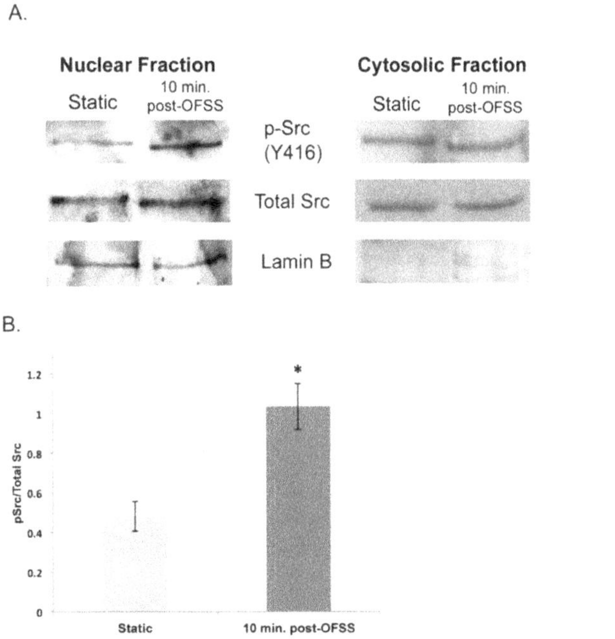

Figure 5. Src activation increases in the nucleus in response to OFSS. (A) Western blot analysis of nuclear fractionation blotted for Src activation (Y416), total Src and lamin B in MLO-Y4 osteocytes exposed to 5 minutes of OFSS or static culture conditions. (B) Graph represents quantification of Src activation (Y416)/total Src in nuclear fractions. Error bars represent standard error. Statistically significant difference between static and 10 minutes post-OFSS (*$p<0.05$). An $n \geq 3$ were used in the repeated experiments.

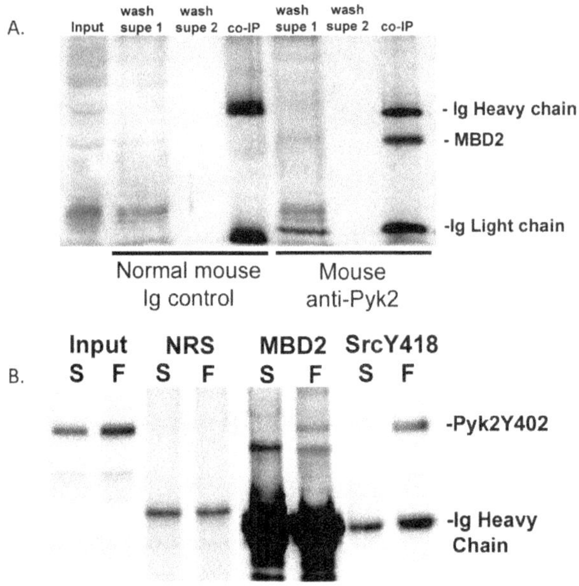

Figure 6. A complex between MBD2 and Pyk2 forms under static conditions in MLO-Y4 osteocytes, while OFSS-induces the association of MBD2 and Pyk2 (Y402) and Src (Y418) and Pyk2 (Y402) in MLO-Y4 osteocytes. (A) Co-immunoprecipitation between MBD2 and Pyk2 was performed from MLO-Y4 osteocytes harvested under static conditions. MBD2 was not associated with Pyk2 when control normal mouse Ig was used in the immunoprecipitation. Anti-MBD2 antibody was used to probe the blot. (B) Co-immunoprecipitation was performed in MLO-Y4 osteocytes harvested under static (S) or OFSS (F) conditions. Normal rat serum (NRS), MBD2, and Src (Y418) were the antibodies used for the immunoprecipitation. Anti-Pyk2 (Y402) specific antibody was used to probe the blot.

results suggest Src normally functions to suppress osteocalcin expression under conditions of both static culture and OFSS. Osteocalcin is an important protein associated with bone formation and its levels in serum directly correlate with measurements of bone mineral density [59,60]. Osteocalcin expression is increased in response mechanical loading in both *in vivo* and *in vitro* models [61,62]. We also analyzed expression of cyclooxygenase-2, runx2, osterix, and osteopontin and found inhibition of Src had no impact on OFSS-induced increases in their expression (data not shown). Our data suggests that while Src affects the basal expression of RunX2, osterix and osteopontin, as previously reported, OFSS-induced changes in osteocalcin expression are Src independent. We used a Src biosensor to demonstrate that Src activity increased in the nucleus of MLO-Y4 osteocytes in response to OFSS; this was further confirmed using nuclear fractionation. Together these results support the novel concept that Src plays a role in osteoblastogenesis by functioning to curb the anabolic response of MC3T3 osteoblasts and MLO-Y4 osteocytes to OFSS via a mechanism that involves a mechanically-induced increase in nuclear Src activity.

Taken together our immunolocalization, FRET microscopy and nuclear fractionation studies suggest that exposure of MLO-Y4 cells to OFSS results in an increase in the amount of activated Src (Y416 phosphorylation) in the perinuclear/nuclear regions and an increase in Src tyrosine kinase activity in the nucleus in response to OFSS. A subtle increase in total Src in the perinulear/nuclear region was seen in response to OFSS. In contrast, a more pronounced increase in activated Src (Y416) was seen in the perinuclear and/or nuclear regions of MLO-Y4 osteocytes (Figure 3B) suggesting that the population of Src that accumulates in this region is activated (as assessed by Y416 phosphorylation). Our nuclear fractionation and FRET data directly demonstrate that Src tyrosine kinase activity increased in the nucleus in response to OFSS. This novel result suggests a previously unrecognized role for Src tyrosine kinase activity in regulating the transcriptional response of MLO-Y4 osteocytes to OFSS. There is not a widely accepted mechanism to explain how Src translocates into the nucleus, however myrstoylation has been suggested to function in regulating transport of Src to the nucleus [63].

Further studies will be needed to determine the detailed molecular mechanism(s) by which a Pyk2 and Src complex and its nuclear binding have the capacity to directly alter transcription and the epigenome.

Supporting Information

Figure S1 Mutant Src biosensor does not respond xxto OFSS in MLO-Y4 osteocytes. (A) Phasor plot overlay of static mutant Src biosensor lifetime and mutant Src biosensor lifetime exposed to OFSS. (B) Lifetime maps of the same MLO-Y4 osteocyte at static and 20 minute post-OFSS time points.

Acknowledgments

We would like to thank Amanda Siegel and Suzanne Young for their thoughtful suggestions.

Author Contributions

Conceived and designed the experiments: JMH RND JPB YW FMP. Performed the experiments: JMH RND FMP. Analyzed the data: JMH FMP. Contributed reagents/materials/analysis tools: JMH RND YW FMP. Wrote the paper: JMH FMP.

References

1. Gil-Henn H, Destaing O, Sims NA, Aoki K, Alles N, et al. (2007) Defective microtubule-dependent podosome organization in osteoclasts leads to increased bone density in Pyk2(−/−) mice. The Journal of cell biology 178: 1053–1064.
2. Boutahar N, Guignandon A, Vico L, Lafage-Proust MH (2004) Mechanical strain on osteoblasts activates autophosphorylation of focal adhesion kinase and proline-rich tyrosine kinase 2 tyrosine sites involved in ERK activation. The Journal of biological chemistry 279: 30588–30599.
3. Guignandon A, Boutahar N, Rattner A, Vico L, Lafage-Proust MH (2006) Cyclic strain promotes shuttling of PYK2/Hic-5 complex from focal contacts in osteoblast-like cells. Biochemical and biophysical research communications 343: 407–414.
4. Avraham H, Park SY, Schinkmann K, Avraham S (2000) RAFTK/Pyk2-mediated cellular signalling. Cellular signalling 12: 123–133.
5. Hall JE, Fu W, Schaller MD (2011) Focal adhesion kinase: exploring Fak structure to gain insight into function. International review of cell and molecular biology 288: 185–225.
6. Okigaki M, Davis C, Falasca M, Harroch S, Felsenfeld DP, et al. (2003) Pyk2 regulates multiple signaling events crucial for macrophage morphology and migration. Proceedings of the National Academy of Sciences of the United States of America 100: 10740–10745.
7. Buckbinder L, Crawford DT, Qi H, Ke HZ, Olson LM, et al. (2007) Proline-rich tyrosine kinase 2 regulates osteoprogenitor cells and bone formation, and offers an anabolic treatment approach for osteoporosis. Proc Natl Acad Sci U S A 104: 10619–10624.
8. Gil-Henn H, Destaing O, Sims NA, Aoki K, Alles N, et al. (2007) Defective microtubule-dependent podosome organization in osteoclasts leads to increased bone density in Pyk2(−/−) mice. J Cell Biol 178: 1053–1064.
9. Young SR, Gerard-O'Riley R, Kim JB, Pavalko FM (2009) Focal adhesion kinase is important for fluid shear stress-induced mechanotransduction in osteoblasts. J Bone Miner Res 24: 411–424.
10. Young SR, Hum JM, Rodenberg E, Turner CH, Pavalko FM (2011) Non-overlapping functions for Pyk2 and FAK in osteoblasts during fluid shear stress-induced mechanotransduction. PLoS One 6: e16026.
11. Calalb MB, Polte TR, Hanks SK (1995) Tyrosine phosphorylation of focal adhesion kinase at sites in the catalytic domain regulates kinase activity: a role for Src family kinases. Mol Cell Biol 15: 954–963.
12. Frame MC, Fincham VJ, Carragher NO, Wyke JA (2002) v-Src's hold over actin and cell adhesions. Nat Rev Mol Cell Biol 3: 233–245.
13. Schaller MD, Hildebrand JD, Shannon JD, Fox JW, Vines RR, et al. (1994) Autophosphorylation of the focal adhesion kinase, pp125FAK, directs SH2-dependent binding of pp60src. Molecular and cellular biology 14: 1680–1688.
14. Xing Z, Chen HC, Nowlen JK, Taylor SJ, Shalloway D, et al. (1994) Direct interaction of v-Src with the focal adhesion kinase mediated by the Src SH2 domain. Molecular biology of the cell 5: 413–421.
15. Soriano P, Montgomery C, Geske R, Bradley A (1991) Targeted disruption of the c-src proto-oncogene leads to osteopetrosis in mice. Cell 64: 693–702.
16. Marzia M, Sims NA, Voit S, Migliaccio S, Taranta A, et al. (2000) Decreased c-Src expression enhances osteoblast differentiation and bone formation. The Journal of cell biology 151: 311–320.
17. Lowe C, Yoneda T, Boyce BF, Chen H, Mundy GR, et al. (1993) Osteopetrosis in Src-deficient mice is due to an autonomous defect of osteoclasts. Proc Natl Acad Sci U S A 90: 4485–4489.
18. Boyce BF, Yoneda T, Lowe C, Soriano P, Mundy GR (1992) Requirement of pp60c-src expression for osteoclasts to form ruffled borders and resorb bone in mice. The Journal of clinical investigation 90: 1622–1627.
19. Horne WC, Neff L, Chatterjee D, Lomri A, Levy JB, et al. (1992) Osteoclasts express high levels of pp60c-src in association with intracellular membranes. The Journal of cell biology 119: 1003–1013.
20. Lowe C, Yoneda T, Boyce BF, Chen H, Mundy GR, et al. (1993) Osteopetrosis in Src-deficient mice is due to an autonomous defect of osteoclasts. Proceedings of the National Academy of Sciences of the United States of America 90: 4485–4489.
21. Missbach M, Jeschke M, Feyen J, Muller K, Glatt M, et al. (1999) A novel inhibitor of the tyrosine kinase Src suppresses phosphorylation of its major cellular substrates and reduces bone resorption in vitro and in rodent models in vivo. Bone 24: 437–449.
22. Hannon RA, Finkelman RD, Clack G, Iacona RB, Rimmer M, et al. (2012) Effects of Src kinase inhibition by saracatinib (AZD0530) on bone turnover in advanced malignancy in a Phase I study. Bone 50: 885–892.
23. Hannon RA, Clack G, Rimmer M, Swaisland A, Lockton JA, et al. (2010) Effects of the Src kinase inhibitor saracatinib (AZD0530) on bone turnover in healthy men: a randomized, double-blind, placebo-controlled, multiple-ascending-dose phase I trial. Journal of bone and mineral research: the official journal of the American Society for Bone and Mineral Research 25: 463–471.
24. Id Boufker H, Lagneaux L, Najar M, Piccart M, Ghanem G, et al. (2010) The Src inhibitor dasatinib accelerates the differentiation of human bone marrow-derived mesenchymal stromal cells into osteoblasts. BMC Cancer 10: 298.
25. Miller JD, McCreadie BR, Alford AI, Hankenson KD, Goldstein SA (2007) Form and Function of Bone. In: Einhorn TA, Buckwalter JA, O'Keefe RJ, editors. Orthopaedic Basic Science: foundations of clinical practice. 3 ed. Rosemont: American Academy of Orthopaedic Surgeons. 129–157.
26. Robling AG, Turner CH (2009) Mechanical signaling for bone modeling and remodeling. Crit Rev Eukaryot Gene Expr 19: 319–338.
27. Nicolella DP, Feng JQ, Moravits DE, Bonivitch AR, Wang Y, et al. (2008) Effects of nanomechanical bone tissue properties on bone tissue strain: implications for osteocyte mechanotransduction. Journal of musculoskeletal & neuronal interactions 8: 330–331.
28. Resh MD (1994) Myristylation and palmitylation of Src family members: the fats of the matter. Cell 76: 411–413.
29. Buss JE, Kamps MP, Gould K, Sefton BM (1986) The absence of myristic acid decreases membrane binding of p60src but does not affect tyrosine protein kinase activity. Journal of virology 58: 468–474.
30. Montgomery RJ, Sutker BD, Bronk JT, Smith SR, Kelly PJ (1988) Interstitial fluid flow in cortical bone. Microvasc Res 35: 295–307.
31. Smalt R, Mitchell FT, Howard RL, Chambers TJ (1997) Mechanotransduction in bone cells: induction of nitric oxide and prostaglandin synthesis by fluid shear stress, but not by mechanical strain. Adv Exp Med Biol 433: 311–314.
32. Knothe Tate ML, Knothe U, Niederer P (1998) Experimental elucidation of mechanical load-induced fluid flow and its potential role in bone metabolism and functional adaptation. Am J Med Sci 316: 189–195.
33. Turner CH, Pavalko FM (1998) Mechanotransduction and functional response of the skeleton to physical stress: the mechanisms and mechanics of bone adaptation. J Orthop Sci 3: 346–355.
34. Plotkin LI, Mathov I, Aguirre JI, Parfitt AM, Manolagas SC, et al. (2005) Mechanical stimulation prevents osteocyte apoptosis: requirement of integrins, Src kinases, and ERKs. American journal of physiology Cell physiology 289: C633–643.
35. Rangaswami H, Schwappacher R, Marathe N, Zhuang S, Casteel DE, et al. (2010) Cyclic GMP and protein kinase G control a Src-containing mechanosome in osteoblasts. Science signaling 3: ra91.
36. Rangaswami H, Schwappacher R, Tran T, Chan GC, Zhuang S, et al. (2012) Protein kinase G and focal adhesion kinase converge on Src/Akt/beta-catenin signaling module in osteoblast mechanotransduction. The Journal of biological chemistry 287: 21509–21519.
37. Pavalko FM, Gerard RL, Ponik SM, Gallagher PJ, Jin Y, et al. (2003) Fluid shear stress inhibits TNF-alpha-induced apoptosis in osteoblasts: a role for fluid shear stress-induced activation of PI3-kinase and inhibition of caspase-3. J Cell Physiol 194: 194–205.
38. Inoue D, Kido S, Matsumoto T (2004) Transcriptional induction of FosB/DeltaFosB gene by mechanical stress in osteoblasts. The Journal of biological chemistry 279: 49795–49803.
39. Kido S, Kuriwaka-Kido R, Imamura T, Ito Y, Inoue D, et al. (2009) Mechanical stress induces Interleukin-11 expression to stimulate osteoblast differentiation. Bone 45: 1125–1132.
40. Sakai K, Mohtai M, Shida J, Harimaya K, Benvenuti S, et al. (1999) Fluid shear stress increases interleukin-11 expression in human osteoblast-like cells: its role in osteoclast induction. Journal of bone and mineral research: the official journal of the American Society for Bone and Mineral Research 14: 2089–2098.
41. Sheffield JB, Graff D, Li HP (1987) A solid-phase method for the quantitation of protein in the presence of sodium dodecyl sulfate and other interfering substances. Anal Biochem 166: 49–54.
42. Wang Y, Botvinick EL, Zhao Y, Berns MW, Usami S, et al. (2005) Visualizing the mechanical activation of Src. Nature 434: 1040–1045.
43. Cole KS, Cole RH (1941) Dispersion and absorption in dielectrics I. Alternating current characteristics Journal of Chemical Physics 9: 341–351.
44. Redford GI, Clegg RM (2005) Polar plot representation for frequency-domain analysis of fluorescence lifetimes. Journal of fluorescence 15: 805–815.
45. Luo SW, Zhang C, Zhang B, Kim CH, Qiu YZ, et al. (2009) Regulation of heterochromatin remodelling and myogenin expression during muscle differentiation by FAK interaction with MBD2. The EMBO journal 28: 2568–2582.
46. Bidwell JP, Pavalko FM (2010) The Load-Bearing Mechanosome Revisited. Clinical reviews in bone and mineral metabolism 8: 213–223.
47. Bidwell JP, Pavalko FM (2011) Mechanosomes carry a loaded message. Sci Signal 3: pe51.
48. Pavalko FM, Norvell SM, Burr DB, Turner CH, Duncan RL, et al. (2003) A Model for mechanotransduction in bone cells: The load-bearing mechanosomes. J Cell Biochem 88: 104–112.
49. Faure C, Corvol JC, Toutant M, Valjent E, Hvalby O, et al. (2007) Calcineurin is essential for depolarization-induced nuclear translocation and tyrosine phosphorylation of PYK2 in neurons. Journal of cell science 120: 3034–3044.

50. Faure C, Ramos M, Girault JA (2013) Pyk2 cytonuclear localization: mechanisms and regulation by serine dephosphorylation. Cellular and molecular life sciences: CMLS 70: 137–152.
51. Lim ST, Chen XL, Lim Y, Hanson DA, Vo TT, et al. (2008) Nuclear FAK promotes cell proliferation and survival through FERM-enhanced p53 degradation. Molecular cell 29: 9–22.
52. Lim ST, Miller NL, Nam JO, Chen XL, Lim Y, et al. (2010) Pyk2 inhibition of p53 as an adaptive and intrinsic mechanism facilitating cell proliferation and survival. The Journal of biological chemistry 285: 1743–1753.
53. Ossovskaya V, Lim ST, Ota N, Schlaepfer DD, Ilic D (2008) FAK nuclear export signal sequences. FEBS letters 582: 2402–2406.
54. Hendrich B, Bird A (1998) Identification and characterization of a family of mammalian methyl-CpG binding proteins. Molecular and cellular biology 18: 6538–6547.
55. Boeke J, Ammerpohl O, Kegel S, Moehren U, Renkawitz R (2000) The minimal repression domain of MBD2b overlaps with the methyl-CpG-binding domain and binds directly to Sin3A. The Journal of biological chemistry 275: 34963–34967.
56. Ng HH, Zhang Y, Hendrich B, Johnson CA, Turner BM, et al. (1999) MBD2 is a transcriptional repressor belonging to the MeCP1 histone deacetylase complex. Nature genetics 23: 58–61.
57. Bird AP, Wolffe AP (1999) Methylation-induced repression–belts, braces, and chromatin. Cell 99: 451–454.
58. Leonhardt H, Cardoso MC (2000) DNA methylation, nuclear structure, gene expression and cancer. Journal of cellular biochemistry Supplement Suppl 35: 78–83.
59. Wolf G (1996) Function of the bone protein osteocalcin: definitive evidence. Nutrition reviews 54: 332–333.
60. Delmas PD, Price PA, Mann KG (1990) Validation of the bone Gla protein (osteocalcin) assay. Journal of bone and mineral research: the official journal of the American Society for Bone and Mineral Research 5: 3–4.
61. Raab-Cullen DM, Thiede MA, Petersen DN, Kimmel DB, Recker RR (1994) Mechanical loading stimulates rapid changes in periosteal gene expression. Calcified tissue international 55: 473–478.
62. Kannus P, Jozsa L, Kvist M, Jarvinen TL, Maunu VM, et al. (1996) Expression of osteocalcin in the patella of experimentally immobilized and remobilized rats. Journal of bone and mineral research: the official journal of the American Society for Bone and Mineral Research 11: 79–87.
63. David-Pfeuty T, Bagrodia S, Shalloway D (1993) Differential localization patterns of myristoylated and nonmyristoylated c-Src proteins in interphase and mitotic c-Src overexpresser cells. Journal of cell science 105 (Pt 3): 613–628.

17

Dynamics of Polymer Molecules with Sacrificial Bond and Hidden Length Systems: Towards a Physically-Based Mesoscopic Constitutive Law

Ahmed E. Elbanna[1,2]*, **Jean M. Carlson**[3]

1 Department of Physics, University of California Santa Barbara, Santa Barbara, California, United States of America, **2** Department of Civil and Environmental Engineering, University of Illinois at Urbana- Champaign, Urbana, Illinois, United States of America, **3** Department of Physics, University of California Santa Barbara, Santa Barbara, California, United States of America

Abstract

We investigate the entropic force-elongation behavior of a polymer chain in the presence of the sacrificial bond and hidden length (SBHL) system observed experimentally in many biomaterials. We show that in most cases the SBHL system leads to a significant increase in toughness. However, the presence of a large number of bonds or relatively strong bonds in the SBHL system can reduce the net gain in toughness. We also incorporate the polymer model into a network of polymers with random properties (e.g., contour length, number and strength of sacrificial bonds, length of hidden loops). This allows us to derive a physically-based mesoscopic force-displacement law that governs the collective behavior.

Editor: Jie Zheng, University of Akron, United States of America

Funding: This work was supported by the David and Lucile Packard Foundation and the Institute for Collaborative Biotechnologies through contract no. W911NF-09-0001 from the U.S. Army Research Office. The content of the information does not necessarily reflect the position or the policy of the Government, and no official endorsement should be inferred. The funders had no role in study design, data collection and analysis, decision to publish, or preparation of the manuscript.

Competing Interests: The authors have declared that no competing interests exist.

* E-mail: elbanna2@uiuc.edu

Introduction

Entropy based energy dissipation mechanisms were shown to play an important role in the dynamics of many physical systems. These include granular materials [1], glassy materials [2], thin film lubricants [3], and hard spheres [4]. Laws of statistical thermodynamics provide a framework for tracking the evolution of entropy and energy flow across different scales in these systems enabling a physically based description of the constitutive response [5–7]. In this paper, we use this framework to construct the force extension law for bone deformation at the scale of mineralized collagen fibrils (~1 μm).

The mineralized collaged fibrils constitute the building blocks of the bone hierarchical structure at the sub micrometer scale. Studies on bone structure show that it is a hierarchical composite of collagen and hydroxyapatite [8–9] with mechanisms to resist fracture at different size scales [10]. These size scales relate to the characteristic structural dimensions in bone, which vary from twisted peptide chains at the nanometer scale to the (secondary) osteon (haversian) structures, which are several hundred micrometers in size. The hierarchical structure at the intermediate scales includes (i) hydroxyapatite-impregnated twisted collagen fibrils at the scale of tens of nanometers; (ii) collagen fibers that are typically a micrometer in diameter and (iii) the lamellar structure of collagen fibers at several micrometer dimensions. It is the simultaneous operation of the fracture-resistance mechanisms at these various length scales that provides bone with its enduring strength and toughness.

Here, we focus on the mechanics of deformation at the scale of the mineralized collagen fibrils. Atomic Force Microscope (AFM) experiments done at this scale [11–12] showed that the fibrils are interconnected by a special type of glue that is composed of polymer chains with sacrificial bonds and hidden length (SBHL) systems. The basic structure and operation mechanism of the SBHL system are shown in Fig. 1. The assembled glue molecule (insert in Fig. 1a) may include more than one polymer chain with sacrificial bonds forming within the chain itself, crosslinking the different chains and connecting the chains to the collagen fibrils. The large scale separation of the collagen fibrils is resisted by an array of parallel gel molecules as shown in Fig. 1a. We use the worm-like chain model [13–15] (WLC) to describe the mechanical response of the glue molecules and to identify the relationship between the SBHL system internal variables and macroscopic observables such as toughness and strength. We also examine the mechanical response of the array of parallel molecules.

The operation of the SBHL system depends on the state of the sacrificial bond. As long as the bond is intact, it shields parts of the polymer length from contributing to the end-to-end distance. This corresponds to a reduction in the chain entropy (the possible number of configurations resulting in the same end-to-end distance) and a corresponding increase in the initial stiffness of the polymer chain. The increased stiffness means that a larger force is required to extend the polymer chain any finite distance, compared to that required in the case of a polymer with no SBHL system. After the sacrificial bond is broken, the shielded loop unfolds and significant energy is dissipated in reducing the chain entropy as it straightens out. Atomic Force Microscope (AFM)

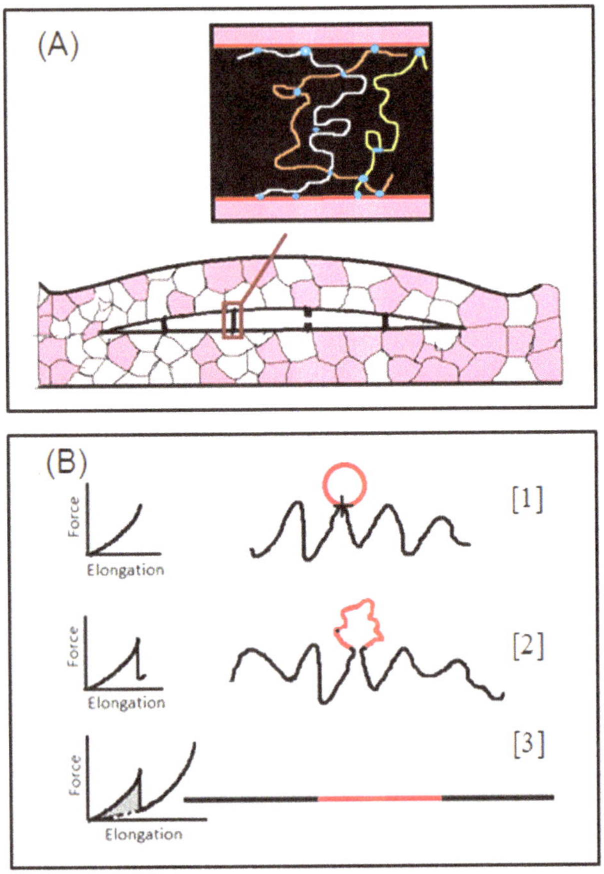

Figure 1. The structure and the basic operation principles of the SBHL system. (A) Hypothesized structures of assembled glue molecules, with sacrificial bonds (represented by blue circles) along the backbone of the polymer molecules resisting rupture of the molecules as they are stretched during microcracking. There are three types of bonds: (i) bonds within the polymer chain, (ii) bonds between different chains, and (iii) bonds connecting the chains to the backbone. (Adapted from Figure 3 in Fantner *et al.* Nature Materials 2005; 4:612–616.) (B) Schematic drawing of the basic principles of the sacrificial bond-hidden length mechanism. [1] Before a sacrificial bond is broken, only the black length of the molecule contributes to the entropic configurations and to the force with which the molecule resists stretching. The red length of the molecule is hidden from the force by the sacrificial bond. [2] When the bond fracture threshold is reached, the bond breaks and the whole length of the polymer (black plus red) contributes to its entropy. The force supported by the polymer molecule abruptly drops in response to this sudden increase in entropy. [3] As the polymer molecule is further stretched the force supported by it increases. This continues until the molecule becomes straight and breaks. The grey area represents the extra work done in stretching a polymer with SBHL system relative to a polymer of the same length but without the SBHL system.

indentation [11], pulling [11], and imaging [16] experiments support this understanding. Moreover, these experimental results suggest that SBHL system, found in gel molecules binding the mineralized collagen fibrils together, may play a substantial mechanical role in bone [12,17–19]. Order of magnitude calculations show that less than 1% by weight of this "glue" can have profound effects on the fracture resistance [12]. This challenges the conventional belief that collagen fibrils and mineral plates are the only components of bone with a strengthening mechanical role [20].

Interestingly, the SBHL system is not limited to bone. Rather, it is widespread in many remarkably tough nano-composite biomaterials such as abalone shell and diatoms [21-27]. Abalone shell, for example, is 97% crystalline calcium carbonate plates by weight, but is 3,000 times more fracture resistant than pure calcium carbonate [21–22]. The other 3% is an interstitial organic matrix, which contains extremely efficient "glue" that incorporates the SBHL system [17]. Adhesive nanofibers from live diatoms exhibit the signature of modular proteins and they show remarkable toughness [27]. The saw-tooth behavior in their force extension response corresponds to unfolding and detachment events similar to the SBHL systems mechanism [27]. A similar behavior has been reported for parallel polyprotein dimers [28] and spider capture silk [29]. A more complete understanding of the SBHL system mechanics may be useful in developing innovative therapeutic procedures as well as designing bio-inspired composite materials with improved strength and toughness.

This paper is organized as follows. In Section II we use the worm like chain model to describe the mechanics of a polymer with the SBHL system and compare the model predictions with AFM experimental observations. In Section III we investigate the influence of the SBHL internal variables, such as the number of bonds and the strength of bonds, on the macroscopic observables such as the increase in toughness. In Section IV we use the polymer force law discussed in Section II in a model of an ensemble of parallel polymers to predict the collective force-elongation behavior at mesoscopic scales. We also examine the effect of the polymer density on the collective behavior. Finally we summarize our conclusions and discuss future directions in Section V.

Review of The Basic Mechanical Properties of Polymers with Sacrificial Bonds and Hidden Length

Polymer elasticity is essentially entropic [30–31]. The relationship between the chain force (f) and its end-to-end distance (x) is controlled by the multiplicity of the number of configurations the chain can take consistent with this given end-to-end distance. The higher the multiplicity, the higher the chain entropy, and the lower the force it can support. As the polymer chain is stretched, its entropy decreases and higher forces are required corresponding to a given end-to-end distance. The end-to-end distance x cannot exceed the contour length of the polymer chain (L_c). (They coincide only when the polymer is completely straight).

The presence of the sacrificial bonds makes the length of the polymer available for entropic fluctuations smaller than the contour length (the difference is the total length of the hidden loops). In this paper, we assume that the bonds break according to a threshold fracture criterion. This is a reasonable assumption in the limit of slow pulling rates [32]. Once a bond breaks, the length of the polymer available for entropic fluctuations increases by an amount equal to the length of the freed loop. This instantaneously increases the chain entropy and leads to an abrupt drop in the force supported by the polymer molecule. With further stretching, the chain entropy decreases and the force in the chain increases.

To quantitatively describe the force-elongation response we use the worm like chain model. We show in Supporting Information Part A in File S1 that this represents a good fit for the experimental data available in the literature on bone glue [11] in the limit of large extension (Fig. S1 in File S1). The force extension relationship is given by:

$$f = \frac{k_B T}{b}\left[\frac{1}{4}\left(1-\frac{x}{L_c}\right)^{-2} - \frac{1}{4} + \frac{x}{L_c}\right], \quad (1)$$

where f is the force, x is the end-to-end distance, b is the persistence length, k_B is Boltzmann' constant and T is the temperature. In the presence of sacrificial bonds, the contour length in Eqn. (1) is replaced by the available length L_a. The available length is the total length of the polymer segments that can contribute to entropic elasticity. The contour and the available lengths are related by:

$$L_a = L_c - \sum_{i=1}^{n} l_i, \quad (2)$$

where l_i is the length of loop i shielded by the sacrificial bond i and n is the number of sacrificial bonds that are not broken yet. Accordingly, Eqn. (1) takes the form:

$$f = \frac{k_B T}{b}\left[\frac{1}{4}\left(1-\frac{x}{L_a}\right)^{-2} - \frac{1}{4} + \frac{x}{L_a}\right]. \quad (3)$$

In this section we review the key features describing the force extension curves observed in AFM experiments on bone glue [11] and discuss their mechanical implications. We follow a computational procedure similar to the one used by Fantner et al., 2006b [19]. In carrying out the numerical simulations, we keep track of the available length. Each time a sacrificial bond is broken, the available length increases by the length of the loop segment that is freed after the bond breakage.

We assume that a bond breaks when it is subjected to a force that exceeds a threshold value taken to be the bond strength. From the AFM experiments, the bond strength is estimated to be of the order of few 100 pN [33]. Several factors can affect this estimate including the bond chemical composition, its interaction with the surrounding solution, and other environmental and loading conditions such as the thermodynamic temperature and the pulling rate. Moreover, a given hidden loop may be shielded by more than one bond. Models based on the transition state theory can be used to account for some of these factors. They have been used to describe unfolding of polymer molecules [34] and strength of molecular adhesion bonds [32].

In this paper we do not account for such details explicitly. Instead, we will make the assumption that the bond strength is a random variable drawn from a uniform distribution between 1 pN and 1 nN (to account roughly for the different sources of variability). This should be a good approximation within the quasistatic loading limit we are considering here. The current framework can be extended to account for the effects of higher loading rates where the details of bond dynamics become significant.

An example of the force-extension behavior generated by Eqn. (2) for a polymer with a single sacrificial bond is shown in Fig. 2. The figure also defines several key concepts including chain stiffness, ductility, and toughness.

The chain stiffness indicates the ability of the chain to resist deformation. It is given by the slope of the tangent to force-extension curve. By differentiating Eqn. (2) with respect to x, we obtain the following expression for the chain stiffness:

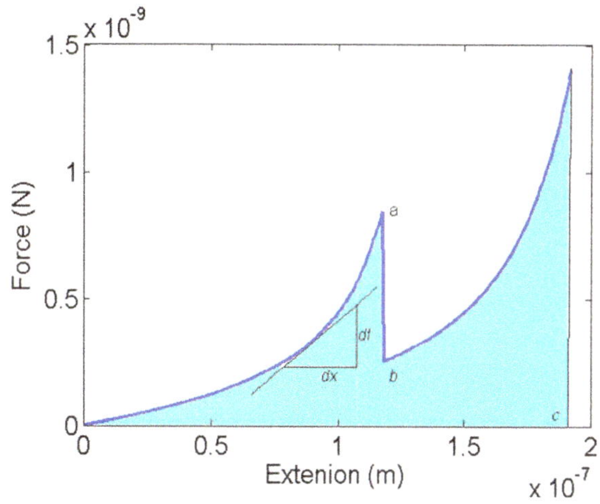

Figure 2. The force-extension behavior of an idealized polymer chain with a single sacrificial bond. The grey-filled area represents the work done in stretching the polymer to its fullest. This is equal to the polymer toughness. Point a, corresponding to the first force peak, represents the strength of the sacrificial bond. Point b represents the force supported by the chain just after the bond has broken. Point c represents the maximum extension to which the polymer chain can be stretched. This is the measure of the chain ductility. The stiffness of the chain at any given displacement is given by the slope of the straight line tangential to the force-extension curve at that displacement ($k = df/dx$).

$$k = df/dx = \frac{k_B T}{b}\left[\frac{1}{2L_a}\left(1-\frac{x}{L_a}\right)^{-3} + \frac{1}{L_a}\right]. \quad (4)$$

That is (i) the chain stiffness decreases as the available length increases, and (ii) the chain stiffness increases as the chain extension x increases. The presence of a sacrificial bond reduces the available length and hence increases the chain stiffness, making the chain stronger at smaller extensions. The saw tooth shape in Fig. 2 is characteristic of sacrificial bond breakage. The peak a corresponds to the bond strength. The magnitude of the force drop Δf is readily computed as:

$$\Delta f = f(x_b, L_a^o) - f(x_b, L_a^o + l_i), \quad (5)$$

where $f(x_b, L_a^o)$ and $f(x_b, l_a^o + l_i)$ are the forces in the chain (Eqn. (2)) just before and after the breakage of the sacrificial bond respectively, x_b is the displacement at which the bond breaks, L_a^o is the available length before the sacrificial bond breakage and l_i is the length of the loop freed by the breakage of the sacrificial bond i.

Two other important concepts, ductility and toughness, are introduced in Fig. 2. The ductility of the polymer is indicative of its ability to deform and stretch without breakage. It is measured by the maximum end-to-end distance the polymer can be stretched to before its failure or detachment from the back bone. The end-to-end distance is always less than or equal to the contour length (the equality holds only when the polymer chain becomes fully straight). Hence, the ductility of the chain cannot exceed its contour length. On the other hand, the toughness represents the work done in stretching the polymer to its maximum end-to-end distance. It is measured by the area under the force-extension line (the hatched area).

Figure 3(a) shows an example force-elongation curve from an AFM experiment [11]. In these experiments, two pieces of the fibril plates placed in a solution are used. One piece is glued to the AFM cantilever tip and the other one is kept fixed at the base. The two pieces are connected together by the polymeric gel filaments. The pieces can be pressed together and then pulled apart to simulate the molecular interactions that occur during the separation of mineralized fibrils within bone. Experiments can be carried out either under displacement-controlled conditions or force-controlled conditions. Figure 3a shows an example from a displacement- controlled AFM experiment. After the two pieces of bone are put in contact, a force is required to separate them. The force as a function of distance during the separation phase is given by the upper line in Fig. 3(a) which consists of a number of smooth increases of the force interrupted by sudden drops. Each force drop corresponds to the breakage of a sacrificial bond or the detachment of a polymer chain from the backbone. The maximum force reported is typically of the order of nanonewtons and the maximum extension is of the order of hundreds of nanometers. As the two ends approach each other, the force in the chain relaxes and the response is described by the smoother lower line in Fig. 3(a). (No bond breakage or polymer detachment occurs during retraction).

Figures 3(b) and 3(c) illustrate our corresponding numerical results for the model when multiple sacrificial bonds and hidden loops are included. The arrangement of the force peaks in the plots depends on the topology of the polymer chain (shown to the right of the plots). In particular, we identify two cases:

Case 1 illustrates the response of a polymer with the SBHL system in which the force peaks are monotonically increasing (Fig. 3(b)). This occurs when each sacrificial bond shields only one hidden loop. With the strength of sacrificial bonds drawn from a random distribution, the weakest sacrificial bonds in this case breaks first.

Case 2 illustrates a situation in which the force peaks are not arranged monotonically (Fig. 3(c)). This latter case is more consistent with AFM experiment (Fig. 3(a)). Possible mechanisms for this non-monotonic variability in the force peaks within the force-elongation response include: (i) weak bonds contained within hidden loops [shown here] and (ii) more than one polymer chain is pulled simultaneously. We will further discuss the case of having multiple parallel connections between the fibrils in Section IV.

The discussion in this section reveals the mechanical role of the SBHL system which improves both the polymer stiffness and toughness. This leads to two key contributions to the intrinsic mechanical response of the bio-material in which the SBHL system exists:

1) Increased resistance to crack initiation: The strength of the polymer chain with sacrificial bonds is always higher at low and intermediate values of displacement. Hence, larger forces will be required to initiate a tear or increase a crack opening in the presence of the SBHL system.
2) Improved energy dissipation: The SBHL system increases polymer toughness. Tougher materials are more ductile and more resistant to brittle (catastrophic) failure. This is particularly important in cases of impact loading where the presence of sacrificial bonds will facilitate the dissipation of the impact energy in inelastic deformation and will reduce the probability of bone breakage.

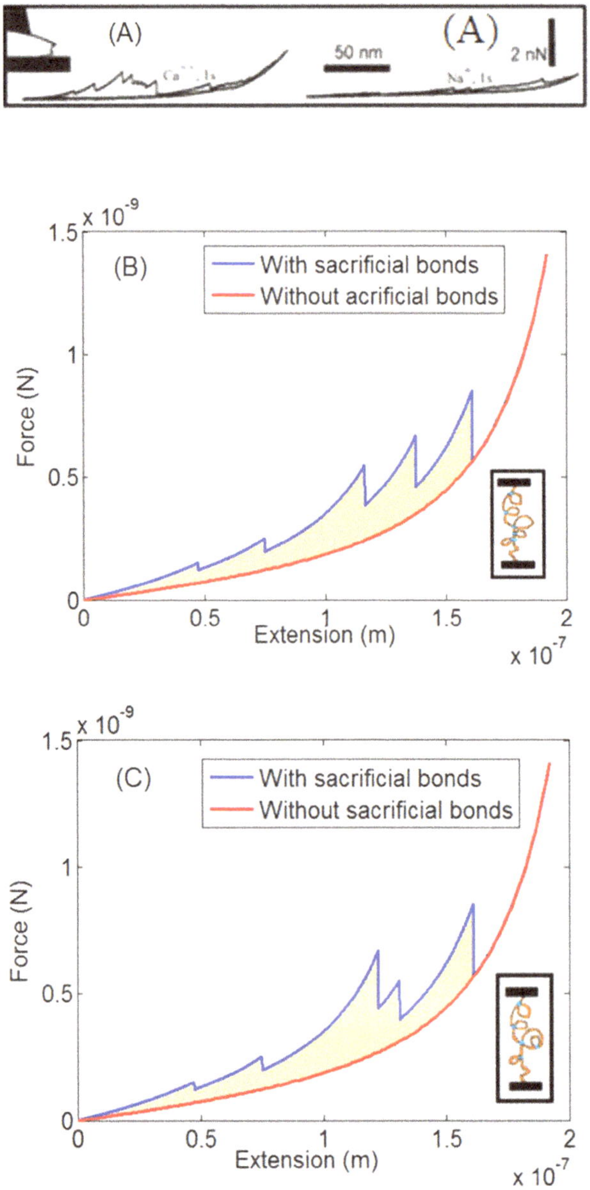

Figure 3. Experimental and numerical results for the force-extension response of polymer chains with SBHL system. (a) The force-extension response typically observed in AFM experiments (Reprinted with permission from [33]), (b) The force-extension response generated by the WLC model Eqn. (2) showing force peaks that are monotonically increasing (Case 1). In this case the weakest sacrificial bond breaks first. (c) The force-extension response generated by the WLC model Eqn. (2) showing force peaks that are non-monotonic (Case 2). This is consistent with the AFM experimental results (shown in Fig. 3(a)). A possible mechanism is that the weaker bond (bond no. 4 from the top) is shielded within a stronger bond loop (bond no.3 from top) and will become exposed only if the third bond breaks and its attached loop unfolds. In both Figs. 3(b) and 3(c), the blue lower line represents a polymer chain with the same contour and persistence length but with no SBHL system. The filled area between the lower blue and upper red lines represents the increase in toughness due to the presence of the SBHL system. ($L_c = 235\,nm$, $b = 0.02$ nm. It is more probable in these experiments that a single connection between the fibrils consist of a number of polymers interconnected with each other and pulled simultaneously. In this case, our model could be understood as being representative of the equivalent polymer chain with the same peak force and maximum extension).

Limitations of The Sacrificial Bonds and Hidden Length System

In this section, we investigate the relationship between the SBHL system internal variables (bond strength and density) and the macroscopic response of the polymer chain in terms of its strength, ductility, and toughness. These factors are expected to play a key role in designing bio-inspired composite materials and in developing therapeutic interventions for improving bone health.

To investigate the effect of the number of sacrificial bonds (i.e. bond density per polymer) on the polymer toughness, we consider a polymer chain with a given contour lengthL_c and n sacrificial bonds. Each bond hides a loop with length l. For the purpose of this estimate, we consider an idealized case in which $l = L_c/(2n+1)$(i.e. all loops have the same length). The available length of the polymer is then readily calculated as

$$L_a = L_c - nl = L_c - \frac{nL_c}{2n+1}. \tag{6}$$

The increase in toughness is the difference in the work done to extend the polymer chain with and without the sacrificial bonds. We calculate the increase in toughness for different values of n. The results are shown in Fig. 4 ($L_c = 240\,nm$and$b = 0.02\,nm$).

In generating the numerical results, each point represents the average of 5000 realizations with randomly varying bonds strength. As the number of bonds increases there is a large increase in the toughness after which the curve eventually levels off.

One of the factors affecting the number of sacrificial bonds is the type of the solution in which the polymer is placed. Negative charges on the chains can combine with free cations in the solution to form sacrificial bonds [35]. Fig. 3a suggests that during the separation of fibrils, more energy is dissipated when filaments are pulled in Ca^{2+} solutions than in Na^{+} solutions. A possible explanation for this difference, in the light of the curves in Fig. 4, is that more sacrificial bonds are formed in the former (with the divalent calcium ion in the solution combining with two negative ions on the polymer backbone) than in the latter enabling a larger increase in toughness.

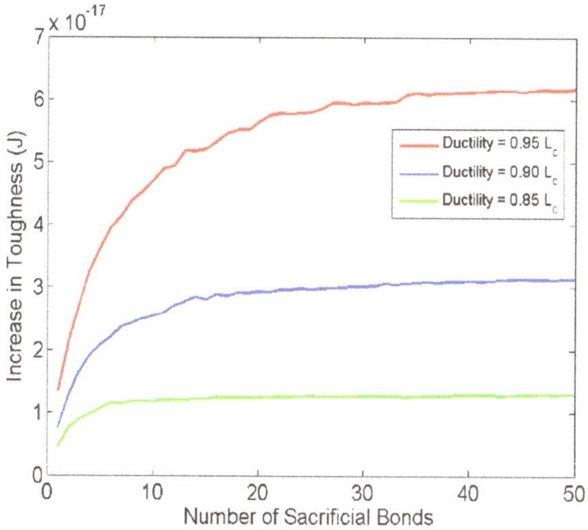

Figure 4. Effect of varying the number of sacrificial bonds on the increase in toughness of the polymer chain. Different curves correspond to different ductility values.

The asymptotic results represented by the curves in Fig. 4 can be understood from the continuum limit of the SBHL system chain as the number of bonds becomes large. For a fixed contour length, as the number of sacrificial bonds increases, the initial value of the available length approaches$L_c/2$asymptotically (Eqn. (6)).In this limit, the instantaneous stiffness of the chain varies weakly with the breakage of sacrificial bonds (Supporting Information Part B in File S2) and the force-extension curves become indistinguishable from each other (Fig. S2 in File S2). Since toughness is measured by the area under the force-extension curve, this implies that there will be little or no change in toughness due to the change in the number of bonds.

The number of bonds at which the increase in toughness levels off depends on the ductility of the polymer chains. As the ductility increases, the increase in toughness for each additional (extra) bond decreases at a smaller rate. The ductility depends on the strength of the bonds connecting the chain to the collagen fibrils as we shortly discuss.

Another important control parameter for the SBHL system is the strength of the sacrificial bonds. Two types of sacrificial bonds are considered: sacrificial bonds within the polymer chain (internal bonds) and sacrificial bonds connecting the polymer to the collagen fibrils (end bonds). This distinction between the two types of bonds is important as they can be structurally different and hence can have different values of strength.

In order for the SBHL system to enhance the polymer toughness, the strength of both types of sacrificial bonds must be such that the polymer can extend to its fullest length. This implies that the strength of end bonds should be, at least, larger than the strength of all the internal sacrificial bonds. This can be explained as follows.

The force in the polymer chain (Eqn. (3)) depends on the x/L_aratio (where x is the end-to-end distance and L_a is the available length). Sacrificial bonds reduce the available length and hence higher forces develop in the chain at smaller extensions. If the internal bond is stronger than the polymer, the polymer breaks first. On the other hand, if the end bonds are weaker than the polymer, this leads to the premature detachment of the polymer chain from the collagen fibrils (Section IV). In both cases, the system fails before the polymer achieves its full extension (corresponding to its contour length). Accordingly, both the ductility and toughness are reduced.

Efforts to enhance the bone mechanical response, whether by stimulating the bone production of or by injecting the bone with gel molecules, must account for these effects. Our results suggest density of internal bonds and constraints on the strength of the internal and end bonds will be factors affecting the SBHL system performance.

A Mesoscopic Cohesive Law for The Polymeric System

AFM experiments [12] suggest that the force supported by a fibril is of the order of a few micronewtons whereas the strength of the single polymer is of the order of several hundred piconewtons to a few nanonewtons. This means that on average 1000 polymers per fibril are required, in a healthy individual, to assure the full transfer of the force by the fibril plate.

We incorporate this in our models of the mechanical response by analyzing a group of polymer chains placed parallel to each other and constrained by the same displacement-controlled loading conditions considered previously. This setup is relevant to a wide range of applications. For example, the mechanical signature of modular proteins in diatoms [27] and parallel polyprotein dimers [28] have been previously identified in AFM experiments. Another example is quasi-brittle cracking in crystalline solids. There, the crack proceeds by breaking arrays atomic bonds intersecting with its path [36].

For the purpose of the current investigation, we consider the contour length of different polymer chains as an additional variable that is drawn from a uniform random distribution. The length of a single polymer is typically 200–350 nm. In reality, however, polymers connect with each other to form chains of much longer length enabling end-to-end extension of the order of micrometers. We assume that the total length of the chain is a random variable with a maximum value of 5 μm.

The strength of sacrificial bonds is drawn from the same random variable distribution used in Sections II and III. Each individual polymer chain deforms according to the worm like chain model (Eqn. (3)). We investigate the collective behavior of the group of polymer chains represented by the overall force-displacement response and how this response changes as a function of the number of polymer chains (N_p).

At any given instant of time, all surviving polymers are constrained by the same end-to-end distance. This is achieved by envisioning a loading apparatus of infinite rigidity. In this limit, the stress disturbance, resulting from the detachment of individual polymers, equilibrates instantaneously and does not affect the force distribution on neighboring polymers.

The force-extension response for different number of polymer chains is shown in Fig. 5. A representative pulling curve observed in AFM experiments on dintin molecules [35] is illustrated in Fig. 5a The case of small number ($N_p = 5$, 10, 20) is shown in Fig. 5(b) while that for the large number ($N_p = 50$, 100, 200) is shown in Fig. 5(c).

For small number of chains ($N_p < 20$) the discrete effects of sacrificial bond breakage and polymer detachment are pronounced. In this range, the results are intrinsically stochastic and sample dependent. These features have been observed in AFM experiments on blobs of dentin molecules (Fig. 5a) suggesting that a small number of chains (~10 molecules) is being pulled in such experiments. On the other hand, when the number of polymer chains becomes sufficiently large ($N_p > 50$) the response is increasingly well approximated by relatively smooth force-extension curves, similar to the cohesive laws routinely used in fracture mechanics [36–37].

We identify two distinct regimes in the force-extension plots shown in Fig 5. For small displacements, the force peaks tend to increase in magnitude as the extension increases. This is the displacement-strengthening regime which is expected to play a significant role in resisting crack initiation and controlling stable crack growth. On the other hand, for large displacements the force peaks tend to decrease with increasing extension corresponding to failure of end bonds and the detachment of polymer chains. This is the displacement-weakening regime which is expected to allow for the growth of instabilities and dynamic crack propagation. This displacement weakening instability is a collective effect of the polymer network and is qualitatively different from the continuing upward trend observed for a single polymer in Fig. 3(b) and 3(c).

The magnitude of the force drops in Fig. 5(b) relative to the overall force scale is large compared to the force fluctuations in Fig. 5(c) where the curves are much smoother. While small scale roughness persists in Fig. 5(c), these irregularities are in most cases of the order of 5% of the maximum force.

Another important difference is the variability in size of the force drops of significantly in Fig. 5(b) compared with Fig. 5(c) or

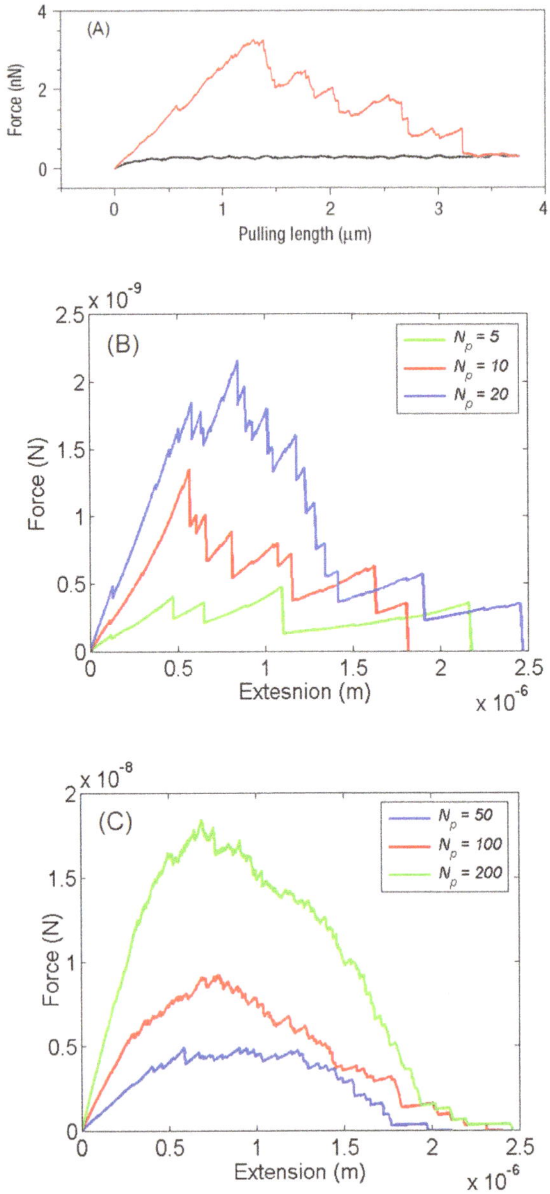

Figure 5. The force-extension response for different number of polymers under controlled displacement loading conditions. (a) Representative pulling curve observed in AFM experiments on dentin molecules (reprinted with permission from [35]) (b) Representative curves illustrating force-extension response for 5, 10 and, 20 polymers. The smaller force drops correspond in most cases to the breakage of sacrificial bonds while the larger force drops typically represent the detachment of polymer chains. The curve shows similar features to the plot in (a) suggesting that only a few chains are being pulled simultaneously during the AFM experiment. (c) The force extension plot for the polymeric gel when the number of polymer chains is large. The curves look much smoother than the curves in (b).

Fig 3(b) and 3(c). The force drops of smaller magnitude correspond in most cases to the breakage of individual sacrificial bonds and unfolding of the hidden loops, whereas the force drops of larger magnitude typically represent detachment of polymers from the backbone. This is because the breakage of an internal sacrificial bond leads to the unfolding of a single hidden loop. This only reduces the stiffness of the system slightly and causes a small force drop. However, once the polymer chain detaches, the force supported by it drops to zero. The force drop in this case is usually bigger especially if the chain is close to its maximum extension.

The detachment of the polymer chain can occur either because the bond connecting it to the fibril breaks (weak end bond) or because the force in the polymer chain exceeds the polymer strength. While polymers also detach from the backbone in Fig. 5(c), the number of polymers is large enough that detachment of single polymer does not significantly impact the system as a whole.

If the number of polymers contributing to the polymeric gel system is small, the accuracy of large-scale models of fracture in mineralized collagen fibrils may depend critically on modeling these discrete effects characteristic of the force-extension curves. However, if the number of polymers is sufficiently large, the interfacial description may be greatly simplified. Our results suggest that the quasi-static cohesive law in this case may be represented by a smooth curve parameterized by three variables: (i) the magnitude of the maximum force that the interface can resist ($F_{\max}$), (ii) the magnitude of the maximum displacement at complete separation ($\delta_{\max}$) and (iii) the displacement corresponding to $F_{\max}$. The self-similarity of the force extension curves (in the limit of large number of polymers) enabled such parameterization. We have found that an expression of the form $F = A\sin(b\delta)\exp(-c\delta)$, fits the results fairly well ($R>0.97$). In this expression$F$and δ are the force and displacement normalized by their maximum values respectively. A,b,and$c$ are fitting constants. For a good approximation: $b=\delta_c^{-1}$, $c=2\delta_c^{-1}$ and $A=\sin(1)\exp(-1/2)$. δ_c is the normalized displacement at maximum force.

Examination of the trends in Figs. 5(b) and 5(c) suggest that the maximum force F_{max} is proportional to the number of polymers while the maximum displacement $\delta_{\max}$ is weakly dependent on the number of polymers. This is verified quantitatively in Fig. 6 which illustrates statistical results for these parameters as a function of the number of polymers N_p. For each value of N_p the numerical experiment was repeated for 1500 realizations. The distribution of the maximum force, for a fixed value of N_p , is non-Gaussian. It can be represented, however, by a finite sum of Gaussian functions. On the other hand, the maximum extension distribution was found to be approximately Gaussian.

The increase in the maximum force with the increase in the number of polymers follows directly from the parallel arrangement of the polymers. At any given displacement x the total force supported by the system is given by:

$$F(x) = \sum_{i}^{N \leq N_p} f_i(x), \quad (7)$$

where$F$is the total force, f_i is the force in the ith polymer chain computed by Eqn.(3) and N is the number of unbroken polymer chains at displacement x. In the displacement strengthening regime,$N\tilde{N}_p$, so that the largerN_p the higher the maximum force F.

On the other hand, the approximate independence of the maximum extension on the number of polymers follows from the fact that the maximum displacement depends only on the contour length of the last surviving polymer chain. This is taken to be a random variable independent of the number of polymers.

Finally we examine the effect of the strength of the end bonds on the macroscopic properties of the polymeric system. End bonds may have different structure from internal bonds and hence the two groups might differ in their strength. The distinction is then important as it impacts the dynamics of the SBHL and could have potential therapeutic implications.

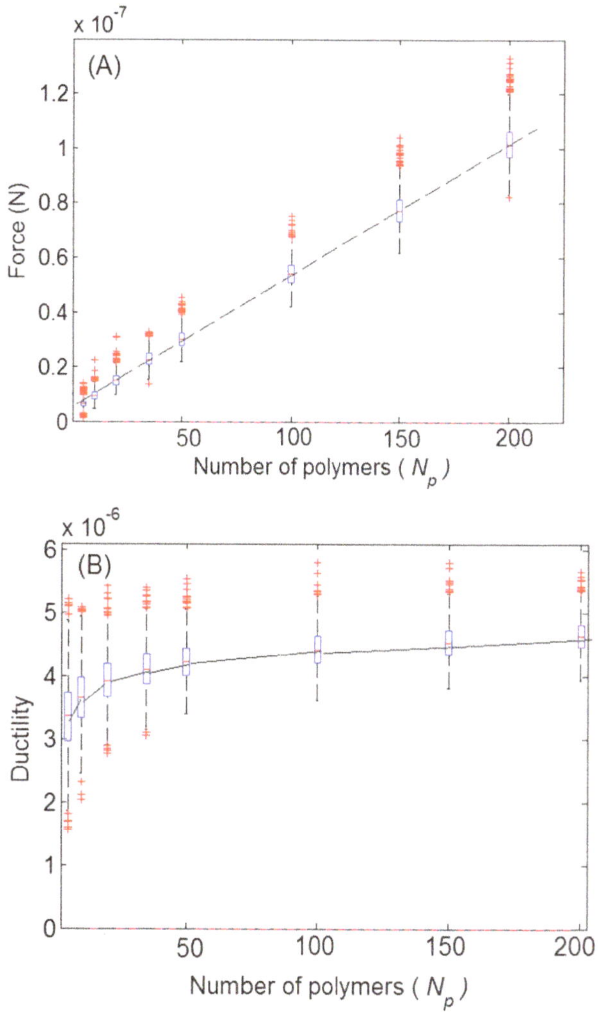

Figure 6. The effect of the number of polymers (N_p) on the maximum force and ductility (maximum extension) of the polymer group. On each box, the central mark is the median, the edges of the box are the 25th and 75th percentiles, the whiskers extend to the most extreme data points not considered outliers, and outliers are plotted individually. (a) The maximum force increases linearly with increasing the number of polymers and (b) the maximum extension is weakly dependent on the number of polymers.

Following the discussion in Section III, if the strength of the end bonds is less than the polymer chain strength, the bonds will break and the polymers will prematurely detach before the SBHL system is fully utilized. This lowers both the strength and toughness of the system. On the other hand, if the end bonds are stronger than the polymer, all the internal sacrificial bonds in each chain will break before detachment and each polymer will extend to its fullest. This, in turn, enables maximal contribution of each polymer to the overall system strength and toughness.

We investigated the two scenarios of weak and strong end bonds by simulating 1500 realizations of polymers with the SBHL system. In both cases, the geometric properties of the polymer chains, such as the contour length and the length of the hidden loops, are drawn from the same random distribution. In one group of simulations, the strength of the end bonds is chosen from the same probability distribution governing the bonds. In this case, the strength of both types of bonds is drawn from a uniform distribution of force thresholds ranging from a minimum value of 1pN to a maximum value of 1nN. In another group of simulations, the strength of the end bonds is chosen greater than the strength of the polymer chain (> 1nN) so that only when the polymer is fully extended it detaches by breaking internally. The results of the numerical investigation are shown in Fig. 7. The cases with strong end bonds (circles) attain on average higher maximum forces, longer extensions and larger toughness values than the cases with nominal (weak) end bonds (squares).

By preventing premature detachment of the polymer chains, the mechanical performance of the polymer group, as measured by strength, ductility and toughness, is significantly enhanced. This suggests that development of therapies which target enhancement of end bonds may play an important role in reducing bone health problems, especially in the elderly.

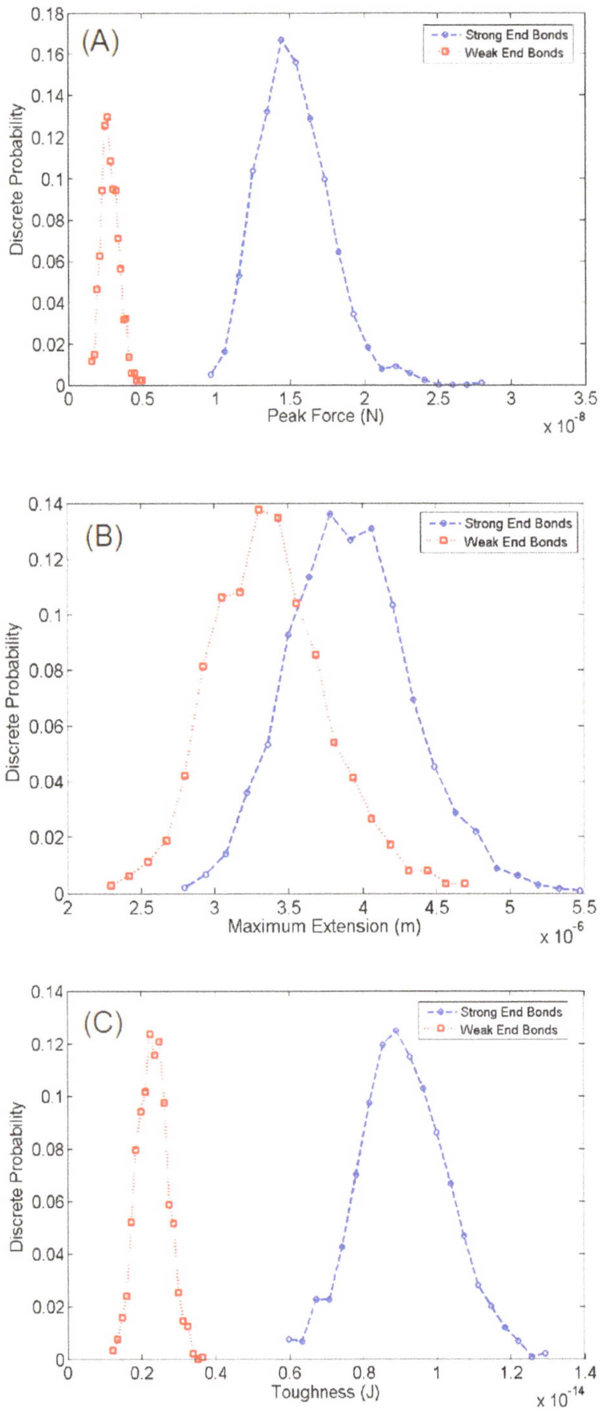

Figure 7. Effect of the strength of the bonds connecting the polymer chains to the mineralized collagen fibrils. Polymers with strong end bonds (blue circles) lead systematically to (a) higher strength, (b) ductility, and (c) toughness, compared to cases where the end bonds are weaker than the polymer itself (red squares). [Depicted probabilities are discrete].

Conclusion

Problems involving dynamics of cohesively held interfaces arise broadly in biological [Martin *et al.*, 1998] as well as in Engineering [36,38] and geophysical [39–40] applications. Common to all of these applications are fundamental physical processes involving deformation, rupture nucleation, propagation and arrest. In strongly nonlinear problems, like dynamic fracture, small scale instabilities can lead to large scale system fragilities [1,41–43] and it is imperative to understand how the microscopic processes influence the crack macroscopic response. In the case of bone, the internal interfaces between the mineralized collagen fibrils may fail under different loading conditions, and the details of the resulting dynamic rupture can determine whether only a part or the whole of the body part (e.g. knee) will fracture.

The separation of the mineralized collagen fibrils under shear or tension is resisted by a special type of polymeric glue that is composed of polymers with sacrificial bonds and hidden length (SBHL) system. The constitutive response of this glue controls the strength and ductility of the fibril plates.

Several mathematical models have been proposed to explain polymer nonlinear elasticity. Of these models, the worm like chain (WLC) and the freely jointed chain (FJC) models are the most widely used [13–15,36]. The two models differ in their idealization of the polymer chain and their prediction of the force extension response.

In this paper we investigated the mechanics and implications of entropy-based energy dissipation in polymer chains with SBHL system using the worm like chain model. Our primary focus was on the influence of the SBHL system on the larger scale mechanical observables such as toughness, ductility and mescoscopic constitutive response.

Our numerical results indicate that the SBHL system generally enhances the toughness and the strength of the polymeric system and this should allow for better resistance to crack initiation and propagation as well as better performance under dynamic loading. These properties can be used in designing base isolators to damp vibrations in structures subjected to ground motions [44].

Investigation of the dependence of polymer toughness and ductility on the internal variables of the SBHL system reveals constraints on the optimum number of sacrificial bonds as well as the strength of the bonds in order for the SBHL system to be fully utilized. In particular, the net gain in toughness may not increase in the presence of a larger number of bonds. Moreover, we show that the presence of strong internal sacrificial bonds can reduce the polymer ductility and toughness. Unlike the strength requirements for the internal bonds, strong end bonds are required to prevent premature detachment of the polymer chain and to allow the SBHL system to fully operate. These observations must be taken into account in developing therapeutic procedures that aim to enhance bone mechanical behavior or in designing bio-inspired composites with improved fracture resistance properties.

We also investigated the collective behavior of a system of parallel polymers constrained by the same displacement controlled loading. In real elastomeric networks, polymers can develop crosslinks with each other. This crosslinking will definitely affect the force distribution and ductility in the polymeric system [45]. The study of the parallel setup, however, acts as a starting point for understanding the constitutive response at larger scales. It is also relevant to a wide range of applications such as modeling diatoms [27], and parallel polyprotein dimers [28]. Moreover, it serves as a good approximation for the glue between the bone fibrils in young healthy individuals. Aging increases the crosslinking between polymers and reduces their toughness and ductility. This effect will be investigated further in our future work.

For a small number of polymer chains, we show that the cohesive law describing the force- extension response carries a clear signature of the microscopic processes of bond breakage and polymer detachment. This is manifested in the existence of force drops of magnitude comparable to the magnitude of the maximum force supported by the system. The implementation of these details in any large scale model of fracture is required because they can significantly affect crack initiation and propagation. We also showed that these details agree with observations from AFM experiments done on dentin molecules [35].

For a large number of polymer chains, however, the force fluctuations due to these microscopic processes are small compared to the amplitude of the maximum forces achieved in the system. The cohesive law in this case is greatly simplified and can be approximated by a smooth curve characterized by two numbers: the maximum force and the maximum extension.

Our results show that the maximum force supported by the polymeric system is proportional to the polymer density (number of polymer chains per unit area) and so is the system toughness. These results are relevant for understanding changes in the bone mechanical response with aging. Since the number of polymers produced by the osteocytes may decrease as the individual ages, this investigation reveals possible mechanisms for bone toughness degradation with age other than loss of bone density. It also suggests that therapeutic interventions that stimulate the production of the polymeric gel can help enhance bone health especially in the elderly [9,20].

A future extension of this study will involve use of the derived cohesive law as a boundary condition for individual elements in large scale dynamical models of bone hierarchal structure. These models will ultimately incorporate the structural complexity of the human bone at different scales to determine the combined effects of microscopic mechanisms of the SBHL system with material and geometric heterogeneities in resisting fracture. Multiscale modeling is a critical ingredient in understanding the fracture toughness in bone as well as in designing new composite materials with high levels of strength and toughness.

Supporting Information

File S1 Supporting Information Part A and Figure S1. Representative Force extension data (dots) from AFM experiments on bone glue. Different colors correspond to retraction curves in Calcium ion solutions after different delay [Source: Thompson et al., 2001]. The data is fitted by the worm like chain model (smooth curves). [Force is normalized by 70 pN and extension is normalized by 2.35 nm].

File S2 Supporting Information Part B and Figure S2. Force-extension plots of a polymer chain ($L_c = 240nm, b = 0.02nm$) with different numbers of sacrificial bonds *n*.

Acknowledgments

The authors are grateful for the comments of two anonymous reviewers that were very useful in improving the manuscript. They are also grateful to Paul Hansma, Jim Langer and Dan Morse for numerous, insightful discussions.

Author Contributions

Conceived and designed the experiments: AE JC. Performed the experiments: AE. Analyzed the data: AE JC. Wrote the paper: AE.

References

1. Daub E, Carlson JM (2010) Friction, Fracture and Earthquakes. Ann. Rev. Cond. Mat. Phys. 1: 397–418.
2. Falk M, Langer JS (1998) Dynamics of viscoplastic deformation in amorphous solids. Phys. Rev. E 57: 7192–7205.
3. Lieou CKC, Langer JS (2012) Nonequilibrium thermodynamics in sheared hard-sphere materials. Phys. Rev. E 85: 061308.
4. Lemaitre A, Carlson JM (2004) Boundary lubrication with a glassy interface. Physical Review E 69: 61611.
5. Bouchbinder E, Langer JS (2009a) Nonequilibrium thermodynamics of driven amorphous materials. Phys. Rev. E. 80, 031131.
6. Bouchbinder E, Langer JS (2009b) Nonequilibrium thermodynamics of driven amorphous materials. II. Effective-temperature theory. Phys. Rev. E. 80, 031132.
7. Bouchbinder E, Langer JS (2009c) Nonequilibrium thermodynamics of driven amorphous materials. III. Shear-transformation-zone plasticity. Phys. Rev. E. 80, 031133.
8. Koester KJ, Ager JW, Ritchie RO (2008) The true toughness of human cortical bone measured with realistically short cracks. Nature Materials 7: 672–677.
9. Nallaa RK, Kruzica JJ, Kinney JH, Ritchie RO (2004) Effect of aging on the toughness of human cortical bone: evaluation by R-curves. Bone 35:1240–1246.
10. Ritchie RO, Beuhler M, Hansma P (2009) Plasticity and toughness in bone. Physics Today: 41–47.
11. Thompson JB, Kindt JH, Drake B, Hansma HG, Morse DE, et al. (2001) Bone Indentation Recovery Time Correlates with Bond Reforming Time. Nature 414:773–775.
12. Fantner GE, Hassenkam T, Kindt JH, Weaver JC, Birkedal H (2005) Sacrificial bonds and hidden length dissipate energy as mineralized fibrils separate during bone fracture. Nature Materials 4: 612–616.
13. Wang MD, Yin H, Landick R, Gelles J, Block SM (1994) Stretching DNA with optical tweezers. Biophys. J. 72:1335–1346.
14. Marko JF, Siggia ED (1995) Stretching DNA. Macromolecules 28: 8759–8770.
15. Bouchiat C, Wang MD, Allemand JF, Strick T, Block SM, et al. (1999) Estimating the Persistence Length of a Worm-Like Chain Molecule from Force-Extension Measurements. Biophys J. 76, No. 1, 409–413.
16. Hassenkam T, Fantner GE, Cutroni JA, Weaver JC, Morse DE, et al. (2004) High-resolution AFM imaging of intact and fractured trabecular bone. Bone 35: 4–10.
17. Smith BL, Schaeffer TE, Viani M, Thompson JB, Frederick NA, et al. (1999) Molecular mechanistic origin of the toughness of natural adhesives, fibres and composites. Nature 399: 761–763.
18. Fantner GE, Oroudjev E, Schitter G, Golde LS, Thurner P, et al. (2006a) Sacrificial Bonds and Hidden Length: Unraveling Molecular Mesostructures in Tough Materials. Biophysical Journal 90 (4): 1411–1419.
19. Fantner GE, Rabinovych O, Schitter G, Thurner P, Kindt JH, et al., (2006b) Hierarchical interconnections in the nano-composite material bone: Fibrillar cross-links resist fracture on several length scales. Composites Science and Technology 66: 1205–1211.
20. Gass M, Dawson-Hughes B (2006) Preventing osteoporosis-related fractures: an overview. Am. J. Med. 119, S3–S11.
21. Currey JD (1977) Mechanical Properties of Mother of Pearl in Tension. Proceedings of the Royal Society of London Series B-Biological Sciences 196: 443–463.
22. Jackson AP, Vincent JFV, Turner RM (1988) The Mechanical Design of Nacre. Proceedings of the Royal Society of London Series B-Biological Sciences 234: 415–440.

23. Gebeschuber IC, Kindt JH, Thompson JB, Del Amo Y, Stachelberger H, et al. (2003) Atomic force microscopy study of living diatoms in ambient conditions. J. Microsc 212: 292–299.
24. Higgins MJ, Crawford SA, Mulvaney P, Wetherbee R (2002) Characterization of the adhesive mucilages secreted by live diatom cells using atomic force microscopy. Protist 153: 25–38.
25. Higgins MJ, Sader JE, Mulvaney P, Wetherbee R (2003) Probing the surface of living diatoms with atomic force microscopy: the nanostructure and nanomechanical properties of the mucilage layer. J. Phycol. 39: 722–734.
26. Higgins MJ, Molino JP, Mulvaney P, Wetherbee R (2003) The structure and nanomechanical properties of the adhesive mucilage that mediates diatom: substratum adhesion and motility. J. Phycol. 39: 1181–1193.
27. Dugdale TM, Degastine R, Chiovitti A, Mulvaney P, Wetherbee R (2005) Single adhesive nano-fibers from a live diatom have the signature fingerprint of modular proteins. Biophysical Journal 89: 4252–4260.
28. Sarkar A, Caamano S, Fernandez J (2007) The Mechanical Fingerprint of a Parallel Polyprotein Dimer. Biophysical Journals, L36-L38, doi: 10.1529/biophysj.106.097741.
29. Becker N, Oroudjev E, Mutz S, Cleveland JP, Hansma PK, et al. (2003) Molecular nanosprings in spider capture-silk threads. Nature Materials 2, no. 4: 278–283.
30. Bustamante C, Marko JF, Siggia ED, Smith S (1994) Entropic elasticity of lambda-phage DNA. Science 265: 1599–1600.
31. Rubenstein M (2003) Polymer Physics. Oxford University Press, USA.
32. Evans E, Ritchie K (1997) Dynamic strength of molecular adhesion bonds. Biophysical Journal 72(4): 1541–1555.
33. Hansma PK, Fantner GE, Kindt JH, Thurner PJ, Schitter G, et al. (2005) Sacrificial bonds in the interfibrillar matrix of bone. J. Musculoskelet Neuronal Interact 5(4): 313–315.
34. Rief M, Fernandez JM, Gaub HE (1998) Elastically Coupled Two-Level Systems as a Model for Biopolymer Extensibility. Phys. Rev. Lett. 81: 4764–4767.
35. Adams J, Fantner GE, Fisher LW, Hansma PK (2008) Molecular energy dissipation in nanoscale networks of Dentin Matrix Protein 1 is strongly dependent on ion valence. Nanotechnology 19: 384008.
36. Barenblatt GI (1962) Mathematical theory of equilibrium cracks in brittle fracture. Advances in Applied Mechanics VII: 55–129.
37. Xu XP, Needleman A (1993) Void nucleation by inclusion debonding in a crystal matrix. Materials Science and Engineering A129: 111–132.
38. Xia K, Chalivendra VB, Rosakis AJ (2006) Spontaneous Mixed-Mode Fracture in Bonded Similar and Dissimilar Materials. Experimental Mechanics 46:163–171.
39. Scholz C (2002) Earthquakes and faulting. Cambridge University Press 2nd edition.
40. Lapusta N (2009) Seismology: The roller coaster of fault friction. Nature Geoscience 2: p. 676–677.
41. Kolmogrov AN (1991) The Local Structure of Turbulence in Incompressible Viscous Fluid for Very Large Reynolds Numbers. Proceedings of the Royal Society of London, Series A: Mathematical and Physical Sciences 434: 9–13.
42. Rice JR (1983) Constitutive Relations for Fault Slip and Earthquake Instabilities. Pure and Applied Geophysics 121: 443–475.
43. Carlson JM, Langer JS (1989) Properties of earthquakes generated by fault dynamics. Phys. Rev. A. 40: 6470–6484.
44. Yang HT, Lin CH, Bridges D, Randall CJ, Hansma PK (2010) Bio-inspired passive actuator simulating an abalone shell mechanism for structural control. Smart Materials and Structures 19(10), 105011.
45. Sbrana F, Lorusso M, Canale C, Bochicchio B, Vassalli M (2011) Effect of chemical cross-linking on the mechanical properties of elastomeric peptides studied by single molecule force spectroscopy. Journal of Biomechanics 44(11): 2118–2122.

18

Distinct Cyclosporin A Doses Are Required to Enhance Bone Formation Induced by Cyclic and Rest-Inserted Loading in the Senescent Skeleton

Sundar Srinivasan*, Dewayne Threet, Leah E. Worton, Brandon J. Ausk, Steven D. Bain, Edith M. Gardiner, Ronald Y. Kwon, Ted S. Gross

Department of Orthopaedics and Sports Medicine, University of Washington, Seattle, Washington, United States of America

Abstract

Age-related decline in periosteal adaptation negatively impacts the ability to utilize exercise to enhance bone mass and strength in the elderly. We recently observed that in senescent animals subject to cyclically applied loading, supplementation with Cyclosporin A (CsA) substantially enhanced the periosteal bone formation rates to levels observed in young animals. We therefore speculated that if the CsA supplement could enhance bone response to a variety of types of mechanical stimuli, this approach could readily provide the means to expand the range of mild stimuli that are robustly osteogenic at senescence. Here, we specifically hypothesized that a given CsA supplement would enhance bone formation induced in the senescent skeleton by both cyclic (1-Hz) and rest-inserted loading (wherein a 10-s unloaded rest interval is inserted between each load cycle). To examine this hypothesis, the right tibiae of senescent female C57BL/6 mice (22 Mo) were subjected to cyclic or rest-inserted loading supplemented with CsA at 3.0 mg/kg. As previously, we initially found that while the periosteal bone formation rate (p.BFR) induced by cyclic loading was enhanced when supplemented with 3.0 mg/kg CsA (by 140%), the response to rest-inserted loading was not augmented at this CsA dosage. In follow-up experiments, we observed that while a 30-fold lower CsA dosage (0.1 mg/kg) significantly enhanced p.BFR induced by rest-inserted loading (by 102%), it was ineffective as a supplement with cyclic loading. Additional experiments and statistical analysis confirmed that the dose-response relations were significantly different for cyclic versus rest-inserted loading, only because the two stimuli required distinct CsA dosages for efficacy. While not anticipated *a priori*, clarifying the complexity underlying the observed interaction between CsA dosage and loading type holds potential for insight into how bone response to a broad range of mechanical stimuli may be substantially enhanced in the senescent skeleton.

Editor: João Costa-Rodrigues, Faculdade de Medicina Dentária, Universidade do Porto, Portugal

Funding: This study was supported, in part, by funding from the National Institutes of Health (SS: AR056235; TSG: AR056652), the Sigvard T. Hansen, Jr. Endowed Chair (TSG) and the Zimmer Fracture Biology Professorship (SDB). The funders had no role in study design, data collection and analysis, decision to publish, or preparation of the manuscript.

Competing Interests: The authors have declared that no competing interests exist.

* E-mail: sundars@uw.edu

Introduction

Age-related bone loss markedly compromises skeletal integrity and increases fracture risk [1,2]. While interventions against osteoclastic bone resorption have proved successful [3], anabolic therapies that can initiate *de novo* bone formation and thereby compensate for accumulated loss of bone mass over age are currently under consideration (e.g., PTH, sclerostin antibodies) [4]. Physical exercise and mechanical loading are also anabolic for bone and hold therapeutic potential to focally buttress weakened skeletal structures [5], particularly given the ability of mechanical loading to substantially influence bone size via periosteal expansion [6]. However, when exercise based trials have been applied to the elderly, they have proven ineffective in influencing bone mass and strength [7]. While many differences exist between the aged and young skeleton, two factors clearly hold potential to limit the effectiveness of exercise in the elderly: 1) age-related alterations in cell function [8,9,10,11,12], and/or 2) poor compliance with the high-intensity types of exercise most capable of periosteal expansion [13,14].

Pre-clinical animal models have unique potential to explore age-related mechanotransduction deficits. However, there is controversy in the literature regarding the degree to which aging alters the responsiveness of the periosteal surface to mechanical stimuli [15,16,17,18]. We have previously reviewed this issue extensively [19], and under controlled conditions, aged animal models can be used to explore the muted periosteal adaptation to physical exercise typically encountered in the elderly [15,16]. For example, our studies in senescent C57BL/6 mice (22 Mo) suggest that bone adaptation to mechanical stimuli is substantially decreased versus that in young [20], and attempts to enhance the low-level bone formation by doubling strain magnitude, increasing cycle numbers and rest-insertion were all ineffective in the senescent skeleton [21]. In contrast, bone formation is differentially enhanced by each of these [22] and other types of perturbations of a 'control' mechanical stimulus in young animals [23,24,25,26]. The consequence of this loss of differential tissue responses in the context of low-level periosteal adaptation is a marked reduction in the range of mild, readily complied with mechanical stimuli

Table 1. Estimated strains (με; mean ± s.e.) induced in animals across the CsA dosages by cyclic and rest-inserted loading.

	CsA dosage (mg/kg)					
	0.0	0.03	0.1	0.3	3.0	6.0
Cyclic	1745±47	-	1670±70	1638±94	1760±47	1848±86
Rest	1736±53	1658±65	1696±55	1813±44	1926±127	-

options capable of robustly influencing periosteal adaptation in the senescent skeleton.

Recently, in a computational model of acute signaling pathway activation during mechanical loading, we observed that specific deficits in activation and nuclear binding of transcription factors were sufficient to account for the muted response of the senescent periosteum to a variety of mechanical stimuli [20]. Based upon model derived insights, we performed a follow-up experiment in which senescent animals were subjected to cyclically applied mechanical stimuli with or without low dose Cyclosporin A (CsA; either 0.3 or 3.0 mg/kg). We found that when cyclical loading was supplemented with CsA, the ensuing bone formation was substantially increased and equivalent to that induced in young animals by loading alone [20].

Given this outcome, we speculated that supplementation with CsA could substantially enhance bone formation induced in senescent animals by different types of mechanical stimuli. As a starting point, we specifically hypothesized that a given CsA supplement would enhance bone formation induced in the senescent skeleton by both cyclic (1-Hz) and rest-inserted loading (wherein a 10-s unloaded rest is inserted between each load cycle). We examined our hypothesis by subjecting the right tibiae of senescent female C57BL/6 mice (22 Mo) to cyclic or rest-inserted loading supplemented with CsA at a dosage (3.0 mg/kg) previously found to be maximally efficacious [20]. However, based upon findings contrary to expectations, we were then compelled to explore the possibility that the two different mechanical loading stimuli (i.e., cyclic, rest-inserted) required distinct CsA dosages in order to significantly enhance bone formation response in senescent animals.

Methods

Ethics Statement

All experiments and protocols were approved by the University of Washington, Institutional Animal Care and Use Committee (IACUC 3306-02).

Methods Overview

All together, we performed a series of three experiments in this study. In each experiment, senescent female C57BL/6 mice (22 Mo; obtained from NIH aged rodent colonies) were subject to mechanical loading with or without CsA supplementation. Mechanical loading was exogenously applied to the right tibiae of anesthetized mice (2% isoflurane) using the noninvasive murine tibia-loading device [27]. Animals were subject to 50 cycles/d of mechanical loading on M, W, F for 3 weeks (9 total bouts), with protocols calibrated to induce peak longitudinal normal strain of 1700 με at the tibia mid-shaft. The loading was applied as either a cyclic (1-Hz) or a rest-inserted waveform (10-s unloaded rest between each load cycle). Prior to the experiments, the right tibia mid-shaft was scanned via *in vivo* microCT (SCANCO vivaCT-40), and animal specific longitudinal normal strains induced by the loading protocols were determined for individual animal mid-shaft cross-sections via beam theory [22]. In addition, animals received CsA supplements s.c. 30 mins prior to each loading bout (Sandimmune, Novartis Pharma), at concentrations specified within each experimental design. Stock solutions were prepared at different dilutions (in physiologic saline), such that experimentally specified concentrations (e.g., 3.0 mg/kg) were re-constituted within each 200 μl s.c. injection (dilutions were prepared by assuming an average mouse weight of 28 gm).

Animal weights were measured prior to loading/CsA administration on each of 9 loading days. Animals were permitted food and water ad libitum. All animals received Calcein labeling i.p. (10 mg/kg) on day 10, 19, and were sacrificed on day 22. Upon sacrifice, the right loaded and left contralateral tibia were dissected of soft tissue and 300 μm thick sections were obtained about the tibia mid-shaft. The sections were hand ground to 90 μm, cover slipped and imaged via an epifluorescent microscope (Nikon, 20x). As previously [22], composite images were assembled, anatomically oriented and standard dynamic histomorphometry measures of mineral apposition rate (MAR, μm/d), surface referent mineralizing surface (MS/BS%) and bone formation rate (BFR, $\mu m^3/\mu m^2/d$) were determined at the periosteal surface using custom software within Image J.

Experiment 1. We first performed an experiment in order to examine our hypothesis that a given CsA supplement would enhance bone formation induced in the senescent skeleton by both cyclic (1-Hz) and rest-inserted loading. For this, the right tibiae of senescent female mice were exposed to cyclic or rest-inserted mechanical loading with/without CsA supplementation. Separate groups of senescent animals received cyclically applied loading with CsA supplementation at 0.0 mg/kg (n = 9), or 3.0 mg/kg (n = 10), or rest-inserted loading supplemented with CsA at 0.0 mg/kg (n = 8) or 3.0 mg/kg (n = 7). One (out of 10) animal in the cyclic loading group supplemented with 3.0 mg/kg died during the experiment and was not included in the analysis.

Experiment 2. Based upon the outcomes of Experiment 1, and a synthesis of the literature on the mechanisms of action of CsA and putative interactions with mechanotransduction pathways, we performed a second experiment. We explored the possibility that rest-inserted loading required a lower dose CsA supplement in order to enhance loading induced bone formation. For this, senescent C57BL/6 mice were exposed to rest-inserted loading supplemented with CsA at 0.1 mg/kg (n = 9) or 0.3 mg/kg (n = 7). As comparative controls, animals were also exposed to cyclic loading supplemented with CsA at 0.1 mg/kg (n = 10), or 0.3 mg/kg (n = 8). Lastly, to examine whether CsA supplementation enhanced bone formation versus that induced by loading alone, and to minimize use of experimental animals, the data from animals receiving loading but not CsA from Experiment 1 was also included in the analysis. One animal each that was exposed to cyclic loading supplemented with CsA at 0.1 mg/kg and 0.3 mg/kg died during the experiment and were therefore not included in the analysis.

Experiment 3. The results of Experiments 1 and 2 suggested the possibility of a different dose response relation for rest-inserted vs cyclic stimuli when supplemented with CsA. Specifically, it appeared that response to cyclic loading supplemented with CsA could be linear, while response to rest-inserted loading supplemented with CsA could be bi-phasic. To more rigorously confirm this possibility while minimizing use of senescent experimental animals, we included two additional experimental groups where CsA dosages were biased based upon the loading waveform

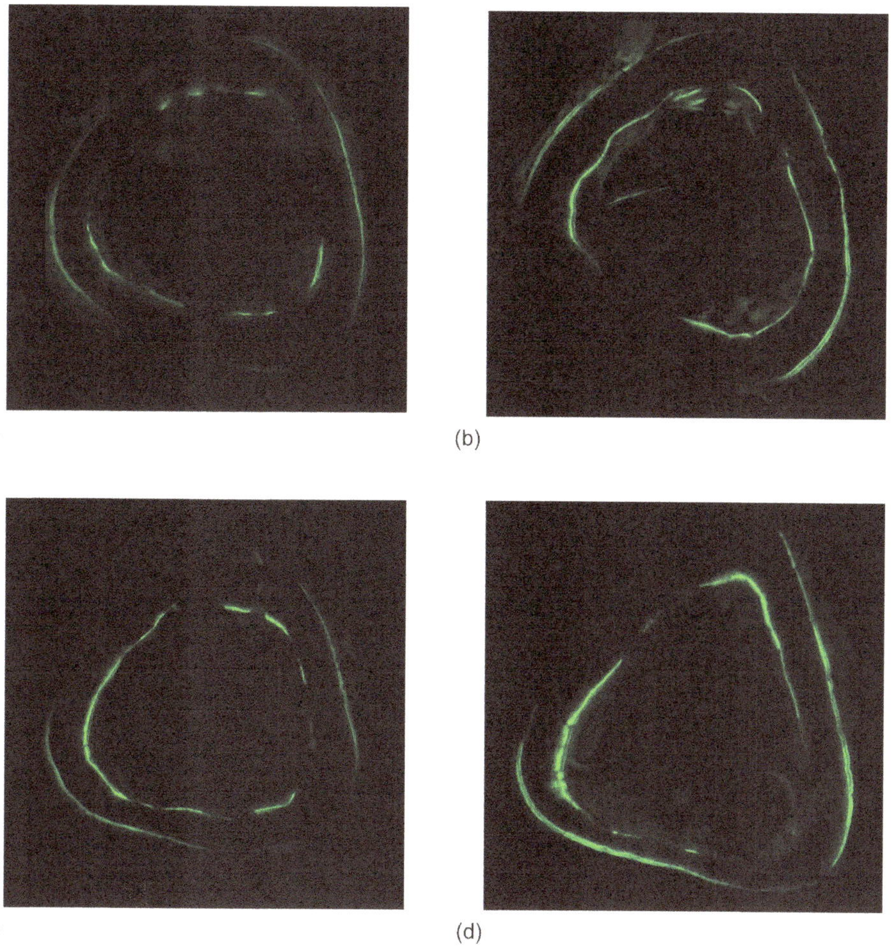

Figure 1. Bone response at the mid-shaft tibiae from animals subject to loading with or without CsA supplementation. Illustrative fluorescent images from animals subject to cyclic loading (a) and supplemented with 3.0 mg/kg CsA (b), or subject to rest inserted loading (c) and supplemented with 0.1 mg/kg CsA (d).

implemented (i.e., higher dose for cyclic and lower dose for rest-inserted loading than those previously implemented in Experiments 1, 2). Specifically, a group of animals were exposed to cyclic loading supplemented with CsA at 6.0 mg/kg (n = 8). A separate group of animals (n = 7) were subject to rest-inserted loading and supplemented with 0.03 mg/kg CsA. The data from Experiments 1 and 2 were included along with the data generated in Experiment 3 for analysis of dose-response relations. One animal exposed to cyclic loading supplemented with CsA at 6.0 mg/kg died prematurely and was therefore not included in the analysis.

To analyze whether the dose-response relation was significantly different for cyclic vs rest-inserted loading, we determined relative measures of periosteal bone response. Specifically, we determined relative periosteal MS/BS (rp.MS/BS), MAR (rp.MAR), and BFR (rp.BFR) as responses measured in the experimentally loaded – contralateral limbs. Given that the consolidated data appeared to follow a biphasic pattern, we developed a non-linear model, similar in functionality to hormesis models [28,29,30], to explore and analyze the dose-response relation. Specifically, we implemented a model of the form:

$$y(x) = y_0 + y_{\max} \times [S(x,\delta_{Max},0) - S(x,\delta_{Inhibit},\delta_{Max})] \quad (1a)$$

where,

$$S(x,\delta_2,\delta_1) = \frac{\left(\dfrac{1}{1+e^{\left(-\frac{x-0.5(\delta_2+\delta_1)}{0.1(\delta_2-\delta_1)}\right)}} - S_0\right)}{S_1 - S_0} \quad (1b)$$

$$S(x \le \delta_1) = 0,\ S(x \le \delta_1) = 0,\ S(x \ge \delta_2) = 1,\ S_1 = \frac{1}{1+e^{-5}},\ S_0 = \frac{1}{1+e^{+5}} \quad (1c)$$

and, 'y' is the bone response measure (i.e., rp.MS, rp.MAR, or rp.BFR), and 'x' is the CsA dosage in mg/kg. Each of the implemented parameters of the current model (n = 4) had a biological relevance. The four parameters modeled the baseline response induced by loading in the absence of CsA (y_0), the maximal quantity by which the response is increased beyond baseline (y_{Max}) when loading is supplemented with the optimal dosage of CsA (δ_{Max}), and the dosage at which the response 'y' returns to baseline ($\delta_{Inhibit}$). This model then permitted us to examine whether the dose-response relations (and aspects within)

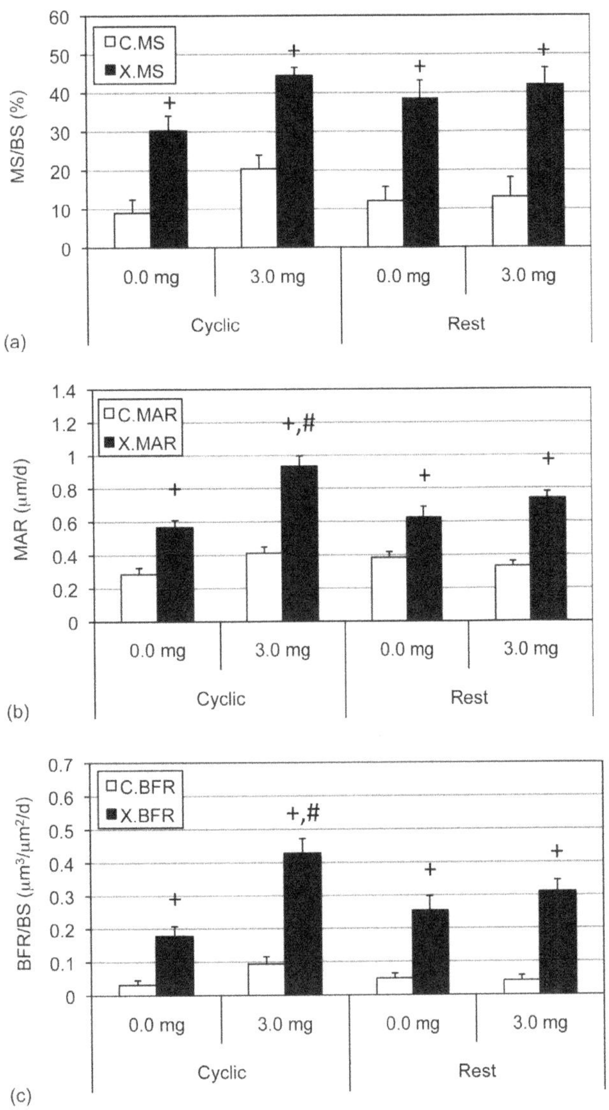

Figure 2. CsA supplementation significantly amplified bone response to cyclic loading. Periosteal MS/BS (a), MAR (b), and BFR/BS (c; mean+s.e.) were significantly increased in experimentally loaded (X) versus contralateral controls (C; '+'). Supplementing cyclic loading with CsA (at 3.0 mg/kg) significantly enhanced MAR and BFR/BS compared with that induced by loading alone ('#').

were equivalent or not between cyclic and rest-inserted loading supplemented with CsA.

Statistical Analysis

Data were primarily analyzed via factorial MANOVA with cyclic vs rest-inserted loading, experimentally loaded vs contralateral tibiae, and CsA dosage as independent factors and with MS/BS, MAR and BFR at the periosteal surface as the dependent variates. Where main effects were significant (and post-hoc analysis required), Dunnett's control test were performed to examine whether CsA supplementation significantly enhanced bone formation compared to that induced by loading alone. All test were performed using SPSS statistical software, and $p \leq 0.05$ was considered to be statistically significant.

To explore dose-response relations, we calibrated the parameters of the non-linear model (eq 1) against the *in vivo* relative bone response measures (rp.MS, rp.MAR, rp.BFR). For this, we used a previously implemented method of maximum likelihood estimation (MLE) and likelihood ratio testing (LRT) [20,31]. Briefly, the method of MLE attempts to determine the model parameters that best simulate experimental data means given experimental variance. Upon parameter estimation, the approach then permits a determination of whether the model (and hence, the dose-response relations) are significantly different between cyclic and rest-inserted loading, as well as a determination of which aspects of the model contribute to the differences in dose-response relations. To implement this approach, we assumed that the data were normally distributed and maximized the likelihood estimate for the non-linear model (eq 1) using the simulated annealing algorithm (SA; 100,000 iterations with 10 random restarts). The MLE and LRT analyses were performed within MATLAB software.

Using this statistical approach, we first explored the null hypothesis that a single model ($n = 4$ parameters) could simulate the dose-response relation for both cyclic and rest-inserted loading supplemented with CsA. If so, we additionally examined whether constraining parameter $y_{Max} = 0$ (i.e., is there a benefit with CsA administration?) permitted simulation of the experimental data. Second, for response measures where the first analysis failed, we explored the null hypothesis that 2 separate models ($n = 8$ parameters) could simulate the dose-response relation for cyclic and rest-inserted loading with CsA. Subsequent analyses were then performed for response measures where the second analysis was successful (i.e., the null hypothesis was accepted). Third, we explored whether null hypotheses constraining each of the 4 modeled parameters to be the same between the cyclic and rest-inserted model, when considered individually and in combinations, could be accepted or rejected. Lastly, we examined whether null hypotheses constraining parameter $y_{Max} = 0$ was within the 95% confidence interval of the MLE for the cyclic and rest-inserted models. We used LRTs to either accept ($p > 0.05$) or reject ($p \leq 0.05$) each of the null hypotheses posed above against alternate models. For the first two analyses above, the alternate model comprised a fully saturated model who's 'global' maximum likelihood estimate (GMLE) was determined by assigning the model means to be equal to the experimental means for each of the experimental groups [20]. For subsequent analyses, the alternate models for null hypotheses contrasts were the MLE's for either the 4 parameter or 8 parameter models described above [20].

Results

Loading induced animal specific strains of groups included in Experiment 1, 2 and 3 were not significantly different across comparisons (Table 1; $p \geq 0.2$).

Experiment 1

In our initial experiment, we sought to determine whether CsA supplementation at a previously efficacious dosage for cyclic loading (3.0 mg/kg), could also enhance bone formation induced by rest-inserted loading. We found that in the contralateral bones, the main effect of loading (cyclic, rest) or CsA did not attain significance for MS ($p = 0.27$), MAR ($p = 0.13$), and BFR ($p = 0.17$). In animals subject to cyclic loading MS, MAR and BFR were significantly increased in the experimentally loaded vs contralateral bones when supplemented by 0.0 mg/kg CsA ($p \leq 0.001$), and by 3.0 mg/kg CsA ($p \leq 0.001$; Fig. 1, 2). In animals subject to rest-inserted loading MS, MAR and BFR were significantly increased in the experimentally loaded vs contralateral bones when supplemented by 0.0 mg/kg CsA ($p \leq 0.01$), and by 3.0 mg/kg CsA ($p \leq 0.001$; Fig. 2).

In the experimentally loaded bones, the main effect of cyclic versus rest-inserted loading supplemented with CsA (0.0, 3.0 mg/kg) attained significance for MAR ($p = 0.001$) and BFR ($p < 0.01$), but not for MS ($p = 0.07$; therefore, influence upon MS was not further analyzed). In the experimental limbs of cyclically loaded animals, CsA supplementation at 3.0 mg/kg significantly enhanced MAR ($p = 0.001$) and BFR ($p < 0.01$) vs that induced by cyclic loading alone (Fig. 1, 2). In the experimental limbs of rest-inserted loaded animals, neither MAR nor BFR were significantly influenced by CsA supplementation ($p \geq 0.17$). Lastly, the bone response parameters were not significantly different in the experimentally loaded bones of animals exposed to cyclic vs rest-inserted loading without or with CsA supplementation ($p = 0.29$).

Experiment 2

We next examined whether lower dosage CsA supplements (0.1 or 0.3 mg/kg) could enhance bone formation induced by rest-inserted loading (and cyclic loading as comparative controls). We found that in the contralateral bones, the main effects of dosage (0.0 vs 0.1 vs 0.3 mg/kg CsA) or protocol type (cyclic, rest-inserted) did not alter outcome measures ($p = 0.29$; Fig. 3). In animals subject to cyclic loading, MS, MAR and BFR were significantly increased in the experimentally loaded vs contralateral bones when supplemented with 0.1 mg/kg CsA ($p \leq 0.02$) and by 0.3 mg/kg CsA ($p \leq 0.01$; Fig. 3). In animals subject to rest-inserted loading MS, MAR and BFR were significantly increased in the experimentally loaded vs contralateral bones when supplemented by 0.1 mg/kg CsA ($p \leq 0.001$) and by 0.3 mg/kg CsA ($p \leq 0.01$; Fig. 3).

In the experimentally loaded bones, the main effect of cyclic versus rest-inserted loading supplemented with CsA (0, 0.1, 0.3 mg/kg) attained significance for MAR ($p < 0.01$) and BFR ($p < 0.01$), but not for MS ($p = 0.14$). In bone exposed to cyclical loading, neither MAR nor BFR were significantly influenced across the CsA dosages ($p \geq 0.32$; Fig. 3). In the experimental limbs of rest-inserted loaded animals, CsA supplementation at 0.1 mg/kg, but not at 0.3 mg/kg significantly enhanced MAR ($p < 0.01$) and BFR ($p = 0.02$) vs that induced in animals subject to rest-inserted loading without CsA (0.0 mg/kg; Fig. 1, 3). Lastly, supplementation with CsA at 0.1 and 0.3 mg/kg CsA significantly enhanced MAR ($p \leq 0.04$) and supplementation with 0.1 mg/kg of CsA significantly enhanced BFR ($p = 0.04$) in animals exposed to rest-inserted vs cyclical loading (Fig. 3).

Experiment 3

In this experiment, we included two additional groups (cyclical loading with 6.0 mg/kg and rest-inserted loading with 0.03 mg/kg CsA) alongside previous data to determine dose-response relations. In the contralateral bones, we found that the main effect of CsA supplementation and loading (cyclic, rest-inserted) upon the response measures were not significant ($p = 0.33$). In animals subject to cyclic loading supplemented with CsA at 6.0 mg/kg, only MAR was significantly increased in experimentally loaded vs contralateral bones (0.59 ± 0.05 vs 0.39 ± 0.04 μm/d, respectively; $p = 0.01$). In animals subject to rest-inserted loading supplemented with CsA at 0.03 mg/kg, MS (38.3 ± 4.1 vs 15.0 ± 3.8%; $p < 0.001$), MAR (0.84 ± 0.09 vs 0.40 ± 0.06 μm/d; $p < 0.01$) and BFR (0.33 ± 0.06 vs 0.06 ± 0.01 $\mu m^3/\mu m^2/d$; $p = 0.001$) were significantly increased in experimentally loaded vs contralateral bones, respectively.

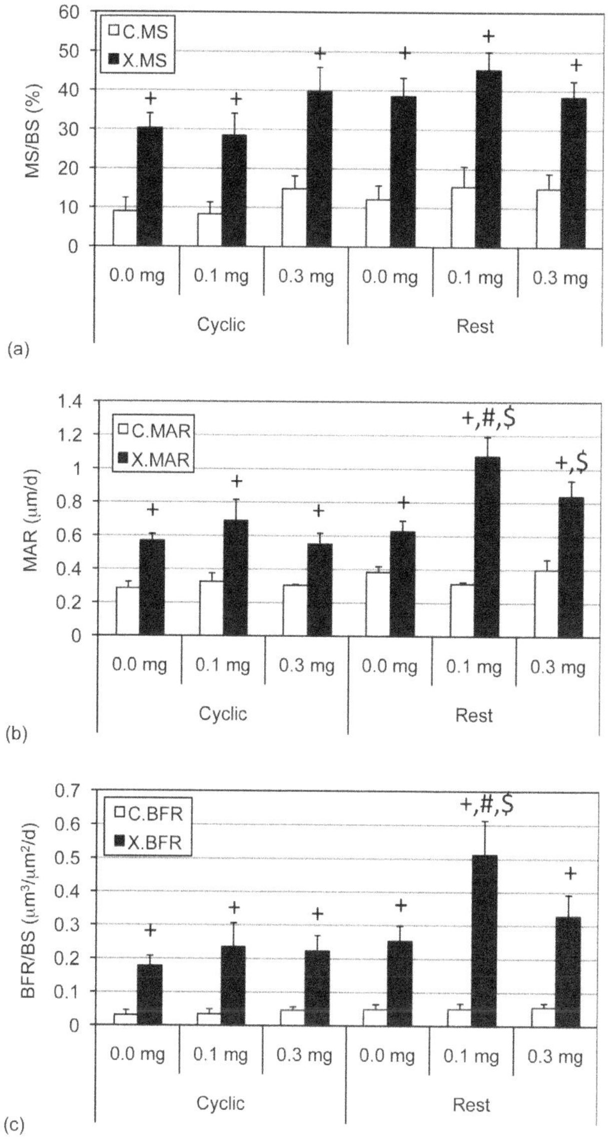

Figure 3. Lower-dose CsA supplementation was required to amplify bone response to rest-inserted loading. Periosteal MS/BS (a), MAR (b), and BFR/BS (c; mean+s.e.) were significantly increased in experimentally loaded (X) versus contralateral controls (C; '+'). Supplementing rest-inserted loading, but not cyclic loading, with low-dose CsA (at 0.1 mg/kg) significantly enhanced MAR and BFR/BS compared with that induced by rest-inserted loading alone ('#'). Additionally, CsA supplementation enhanced MAR (at 0.1, 0.3 mg/kg) and BFR/BS (at 0.1 mg/kg) in animals subject to rest-inserted versus cyclic loading ('$').

To explore dose-response relations, we included these data along side the data from Experiments 1 and 2. We implemented our non-linear model (eq 1) and used relative bone histomorphometry parameters as outcomes (i.e., rp.MAR, rp.MS, rp.BFR). Acceptance (or rejection) of null hypotheses describing the dose-response relations was dependent upon the assayed response. In our analysis of rp.MS, we found that a single model (i.e., parameters constrained to be the same for cyclic and rest-inserted models) including the null hypothesis that CsA supplementation has no benefit (i.e., $y_{Max} = 0$) could describe the response induced by both cyclic and rest-inserted loading across the CsA dosages

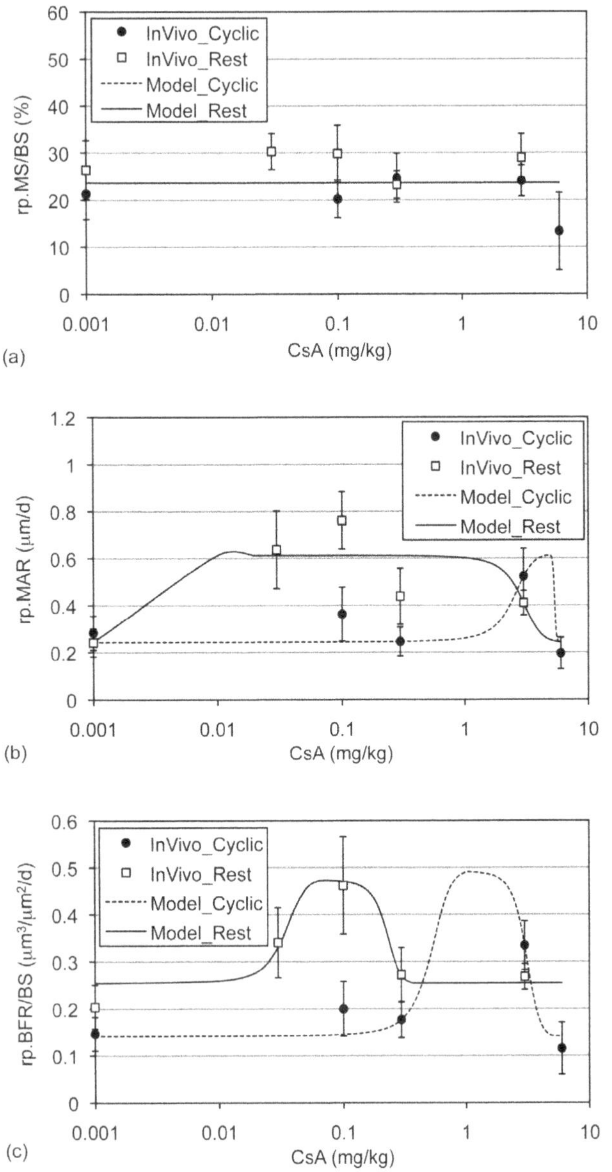

Figure 4. Dose-response relations simulated by the implemented non-linear models. A single model, which assumed that there is no adaptive benefit of loading supplemented with CsA, could simulate the rp.MS/BS data (a; mean ± s.e.). In contrast, two separate models were required to simulate rp.MAR (b) and rp.BFR/BS (c) induced by cyclic and rest-inserted loading supplemented with CsA. Please note that CsA dosage is plotted on a log-scale.

implemented experimentally ($p = 0.32$; Fig. 4; Table 2). In contrast, the single model null hypothesis was rejected for both rp.MAR ($p = 0.03$) and rp.BFR ($p = 0.01$).

As a result, we explored the null hypothesis that two separate models were required to simulate the rp.MAR and rp.BFR data. The null hypotheses that two separate models for cyclic and rest-inserted loading were required to describe the rp.MAR ($p = 0.09$) and rp.BFR response were both accepted ($p = 0.25$; Fig. 4; Table 2). However, the null hypothesis that CsA supplementation has no benefit (i.e., $y_{Max} = 0$) as a supplement for cyclic and rest-inserted loading was rejected for both rp.MAR ($p \leq 0.001$) and rp.BFR ($p \leq 0.03$). Given these findings, further analysis of the modeled parameters suggested that the optimal dosage at which CsA maximally enhances loading induced bone formation (i.e., δ_{Max}) was significantly different between cyclic and rest-inserted loading models ($p = 0.01$ for rp.MAR and $p = 0.03$ for rp.BFR). Null hypotheses constraining the remaining parameters to be the same between the cyclic and rest-inserted models, when considered separately and in combinations, were all accepted for both rp.MAR ($p \geq 0.1$) and rp.BFR response measures ($p \geq 0.06$).

Discussion

The loss of differential responses and the low-level bone response to mechanical signals markedly reduces the types of mild loading stimuli that can be used to robustly influence bone adaptation at senescence. Based upon the previously observed efficacy of cyclical loading supplemented with CsA [20], we began to explore whether CsA supplementation could enhance bone formation induced by different types of mechanical stimuli in the senescent skeleton. We found that CsA supplementation substantially enhanced bone formation induced by both cyclic and rest-inserted mechanical loading, but unexpectedly required distinct dosages for each mechanical stimulus (3.0, 0.1 mg/kg, respectively). Statistical analyses confirmed that CsA supplementation of cyclic and rest-inserted loading resulted in unique dose-bone response relations only at the 'optimal' dosage at which enhanced adaptation was induced. Given this unexpected outcome, a mechanistic understanding of CsA – loading interactions may be required for the optimized design of protocols that enhance bone response to a broad range of mild mechanical stimuli in the senescent skeleton.

Prior to interpreting our data, we discuss some of the limitations of our study. We designed a non-linear model to explore the dose-response relation and to determine whether specific aspects of the relation were different between cyclic and rest-inserted loading supplemented with CsA. While the model was specifically designed to simulate bi-phasic data, alternate models have also been developed for this purpose [28,29,30]. Of note, given the resolution of the model in simulating the data, statistical analysis suggests that model refinement or alternate model implementation will not significantly improve simulation of the current data set. Secondly, we observed premature animal death ($n = 4$) in groups subjected to cyclic loading. We consider these adverse events to be primarily due to the advanced age of these animals, considering the absence of adverse events in animals subject to rest-inserted loading with/without CsA (a protocol that notably required a 2 fold greater duration under anesthesia), as well as a lack of significant weight change in animals across time.

Our current data were inconsistent with our previous observations in one instance [20]. Specifically, here we found that supplementing cyclical loading with CsA at 0.3 mg/kg did not significantly enhance loading induced bone formation as was previously observed (where p.BFR increased from 0.12 ± 0.02 to 0.21 ± 0.02 $\mu m^3/\mu m^2/d$) [20]. In the current study, while CsA supplementation at 0.3 mg/kg induced a similar p.BFR (0.22 ± 0.05 $\mu m^3/\mu m^2/d$), the response in animals subject to cyclic loading alone was 0.18 ± 0.03 $\mu m^3/\mu m^2/d$. Thus the difference in the studies was not in the response to the 0.3 mg/kg CsA supplement, but in the response of the aged mice to cyclically applied loading (of note, the cyclical loading protocols were implemented identically across studies and the loading induced strains in animals were also not significantly different, $p = 0.56$; 1745 ± 47 vs 1703 ± 55 $\mu\varepsilon$ in the previous study). While the p.BFR response to cyclic loading in the previous study was 33% lower than currently, it was within 1 S.D. of the across study means and

Table 2. MLEs for model parameters for p.MS/BS, p.MAR, and p.BFR/BS (+ $p<0.05$ vs cyclic).

		y_0	y_{Max}	δ_{Max}	$\delta_{Inhibit}$
p.MS/BS	Cyclic	23.625	0.0	5.9047	12.649
	Rest	23.625	0.0	5.9047	12.649
p.MAR	Cyclic	0.2437	0.3694	4.9215	5.7544
	Rest	0.2437	0.3694	0.0029+	5.7544
p.BFR	Cyclic	0.1415	0.3498	1.0444	5.1182
	Rest	0.2543	0.219	0.0686+	0.3789

was similar to the experimental variability observed in mice at these advanced ages [21].

In our first experiment, we observed that CsA at the dosage previously found to be maximally efficacious for cyclic loading (3.0 mg/kg) was ineffective as a supplement for rest-inserted loading. This outcome was initially disappointing; it raised the possibility that supplementing loading with CsA was efficacious only in a very limited context (of the implemented cyclic stimulus). To further explore this confounding outcome, we considered mechanisms via which CsA might interact with loading induced activation of signaling pathways. Briefly, while CsA primarily inhibits Calcineurin (Cn) activity, it has off target effects on interacting MAPKs (p38, ERK, JNK), and with GSK-3β signaling [32,33] – competitive pathways also involved in bone mechanotransduction [34,35,36,37,38,39]. Thus, the benefits of supplementing cyclic loading with CsA could emerge via differential suppression of Cn, JNK, p38 and GSK-3β signaling, and a resulting bi-phasic enhancement in ERK activation and AP-1 transcription [33]. However, given reports that rest-inserted stimuli enhance Ca^{2+} signaling [40], and significantly more ERK phosphorylation [41], it was likely that this stimulus would require a larger quantity of uninhibited intermediate kinases and phosphatases vs cyclic stimuli (e.g., Cn, JNK, ERK), in order for augmentation of downstream events. As such, in order for acute signaling induced by rest-inserted loading (vs cyclic loading) to be augmented by CsA, a lower quantity of 'beneficial' intermediates (e.g., JNK, Cn) may 'ideally' need to be inhibited.

This interpretation of the literature suggested the possibility that rest-inserted loading might require CsA supplementation at a lower dosage compared with cyclic stimuli. In support, our in vivo data (Fig. 1–3) and analysis (Fig. 4) confirmed that cyclic and rest-inserted loading require distinct CsA dosages. In particular, a 30-fold lower CsA dosage was required before bone formation induced by rest-inserted loading could also be substantially enhanced in senescent animals. While CsA supplementation significantly augmented responses to both cyclic and rest-inserted loading, the induced adaptation was statistically equivalent between mechanical stimuli. We believe that further protocol refinement that explicitly considers previously unanticipated interactions between CsA dosage and loading type may both augment *and* re-establish differential responses to these stimuli, as observed in young animals [25,26,42,43].

However, the observed interaction between CsA dosage and mechanical stimuli substantially compounds the complexity of attempts at protocol design optimization. Theoretically, every perturbation of a 'control' mechanical stimulus (e.g., increased strain, load cycles, frequency, rest-insertion) may require a unique optimal drug dosage that must be experimentally confirmed. Additionally, given that different types of mechanical stimuli may differentially activate mechanotransduction signaling pathways [5,41], other agents that interact with mechanical stimuli (e.g., PTH, IGF-1) may also exhibit this complexity [27,44]. In this case, alternate approaches such as utilizing mechanistic computational modeling may enable exploration and optimization of such interactions *in silico*, prior to examination of a limited sub-set of protocols in animal studies [20].

In conclusion, periosteal bone response to cyclical and rest-inserted loading induced in senescent animals was significantly enhanced when supplemented with distinct dosages of Cyclosporin A. Despite development as an immunosuppressive agent, the effects of CsA are bi-phasic and at low dosages, CsA has been shown to down regulate osteoblast proliferation while increasing differentiation and mineralization [33]. Consistent with this finding, in our studies, CsA enhances bone formation primarily by increasing mineral apposition rates. Taken together, the effects of CsA in enhancing bone formation (while reducing TRAP-positive osteoclasts) in the trabecular compartment [33], and its ability to enhance loading induced bone formation in the cortical compartment of senescent animals suggest new uses for this inexpensive drug [45]. Given the potential for interaction between systemic drugs and mechanotransduction as observed here, locating optimal effective drug concentrations and supplementation regimens may require implementation of more complex experimental designs. We speculate that approaches that integrate experimental studies with computational tools may be required for the discovery of optimized protocols that enable the deployment of a broad range of mild, yet potently osteogenic regimens in the senescent skeleton.

Author Contributions

Conceived and designed the experiments: SS LEW EMG SDB RYK TSG. Performed the experiments: DT BJA SS. Analyzed the data: DT BJA SS. Contributed reagents/materials/analysis tools: SDB DT BJA SS. Wrote the paper: SS EMG LW SDB BJA RYK TSG.

References

1. Cooper C, Westlake S, Harvey N, Javaid K, Dennison E, et al. (2006) Review: developmental origins of osteoporotic fracture. Osteoporos Int 17: 337–347.
2. Seeman E (2001) Unresolved issues in osteoporosis in men. Rev Endocr Metab Disord 2: 45–64.
3. Hosking D, Chilvers C, Christiansen C, Ravn P, Wasnich R, et al. (1998) Prevention of bone loss with alendronate in postmenopausal women under 60 years of age. Early Postmenopausal Intervention Cohort Study Group. N Engl J Med 338: 485–492.
4. Baron R, Hesse E (2012) Update on bone anabolics in osteoporosis treatment: rationale, current status, and perspectives. J Clin Endocrinol Metab 97: 311–325.
5. Ozcivici E, Luu YK, Adler B, Qin YX, Rubin J, et al. (2010) Mechanical signals as anabolic agents in bone. Nat Rev Rheumatol 6: 50–59.
6. Bass SL, Saxon L, Daly RM, Turner CH, Robling AG, et al. (2002) The effect of mechanical loading on the size and shape of bone in pre-, peri-, and postpubertal girls: a study in tennis players. J Bone Miner Res 17: 2274–2280.
7. Nikander R, Sievanen H, Heinonen A, Daly RM, Uusi-Rasi K, et al. (2010) Targeted exercise against osteoporosis: A systematic review and meta-analysis for optimising bone strength throughout life. BMC Med 8: 47.
8. Pahlavani MA, Harris MD, Richardson A (1995) The age-related decline in the induction of IL-2 transcription is correlated to changes in the transcription factor NFAT. Cell Immunol 165: 84–91.
9. Pahlavani MA, Vargas DM (1999) Age-related decline in activation of calcium/calmodulin-dependent phosphatase calcineurin and kinase CaMK-IV in rat T cells. Mech Ageing Dev 112: 59–74.

10. Manolagas SC, Almeida M (2007) Gone with the Wnts: {beta}-catenin, TCF, FOXO, and oxidative stress in age-dependent diseases of bone, lipid, and glucose metabolism. Mol Endocrinol.
11. Klein-Nulend J, Sterck JG, Semeins CM, Lips P, Joldersma M, et al. (2002) Donor age and mechanosensitivity of human bone cells. Osteoporos Int 13: 137–146.
12. Donahue SW, Jacobs CR, Donahue HJ (2001) Flow-induced calcium oscillations in rat osteoblasts are age, loading frequency, and shear stress dependent. Am J Physiol Cell Physiol 281: C1635–1641.
13. Karinkanta S, Heinonen A, Sievanen H, Uusi-Rasi K, Pasanen M, et al. (2007) A multi-component exercise regimen to prevent functional decline and bone fragility in home-dwelling elderly women: randomized, controlled trial. Osteoporos Int 18: 453–462.
14. Kukuljan S, Nowson CA, Sanders KM, Nicholson GC, Seibel MJ, et al. (2011) Independent and Combined Effects of Calcium-Vitamin D3 and Exercise on Bone Structure and Strength in Older Men: An 18-Month Factorial Design Randomized Controlled Trial. J Clin Endocrinol Metab.
15. Rubin CT, Bain SD, McLeod KJ (1992) Suppression of the osteogenic response in the aging skeleton. Calcif Tissue Int 50: 306–313.
16. Turner CH, Takano Y, Owan I (1995) Aging changes mechanical loading thresholds for bone formation in rats. J Bone Miner Res 10: 1544–1549.
17. Leppanen OV, Sievanen H, Jokihaara J, Pajamaki I, Kannus P, et al. (2008) Pathogenesis of age-related osteoporosis: impaired mechano-responsiveness of bone is not the culprit. PLoS One 3: e2540.
18. Brodt MD, Silva MJ (2010) Aged mice have enhanced endocortical response and normal periosteal response compared with young-adult mice following 1 week of axial tibial compression. J Bone Miner Res 25: 2006–2015.
19. Srinivasan S, Gross TS, Bain SD (2012) Bone mechanotransduction may require augmentation in order to strengthen the senescent skeleton. Ageing Res Rev 11: 353–360.
20. Srinivasan S, Ausk BJ, Prasad J, Threet D, Bain SD, et al. (2010) Rescuing loading induced bone formation at senescence. PLoS Comput Biol 6: e1000924.
21. Srinivasan S, Agans SC, King KA, Moy NY, Poliachik SL, et al. (2003) Enabling bone formation in the aged skeleton via rest-inserted mechanical loading. Bone 33: 946–955.
22. Srinivasan S, Ausk BJ, Poliachik SL, Warner SE, Richardson TS, et al. (2007) Rest-inserted loading rapidly amplifies the response of bone to small increases in strain and load cycles. J Appl Physiol 102: 1945–1952.
23. Qin YX, Rubin CT, McLeod KJ (1998) Nonlinear dependence of loading intensity and cycle number in the maintenance of bone mass and morphology. J Orthop Res 16: 482–489.
24. Mosley JR, Lanyon LE (1998) Strain rate as a controlling influence on adaptive modeling in response to dynamic loading of the ulna in growing male rats. Bone 23: 313–318.
25. Umemura Y, Sogo N, Honda A (2002) Effects of intervals between jumps or bouts on osteogenic response to loading. J Appl Physiol 93: 1345–1348.
26. LaMothe JM, Zernicke RF (2004) Rest insertion combined with high-frequency loading enhances osteogenesis. J Appl Physiol 96: 1788–1793.
27. Gross TS, Srinivasan S, Liu CC, Clemens TL, Bain SD (2002) Noninvasive loading of the murine tibia: an in vivo model for the study of mechanotransduction. J Bone Miner Res 17: 493–501.
28. Belz RG, Piepho HP (2012) Modeling effective dosages in hormetic dose-response studies. PloS one 7: e33432.
29. Calabrese EJ (2008) Hormesis and medicine. Br J Clin Pharmacol 66: 594–617.
30. Brain P, Cousens R (1989) An equation to describe dose responses where there is stimulation of growth at low doses. Weed Res 29: 93–96.
31. Zar JH (1996) Biostatistical Analysis. Upper Saddle River, NJ: Prentice-Hall, Inc.
32. Matsuda S, Koyasu S (2000) Mechanisms of action of cyclosporine. Immunopharmacology 47: 119–125.
33. Yeo H, Beck LH, McDonald JM, Zayzafoon M (2007) Cyclosporin A elicits dose-dependent biphasic effects on osteoblast differentiation and bone formation. Bone 40: 1502–1516.
34. Riddle RC, Taylor AF, Genetos DC, Donahue HJ (2006) MAP kinase and calcium signaling mediate fluid flow-induced human mesenchymal stem cell proliferation. Am J Physiol Cell Physiol 290: C776–784.
35. You J, Reilly GC, Zhen X, Yellowley CE, Chen Q, et al. (2001) Osteopontin gene regulation by oscillatory fluid flow via intracellular calcium mobilization and activation of mitogen-activated protein kinase in MC3T3-E1 osteoblasts. J Biol Chem 276: 13365–13371.
36. Case N, Ma M, Sen B, Xie Z, Gross TS, et al. (2008) Beta-catenin levels influence rapid mechanical responses in osteoblasts. J Biol Chem 283: 29196–29205.
37. Mulkey RM, Endo S, Shenolikar S, Malenka RC (1994) Involvement of a calcineurin/inhibitor-1 phosphatase cascade in hippocampal long-term depression. Nature 369: 486–488.
38. Gomez del Arco P, Martinez-Martinez S, Maldonado JL, Ortega-Perez I, Redondo JM (2000) A role for the p38 MAP kinase pathway in the nuclear shuttling of NFATp. J Biol Chem 275: 13872–13878.
39. Sen B, Styner M, Xie Z, Case N, Rubin CT, et al. (2009) Mechanical loading regulates NFATc1 and beta-catenin signaling through a GSK3beta control node. J Biol Chem 284: 34607–34617.
40. Batra NN, Li YJ, Yellowley CE, You L, Malone AM, et al. (2005) Effects of short-term recovery periods on fluid-induced signaling in osteoblastic cells. J Biomech 38: 1909–1917.
41. Worton LE, Ausk BJ, Downey LM, Bain SD, Gardiner EM, et al. (2013) Systems-based identification of temporal processing pathways during bone cell mechanotransduction. PloS one 8: e74205.
42. Srinivasan S, Weimer DA, Agans SC, Bain SD, Gross TS (2002) Low-magnitude mechanical loading becomes osteogenic when rest is inserted between each load cycle. J Bone Miner Res 17: 1613–1620.
43. Robling AG, Burr DB, Turner CH (2001) Recovery periods restore mechanosensitivity to dynamically loaded bone. J Exp Biol 204: 3389–3399.
44. Sugiyama T, Saxon LK, Zaman G, Moustafa A, Sunters A, et al. (2008) Mechanical loading enhances the anabolic effects of intermittent parathyroid hormone (1–34) on trabecular and cortical bone in mice. Bone 43: 238–248.
45. Chong CR, Sullivan DJ Jr (2007) New uses for old drugs. Nature 448: 645–646.

19

Periarticular Osteophytes as an Appendicular Joint Stress Marker (JSM): Analysis in a Contemporary Japanese Skeletal Collection

Toshiyuki Tsurumoto[1]*, Kazunobu Saiki[1], Keishi Okamoto[1], Takeshi Imamura[2], Junichiro Maeda[2], Yoshitaka Manabe[3], Tetsuaki Wakebe[1]

1 Department of Macroscopic Anatomy, Graduate School of Biomedical Science, Nagasaki University, Nagasaki, Japan, **2** Department of Orthopaedic surgery, Graduate School of Biomedical Science, Nagasaki University, Nagasaki, Japan, **3** Department of Oral Anatomy and Dental Anthropology, Graduate School of Biomedical Science, Nagasaki University, Nagasaki, Japan

Abstract

Objective: The aim of this study was to investigate the possibility that periarticular osteophytes plays a role as a appendicular joint stress marker (JSM) which reflects the biomechanical stresses on individuals and populations.

Methods: A total of 366 contemporary Japanese skeletons (231 males, 135 females) were examined closely to evaluate the periarticular osteophytes of six major joints, the shoulder, elbow, wrist, hip, knee, and ankle and osteophyte scores (OS) were determined using an original grading system. These scores were aggregated and analyzed statistically from some viewpoints.

Results: All of the OS for the respective joints were correlated logarithmically with the age-at-death of the individuals. For 70 individuals, in whom both sides of all six joints were evaluated without missing values, the age-standardized OS were calculated. A right side dominancy was recognized in the joints of the upper extremities, shoulder and wrist joints, and the bilateral correlations were large in the three joints on the lower extremity. For the shoulder joint and the hip joint, it was inferred by some distinctions that systemic factors were relatively large. All of these six joints could be assorted by the extent of systemic and local factors on osteophytes formation. Moreover, when the age-standardized OS of all the joints was summed up, some individuals had significantly high total scores, and others had significantly low total scores; namely, all of the individuals varied greatly in their systemic predisposition for osteophytes formation.

Conclusions: This study demonstrated the significance of periarticular osteophytes; the evaluating system for OS could be used to detect differences among joints and individuals. Periarticular osteophytes could be applied as an appendicular joint stress marker (JSM); by applying OS evaluating system for skeletal populations, intra-skeletal and inter-skeletal variations in biomechanical stresses throughout the lives could be clarified.

Editor: Luca Bondioli, Museo Nazionale Preistorico Etnografico 'L. Pigorini', Italy

Funding: The authors have no funding or support to report.

Competing Interests: The authors have declared that no competing interests exist.

* E-mail: tsurumot@nagasaki-u.ac.jp

Introduction

Marginal osteophytes are small protrusions of bone that may develop around the periphery of joints. These osteophytes emerge and grow gradually throughout a lifetime with the ageing process from physiological reactions to pathological conditions, in what is called degenerative joint disease (DJD). Analyzing the distributions of these alterations throughout the skeletal system can provide insights into a disturbed homeostasis that occurs in joints with DJD [1], but also these periarticular marginal osteophytes in vertebrate articulations can be probable and useful resources for studies on bioarchaeology.

Originally, synovial cartilage on bearing surfaces of most joints is not very strong, and, therefore, the loads being transferred from one bone to the next must be spread out over a rather large area of cartilage. Many vertebrate joints have a large angle of excursion, and the requirement for low stress implies large radii of curvature [2]. Osteophytes formation seems to be associated with these issues and progresses during physical ageing and pathological conditions such as osteoarthritis. Thus, periarticular osteophyte formation itself is a proliferative phenomenon. Moreover, it is one of the most discriminative changes in articular degeneration. Therefore, certainly they reflect the continuous biomechanical stresses placed on appendicular joints throughout one's life.

Periarticular osteophytes around all of the appendicular joints are themselves age-related phenomena. Thus, we thought that they should be evaluated appropriately using an age-standardized osteophyte scoring system. With such an original scoring system, we investigated periarticular marginal osteophytes of six major joints in a sizable skeletal population whose ages-at-death had been exactly recorded. The aim of this study was to investigate whether periarticular osteophytes play a role as an appendicular joint stress marker (JSM) which reflects the biomechanical stresses on individuals and populations. Intra-skeletal and inter-skeletal variations in osteophytes formation were evaluated to clarify the activity patterns and magnitudes among the individuals and the populations.

Materials and Methods

(1) Materials

A total of 366 modern Japanese skeletons (231 males, 135 females) were examined macroscopically. They were obtained from the cadavers that had been provided to Nagasaki University School of Medicine for anatomical dissection by medical students between the 1950s and 1970s, and most of them were voluntarily donated, and nowadays most of them were anonymous subjects.

After they had been dissected, their soft tissues were almost entirely removed from their bodies to produce dry skeletal preparations. Skeletons with some pathological conditions, for example, rheumatoid arthritis, infectious diseases, fractured joints, were excluded from this study. This was because the accidental influences by systemic diseases, metabolic diseases and injuries should be excluded in order to examine the effects of increasing age on the periarticular osteophyte formation. The sex and ages-at-death of all the individuals were registered exactly; the mean age-at-death was 64.4 years old (males: 61.8; females: 68.7 range: from 20 to 89) (Table 1).

In each individual, six major joints, the shoulder, elbow, wrist, hip, knee, and ankle, were visually examined. The evaluated joint components were as follows; i) the humeral head and glenoid fossa for the shoulder joint, ii) the distal humerus, proximal ulna, and proximal radius for the elbow joint, iii) the distal radius and distal ulna for the wrist joint, iv) the acetabulum and femoral head for the hip joint, v) the distal femur, patella, and proximal tibia for the knee joint, and vi) the distal tibia, distal fibula, and the upper surface of talus for the ankle joint.

(2) Osteophyte scoring system

The osteophytes in marginal regions were visually examined and graded 0, 1, 2, 3, or 4 according to criteria assessing osteophyte proliferation and the appearance of the border and surface of the joint (Figure 1). Marginal regions without any eminences were regarded as grade 0. Marginal osteophytes with an obscure border and even surface were graded 1. Marginal osteophytes with a distinct border and uneven surface were graded 2. Marginal osteophytes with a dominant border and rough surface were categorized as grade 3. Marginal osteophytes that displayed severe proliferation both at their border and on their surface were classified as grade 4. To improve the objectivity and stability of the osteophyte scoring system, more than fifty arbitrarily chosen skeletons were examined in a preliminary study, and then the system was reviewed. Finally, all of the skeletons were consecutively evaluated by one of the authors (TT).

Table 1. Age-at-death and sex distribution of the samples.

Age	male	female	total
20–29	8	2	10
30–39	11	3	14
40–49	31	12	43
50–59	39	7	46
60–69	63	28	91
70–79	57	54	111
80–89	22	29	51
Total	231	135	366

(3) Stepwise determination of the osteophyte score (OS)

The marginal regions of each joint component were divided into an appropriate number of segments; for example, the humeral proximal joint margin was divided into eight segments, and the glenoid margin was divided into four segments. The OS for each segment was determined from its osteophyte grades; i.e., grade 0, 1, 2, 3, and 4 resulted in OS of 0, 10, 20, 30, and 40, respectively (*step A* in Figure 2). When a segment contained areas with various grades, its OS was determined by averaging the score for each area within the segment. The OS for each joint component was determined by averaging all of the segmental OS (*step B*). Incomplete joint components; i.e., those for which less than half of their segments were examined, were excluded from the analysis. The OS for all components in a joint were averaged to determine the individual joint score (IJS) (*step C*); for example, the score for the shoulder joint was calculated by averaging the OS for the humeral head and the glenoid fossa of the scapula. The joints missing one or more joint components were excluded from the analysis. Accordingly, 70 individuals (48 males, 22 females) with all of the twelve IJS (six joints on the right and left sides) were selected (*step D*); for them, the averaged IJS (AIJS) was calculated by averaging the IJS for the right and left sides.

(4) Analysis of the individual joint score (IJS) obtained in *step C*

The right and left IJS values of all six joints were analyzed as follows; (i) Comparison of the right and left IJS: For all six joints, the right and left IJS of the both sexes were compared using the paired t-test with $p<0.05$ and $p<0.01$ (two-tailed). (ii) Analysis of the mean IJS for each joint according to decennial age group; For each of the joints, the mean IJS of decennial age groups ranging from 20–29 years old to 80–89 years old were calculated and plotted on line charts. The significance of the differences between the right and left sides was tested using the paired t-test with $p<0.05$ and $p<0.01$ (two-tailed), and the significance of the differences between the values for males and females was tested using the Student's t-test with $p<0.05$ and $p<0.01$ (two-tailed).

(5) Analyses of joint scores obtained in *steps D*

(i) Correlation analysis on IJS; For all of the well-preserved 70 individuals, correlation coefficients in respective IJS values of both right and left sides in six joints were analyzed in a cross table with $p<0.05$ and $p<0.01$. (ii) Calculation of age-standardized IJS values; For all of the 70 individuals examined in step D, "age-standardized IJS" values that took the age of each individual into account were calculated with non-linear equations; these values were equal to the residual errors between the IJS and the prediction values in non-linear regression analysis. (iii) Analysis of 70 individuals with the sum values of age-standardized IJS; For all of the 70 individuals, the sum values of age-standardized IJS were calculated, and these individuals were arranged on a table in the order of these values to distinguish the individuals with extremely high total scores and those with extremely low total scores. (iv) Principal component analysis (PCA) and cluster analysis in 70 individuals; The characteristics in the respective joints were

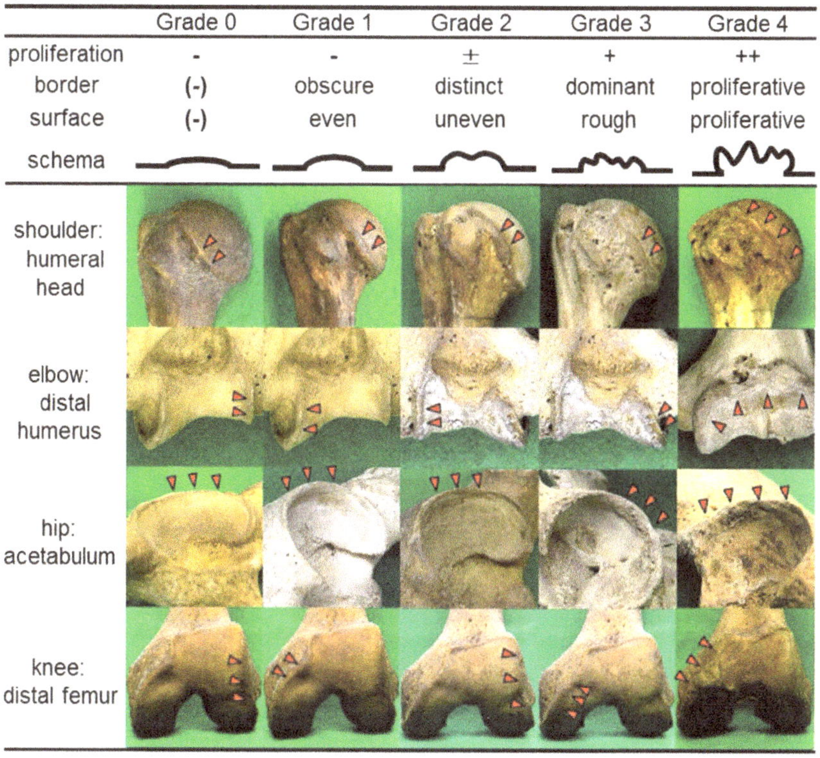

Figure 1. Periarticular marginal osteophytes: criteria for Grade 0, 1, 2, 3, and 4. Schemas and typical four articular components are shown (humeral head in shoulder joint, distal end of humerus in elbow joint, acetabulum in hip joint, and distal femur in knee joint).

evaluated with principal components analysis (PCA); a variety of the combinations of age-standardized AIJS values in six joints of the 70 individuals were evaluated with the statistical software JMP (version 10.0.2) (SAS Institute Inc.). Moreover, cluster analysis using the values of age-standardized IJS in 12 joints of the 70 individuals was applied to assess how individual joints grouped with respect to each other. The open source programming language "R" (version 2.15.1) was used for characterizing cluster dendrogram, and its reliability was assessed with the bootstrap probability (BP) values.

Results

(1) Comparison of the right and left IJS values (table 2)

Both sides of the shoulder joint and hip joint showed relative high IJS values. Some joints in the upper extremities showed the dominancy of the right side; the IJS for the right shoulder in both sexes and those for the right wrist in females were significantly higher than those for the same joints on the left side with the paired t- test. Most people from different geographic regions are right handed; therefore, high IJS values of the right sides in the shoulder and wrist joints were reasonable.

(2) Analysis of the mean IJS values for each joint among decennial groups (Figure 3)

The mean IJS of each joint were analyzed among decennial groups as follows. (i) Shoulder joint: In the 60 to 79-year-old females, the mean IJS values for the right side were higher than those for the left side. The mean IJS values of the males continued to increase steadily until extreme old age and were higher than those of the females in the over sixties age group. (ii) Elbow joint: There were few differences between the right and left sides or between the sexes. (iii) Wrist joint: There were few differences between the mean IJS values of the right and left sides, but in males the mean IJS for both sides were significantly higher than those of the females in the 60 to 79-year-old age group. The distribution of the mean IJS for the wrist joint resembled that of the shoulder joint. These occasional high scores of the right-side upper extremities inferred the right side dominance in most individuals. (iv) Hip joint: The mean IJS values in the males seldom increased after middle age, and those of the females increased gradually. The former were consistently higher than the latter in all age groups. (v) Knee joint: All of the males displayed similar mean IJS after forty years of age, but those of the females continued to increase steadily until extreme old age and overtook the males in the older groups. (vi) Ankle joint: The males displayed similar averages after forty years of age, but those of the females continued to increase steadily until extreme old age. The values for the females were higher than those of the males in the over 70-year-old age group. The distribution of the mean IJS for the ankle joint resembled that of the knee joint.

(3) Calculation of age-standardized IJS values

Considering the result of analysis about the mean IJS values for each joint among decennial groups (Figure 3), the relationships between the IJS and the chronological ages of the individuals approximated with logarithmic non-linear correlations. Natural logarithmic functions in respective joints of the males and females were determined by analyzing the non-linear regression between the chronological ages and the IJS values of each joint ($n = 70$);

Shoulder: $IJS\ (male) = 16.073 \times \log_e(ca) - 42.701 \quad (r = 0.726)$

$IJS\ (female) = 12.472 \times \log_e(ca) - 33.985 \quad (r = 0.620)$

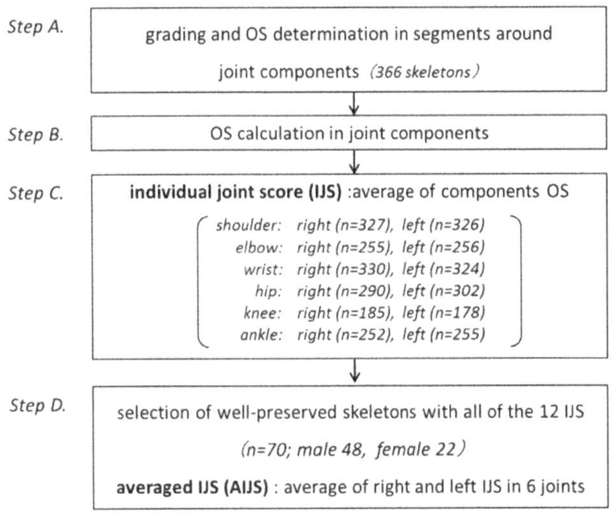

Figure 2. Flow chart describing our method for the steps in determining the osteophyte scores (OS): Step A: The OS for each segment was determined from its osteophyte grades. Step B: The OS for each joint component was determined by averaging all of its segmental scores. Step C: Individual joint scores (IJS) were determined by averaging the scores for all of its components. Step D: Well-preserved 70 individuals were selected, and for them averaged individual joint scores (AIJS) were determined by averaging the IJS of the right and left sides.

Elbow: IJS (male) = $12.224 \times \log_e(\text{ca}) - 29.7$ ($r = 0.531$)
IJS (female) = $8.7015 \times \log_e(\text{ca}) - 17.799$ ($r = 0.669$)
Wrist: IJS (male) = $9.2158 \times \log_e(\text{ca}) - 16.911$ ($r = 0.444$)
IJS (female) = $10.043 \times \log_e(\text{ca}) - 24.81$ ($r = 0.626$)
Hip: IJS (male) = $12.616 \times \log_e(\text{ca}) - 23.563$ ($r = 0.671$)
IJS (female) = $11.402 \times \log_e(\text{ca}) - 21.415$ ($r = 0.796$)
Knee: IJS (male) = $10.574 \times \log_e(\text{ca}) - 24.483$ ($r = 0.534$)
IJS (female) = $15.143 \times \log_e(\text{ca}) - 43.187$ ($r = 0.732$)
Ankle: IJS (male) = $3.4802 \times \log_e(\text{ca}) - 2.462$ ($r = 0.247$)
IJS (female) = $7.2104 \times \log_e(\text{ca}) - 17.624$ ($r = 0.714$)
(ca; chronological age of individual skeletons)

These correlation coefficients in non-linear regression analysis between IJS and chronological age are shown in Figure 4. Regarding these values, five joints (other than the shoulder) showed the dominancy of the female. The shoulder and hip joints, which are located at the proximal positions in the upper and lower extremities, had high values more than 0.7; moreover, the distal joints had lower coefficients. In particular, the ankle joint in the males showed the lowest coefficient, 0.247. On the other hand, all of the female joints had values higher than 0.6; especially the coefficients of all three joints in the lower extremity were as high as 0.7.

(4) Correlation analysis of IJS in 70 individuals

For the well-preserved 70 individuals, the correlation coefficients between AIJS values in respective joints are shown in figure 5. The high values are shown in dark brown boxes and lower values in light brown or white boxes in this cross table. Almost all of the joints (other than the ankle joints) had significantly high correlation coefficients. For all six major joints, the correlation coefficients between the right and left of the respective joints were high. Especially three joints of the lower extremities had high correlations; hip 0.9186, knee 0.8590, ankle 0.7634. Furthermore, between the shoulder joints and the hip joints, between the left shoulder and the left wrist joint, the correlation coefficients were relatively high. On the other hand, the ankle joints showed a low correlation with the others. Furthermore, between the shoulder and knee joints, between the shoulder and ankle joints, between the wrist and ankle joints, the correlation coefficients were rather low.

Table 2. Average values of individual joint scores (IJS) for the right and left sides of the 12 appendicular joints (*$p<0.05$, **$p<0.01$).

		IJS ± S.D.		
		right		left
Shoulder	male	24.9±9.0	>*	23.9±8.7
	female	21.6±9.2	>**	19.5±7.0
Elbow	male	20.6±8.9		21.0±10.4
	female	20.6±8.7		20.0±8.5
Wrist	male	21.3±8.2		21.2±8.0
	female	18.7±6.5	>**	17.6±6.1
Hip	male	28.9±6.1		29.0±6.3
	female	27.6±5.7		27.7±5.6
Knee	male	18.5±7.6		19.5±7.8
	female	19.7±9.0		18.8±8.8
Ankle	male	11.0±5.1		10.5±4.7
	female	13.0±4.7		13.6±5.8

(5) Analysis of 70 individuals with the sum total values of age-standardized IJS

Figure 6 shows all of the age-standardized IJS in the 70 individuals; the high values in each column are shown in red and lower values in blue. The second column from the right listed the sum total values of each individual, and the rightmost column indicates the ranking numbers from the highest to the lowest individuals. There was a wide variability in the sum total values of respective individuals from the highest 84.1 to the lowest −89.8; this result indicated the difference among individuals in periarticular osteophytes formation. Moreover, some individuals had systemically almost equivalent values, and other individuals had uneven distributions. Figure 7 is the scatter chart which indicated the relationship between the sum of age-standardized IJS values of 12 joints and the ranking numbers. The great majority of the individuals showed a linear relationship, but the some individuals with high scores swerved from the line to higher values and, some individuals with low values, whose ranking number was 61 or more, dropped from the line to lower values.

(6) Principal component analysis (PCA) and cluster analysis in 70 individuals

Figure 8 indicates PCA variable loadings; the high values are shown in red boxes and lower values in blue. The first three PCs explained 65.4% of the total variance among taxa, with 44.9% on PC1, 16.8% on PC2, 13.7% on PC3. Loading values in all of the six joints were positive and more than 0.5 in PC 1; this axis was indicated to show the overall tendency of osteophyte formation in individuals. This meant that one of the most influential factors for osteophyte formation was the individual specificity. In PC2, the loading values of the shoulder joint and hip joint were high; both

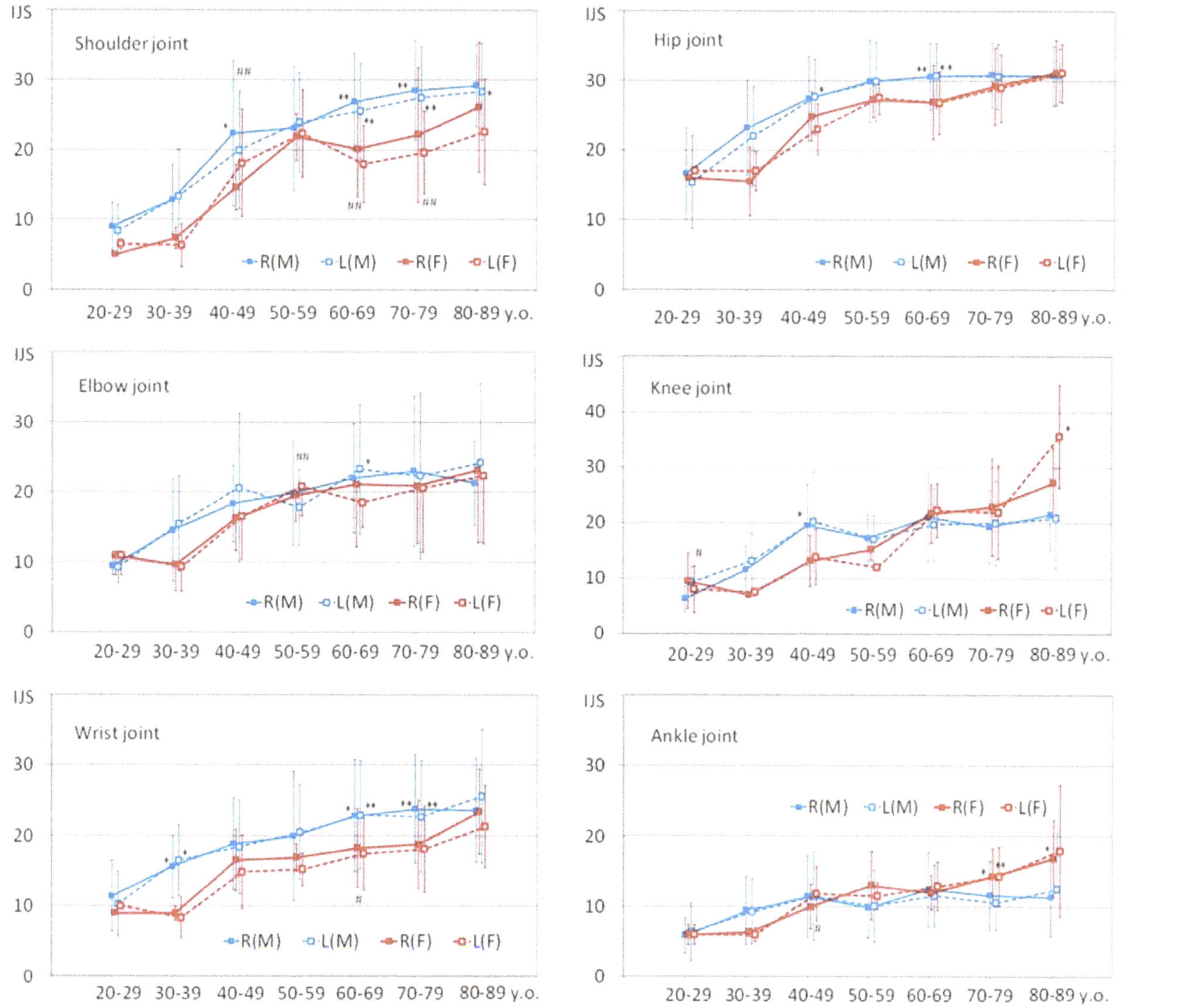

Figure 3. Individual joint scores (IJS) for the shoulder, elbow, wrist, hip, knee, and ankle joints of decennial age groups (mean and standard deviation (bar line) values). R(M) blue full line; males, right L(M) blue dotted-line: males, left. R(F) red full line; females, right L(F) red dotted-line; females, left. Significant difference between right and left sides (# $p<0.05$, ## $p<0.01$). Significant difference between males and females (* $p<0.05$, ** $p<0.01$).

of them take proximal position in the extremities. On the other hand, loadings in the elbow, knee and ankle joints were low. In PC3 and PC4, joints in the upper extremity and joints in the lower extremity were almost decoupled. In PC5, joints in the peripheral position, wrist and ankle showed relatively high values.

Cluster dendrograms in Figure 9 showed several similarities in 12 joints among the well-preserved 70 individuals; Figure 9 shows the dendrogram charts analyzed with ward method (left) and with the group average method (right). Firstly, both dendrogram charts generally confirmed great similarity between right and left sides in respective joints. Especially, in the lower extremity, all of the three joints showed high BP values of 99 or 100%, and extremely close relationships with each opposite side were indicated. Compared with these joints in the lower extremity, both sides of the shoulder, elbow and wrist joints have relatively low BP values from 44 to 71%. Secondly, both dendrograms indicated the unexpected similarity between shoulder joints and hip joints. This similarity was confirmed by the axis 2 of PCA in Figure 8.

Discussion

Osteoarthritis, or DJD, is a gradually progressing degeneration of appendicular joints. Basically, this is a complicated pathological condition which combines proliferative changes of osteophyte formation and often slight inflammations. The osteophyte formation closely resembles the processes of chondrogenesis and endochondral bone formation, which occur during embryogenesis [1]. Periarticular osteophytes emerge through the endochondral ossification of fibrous cartilage at the synovial bone-cartilage junction. In a number of disease conditions, the formation of abnormal calcifications and bony spurs seems to be related to changes in the composition of fibrocartilage in the attachment zone [3].

Both systemic factors and local factors have effects on DJD progression. The former contains age, sex, metabolic factors, nutrition, vascular profusion, endocrine factors and heredity, and the latter contains severe trauma and chronic functional stress

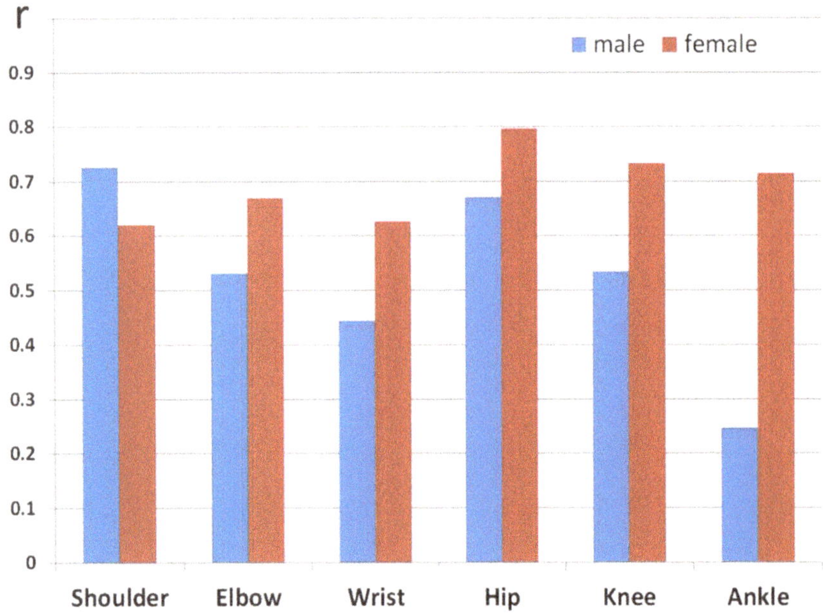

Figure 4. Values of correlation coefficients in non-linear, logarithmic regression analysis between IJS and chronological age (blue: male, red: female).

[4][5]. General obesity is one of the local factors, because it has a great effect on local mechanical stress to the lower extremities. Moreover, osteoporosis is a potent systemic factor, and the degree of inflammation and degeneration itself, which yields debris within articular space, have local effects on these formations. Moreover, some genetic aspects of osteoarthritis have been referred to; for example, the manifestation of generalized OA was shown to be dominant in females and recessive in males [6]. OA is a polygenic disease indeed, and some osteoarthritis susceptibility genes have been reported by many researchers [7][8]. It is possible that these genetic factors work in concert to affect OA onset and progression.

For the purpose of clarification of these DJD developments and features, in this study, the six major appendicular joints of dried skeletons were observed and only the periarticular osteophytes were evaluated. They were strictly investigated by a simple and detailed evaluation system. There have been many studies which dealt with degenerative and proliferative changes of the appendicular joints. Some early studies dealt with the cadaver materials [9]. Then, Jurmain studied a total of 111 skeletons whose ages and

	SR	SL	ER	EL	WR	WL	HR	HL	KR	KL	AR	AL
SR	-	0.7444	0.4376	0.4374	0.5054	0.5015	0.7057	0.7269	0.4556	0.4236	* 0.2697	0.3616
SL	0.7444	-	0.5577	0.5419	0.4580	0.6845	0.6913	0.6896	0.4320	0.4210	* 0.3057	* 0.2447
ER	0.4376	0.5577	-	0.6815	0.5438	0.5112	0.5444	0.5908	0.5854	0.6071	0.4325	0.4794
EL	0.4374	0.5419	0.6815	-	0.4073	0.4098	0.4447	0.5462	0.4766	0.5108	0.3064	0.4200
WR	0.5054	0.4580	0.5438	0.4073	-	0.6308	0.4788	0.4435	0.5580	0.5255	* 0.3058	0.4056
WL	0.5015	0.6845	0.5112	0.4098	0.6308	-	0.5193	0.4838	0.4838	0.5665	* 0.2768	* 0.2509
HR	0.7057	0.6913	0.5444	0.4447	0.4788	0.5193	-	0.9186	0.5889	0.5386	0.4727	0.3818
HL	0.7269	0.6896	0.5908	0.5462	0.4435	0.4838	0.9186	-	0.6220	0.5599	0.4647	0.4146
KR	0.4556	0.4320	0.5854	0.4766	0.5580	0.4838	0.5889	0.6220	-	0.8590	0.4038	0.4608
KL	0.4236	0.4210	0.6071	0.5108	0.5255	0.5665	0.5386	0.5599	0.8590	-	0.4369	0.4931
AR	* 0.2697	* 0.3057	0.4325	0.3064	* 0.3058	* 0.2768	0.4727	0.4647	0.4038	0.4369	-	0.7634
AL	0.3616	* 0.2447	0.4794	0.4200	0.4056	* 0.2509	0.3818	0.4146	0.4608	0.4931	0.7634	-

Figure 5. Correlation coefficients between AIJS values in respective joints among the well-preserved 70 individuals; the high values are shown in dark brown and lower values were in light brown or white (* p<0.05, no mark p<0.01).

sex	age	SR	SL	ER	EL	WR	WL	HR	HL	KR	KL	AR	AL	sum	ranking
M	49	4.1	−0.9	6.1	27.1	10.0	4.0	0.5	3.5	5.3	5.3	6.9	11.9	84.1	1
M	66	3.4	4.4	1.5	8.5	8.3	10.3	0.7	4.7	17.2	15.2	−3.1	−2.1	68.8	2
M	72	−2.0	3.0	7.4	9.4	5.5	9.5	5.6	2.6	10.3	11.3	3.6	2.6	68.7	3
M	71	2.2	8.2	23.6	12.6	3.6	2.6	4.8	4.8	−3.6	−3.6	3.6	4.6	63.5	4
M	52	5.2	6.2	5.4	2.4	4.5	10.5	0.7	1.7	7.7	4.7	1.7	6.7	57.4	5
F	67	−5.5	−5.5	19.2	−0.8	16.6	12.6	−4.5	−4.5	10.5	11.5	2.3	4.3	56.3	6
M	77	3.9	0.9	9.6	25.6	−1.1	−3.1	−1.2	5.8	−1.4	1.6	7.3	8.3	56.0	7
M	83	0.7	0.7	3.7	13.7	−0.8	13.2	2.8	1.8	12.8	13.8	−3.9	−3.9	54.4	8
M	40	20.4	10.4	0.6	−2.4	8.9	8.9	7.0	5.0	1.5	−1.5	−3.4	−2.4	53.1	9
M	60	3.9	2.9	8.7	7.7	10.2	1.2	5.9	6.9	8.2	−3.8	−0.8	1.2	52.1	10
M	53	12.9	7.9	6.2	2.2	3.3	9.3	2.5	2.5	−3.5	0.5	1.6	2.6	48.0	11
F	71	30.8	3.8	−2.3	3.7	1.0	4.0	5.8	2.8	−5.4	−0.4	−2.1	3.9	45.7	12
M	44	0.9	−2.1	−0.6	−0.6	−2.0	4.0	8.8	8.8	4.5	8.5	7.3	4.3	41.9	13
M	63	7.1	2.1	−2.9	0.1	1.7	1.7	4.3	7.3	0.7	9.7	4.0	3.0	38.8	14
M	64	−1.1	−1.1	2.9	1.9	−0.4	2.6	8.1	4.1	0.5	−1.5	17.0	5.0	37.8	15
F	68	7.4	3.4	−0.9	0.1	2.4	0.4	5.3	5.3	8.3	2.3	0.2	1.2	35.3	16
F	73	13.5	2.5	0.5	−6.5	0.7	2.7	3.5	8.5	15.2	1.2	−4.3	−3.3	34.1	17
M	48	3.5	6.5	3.4	5.4	2.2	1.2	3.7	4.7	6.5	5.5	−4.0	−5.0	33.7	18
M	61	2.6	−2.4	4.4	2.4	8.0	10.0	−4.3	−4.3	5.0	8.0	2.2	1.2	32.9	19
F	24	−0.7	1.3	3.1	3.1	1.9	2.9	1.2	2.2	8.1	6.1	1.7	1.7	32.7	20
M	50	3.8	4.8	−1.1	−3.1	−0.1	3.9	11.2	10.2	2.1	2.1	−1.2	−1.2	31.5	21
M	41	7.0	−1.0	5.3	1.3	−1.3	−4.3	3.7	5.7	2.2	1.2	6.5	3.5	29.9	22
M	58	−3.6	−1.6	−0.9	−0.9	26.5	2.5	−5.7	−6.7	5.5	6.5	1.3	5.3	28.4	23
M	23	4.3	2.3	1.4	1.4	9.0	−1.0	2.0	5.0	−0.7	0.3	1.5	2.5	28.1	24
M	75	−8.7	23.3	−4.1	4.9	−8.9	27.1	−1.9	−2.9	−6.2	−2.2	2.4	−2.6	20.4	25
M	49	9.1	7.1	1.1	−2.9	−9.0	−7.0	3.5	7.5	−1.7	1.3	4.9	2.9	17.1	26
M	47	−6.2	−3.2	1.6	1.6	−0.6	−2.6	4.0	3.0	−2.2	−1.2	17.1	5.1	16.4	27
F	74	−7.7	−6.7	−0.7	1.3	2.6	−0.4	4.3	0.3	9.0	8.0	5.6	0.6	16.4	28
M	57	−0.3	3.7	3.3	−1.7	0.7	−4.3	2.6	0.6	4.7	1.7	6.4	−1.6	15.6	29
F	47	3.0	14.0	3.3	5.3	5.1	1.1	−1.5	−0.5	−4.1	−5.1	−3.1	−4.1	13.3	30
F	64	2.1	0.1	3.6	2.6	4.0	0.0	0.0	−1.0	−3.8	−1.8	1.6	2.6	10.2	31
M	20	3.6	1.6	3.1	1.1	4.3	3.3	−0.2	−4.2	−0.2	2.8	−4.0	−4.0	7.1	32
F	50	1.2	−1.8	2.8	3.8	2.5	−2.5	1.8	5.8	−1.1	−4.1	−1.6	−1.6	5.3	33
M	27	0.7	−2.3	−0.6	2.4	−4.5	1.5	1.0	0.0	−0.4	2.6	−1.0	4.0	3.6	34
F	42	−0.6	−0.6	0.3	−1.7	−3.7	−1.7	−1.2	−1.2	1.6	1.6	4.7	5.7	3.0	35
F	70	−2.0	−2.0	3.8	0.8	1.1	−0.9	−5.0	2.0	0.9	−2.1	3.0	3.0	2.6	36
M	71	5.2	−1.8	−6.4	−8.4	4.6	−1.4	1.8	−0.2	5.4	0.4	1.6	0.6	1.5	37
F	25	−1.2	−0.2	−1.2	−1.2	1.5	2.5	0.7	1.7	0.4	−0.6	−0.6	−0.6	1.4	38
F	74	4.3	3.3	−1.7	0.3	2.6	6.6	−5.7	−4.7	−4.0	−4.0	−1.4	4.6	0.4	39
M	45	0.5	−7.5	−4.8	−6.8	3.8	4.8	1.5	5.5	0.2	−0.8	1.2	−1.8	−4.0	40
M	79	−4.5	0.5	−3.7	−3.7	−6.4	−4.4	−2.6	−2.6	8.3	2.3	5.3	2.3	−9.2	41
F	31	0.2	0.2	1.9	0.9	0.3	0.3	−5.7	−2.7	−1.8	−1.8	−1.1	−0.1	−9.6	42
F	42	−1.6	−1.6	−5.7	−0.7	−0.7	−0.7	1.8	−0.2	−0.4	−5.4	−1.3	3.7	−13.0	43
M	81	−9.9	−7.9	5.0	−4.0	−4.6	9.4	−5.9	−3.9	−3.0	13.0	0.2	−1.8	−13.5	44
M	36	−4.9	−4.9	−1.1	−0.1	−1.1	0.9	−2.6	−1.6	2.6	2.6	−2.0	−2.0	−14.4	45
F	64	−1.9	−3.9	−0.4	−1.4	−3.0	−2.0	−1.0	−1.0	2.2	2.2	−4.4	−2.4	−16.8	46
F	70	−7.0	−6.0	2.8	0.8	0.1	−6.9	4.0	−2.0	−0.1	−1.1	−1.0	−2.0	−18.4	47
F	60	−2.1	−3.1	−1.8	−2.8	−6.3	−4.3	−4.3	0.7	−0.8	3.2	2.1	0.1	−19.4	48
M	81	1.1	−5.9	−11.0	−12.0	−1.6	−8.6	−0.9	−2.9	2.0	2.0	6.2	7.2	−24.5	49
F	32	−2.2	−2.2	−5.4	−3.4	−2.0	−5.0	0.9	0.9	−2.3	−1.3	−1.4	−2.4	−25.7	50
M	65	−2.4	−1.4	1.7	2.7	0.4	−9.6	−2.1	−0.1	−4.7	−2.7	−7.1	−3.1	−28.2	51
F	44	0.8	−0.2	−4.1	−3.1	−1.2	−6.2	−0.7	−2.7	−7.1	−2.1	−3.7	−0.7	−31.1	52
M	65	−1.4	−0.4	3.7	3.7	−9.6	−12.6	−1.1	−1.1	0.3	−0.7	−6.1	−7.1	−32.2	53
M	74	10.5	4.5	−8.9	−14.9	0.2	0.2	−2.7	−3.7	−9.0	−9.0	2.5	−3.5	−33.9	54
M	55	−1.7	−1.7	−2.3	−5.3	0.0	0.0	−2.0	−4.0	−4.9	−2.9	−5.5	−5.5	−35.8	55
M	60	−0.1	−0.1	2.7	−5.3	−7.8	1.2	−1.1	−2.1	−4.8	−5.8	−6.8	−5.8	−35.9	56
M	61	−0.4	0.6	−5.6	−2.6	−4.0	−4.0	2.7	4.7	−9.0	−12.0	−5.8	−5.8	−41.1	57
M	37	−6.3	−4.3	−5.4	−3.4	−4.4	−1.4	1.0	−1.0	−4.7	−4.7	−3.1	−4.1	−41.9	58
F	71	−3.2	−6.2	−1.3	−1.3	−8.0	−6.0	0.8	0.8	−8.4	−9.4	−1.1	0.9	−42.3	59
M	87	−1.1	−1.1	−8.9	−10.9	9.8	13.8	−0.8	−4.8	−12.7	−13.7	−4.1	−9.1	−43.6	60
M	65	−0.7	−4.7	−8.6	22.4	−9.0	−10.0	−10.5	−5.5	−5.5	−5.5	−7.0	−8.0	−52.6	61
M	79	−3.5	2.5	−4.7	−6.7	−14.4	−12.4	−1.6	−1.6	−4.7	−5.7	0.3	−2.7	−55.2	62
M	63	−5.9	−6.9	−1.9	−8.9	−10.3	−7.3	−4.7	−3.7	−6.3	−6.3	2.0	−1.0	−61.2	63
M	81	−1.9	−3.9	−10.0	−8.0	−8.6	−8.6	−3.9	−6.9	−6.0	−5.0	−3.8	0.2	−66.5	64
M	32	−8.0	−9.0	−3.7	−2.7	−9.0	−9.0	−10.2	−8.2	−4.2	−4.2	−0.6	1.4	−67.2	65
M	45	−6.5	−9.5	−6.8	−6.8	−3.2	−2.2	−8.5	−6.5	−6.8	−4.8	−5.8	−5.8	−73.0	66
M	25	−6.0	−4.0	−2.6	−3.6	−8.8	−8.8	−14.0	−13.0	−5.6	−4.6	−2.7	−4.7	−78.6	67
F	76	−7.0	−9.0	−6.9	−8.9	−6.7	−7.7	−5.0	−6.0	−7.4	−6.4	−2.6	−6.6	−80.1	68
M	60	−9.1	−10.1	−9.3	−13.3	−11.8	−2.8	−8.1	−5.1	−3.8	−4.8	−4.8	−5.8	−88.9	69
M	59	−12.8	−11.8	−8.1	−9.1	−6.7	−8.7	−0.9	−2.9	−9.6	−4.6	−7.7	−6.7	−89.8	70

Figure 6. Tabulated list of age-standardized IJS in the well-preserved 70 individuals. Individuals are arranged in the order corresponding to the sum values of all of the 12 IJS; higher values in each column are shown in red and lower values in blue. The rightmost column indicated the ranking numbers from the highest as 1 to the lowest individuals as 70. (SR: right shoulder, SL: left shoulder, RE: right elbow, LE: left elbow, RW: right wrist, LW left wrist, RH: right hip, RL left hip, RK: right knee, LK: left knee, RA: right ankle and LA: left ankle).

sexes were relatively precisely known, called the Terry collection; he evaluated DJD in their four major joints by scoring marginal osteophyte and articular surface conditions in some parts of the joints, and this yielded much useful information on DJD [10]. Like Jurmain, some other studies adopted the direct observation techniques for skeletons. Moreover, there have been a lot of studies which evaluated the features in DJD by means of roentgenographic evaluation techniques [11–18], which were proposed originally by Kellgren and Lawrence [19]. X-ray goes through the objects to form two-dimensional images on the films; therefore, concerning the periarticular osteophytes, the evaluated area is only a narrowly restricted tangential portion of the joint margin [20][21].

In this study, periarticular osteophytes were evaluated with our original scoring system. With this system, osteophytes were scored in many small segments in order to calculate a whole joint score. For example, one shoulder joint was divided to a total of 12 segments, and one knee joint was divided to a total of 19 segments. Jurmain once emphasized the significance of a fine grading system while overweighting the importance of osteophyte development to sense the DJD frequencies within different joints. Though quantification of these periarticular osteophytes was relatively easy, it was difficult to evaluate the articular surface condition with unitary criteria; this was because a characteristic degenerative change in one joint might not be observed in another [10]. Merely for the purpose of studying the frequency of DJD in the skeletons, it might be better to evaluate the highest scores in respective joints. However, the purpose of this study was not only the evaluation of DJD frequency in a skeletal population but also the quantification of biomechanical stresses with the evidence in articular regions. Therefore, osteophytes located in periarticular regions were graded from 0 to 4, and the calculated scores were averaged for further evaluation. All of the appendicular joints were evaluated with common simple criteria, which made it possible to compare the different kinds of joints objectively. As described above, the periarticular osteophytes themselves are proliferative changes, and they often emerge as articular degeneration with ageing; they can be good biomechanical stress markers.

A good deal of study presented in the literatures, which discussed DJD prevalence on skeletal series from archaeological contest, were troubled by the fact that the most reliable age-at-death skeletal indicators (such as the changes of the sternal end of the ribs, the auricular surface and the pubic symphysis of the hip bone) were also related to the biomechanical stress during the individual's life [22–29]. On the other hand, in this study, as with Jurmain [10][30] and Waldron et al. [31][32], the skeletal individuals with exact records on sex and age-at-death were targeted, and this made it possible to discuss the features around osteophyte formation and ageing.

By considering the results of age correlation, bilateral correlation and the difference between the right and left sides in this study, the extent to which systemic or local factors got involved in

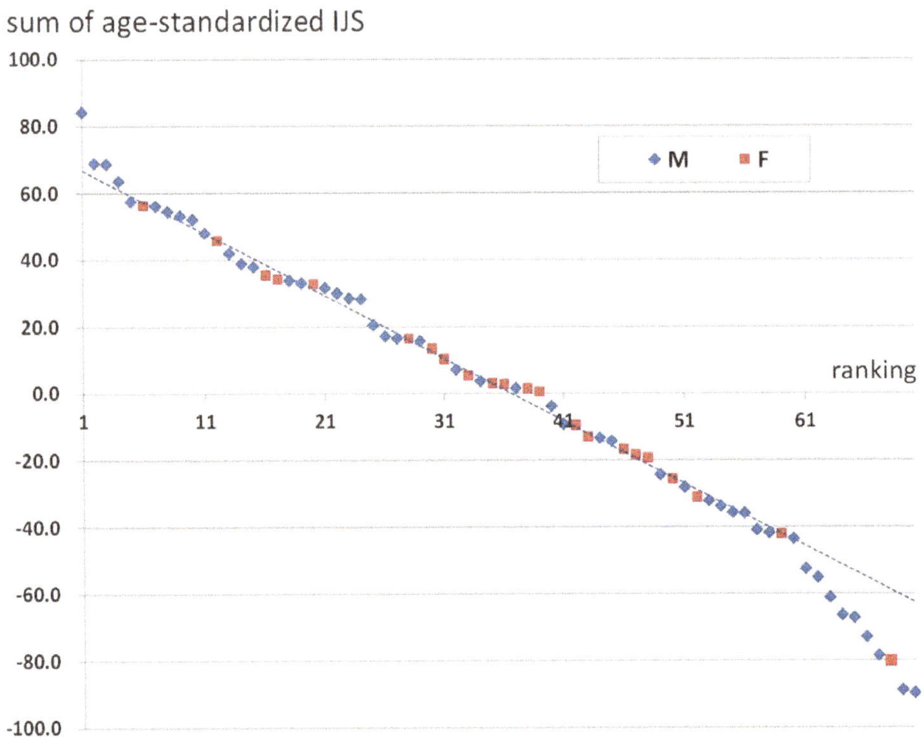

Figure 7. Scatter chart indicating the relationship between the sum of age-standardized IJS values of the 12 joints and the ranking numbers in the well-preserved 70 individuals (blue: male, red: female).

variables	PC1	PC2	PC3	PC4	PC5	PC6
Shoulder	0.62	0.69	−0.03	0.11	0.14	0.32
Elbow	0.70	−0.24	−0.05	0.64	−0.18	−0.07
Wrist	0.70	0.01	−0.56	−0.15	0.35	−0.24
Hip	0.70	0.37	0.37	−0.22	−0.32	−0.28
Knee	0.70	−0.43	−0.22	−0.32	−0.32	0.26
Ankle	0.59	−0.39	0.57	−0.06	0.42	0.05
percent of variance(%)	44.9	16.8	13.7	10.0	9.2	5.3

Figure 8. PCA variable loadings evaluating the characteristics in the respective six joints with age-standardized AIJS values; the high values are shown in red and lower values in blue.

the respective joints was clarified. From the result of the paired-T test, right side dominancy was recognized in the joints of the upper extremities, shoulder and wrist joint. This suggested that upper extremities were generally under the influence of local stress of various sizes. However, in the shoulder joint, the high bilateral correlation indicated the disparities among the individuals; so not only the local stress but also the general osteophyte proliferation tendency might be high in this joint.

The correlation coefficients between the right and left side of the lower extremities were high, especially in females. This could be explained by the fact that the female's scores continued to increase after middle age. One of the reasons might be the high morbidity rate of osteoarthritis in the knee joints of middle-aged and older females in Japan. Conversely, in males, age correlation of scores in knee and ankle joints was low. This meant that the local stresses, for example with trauma or injuries, were high in these male joints. These sex discrepancies in IJS were considered to reflect the differences in lifestyle, habitual activities, body habitus, metabolic/endocrinal condition and the receptivity to DJD among Japanese males and females. The individuals in this study lived their lives between the last decades of nineteenth century and mid-twentieth century, and most of them survived the extreme and hard days before and after World War II. Though the samples in this study were too heterogeneous to elaborate on these differences, all that was certain is that most Japanese women from these generations habitually sat down "Japanese style" with their buttocks on top of the ankles; it must lead to the high prevalence of DJD in the lower extremities.

From the viewpoint of periarticular osteophyte formation, there was a similarity in the shoulder joint and the hip joint; it was inferred that systemic factors were indicated to be relatively large in these two joints. This feature was consistent with the results on both PC2 loading values in PCA and dendrogram in cluster analysis. These two joints are relatively mobile from the biomechanical homologies in that the components are almost spherical, and in that both of them are multiaxial. Moreover, they are similarly located at the proximal positions in the upper and lower extremities. These anatomical and biomechanical analogies might explain the similarly steady progressive pattern in osteophyte formation by ageing. Jurmain reported that the age correlations of the shoulder and hip joints were higher than those of elbow and knee joints in the Terry collection and that the bilateral correlation in the elbow joint was low [10]. By quoting Fischer's [33] observation, Jurmain referred to the asymmetry of elbow joints and great stress in this joint [10]. The results in this study mostly confirmed their finding.

Radiographic changes of DJD, particularly osteophytes, are common in the aged population, but symptoms of joint pain may

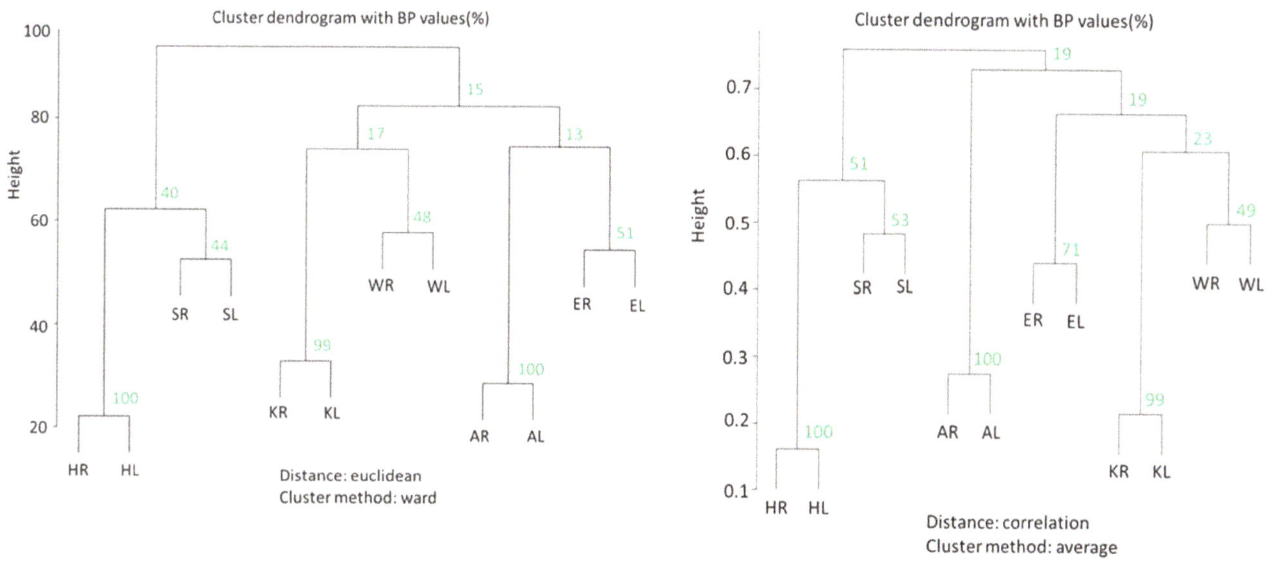

Figure 9. Results of cluster analysis showing the similarities in the 12 joints among the well-preserved 70 individuals (left; dendrogram chart with ward method, right; dendrogram with group average method).

be independent of radiographic severity in many older adults [34]. Indeed, one of the impressive results in this study was the relative high osteophyte scores in shoulder and hip joints of males and females. Clinically the frequency of DJD of the knee is highest among the appendicular joints in Japanese people; on the other hand, generally the hip joint is seldom affected with primary osteoarthritis. Disjunction was noted between these facts and the results of this study; therefore, osteophyte formation must be one of the distinct phenomena in joints with DJD, and it was doubted that all of the formed osteophytes were not related to DJD. In this study, osteophytes scores in almost all of the joints increased logarithmically with ageing. Namely, it was speculated that periarticular osteophytes started to grow rapidly before the symptoms of DJD became apparent. Though most of the joints stopped showing increasing osteophyte scores after middle age, some of the joints in the male's upper extremity and in female's lower extremity continued to increase even in the elderly. In these joints osteophytes formation must be related to DJD progression. Indeed, in Japan, one of the dominant joints with DJD is females' knee joint, though it would be impossible to explain the difference of physical activities. Hernborg et al. confirmed that osteophytes were frequently observed in cases that later on developed osteoarthritis and continue to grow in size in these cases at a faster rate than in cases that did not develop osteoarthritis with structural changes in the joint [35]. On the other hand, there were osteophytes which stopped growing after middle age; they might not be pathological but physiological.

Chronological ages of the individuals are thought to have a profound effect on the degree of periarticular osteophytes. In this study, the age-standardized osteophyte scores were investigated among the individuals; this made it possible to compare the osteophyte proliferation size and grade in different kinds of joints. As indicated in Figure 7, osteophytes proliferation tendency in a whole body showed wide individual variation. Especially on both sides of the scatter chart, there existed some individuals with extremely high or low scores. Rogers et al. pointed out that osteophyte and enthesophyte proliferations are linked; thus, individuals in populations can be classified into "bone formers" and "poor bone formers" [36][37]. Some factors should be pointed out as backgrounds of these individual differences; among the various factors listed above, the systemic factors for DJD progression can have effects on the differences in bone formation. For example, genetic factors might significantly contribute to these tendencies.

Moreover, recently it has been reported that some kinds of calcifying nanoparticles might make ectopic calcifications and trigger some pathological conditions in many organs in human bodies, for example, heart valves [38][39], urinary bladder [40], prostate [41], placenta [42], and synovial joints [43]. If these nanoparticles increased in the synovial joint spaces, ectopic calcification, ossification and osteophyte formation could be accelerated around the joint surfaces. Moreover, Timms et al. confirmed in his review of the genetic potentials in the patients with chondrocalcinosis due to calcium pyrophosphate deposition (CPPD), diffuse idiopathic systemic hyperostosis (DISH) and ossification of posterior longitudinal ligament (OPLL) [44]; and the generalized osteoarthritis (GOA) should be considered in the same category [45]. Some genetic studies targeting the individuals with high or low osteophyte scores in this study might yield a meaningful result in the future.

It has been emphasized that the degenerative changes in peripheral joints could be used as the markers of mechanical stresses; and frequently they have been applied to reconstruct the past lifestyles and activity patterns and to clarify the differences among human groups [46–50]. This study suggests that only in cases in which age is standardized properly can periarticular osteophytes be used as a sensitive biomarker for indicating abnormal phenomena in the appendicular joints, osteoarthritis severity, and the biomechanical stresses placed on individuals and populations. Even if some individuals and some joints dominantly are affected by the influence of systemic factors, they cannot but undergo various local biomechanical stresses. Therefore, osteophytes could play a significant role as a "joint stress marker (JSM)" in a similar manner to "musculoskeletal stress markers (MSM)", which is a term used for the sites of origin and insertion of muscle tendons (entheses) and ligament attachments (syndesmoses) in the skeleton [51–53]. Additional analyses targeting the marginal osteophytes of both joint components and of independent parts in joint surfaces would be useful for studying poorly preserved archeological samples. For these samples, some interesting and valuable findings might be able to be confirmed with some comparison/correlation analyses, PCA and cluster analysis.

Author Contributions

Conceived and designed the experiments: TT TW. Performed the experiments: TT KO JM. Analyzed the data: KS YM TT. Contributed reagents/materials/analysis tools: KS TI TT. Wrote the paper: TT.

References

1. Molnar P, Wim B (2007) Osteophytes: relevance and biology. Osteoarthritis Cartilage 15: 237–244.
2. Currey JD (2002) Bones: Structure and mechanics. New Jersey: Princeton University Press. 225 p.
3. Ralphs JR, Benjamin M (1994) The joint capsule: structure, composition, ageing and disease. J Anat 184: 503–509.
4. Jurmain R (1977) Stress and the Etiology of Osteoarthritis. Am J Phys Anthrop 46: 353–365.
5. Weiss E, Jurmain R (2007) Osteoarthritis revisited: a contemporary review of aetiology. Int J Osteoarchaeol 17: 437–450.
6. Meulenbelt I (2012) Osteoarthritis year 2011 in review: genetics. Osteoarthritis Cartilage 20: 218–222.
7. Dai J, Ikegawa S (2010) Recent advances in association studies of osteoarthritis susceptibility genes. J Hum Genet 55: 77–80.
8. Irlenbusch U, Schaller T (2006) Investigations in generalized osteoarthritis. Part 1: genetic study of Heberden's nodes. Osteoarthritis Cartilage 14: 423–427.
9. Heine J (1926) Uber die Arthritis deformans. Virchow's Arch Pathol Anat 260: 521–663.
10. Jurmain R (1980) The pattern of involvement of appendicular degenerative joint disease. Am J Phys Anthropol 53: 143–150.
11. Jan LCM . van Saase, Leo KJ . van Romunde, Cats A, Vandenbroucke JP, Valkenburg HA (1989) Epidemiology of osteoarthritis: Zoetermeer survey. Comparison of radiological osteoarthritis in a Dutch population with that in 10 other populations. Ann Rheum Dis 48: 271–280.
12. Spector TD, Hart DJ, Byrne J, Harris PA, Dacre JE, et al. (1993) Definition of osteoarthritis of the knee for epidemiological studies. Ann Rheum Dis 52: 790–794.
13. Neame R, Zhang W, Deighton C, Doherty M, Doherty S, et al. (2004) Distribution of radiographic osteoarthritis between the right and left hands, hips, and knees. Arthritis Rheum 50: 1487–1494.
14. Altman RD, Gold GE (2007) Atlas of individual radiographic features in osteoarthritis, revised. Osteoarthritis Cartilage 15: A1–A15.
15. Petersson IF (1996) Occurrence of osteoarthritis of the peripheral joints in European populations. Ann Rheum Dis 55: 659–664.
16. Lanyon P, O'Reilly S, Jones A, Doherty M (1998) Radiographic assessment of symptomatic knee osteoarthritis in the community: definitions and normal joint space. Ann Rheum Dis 57: 595–601.
17. Braga L, Renner B, Schwartz TA, Woodard J, Helmick CG (2009) Differences in radiographic features of knee osteoarthritis in African-Americans and Caucasians: the Johnston country osteoarthritis project. Osteoarthritis Cartilage 17: 1554–1561.
18. Petersson IF (2002) Osteoarthritis of the peripheral joints. Best Pract Res Clin Rheumatol 16: 741–760.
19. Kellgren JH, Lawrence JS. (1957) Radiological assessment of osteoarthrosis. Ann Rheum Dis 16: 494–502.

20. Messent EA, Ward RJ, Tonkin CJ, Buckland-Wright C (2007) Osteophytes, juxta-articular radiolucencies and cancellous bone changes in the proximal tibia of patients with knee osteoarthritis. Osteoarthritis Cartilage 15:179–186.
21. Buckland-Wright JC, Macfarlane DG, Lynch JA (1991) Osteophytes in the osteoarthritic hand: their incidence, size, distribution, and progression. Ann Rheum Dis 50: 627–630.
22. Debono L, Mafart B, Jeusel E, Guipert G (2004) Is the incidence of elbow osteoarthritis underestimated: Insights from paleopathology. Joint Bone Spine 71: 397–400.
23. Jurmain R, Kilgore L (1995) Skeletal evidence ofosteoarthritis: a palaeopathological perspective. Ann Rheum Dis 54: 443–450.
24. Inoue K, Hukuda P, Fardellon P, Yang Z, Nakai M, et al. (2001) Prevalance of large-joint osteoarthritis in Asian and Causcasian skeletal polupations. Rheumatology 40: 70–73.
25. Bridges PS (1991) Degenerative joint disease in hunter-gatherers and agriculturalists from the Southeastern United States. Am J Phys Anthrop 85: 379–391.
26. Waldron HA (1997) Association between osteoarthritis of the hand and knee in a population of skeletons from London. Ann Rheum Dis 56: 116–118.
27. Brickley M, Waldron T (1998) Relationship Between Bone Density and Osteoarthritis in a Skeletal Population from London. Bone 22: 279–283.
28. Klaus HD, Larsen CS, Tam ME (2009) Economic Intensification and Degenerative Joint Disease: Life and Labor on the Postcontact North Coast of Peru. Am J Phys Anthropol 139: 204–221.
29. Watkins R (2010) Variation in Health and Socioeconomic Status within the W. Montague Cobb Skeletal Collection: Degenerative Joint Disease, Trauma and Cause of Death. Int J Osteoarchaeol 22: 22–44.
30. Jurmain RD (1991) Degenerative changes in peripheral joints as indicator of mechanical stress: opportunities and limitations. Int J Osteoarcheol 1: 247–252.
31. Waldron HA, Cox M (1986) Occupational arthropathy: evidence from the past. Br J Ind Med 46: 420–422.
32. Waldron HA (1991) Prevalence and distribution of osteoarthritis in a population from Georgian and early Victorian London. Ann Rheum Dis 50: 301–307.
33. Fischer A (1932) Rheumatismus als Berufskrankeit. Acta Rheumatol 4: 24–28.
34. Anderson AS. (2010) Why is osteoarthritis an age-related disease. Best Pract Res Clin Rheumatol 24: 15–26.
35. Hernborg J, Nilsson N (1973) The relationship between osteoarthritis in the knee joint, osteophyte and aging. Acta Orthop Scand 44: 69–74.
36. Rogers J, Shepstone L, Dieppe P (1997) Bone formers: osteophyte and enthesophyte formation are positively associated. Ann Rheum Dis 56: 85–90.
37. Rogers J, Shepstone L, Dieppe P (2004) Is osteoarthritis a systemic disorder of bone? Arthritis Rheum 50: 452–457.
38. Candermir B, Ertas FS, Kaya CT, Ozdol C, Hasan T, et al. (2010) Association Between Antibodies Against Calcifying Nanoparticles and Mitral Annular Calcification. J Heart Valve Dis 19: 745–752.
39. Bratos-Pe'rez MA, Sa'nchez PD, Cruz SD, Villacorta E, Palacios IF (2008) Association between self-replicating calcifying nanoparticles and aortic stenosis: A possible link to valve calcification. Eur Heart J 29: 371–376.
40. Jelic TM, Roque R, Yasar U, Tomchin SB, Serrato JM, et al. (2008) Calcifying nanoparticles associated encrusted urinary bladder cystitis. Int J Nanomed 3: 385–390.
41. Zhou Z, Hong L, Shen X, Rao X, Jin X, et al. (2008) Detection of nanobacteria infection in type III prostatitis. Urology 71: 1091–1095.
42. Guo Y, Zhang D, Lu H Luo S, Shen X (2012) Association between calcifying nanoparticles and placental calcification. Int J Nanomed 7: 1679–1686.
43. Tsurumoto T, Matsumoto T, Yonekura A, Shindo H (2006) Nanobacteria-Like Particles in Human Arthritic Synovial Fluids. J Prot Res 5: 1276–1278.
44. Timms A., Zhang Y, Russel R, Broum M (2002) Genetic studies of disorders of calcium crystal deposition. Rheumatology 41: 725–729.
45. Copper C, Egger P, Coggon D, Hart DJ, Masud T, et al. (1996) Generalized Osteoarthritis in Women: Pattern of JointInvolvement and Approaches to Definition for Epidemiological Studies. J Rheumatol 23: 1938–1942.
46. Esposito A, Souto SC, Catalano OA, Doria AS, Trigo PBS, et al. (2006) Pattern of osteophytes and enthesophytes in the proximal ulna: an anatomic, paleopathologic, and radiologic study. Skeletal Radiol 35: 847–856.
47. Weiss E (2003) Understanding muscle markers: aggregation and construct validity. Am J Phys Anthropol 121: 230–240.
48. Jurmain RD (1991) Degenerative Changes in Peripheral Joints as Indicators of Mechanical Stress: Opportunities and Limitations. Int J Osteoarchaeol 1: 247–252.
49. Braga L, Renner JB, Schwartz TA, Woodard J, Helmick CG, et al. (2009) Differences in radiographic features of knee osteoarthritis in African-Americans and Caucasians: the Johnston country osteoarthritis project. Osteoarthritis Cartilage 17: 1554–1561.
50. Jurmain RD, Kilgore L (1995) Skeletal evidence of osteoarthritis: a palaeopathological perspective. Ann Rheum Dis 54: 443–450.
51. Hawkey DE, Merbs CF (1995) Activity-induced musculoskeletal stress markers (MSM) and subsistence strategy changes among ancient Hudson Bay Eskimos. Int J Osteoarchaeol 5: 324–338.
52. Molnar P (2006) Tracing prehistoric activities: Musculoskeletal stress marker analysis of a stone-age population on the Island of Gotland in the Baltic Sea. Am J Phys Anthrop 129: 12–23.
53. Molnar P, Ahlstrom TP, Leden I (2011) Osteoarthritis and activity - an analysis of the relationship between eburnation, musculoskeletal stress markers (MSM) and age in two neolithic hunter–gatherer populations from Gotland, Sweden. Int J Osteoarchaeol 21: 283–291.

20

Biomechanics of Forearm Rotation: Force and Efficiency of Pronator Teres

Pere Ibáñez-Gimeno[1], Ignasi Galtés[2,3], Xavier Jordana[4], Assumpció Malgosa[1], Joan Manyosa[5]*

1 Unitat d'Antropologia Biològica, Departament de Biologia Animal, Biologia Vegetal i Ecologia, Universitat Autònoma de Barcelona, Bellaterra, Barcelona, Catalonia, Spain, **2** Centre de Patologia Forense de Collserola, Institut de Medicina Legal de Catalunya, Montcada i Reixach, Barcelona, Catalonia, Spain, **3** Unitat de Medicina Legal i Forense, Departament de Psiquiatria i de Medicina Legal, Universitat Autònoma de Barcelona, Bellaterra, Barcelona, Catalonia, Spain, **4** Departament de Paleobiologia, Institut Català de Paleontologia Miquel Crusafont (ICP), Universitat Autònoma de Barcelona, Bellaterra, Barcelona, Catalonia, Spain, **5** Unitat de Biofísica, Departament de Bioquímica i de Biologia Molecular, and Centre d'Estudis en Biofísica, Universitat Autònoma de Barcelona, Bellaterra, Barcelona, Catalonia, Spain

Abstract

Biomechanical models are useful to assess the effect of muscular forces on bone structure. Using skeletal remains, we analyze pronator teres rotational efficiency and its force components throughout the entire flexion-extension and pronation-supination ranges by means of a new biomechanical model and 3D imaging techniques, and we explore the relationship between these parameters and skeletal structure. The results show that maximal efficiency is the highest in full elbow flexion and is close to forearm neutral position for each elbow angle. The vertical component of pronator teres force is the highest among all components and is greater in pronation and elbow extension. The radial component becomes negative in pronation and reaches lower values as the elbow flexes. Both components could enhance radial curvature, especially in pronation. The model also enables to calculate efficiency and force components simulating changes in osteometric parameters. An increase of radial curvature improves efficiency and displaces the position where the radial component becomes negative towards the end of pronation. A more proximal location of pronator teres radial enthesis and a larger humeral medial epicondyle increase efficiency and displace the position where this component becomes negative towards forearm neutral position, which enhances radial curvature. Efficiency is also affected by medial epicondylar orientation and carrying angle. Moreover, reaching an object and bringing it close to the face in a close-to-neutral position improve efficiency and entail an equilibrium between the forces affecting the elbow joint stability. When the upper-limb skeleton is used in positions of low efficiency, implying unbalanced force components, it undergoes plastic changes, which improve these parameters. These findings are useful for studies on ergonomics and orthopaedics, and the model could also be applied to fossil primates in order to infer their locomotor form. Moreover, activity patterns in human ancient populations could be deduced from parameters reported here.

Editor: David Carrier, University of Utah, United States of America

Funding: This work is supported by grants from the Ministerio de Ciencia e Innovación (grant no. CGL2008-00800/BOS), the Generalitat de Catalunya (grant no. 2009 SGR 566), the Programa de Formación de Profesorado Universitario, Ministerio de Educación, Cultura y Deporte (grant no. AP2009-5102) awarded to Pere Ibáñez-Gimeno and the Programa Juan de la Cierva, Ministerio de Economía y Competitividad (grant no. JCI-2010-08157) awarded to Xavier Jordana. The funders had no role in study design, data collection and analysis, decision to publish, or preparation of the manuscript.

Competing Interests: The authors have declared that no competing interests exist.

* E-mail: joan.manyosa@uab.cat

Introduction

The effect of muscular forces on bone structure can be predicted from osteometric parameters using biomechanical models if the line of action and the origins of the tendon are known [1,2]. The rotational efficiency (E_{rot}) of the pronator teres (PT) is a measure of its rotational capacity as a function of the applied force [3]. The PT E_{rot} can be calculated from several osteometric parameters of the upper-limb skeleton, basically related to the curvature of the diaphysis of the radius bone, the size and shape of the humeral medial epicondyle, and the proximo-distal location of PT radial enthesis [3–5].

During resisted pronation, PT acts as the primary agonist, displaying relatively higher activity levels than pronator quadratus [6]. In contrast to the latter, PT is largely affected by elbow and forearm position [6,7]. The positioning of the forearm may also influence the components of PT force, which in turn can entail structural changes with different functional implications. Therefore, it can be hypothesized that each component influences the skeletal structure in a different way, e.g. a component may enhance the curvature of the radius when it exerts a bending loading on its shaft [3]. However, the biomechanical behavior and structural effects of these components in the pronation-supination and flexion-extension ranges have never been examined.

This study aims to analyze PT E_{rot} for a full range of elbow flexion angles in order to (i) analyze the relationship between the components of the force vector and the skeletal structure, (ii) assess how E_{rot} is modified by changes in several osteometric parameters and (iii) get further knowledge about the functional implications of the variation of this parameter in the flexion-extension range. The results of this biomechanical analysis will lay the foundations for future studies about comparative and evolutionary anatomy, as well as works on applied sciences, such as ergonomics, sports medicine and orthopaedics, providing relevant information about the relationship between the skeletal structure and PT functionality.

Materials and Methods

Materials

The skeletal remains used in this study are part of an osteological collection housed at Unitat d'Antropologia Biològica (Universitat Autònoma de Barcelona). The skeletons in this collection were ceded to Unitat d'Antropologia Biològica (Universitat Autònoma de Barcelona) by Cementiri de Granollers (Ajuntament de Granollers). This cession was subjected to prior agreement between both institutions. Moreover, this study is part of a project (CGL2008-00800/BOS), which was approved by Ministerio de Ciencia e Innovación (Gobierno de España).

Rotational efficiency was calculated for the right upper-limb skeleton (humerus, radius and ulna) of a 32-year-old male from the abovementioned collection. The E_{rot} of the studied individual was previously shown to be within to the human pattern of variation, calculated for full elbow extension (180°) and intermediate flexion (90°) [5]. The biomechanical model used in the current study enables to calculate E_{rot} as function of the elbow flexion angle by using 3D imaging techniques. NextEngine's 3D Scanner was used to obtain a three-dimensional image of the humerus, which was processed with ScanStudio HD software [8]. The image was exported to the modeling software Rhinoceros 4.0 SR1 [9], where planes and axes were defined and measurements were taken.

Calculation of pronator teres rotational efficiency

Galtés et al. [3] developed the biomechanical model to calculate the rotational efficiency (E_{rot}) of the pronator teres (PT), which was initially based on the use of CT scan images of the upper-limb. In accordance with this work, E_{rot} is defined by the expression:

$$E_{rot} = \cos\alpha \times \cos\beta \times \overline{AO'}$$

The biomechanical model was later adapted to calculate E_{rot} using skeletal remains by means of photographs of the distal epiphysis of humerus [4]. Although this methodology was simple and practical, the technique was limited since the spatial representation of the humeral planes was not possible. Therefore, some assumptions about the arm and forearm mechanics and the representation of the geometrical points used to calculate E_{rot} had to be made. The use of 3D imaging, basically to define the humeral planes and axes and to determine important details of the medial epicondyle, enabled to obtain more accurate calculations of E_{rot} [5]. As a matter of fact, the calculation of E_{rot} at any elbow position described in the current paper is based on the approach developed by Galtés et al. [4] and Ibáñez-Gimeno et al. [5]. In order to calculate angles α and β at a given forearm and elbow position, several parameters are required (Table 1) [5]. Two of these parameters, $\boldsymbol{l_1}$ distance and $\overline{O'B'}$ distance, depend on the value of carrying angle (λ) and thus vary throughout the flexion-extension range (Fig. 1) [10]. The carrying angle is the angle between the arm and the forearm long axes (Fig. 1). Assuming a linear variation of this angle between a maximum value (λ_m) in full elbow extension (180°), which is measured on dry bones [11], and $\lambda = 0°$ in full elbow flexion (40°) [10,12–14], and using $\overline{XB}$ and $\overline{XC}$ values (Fig. 1B) obtained from the three-dimensional image of the humerus, we can obtain:

$$\Delta l_1(\lambda_m) = l_1(180°) - l_1(40°) = \overline{CB} \times \sin(\omega + \lambda) - \overline{CB} \times \sin\omega \quad \text{(Eq.1)}$$

$$\Delta\overline{OB'}(\lambda_m) = \overline{OB'}(180°) - \overline{OB'}(40°) = \overline{CB} \times \cos(\omega + \lambda) - \overline{CB} \times \cos\omega \quad \text{(Eq.2)}$$

Distance l_l ($\overline{P_1P_3}$) is the sum of $\overline{P_2P_3}$ and $\overline{P_1P_2}$ (Figs. 1A and 2A). $\overline{P_2P_3}$ can be measured directly on the radius bone (Figs. 1A and 2A, l_{pr}), and $\overline{P_1P_2}$ can be obtained from: (i) geometric parameters obtained from the three-dimensional image of the humerus (R_e, d_e, ε, Fig. 2B); (ii) the position of the humeral medial epicondyle at each flexion angle (Fig. 2B), and (iii) the position of the elbow flexion axis, which depends on the carrying angle (λ) and varies throughout the flexion-extension range (see Fig. 1 and Eq. 1) [10]. Then, the distance l_1 in maximum elbow extension can be calculated as follows:

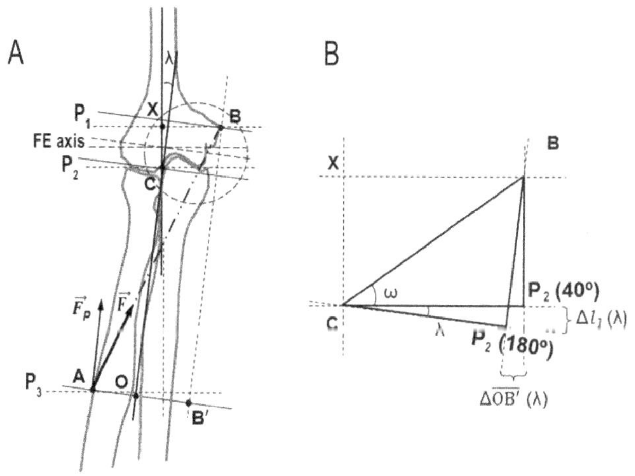

Figure 1. Representation of the influence of carrying angle (λ) on several parameters used to calculate rotational efficiency. A: Anterior view of right distal arm and forearm bones in supination position. Humeral and forearm axes, the flexion-extension axis (FE axis), as well as the force exerted by pronator teres muscle ($\vec{F}$, from point A to point B), are represented. $\vec{F}_P$ is the vertical component of pronator teres force. Point A indicates pronator teres distal enthesis just at the apex of radial curvature. Point B indicates its proximal attachment site, just at the apex of the medial epicondyle, and point B′ is the projection of point B on plane P_3. Planes P_1, P_2 and P_3 are parallel to each other and perpendicular to the forearm axis. P_1 passes through point B, P_2 passes through the most proximal point of the radial head and P_3 passes through point A. Point X is the intersection between humeral axis and a plane perpendicular to the humeral axis that passes through point B. Point C is the most distal humeral point of the humeral axis. Point O is the intersection between plane P_3 and the forearm axis. The dashed circle indicates the zoomed-in area of the right image. **B:** Detail of the left image. Plane P_2 is represented for a position of full elbow extension (P_2 (180°)) and for a position of full elbow flexion (P_2 (40°)). The variation of this plane is caused by the variation of the carrying angle (λ). This causes a variation in l_l and in $\overline{OB'}$ (Δl_l (λ) and $\Delta\overline{OB'}$ (λ)), which depends on the elbow angle. Angle ω is the angle between plane P_2 (40°) and $\overline{CB}$ segment.

Table 1. Osteometric and geometric parameters used to calculate forearm rotational efficiency.

Parameter	Value	Definition
d_r	1.10	Radial head radius
d_c	1.10	Ulnar distal epiphysis radius
l_f	23.00	Physiological length of the radius
l_{pr}	9.70	Distance between P_2 and P_3 planes
λ_{180}	10.00°	Carrying angle in full elbow extension
ε	45.65°	Angle between the positive *x*-axis and the position vector of point B
d_e	0.75	Distance between flexion-extension axis and point B
R_c	1.14	Humeral capitulum radius
B	(0.52, −0.53)	Coordinates of point B
$\overline{XB}$	3.93	Distance between point B and humeral axis
$\overline{XC}$	1.34	Distance between P_1 and P_2 planes
$\overline{AO}$	2.60	Curvature of the radius

Distance values are in centimeters. See Materials and Methods and Figures 1, 2 and 3 for further information about the parameters definition.

$$l_1(180^\circ) = l_{pr} + R_c + d_e \times \cos\varepsilon + \Delta l_1(\lambda_{180})$$

where $\Delta l_1(\lambda_{180})$ is obtained from Eq. 1. Distance $\overline{AO}$ is the curvature of the radius, measured on dry bone [4,15]. Distance $\overline{OB'}$ (projection of $\overline{CB}$ segment on plane P_3), is dependent on λ value and can be obtained for each position of the elbow using Eq. 2.

Then, $\overline{AO'}$ and $\overline{O'B'}$ can be respectively calculated from $\overline{AO}$ and $\overline{OB'}$ by determining distance $\overline{OO'}$ [4]. Knowing the position of point B and its projection on plane P_3 (Fig. 3), we can calculate, at any flexion angle of the elbow, distance $\overline{AB'}$, angle β, $\vec{F}''$ and $\vec{F}r$ and, therefore, the value of E_{rot}.

Results

Figure 4 shows PT E_{rot} throughout the flexion-extension and the pronation-supination ranges. Rotational efficiency for each elbow position is maximal when the forearm is close to the neutral position (position attained when the thumb points superiorly and the palm faces medially, at 0° of pronation-supination [10]) and is minimal in the extremes of the pronation-supination range. Maximum E_{rot} for each elbow position undergoes a nonlinear growth of 18% from full extension (180°) to full flexion (40°). The position of maximum E_{rot} displaces from −11° of pronation at 180° of elbow extension towards 6° of supination at 40° of elbow flexion (40°) (Fig. 4B). At 120° of elbow flexion, E_{rot} reaches its maximum when the forearm is in the neutral position.

The force that PT exerts on the radius is represented by $\vec{F}$ (Fig. 1). The projection of this vector on the axial plane P_3 is

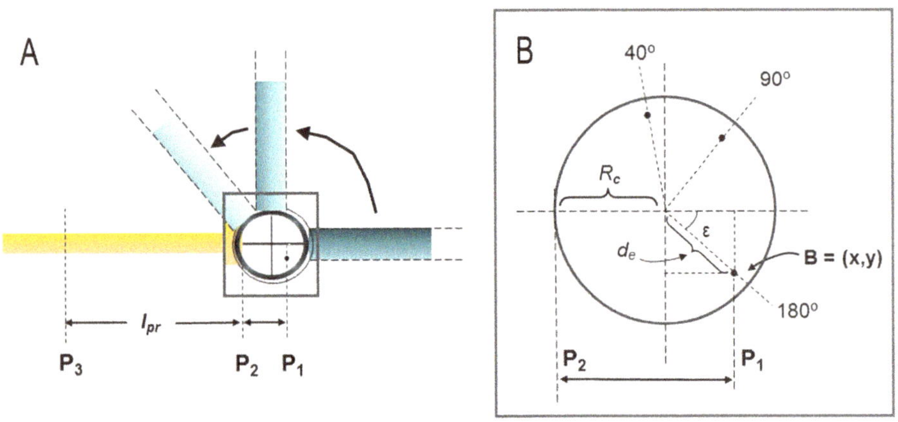

Figure 2. Representation of the changes in position of point B as a function of the elbow angle. A: Representation of the elbow in full extension (180°), an intermediate position (90°) and full flexion (40°) from a lateral view. A static radius (yellow) is represented with the humerus in the three positions (blue). Planes P_1, P_2 and P_3 are represented. The point (point B), and so plane P_1, are shown for 180° of elbow extension. Distance l_{pr} is the distance between planes P_2 and P_3. The distance between planes P_1 and P_2 depends on the elbow position. The square indicates the zoomed-in area of the right image. **B:** Change in the position of point B and in the distance $\overline{P_1P_2}$ as a function of the elbow angle. The position of point B for the three elbow angles is represented. Point B is positioned in a coordinates system (*x*, *y*) which center is the flexion-extension axis from a lateral point of view. R_c is the radius of the humeral condyle. d_e is the distance between the center of coordinates and point B. Angle ε is the angle between the positive *x*-axis and the position vector of point B.

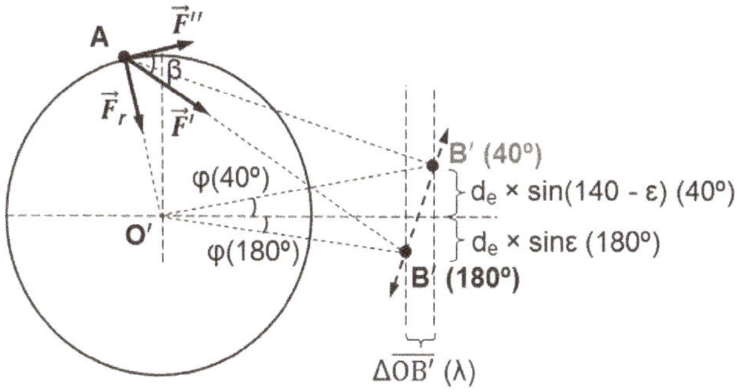

Figure 3. Diagram of plane P_3 with the main parameters to calculate rotational efficiency. Two elbow positions (180° and 40°) are represented. $\overrightarrow{F}'$ is the projection of the pronator teres force on plane P_3. $\overrightarrow{F}r$ is the radial component of $\overrightarrow{F}'$. $\overrightarrow{F}''$ is the component of $\overrightarrow{F}'$ tangential to the rotational movement. Angle β is the angle between $\overrightarrow{F}''$ and $\overrightarrow{F}'$. Point A is the radial attachment site of pronator teres. Point O′ is the center of the rotational movement. Point B′ is the projection of point B on plane P_3. The position of this point varies as a function of the carrying angle of the elbow ($\Delta\overline{OB'}$ (λ), see Fig. S1) and it is assessed with regards to the horizontal axis by φ angle. The displacement of point B′ from the horizontal axis can be calculated from the variation of point B position as a function of the elbow angle (see Fig. 2).

represented by $\overrightarrow{F}'$ (Fig. 3), whereas the projection on the vertical axis is named $\overrightarrow{F}p$ (Fig. 1). $\overrightarrow{F}'$ can be decomposed into two vectors: $\overrightarrow{F}''$, which is tangent to the trajectory of the radial rotational movement, and $\overrightarrow{F}r$, which is directed to the rotation center (Fig. 3). Figure 5 shows the relative values for these components at three elbow angles (40°, 90° and 180°). $\overrightarrow{F}'$ is greater in supination than in pronation, regardless of the elbow angle. The modulus for the perpendicular component of $\overrightarrow{F}$ (F_p) displays values that vary between the 86% and 99% of F value, depending on the pronation-supination and flexion-extension angles. This component increases as the forearm pronates, regardless of the elbow position. It is also slightly greater in extension than in flexion of the elbow.

Concerning the radial component ($\overrightarrow{F}r$), its modulus values are approximately the 50% of F value in a full supination position for the entire flexion-extension range. These values decrease as the forearm pronates, reaching negatives values in pronation. The forearm position where $F_r = 0$ depends on the elbow angle. At 180° of elbow extension, the modulus for $\overrightarrow{F}r$ reaches 0 at −46° of pronation, whereas in full elbow flexion this occurs at −25° of pronation. Therefore, this component reaches lower negative values, i.e. higher values for its modulus being the vector negative, as the elbow flexes (up to 15% in full flexion). Regarding $\overrightarrow{F}''$, which modulus does not reach the 40% of F, its values change in a similar way to the values of E_{rot}. The pronation-supination angle where $F'' = F_r$ is dependent on the elbow position. At 180°, it is close to the neutral position of the forearm (at 11° of supination). As the elbow flexes, it displaces towards a more supinated position of the forearm, reaching 31° of supination in full flexion.

Several simulations were carried out to assess how E_{rot} and $\overrightarrow{F}$ components are modified by changes in some osteometric parameters. From the mathematic expression to calculate E_{rot} (see Materials and Methods and Figures 1, 2 and 3), it is easily inferable that a greater curvature of the radius ($\overline{AO}$), and so a greater rotational radius ($\overline{AO'}$), leads to a proportional increase in

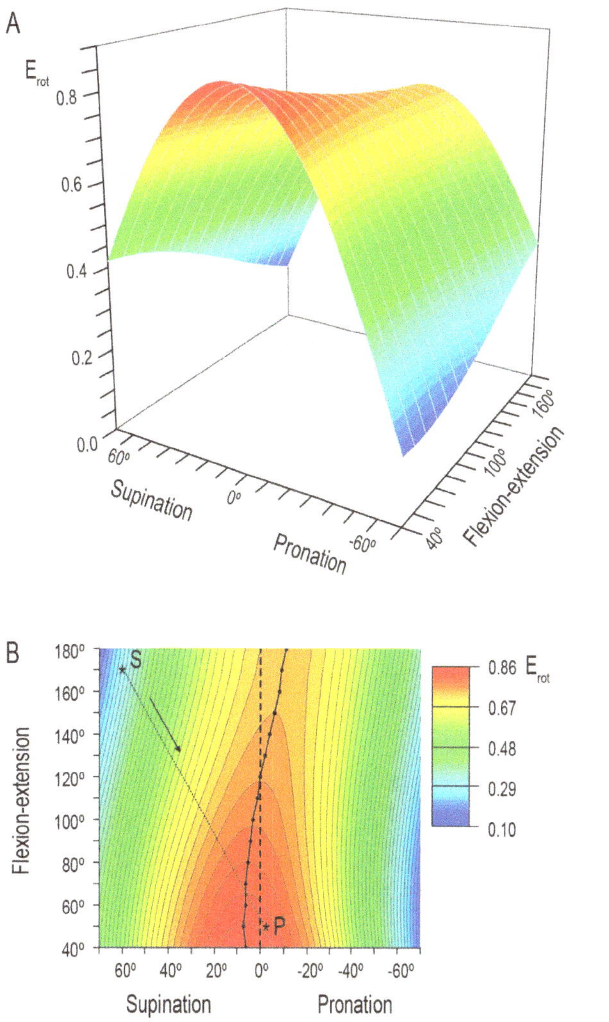

Figure 4. Forearm rotational efficiency (E_{rot}) as a function of pronation-supination and flexion-extension angles. A: Three-dimensional surface showing efficiency values at each forearm and elbow angles. **B:** Projection of the three-dimensional surface on XY plane showing efficiency ranges at each forearm and elbow angles. The points connected by a continuous line indicate the forearm positions where efficiency is maximal for each elbow angle. The dashed line indicates the neutral position of the forearm. The dotted line shows a trajectory followed by the forearm to reach an object with the elbow almost fully extended (170°) and the forearm supinated (60°) (asterisk S) and to bring it close to the face (50° of elbow flexion and −5° of pronation) (asterisk P). This trajectory, which direction is indicated by the arrow, is the shortest and entails an increase of about 190% in the efficiency value.

the E_{rot} values (Fig. 6A). Moreover, any change in one or several osteometrical parameters that causes an increase of α and/or β angles will consequently enhance E_{rot} (see Materials and Methods). Hence, the moment of force can be improved by rising either the tangential force ($\overrightarrow{F}''$) or the curvature of the radius ($\overline{AO}$). Although both scenarios would cause an increase in E_{rot}, they are related to different structural characteristics. A 10% rise of $\overline{AO}$ has a minor effect on the components of $\overrightarrow{F}$, being $\overrightarrow{F}''$ modulus constant (Fig. 6A) and slightly reducing $\overrightarrow{F}r$ modulus at −70° of pronation, from 8–15% to 6–13% of F value, depending on elbow position. When a similar increase in E_{rot} is simulated by a 10%

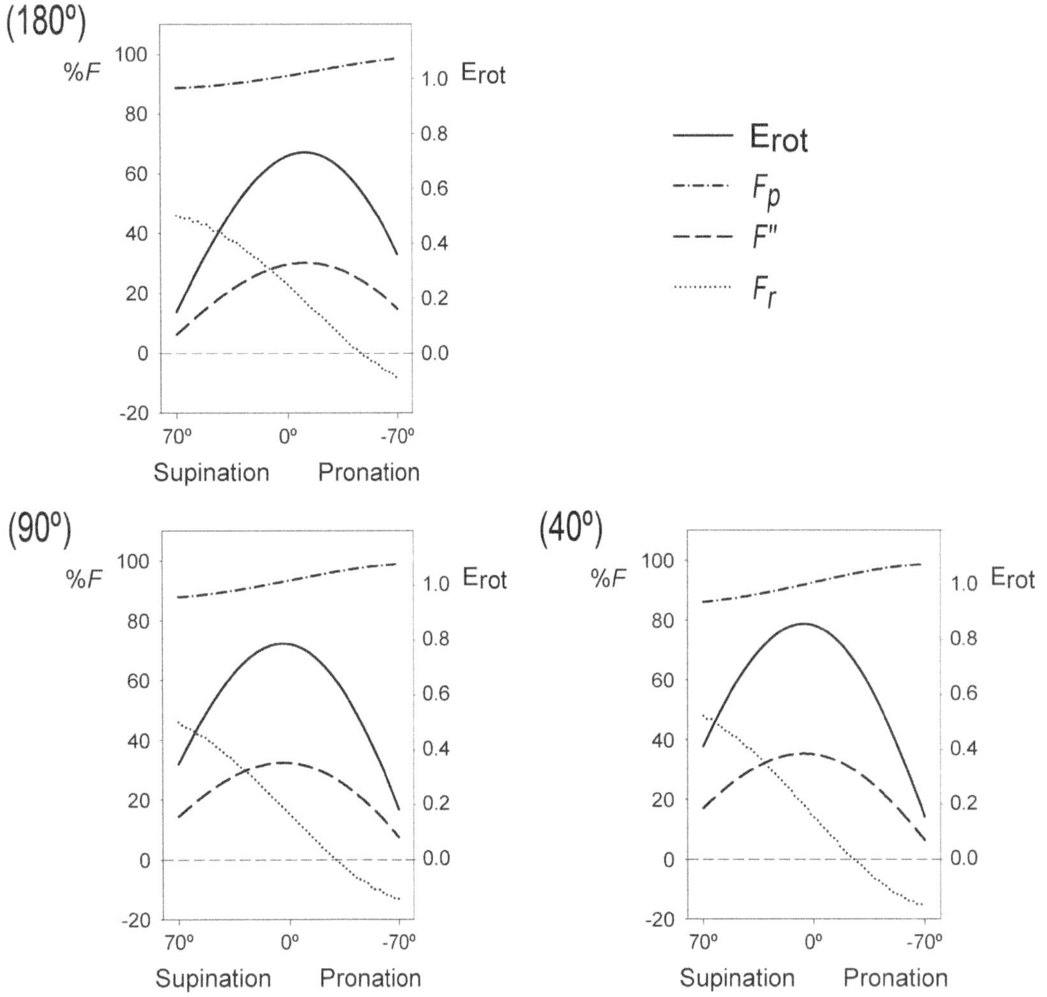

Figure 5. Relative values for $\vec{F}$ components and forearm rotational efficiency (E_{rot}) in three elbow positions. Full extension (180°), intermediate position (90°) and full elbow flexion (40°) scenarios are shown.

decrease of l_{pr}, a completely different behavior of $\vec{F}$ vectors can be observed: $\vec{F}''$ modulus increases proportionally to E_{rot} during the entire flexion range (Fig. 6B), whereas $\vec{F}r$ modulus rises from 46–48% to 49–51% of F value at 70° of supination and from 8–15% to 10–19% at −70° of pronation. A 10% increase of $\overline{XB}$ has broadly the same effect on E_{rot} and $\vec{F}''$ and $\vec{F}r$ moduli than the reported 10% decrease of l_{pr}. $\vec{F}p$ is not meaningfully modified by changes in the abovementioned parameters, whereas the forearm positions where $\vec{F}r$ modulus reaches 0, where $\vec{F}''$ and $\vec{F}r$ become equal and where E_{rot} is maximal are considerably affected by these changes. All this information is summarized in Table 2.

Conversely to the abovementioned simulations, the direction of the change in E_{rot} and $\vec{F}''$ modulus (increase or decrease) caused by a change in the position of point B depends on the elbow angle (Fig. 6C). When coordinate x increases, maximal E_{rot} and $\vec{F}''$ modulus rise in flexion of the elbow and decrease in extension. When this coordinate is lower, the values for these parameters decrease in flexion and rise in extension. When coordinate y is closer to 0, E_{rot} and $\vec{F}''$ modulus increase in flexion and fall in extension, whereas when this coordinate is lower, these parameters decrease in flexion and rise in extension.

Efficiency is also lower when the carrying angle (λ) is greater. A change of 5° in this angle leads to a variation of about 6.5% of the maximum E_{rot} value at 180° of elbow extension. This effect is lesser as the elbow flexes and it is null in full flexion (40°).

Discussion

Rotational efficiency, force components and structural implications

In the current study, PT E_{rot} has been assessed throughout the entire flexion-extension range using three-dimensional technology. The variation of E_{rot} obtained from our innovative biomechanical model is in agreement with the results of kinematic studies using cadaveric specimens [16,17] and virtual and resin models of the upper-limb skeleton [18–20], as well as with analysis on forearm discomfort [21] and on electromyographic signals of the forearm pronators [7].

Pronator teres E_{rot} is dependent on the skeletal structure of the arm, elbow and forearm, which in turn can be modified by the usage of this muscle. In this regard, the analysis of E_{rot} has enabled to study the effect of the components of PT force vector on the

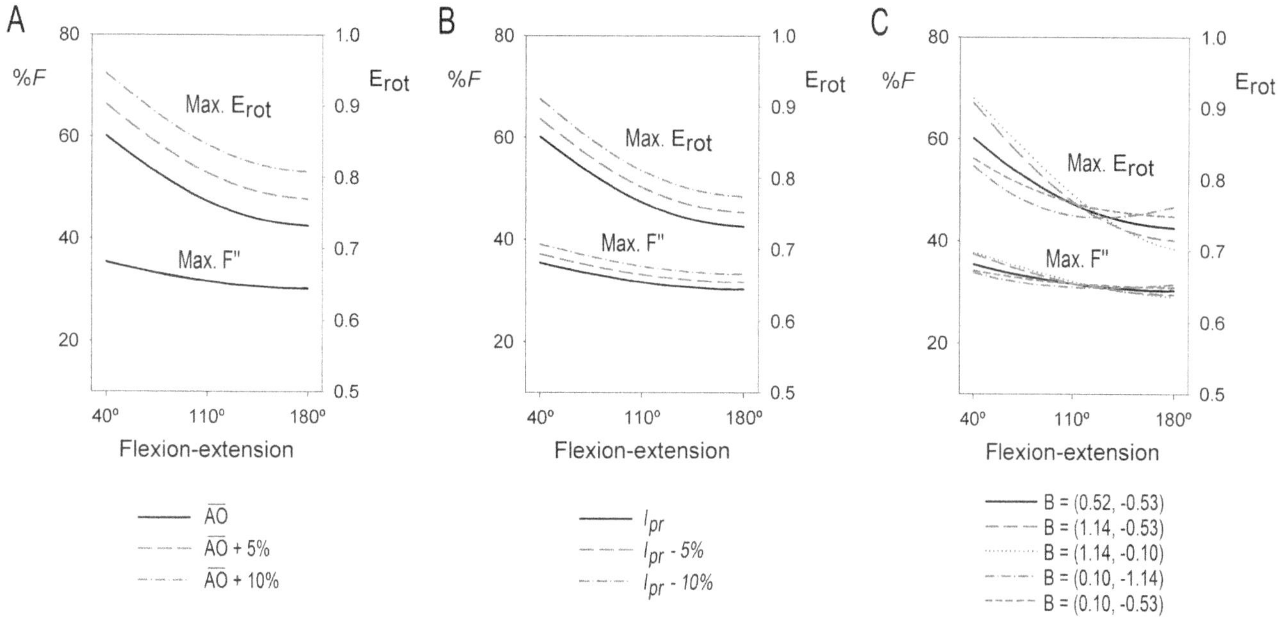

Figure 6. Simulated changes on maximum rotational efficiency (Max. E_{rot}) and maximum F'' value (Max. F''). Simulations are shown throughout the flexion-extension range. **A:** Simulations of an increase in $\overline{AO}$. Note that the relative values for F'' of the three simulations overlap. **B:** Simulations of a decrease in l_{pr}. The effect caused by an increase in $\overline{XB}$ is similar to the effect caused by the decrease in l_{pr} shown here. **C:** Simulations with different coordinates of point B (cm).

upper-limb skeleton. The perpendicular component of this vector ($\vec{F}p$) shows high relative values, which indicates that an important part of PT force is employed in a direction parallel to the rotational axis of the forearm, i.e. compressing the radius lengthwise towards the distal epiphysis of the humerus. This compression is also produced during the contraction of other upper-limb muscles, such as biceps brachii and the wrist and fingers flexors. As regards PT, the compressive effect on the radius is higher in pronation than in supination and slightly decreases from elbow extension to maximum flexion. Although the differences are slight, this indicates that pronated positions of the forearm enhance the curvature of the radius through radial compression in a greater degree than supinated positions. This effect is independent of the skeletal structure, as $\vec{F}p$ is broadly unaffected by changes in the parameters used to calculate E_{rot}.

When the forearm is pronated, biceps brachii is reflexly inhibited and plays little if any role in flexion, because it would supinate the forearm during contraction [22–24]. As mentioned, the perpendicular component of PT force is greater on the prone forearm. This increase may partially compensate the lack of action of biceps brachiii, enhancing the assisting role of PT as elbow flexor and joint stabilizer in this position.

The component $\vec{F}r$, which directs to the rotation center, reaches negative values in forearm pronation. When this component is negative, the vector directs opposite to the rotational center, and so it enhances the curvature of the radius. Negative values are reached in a position of the forearm that gets closer to the neutral position as the elbow flexes. Therefore, the curvature of the radius ($\overline{AO}$) is enhanced during pronation in flexion rather than in extension of the elbow. In any case, the relative values for $\vec{F}r$ responsible for the curvature of the radius are low when compared to values for $\vec{F}p$, which suggests that radii with marked curvatures are more probably associated to compression forces from PT, among other muscles, than to forces applied perpendicularly to the forearm axis. These findings are in agreement with a previous empirical study that revealed that the pattern of muscular loading exerted on the apex of the radial shaft curvature by the PT muscle plays an important role as a mechanical stimulus involved in diaphyseal bowing [15].

Table 2. Effect of the simulations on $\vec{F}$ components and rotational efficiency (E_{rot}) for three elbow positions (180°, 90° and 40°).

Simulation	Forearm position where F_r=0			Forearm position where F'' = F_r			Forearm position where E_{rot} is maximal		
	180°	90°	40°	180°	90°	40°	180°	90°	40°
Original values	−47°	−29°	−25°	11°	28°	31°	−11°	4°	6°
$\overline{AO}$ increase (+10%)	−52°	−34°	−30°	8°	25°	28°	−11°	4°	6°
l_{pr} decrease (−10%)	−44°	−27°	−23°	13°	29°	34°	−11°	3°	5°
$\overline{XB}$ increase (+10%)	−42°	−26°	−23°	14°	29°	33°	−10°	3°	5°

The effect that the skeletal structure and form have on E_{rot} and on the force vectors has also been assessed. The results show that a greater bowing of the radius entails an increase of E_{rot}. This is consistent with previous studies suggesting an enhancement of PT action and forearm rotational power by a markedly bowed radius [3,25–28]. An increase of the radial curvature also causes that $\vec{F}r$ becomes negative in a more pronated position of the forearm, and so its modulus reach lower values in full pronation. Therefore, the radius is more easily bowed when its curvature is low.

The radial location of PT muscle also affects E_{rot}: at any elbow angle, E_{rot} increases when this enthesis is more proximally located, which is consistent with previous observations in full elbow extension [3]. Moreover, radii with a more proximal enthesis for PT muscle lead to the reach of negative values of $\vec{F}r$ closer to the neutral position of the forearm. Therefore, these radii entail lower negative values for this component, i.e. higher values for its modulus being the vector negative, which stimulates radial curvature.

Concerning the humeral medial epicondyle, E_{rot} also tends to increase in all elbow positions as this structure enlarges. Even though the current analysis uses a different approach to quantify humeral medial epincondylar projection ($\overline{XB}$), the results are consistent with previous studies [3,5,29]. Moreover, an enlargement of the medial epicondyle has the same effect on $\vec{F}r$ than a more proximally located radial enthesis for PT, and therefore a more medially projected epicondyle enhances radial curvature.

The orientation of the medial epicondyle is also relevant for the determination of E_{rot}. The alteration of this orientation causes changes in $\vec{F}''$ that lead to changes in E_{rot}. A more posteriorly oriented epicondyle, i.e. more retroflexed [5,30], is associated with a greater E_{rot} in full extension of the elbow, whereas an epicondyle with a lower degree of retroflexion has greater values of E_{rot} in full flexion. Moreover, a more proximally oriented epicondyle enhances E_{rot} in full flexion, whereas when it is more distally oriented, E_{rot} increases in extension. The orientation of the medial epicondyle was reported to present a partially activity dependent plasticity, and so it was hypothesized that it can be modified to enhance certain abilities [30]. In this regard, and in agreement with the abovementioned relationship between E_{rot} and epicondylar orientation, a simple observation of the upper-limb positioning shows that a habitual and continued contraction of PT in full elbow flexion would reorient the epicondyle towards a more proximal position. Conversely, this reorientation would occur distally in full elbow extension. The reported association between the orientation of the medial epicondyle and E_{rot} may have important implications on the evolutionary pathway of the upper-limb skeleton, as this structure plays a central role in the locomotor diversity of primates [5,31–33].

Regarding the carrying angle of the elbow [11], this is the first quantitative insight into its biomechanical implications on forearm rotation. An increase in this angle leads to lower values of E_{rot}. This effect is the greatest in full elbow extension and becomes lower as it is flexed, given that carrying angle is maximal in full extension, decreases during flexion and reaches 0° when the elbow is completely flexed [10,12–14].

Functional implications of forearm rotation

The biomechanical model described here enables to make a thorough quantitative approach to clarify some mechanical aspects about the relationship between PT and forearm and elbow motion. For instance, the results indicate that maximal E_{rot} for each elbow angle is close to the neutral position of the forearm. This position has been commonly associated to the functional position, which minimizes the expenditure of muscular energy as it implies a natural equilibrium between antagonist muscles [10]. Moreover, it entails an enhancement of the precision of the grip, because the forearm axis is in line with the pronation-supination axis [10,34].

Although skeletal structures with different morphologies can have the same E_{rot}, they do not have to imply the same abilities in terms of precision. For instance, if the same force is exerted by PT on two upper-limbs with the same E_{rot}, the one with the greatest curvature will be able to reach a lower rotational angle (File S1 and Fig. S1), and thus a greater rotational precision.

The stability of the elbow joint has relevant implications for sports medicine and other pathological conditions [14,35,36]. During pronation, $\vec{F}'$ plays an important role in the stability of the radio-ulnar joint (see File S1 and Fig. 3), whereas $\vec{F}p$ participates in the radio-humeral stability (see Fig. 1A). The global stability of the elbow is thus enhanced by the combination of both components. Although $\vec{F}p$ is slightly lower when the forearm is supinated, the great $\vec{F}'$ value in this position leads to a better fitting between the radius and the ulna than in pronation [37].

Rotational efficiency and the forces that act during pronation may be associated to the estimations of the discomfort levels done by Mukhopadhyay et al. [38], as the movements implying a high level of discomfort correspond to positions where E_{rot} is low. Moreover, the concept "efficiency" provides information about the rotational stability of a given position, as the work needed to modify the forearm rotational angle depends directly on the value of E_{rot} in each position (see File S1). For a given pronation movement, the model can be used to determine the trajectories of the hand that entail the minimal expenditure of energy for PT. In humans, pronation is usually performed when an object has been reached with the hand supinated and the elbow extended and is then brought closer to the body. The final position of this movement will entail a full flexion of the elbow and a close-to-neutral position of the forearm. This movement implies an increase of PT E_{rot}, which indicates that the energy expenditure of this muscle diminishes when the elbow is flexed (see Fig. 4B). The results show that a great part of this trajectory entails upper-limb positions where $\vec{F}''$ and $\vec{F}r$ have a similar value, i.e. around the forearm position where $F'' = F_r$. This indicates that during this trajectory the forces that the elbow joint is submitted to are quite equilibrated.

These two conditions (equilibrium between forces and increase of E_{rot}) are not observed for other trajectories, such as those where the end point is close to full pronation with the elbow flexed. In this case, the final part of the trajectory entails a decrease of E_{rot} and very different values of these two force components. If the forearm was very regularly used to perform this movement with important mechanical loads, the disequilibrium could have pathological consequences, as a result of heavy tensions in the radio-ulnar proximal joint. In order to minimize the expenditure of energy and to rebalance the forces, the radial curvature could increase. As reported by our simulations, a rise of the curvature of the radius causes an increase of E_{rot} and a displacement of the position where $F_r = 0$ towards full pronation, as well as a displacement of the position where $\vec{F}r$ and $\vec{F}''$ become equal from supination towards a position closer to the neutral.

Therefore, the results of the current study also indicate that the upper-limb skeleton may experience plastic changes as a result of PT activity when it is used in positions where E_{rot} is low and forces are not equilibrated. These changes entail an improvement of these parameters, in order to adjust to the unfavorable conditions.

Conversely, if the upper-limb is mainly used in positions with high E_{rot} values, PT will not trigger changes in the skeletal structure. Overall, E_{rot} and its relationship with energy expenditure and rotational stability, as well as the relative values of the force components, which are linked to the joint stability, provide a global insight into pronation and its association to the forearm skeletal structure. These findings will be useful for future analyses on ergonomics and orthopaedics of the upper-limb skeleton, as they provide relevant information about the relationship between PT functionality and the skeletal structure.

Applying this biomechanical model on studies about comparative anatomy of primate taxa would provide valuable information about the functional meaning of the upper-limb skeletal interspecific differences, which will probably be associated to the locomotor abilities of each taxon. Moreover, an analysis of PT E_{rot} and force components on a fossil primate would very useful for inferring its upper-limb involvement in locomotion.

Some skeletal parameters essential for the determination of PT functionality, such as the radial curvature and the medial epicondylar form, are reported to be plastic and related to the usage of PT muscle [15,30]. Therefore, this biomechanical model would also be of great interest if applied to ancient human populations. Differences in parameters derived or related to E_{rot} between sexes, groups or populations would account for differences in occupational and habitual activities.

Supporting Information

Figure S1 Diagrams showing the displacement caused by a force in different scenarios. A: Linear displacement (Δs) and rotational angle ($\Delta\theta$) caused by a force $\vec{F}$ on a rotating body, being the center of rotation O and the rotational radius R. **B:** Representation of the differences in the force ($\vec{F}_1$ and $\vec{F}_2$) that are needed to obtain the same rotational angle when the rotation performed by pronator teres muscle starts at a different point (A_1 and A_2) (see Fig. 3). **C:** Representation of the differences in the rotational angle ($\Delta\theta_1$ and $\Delta\theta_2$) obtained when the same force ($\vec{F}$) is applied by pronator teres muscle on two radii with different rotational radius (r_1 and r_2) (see Fig. 3). Note that the same linear displacement (Δs) is obtained in both cases.

Acknowledgments

The authors are grateful to Antoni Morros for his assistance in the preparation of the artwork. They are also indebted to the Academic Editor, David Carrier, and an anonymous reviewer for their comments on an earlier version of the manuscript.

Author Contributions

Conceived and designed the experiments: PI IG JM. Performed the experiments: PI JM. Analyzed the data: PI IG XJ AM JM. Contributed reagents/materials/analysis tools: XJ AM. Wrote the paper: PI JM. Revised the paper: PI IG XJ AM JM.

References

1. Murray WM, Buchanan TS, Delp SL (2002) Scaling of peak moment arms of elbow muscles with upper extremity bone dimensions. J Biomech 35: 19–26.
2. Tsaopoulos DE, Maganaris CN, Baltzopoulos V (2007) Can the patellar tendon moment arm be predicted from anthropometric measurements? J Biomech 40: 645–651.
3. Galtés I, Jordana X, Cos M, Malgosa A, Manyosa J (2008) Biomechanical model of pronation efficiency: New insight into skeletal adaptation of the hominoid upper limb. Am J Phys Anthropol 135: 293–300.
4. Galtés I, Jordana X, Malgosa A, Manyosa J (2009) Technical note: Forearm pronation efficiency analysis in skeletal remains. Am J Phys Anthropol 140: 589–594.
5. Ibáñez-Gimeno P, Jordana X, Manyosa J, Malgosa A, Galtés I (2012) 3D analysis of the forearm rotational efficiency variation in humans. Anat Rec 295: 1092–1100.
6. Gordon KD, Pardo RD, Johnson JA, King GJW, Miller TA (2004) Electromyographic activity and strength during maximum isometric pronation and supination efforts in healthy adults. J Orthop Res 22: 208–213.
7. O'Sullivan LW, Gallwey TJ (2002) Upper-limb surface electro-myography at maximum supination and pronation torques: the effect of elbow and forearm angle. J Electromyogr Kines 12: 275–285.
8. ScanStudio HD 1.2.1 (2006) Software for Windows. Santa Monica: NextEngine, Inc.
9. Rhinoceros 4.0 SR1 (2007) Educational Edition for Windows. Seattle: Robert McNeel & Associates.
10. Kapandji AI (2002) Fisiología articular, miembro superior. Madrid: Editorial Médica Panamericana.
11. Knussmann R (1967) Humerus, ulna und radius der Simiae. Bibl Primatol 5: 1–399.
12. Morrey BF, Chao EYS (1976) Passive motion of the elbow joint. J Bone Joint Surg Am 58: 501–508.
13. Rouvière H, Delmas A (1988) Anatomía humana: Descriptiva, topográfica y funcional, tomo III, 9th ed. Barcelona: Masson.
14. Goto A, Moritomo H, Murase T, Oka K, Sugamoto K, et al. (2004) In vivo elbow biomechanical analysis during flexion: Threedimensional motion analysis using magnetic resonance imaging. J Shoulder Elbow Surg 13: 441–447.
15. Galtés I, Jordana X, Manyosa J, Malgosa A (2009) Functional implications of radial diaphyseal curvature. Am J Phys Anthropol 138: 286–292.
16. Murray WM, Delp SL, Buchanan TS (1995) Variation of muscle moment arms with elbow and forearm position. J Biomech 28: 513–525.
17. Haugstvedt JR, Berger RA, Berglund LJ (2001) A mechanical study of the moment-forces of the supinators and pronators of the forearm. Acta Orthop Scand 72: 629–634.
18. Lan N, Baker L (2004) Biomechanical couplings between elbow and forearm movements. Conf Proc IEEE Eng Med Biol Soc 6: 4661–4664.
19. Bremer AK, Sennwald GR, Favre P, Jacob HAC (2006) Moment arms of forearm rotators. Clin Biomech 21: 683–691.
20. Hale R, Dorman D, Gonzalez RV (2011) Individual muscle force parameters and fiber operating ranges for elbow flexion-extension and forearm pronation-supination. J Biomech 44: 650–656.
21. O'Sullivan LW, Gallwey TJ (2001) Forearm discomfort for repeated isometric torque exertions in pronation and supination. In: Hanson MA, editor. Contemporary ergonomics 2001. London: Taylor and Francis. pp. 79–83.
22. Basmajian JV, Latif A (1957) Integrated actions and functions of the chief flexors of the elbow: A detailed electromyographic analysis. J Bone Joint Surg Am 39-A: 1106-1118.
23. Naito A, Shimizu Y, Handa Y, Ichie M, Hoshimiya N (1991) Functional anatomical studies of the elbow movements I: Electromyographic (EMG) analysis. Okajimas Folia Anat Jpn 68: 283–288.
24. Latarjet M, Ruiz Liard A, Pró E (2004) Anatomía humana. Buenos Aires: Médica Panamericana.
25. Trinkaus E, Churchill SE (1988) Neandertal radial tuberosity orientation. Am J Phys Anthropol 75: 15–21.
26. Aiello L, Dean C (1990) An introduction to human evolutionary anatomy. London: Academic Press.
27. Tuttle RH, Hollowed JR, Basmajian JV (1992) Electromyography of pronators and supinators in great Apes. Am J Phys Anthropol 87: 215–226.
28. Rose MD (1993). Functional anatomy of the elbow and forearm in primates. In: Gebo DL, editor. Postcranial adaptation in nonhuman primates. DeKalb: Northern Illinois University Press. pp. 70–95.
29. Jablonski NG, Leakey MG, Kiarie C, Antón M (2002) A new skeleton of *Theropithecus brumpti* (Primates: Cercopithecidae) from Lomekwi, West Turkana, Kenya. J Hum Evol 43: 887–923.
30. Ibáñez-Gimeno P, Galtés I, Jordana X, Fiorin E, Manyosa J, et al. (2013) Entheseal changes and functional implications of the humeral medial epicondyle. Int J Osteoarchaeol 23: 211–220.
31. Seiffert ER, Simons EL, Fleagle JG (2000) Anthropoid humeri from the late Eocene of Egypt. Proc Natl Acad Sci 97: 10062–10067.
32. Ciochon RL, Gunnell GF (2004) Eocen large-bodied primates of Myanmar and Thailand: Morphological considerations and phylogenetic affinities. In: Ross CF, Kay RF, editors. Anthropoid origins: New visions. New York: Kluwer Academic/Plenum Publishers. pp. 249–282.
33. MacPhee R, Meldrum J (2006) Postcranial remains of the extinct monkeys of the Greater Antilles, with evidence for semiterrestriality in *Paralouatta*. Am Mus Novit 3516: 3–65.

34. Marzke MW (1997) Precision grips, hand morphology, and tools. Am J Phys Anthropol 102: 91–110.
35. Shiba R, Sorbie C, Siu DW, Bryant JT, Cooke TDV, et al. (1988) Geometry of the humeroulnar joint. J Orthop Res 6: 897–906.
36. Richards RR (1996) Chronic disorders of the forearm. J Bone Joint Surg Am 78: 916–930.
37. Morrey BF, An KN, Stormont TJ (1988) Force transmission through the radial head. J Bone Joint Surg Am 70: 250–256.
38. Mukhopadhyay P, O'Sullivan L, Gallwey TJ (2007) Estimating upper limb discomfort level due to intermittent isometric pronation torque with various combinations of elbow angles, forearm rotation angles, force and frequency with upper arm at 90° abduction. Int J Ind Ergonom 37: 313–325.

Multiscale, Converging Defects of Macro-Porosity, Microstructure and Matrix Mineralization Impact Long Bone Fragility in NF1

Jirko Kühnisch[1,2]*, Jong Seto[3,4], Claudia Lange[3,5], Susanne Schrof[6], Sabine Stumpp[1], Karolina Kobus[2], Julia Grohmann[2], Nadine Kossler[2], Peter Varga[6], Monika Osswald[2], Denise Emmerich[1,2], Sigrid Tinschert[7,8], Falk Thielemann[9], Georg Duda[6,10], Wenke Seifert[11], Thaqif el Khassawna[12], David A. Stevenson[13], Florent Elefteriou[14], Uwe Kornak[1,2], Kay Raum[6], Peter Fratzl[3,10], Stefan Mundlos[1,2,10], Mateusz Kolanczyk[1,2]*

1 Institute for Medical Genetics and Human Genetics, Charité - Universitätsmedizin Berlin, Berlin, Germany, **2** FG Development & Disease, Max Planck Institute for Molecular Genetics, Berlin, Germany, **3** Department of Biomaterials, Max Planck Institute for Colloids and Interfaces, Potsdam, Germany, **4** Department of Chemistry, Universität Konstanz, Konstanz, Germany, **5** Institut für Physiologische Chemie, MTZ, Medizinische Fakultät Carl Gustav Carus, Technische Universität Dresden, Dresden, Germany, **6** Julius Wolff Institute & Brandenburg School of Regenerative Therapies, Charité - Universitätsmedizin Berlin, Berlin, Germany, **7** Division für Humangenetik, Medizinische Universität Innsbruck, Innsbruck, Austria, **8** Institut für Klinische Genetik, Medizinische Fakultät Carl Gustav Carus, Technische Universität Dresden, Dresden, Germany, **9** Klinik für Orthopädie, Medizinische Fakultät Carl Gustav Carus, Technische Universität Dresden, Dresden, Germany, **10** Berlin-Brandenburg Center for Regenerative Therapies, Berlin, Germany, **11** Institute for Vegetative Anatomy, Charité - Universitätsmedizin Berlin, Berlin, Germany, **12** Laboratory of Experimental Trauma Surgery Giessen, Justus-Liebig University Giessen, Giessen, Germany, **13** University of Utah, Department of Pediatrics, Division of Medical Genetics, Salt Lake City, Utah, United States of America, **14** Department of Medicine, Pharmacology and Cancer Biology, Center for Bone Biology, Vanderbilt University - Medical Center, Nashville, Tennessee, United States of America

Abstract

Bone fragility due to osteopenia, osteoporosis or debilitating focal skeletal dysplasias is a frequent observation in the Mendelian disease Neurofibromatosis type 1 (NF1). To determine the mechanisms underlying bone fragility in NF1 we analyzed two conditional mouse models, Nf1Prx1 (limb knock-out) and Nf1Col1 (osteoblast specific knock-out), as well as cortical bone samples from individuals with NF1. We examined mouse bone tissue with micro-computed tomography, qualitative and quantitative histology, mechanical tensile analysis, small-angle X-ray scattering (SAXS), energy dispersive X-ray spectroscopy (EDX), and scanning acoustic microscopy (SAM). In cortical bone of Nf1Prx1 mice we detected ectopic blood vessels that were associated with diaphyseal mineralization defects. Defective mineral binding in the proximity of blood vessels was most likely due to impaired bone collagen formation, as these areas were completely devoid of acidic matrix proteins and contained thin collagen fibers. Additionally, we found significantly reduced mechanical strength of the bone material, which was partially caused by increased osteocyte volume. Consistent with these observations, bone samples from individuals with NF1 and tibial dysplasia showed increased osteocyte lacuna volume. Reduced mechanical properties were associated with diminished matrix stiffness, as determined by SAM. In line with these observations, bone tissue from individuals with NF1 and tibial dysplasia showed heterogeneous mineralization and reduced collagen fiber thickness and packaging. Collectively, the data indicate that bone fragility in NF1 tibial dysplasia is partly due to an increased osteocyte-related micro-porosity, hypomineralization, a generalized defect of organic matrix formation, exacerbated in the regions of tensional and bending force integration, and finally persistence of ectopic blood vessels associated with localized macro-porotic bone lesions.

Editor: Valérie Geoffroy, INSERM U606 - university Paris 7, France

Funding: MK and NK were supported by the Young Investigator Award from Children Tumour Fundation – New York, Grant 2007-01-038 and by Bundesministerium für Bildung und Forschung, Grant NF1-01GM0844 (MK, SM). This work was also supported by the Sixth Framework of the European Commission, EuroGrow project LSHM-CT-2007-037471, and by grant from Berlin-Brandenburg Center for Regenerative Therapies: ("Optimisation and application of a mouse cortical injury system for the survey of new bone anabolic therapies and delivery systems" - Platform A nr-30). DS was supported by a Doris Duke Charitable Foundation Clinical Scientist Development Award and the Thrasher Research Fund. The funders had no role in study design, data collection and analysis, decision to publish, or preparation of the manuscript.

Competing Interests: The authors have declared that no competing interests exist.

* E-mail: jirko.kuehnisch@gmx.de (JK); kolanshy@molgen.mpg.de (MK)

Introduction

Neurofibromatosis type 1 (NF1) is an autosomal dominant disease caused by loss of function mutations in the *NF1* gene, which encodes the Ras-GAP protein neurofibromin. NF1 is frequently associated with skeletal manifestations such as osteopenia, osteoporosis or debilitating focal skeletal dysplasias [1,2,3,4,5]. *NF1* ablation results in activation of canonical mitogen-activated protein kinase (MAPK) signaling. Activation of MAPK signaling modifies PI3K-mTOR, c-Jun N-terminal kinase (JNK), or JAK-

STAT3 signaling, dependent on the cellular context [6,7]. Loss of *NF1* also impacts cAMP-PKA [8], Rho-ROCK-LIMK2-Cofilin [9], and Rac1-Pak1-LIMK1-Cofilin [10] pathways. We have previously shown that conditional inactivation of *Nf1* in mesenchymal progenitor cells of developing limbs (Nf1Prx1) results in diminished long bone growth, tibial bowing, hip joint fusion, and muscle dystrophy [11,12]. Skeletal dysplasia in Nf1Prx1 mice is primarily caused by decreased proliferation and premature hypertrophy of the growth plate chondrocytes and secondly by increased osteoblast proliferation and impaired differentiation [11]. The muscle abnormalities and weakness we observed appear to aggravate the tibial dysplasia phenotype in Nf1Prx1 mice [12]. A much milder bone phenotype, characterized by hyperosteoidosis and high bone turnover, is observed in Nf1Col1 mice. Ablation of *Nf1* in Nf1Col1 mice occurs at the pre-osteoblast stage and is restricted to bone forming cells [13]. Our current view of the NF1 bone pathology, based on the analysis of growth plate chondrocyte, osteoblast and osteoclast dysfunction, is that increased bone turnover and an imbalance between extracellular matrix (ECM) synthesis and mineralization cause the NF1 skeletal manifestations [11,13,14,15]. However, our understanding of the mechanisms underlying long bone fragility in NF1 remains incomplete.

The ultimate strength of individual skeletal elements is determined by several factors, including organ morphology, microscopic tissue structure and molecular organic/inorganic matrix composition [16,17,18]. Long bones typically develop through the process of endochondral ossification, where a cartilaginous template is progressively replaced by trabecular and cortical bone [19,20]. During embryogenesis, bone formation is preceded by blood vessel invasion of the cartilaginous template and consecutive infiltration by mesenchymal and haematopoietic progenitor cells [21,22]. Subsequently, soft tissue templates are entirely replaced with mineralized matrix and most blood vessels are removed [19]. In adult human bones the Haversian system, a network of ~50–100 μm diameter wide channels, facilitates blood supply. These structures are continuously remodeled and account for an estimated macro-porosity of about 5% in the diaphyseal human bone cortex volume [20].

Osteoclast- and osteoblast-driven remodeling of the lacuno-canallicular system is coordinated by osteocytes, the predominant cell type in adult cortical bone (>90%), conferring bone its capability to sense and to respond to mechanical stimuli. Thus, bone strength is critically controlled by osteocytes, which determine micro-porosity, degree of bone matrix formation and quantity as well as properties of deposited mineral [16,17,23,24,25]. Depending on species and age, the volume fraction of osteocyte lacunae in the mammalian cortical bone can vary between 1 and 4% [24,26]. Results of mechanical testing suggest a strong correlation between the osteocyte fraction volume and the elastic modulus [24,26]. However, larger defects originating from bone mineral lesions, or abundant blood vessels, exert a presumably higher impact on the elastic modulus and ultimate strength. On the micro-structural level, bone tissue is a composite of a collagenous framework, integrated small proteins, and the mineral phase formed by carbonated hydroxyapatite (HA) [18,20,23]. The HA mineral phase provides strength and stiffness, while the collagen framework mainly confers toughness [27]. Defects in any one of these components can cause low bone mass and/or diminished bone quality, resulting in bone fragility and increased fracture risk.

Here we apply a combination of biophysical, histological and molecular techniques to give insights into bone structure, micromechanical parameters and material properties. We also assess the underlying cellular changes of bone fragility in the context of *Nf1* deficiency in the mesenchymal lineage. Our analysis sheds light on the previously unrecognized role of osteocytes and blood vessels in the etiology of bone micro-structure and focal cortical bone mineralization defects in Nf1Prx1 mice. These findings suggest that interactions of *Nf1* deficient osteoblasts, osteocytes and blood vessels are important to the development of fragility in NF1 long bone dysplasia.

Materials and Methods

Mouse breeding and genotyping

Nf1Prx1 and Nf1Col1 mice were bred and genotyped as described previously [11,13]. All experimental procedures were approved by the 'Landesamt für Gesundheitsschutz und Technische Sicherheit (LaGeTSi), Berlin, Germany (protocol number ZH 120) and the Institutional Animal Care and Use Committee (IACUC) at the Vanderbilt University Medical Center (protocol number M/06/508).

Histology

For histological analysis, adult limbs were fixed in buffered 4% PFA, dehydrated in subsequent ethanol steps and embedded in methyl methacrylate (MMA) according standard laboratory procedures [28]. For histological assessment, 5 μm plastic sections (RM2255, Leica, Germany) were stained with a combined von Kossa/Masson&Goldner or von Kossa/Toluidin procedure. Bright light microscopy was performed with an Olympus BX60 (Olympus, Japan). To analyze presence of acid bone matrix proteins, sections were stained with AgNOR [29]. Deposited acidic matrix proteins appear brown with AgNOR staining, while negative regions remain unstained. The collagenous bone matrix was assessed with bright or polarized light microscopy after picrosirius red staining [30,31] (Leica DMRB, Germany). Linear polarization microscopy was performed with a Leica DMRB at which the polarization and analyst filters were set with 90° to each other. In bright light, picrosirius red stains all collagenous connective tissue (e.g. bone) red. By polarized microscopy, collagen fibers appear in shades of green, yellow and red. The polarization color indicates fiber thickness and degree of packaging [30,31]. Red colored collagen fibers are highly packed and thick, while green colored fibers are less packed and disorganized [31]. Histomorphometric analysis was performed with AxioVision Software (Zeiss, Germany). Nomenclature was used according to ASBMR guidelines [32]. The ASBMR nomenclature does not provide a term for blood vessels, we used BlVes. Statistical analysis was performed with the unpaired t-test, * $p \leq 0.05$, ** $p \leq 0.01$.

Immunohistology

Immunodetection of proteins within mineralized cortical bone was achieved according to standard procedure [33]. Frozen tissue was sectioned (5 μm) on a cryostat (Leica CM3050 S, Wetzlar, Germany). Sections were fixed in PBS buffered 4% PFA, then permeabilized with 0.1% saponin in PBS buffered 3% BSA, and blocked with 5% donkey serum. Antibodies were incubated in PBS buffered 3% BSA. The following antibodies were used for immunodetection: panendothelial cell antigen (550563, BD Pharmingen, USA) and anti-ratAlexa555 (A11081, Invitrogen, USA). Sections were analyzed with confocal microscopy (lsm 510, Zeiss, Germany).

Micro computed tomography (microCT) analysis

Bone samples were analyzed with low (6 μm voxel) or high (up to 1 μm voxel) resolution microCT from skyscan 1172 (skyscan,

Belgium). For BMD analysis, samples were measured with a multi-sample holder at a 6 μm pixel size, 180° degree rotation, rotation angle 0.3°, filter Al 0.5 mm, averaging 4, random movement 3, voltage 80 kV, and current 120 μA. Raw data reconstruction occurred with NRecon, with a defined threshold of 0.00 to 0.10, smoothing 3, ring artefact correction 9, and beam hardening correction 30%. Quantitative evaluation was performed with CTan after definition of appropriated regions of interest (ROIs). For analysis of cortical bone porosity, samples were measured as single samples at 1 μm pixel size, 180° degree rotation, rotation angle 0.3°, filter Al 0.5 mm, averaging 4, random movement 10, voltage 80 kV, and current 120 μA. Quantitative evaluation was performed with CTan within a ROI comprising 1300 slices. Nomenclature was used according ASBMR guidelines [32]. We used the terminology micro-porosity for Ot. lacunae (lacunae range from 100–4000 μm^3) and macro-porosity (lacunae range 0.05–1*10^6 μm^3) for large non-mineralized structures. Volumes for large pores comprise volumes occupied by blood vessels and non-mineralized bone tissue. Statistical analysis was performed with the unpaired t-test, * $p \leq 0.05$, ** $p \leq 0.01$.

Sample preparation for mechanical tensile measurements

Bone samples were sectioned from the mid-diaphysis of femora of three-month old mice and at other time points (Table S2). Femora were sectioned along the tangential-longitudinal plane. Each half of the femoral cortex was polished mechanically from both sides in an automatic polisher (Logitech PM5, Logitech Ltd., Glasgow, UK) until the sample was planar. Care was taken to make sure the samples' longitudinal axes were parallel to the main longitudinal bone axis. Polishing was performed using sequentially 5, 3, and 1 μm grit-sized diamond particles (DP-Spray P, Struers A/S, Ballerup, Denmark) until the final sample thickness of 50 μm was achieved. Gross sectioning of cortical bones was performed with a slow speed saw (Isomet Low Speed Saw, Buehler Ltd., Lake Bluff, IL, USA) and further processed by UV laser micro-dissection, prior to spectroscopic and micro-mechanical probing of the tissues. The samples were further sectioned in an UV laser micro-dissection system (PALM MicroBeam C, P.A.L.M. Micro-laser Technologies GmbH, Bernried, Germany) to isolate sections with the dimension of 150 μm width×50 μm thickness ×2.5 mm length. All sectioning and micro-dissection were performed on hydrated samples.

Mechanical Tensile analysis

Tensile analysis was performed as described elsewhere [34]. Tensile experiments were performed with a custom-made micro-tensile testing apparatus with a translation motor (M-126.DG, Physik Instrumente, Karlsruhe, Germany) and a 250 g load cell (ALD-MINI-UTC-250, A.L. Design Inc., Buffalo, NY, USA) at a constant strain rate of 0.2 μm s^{-1} to simulate quasi-static loading. Each sectioned sample was glued to stiff teflon foils with cyanoacrylate (Loctite Deutschland GmbH, Munich, Germany) and mounted into the tensile apparatus so that the tensile axis was parallel to the longitudinal axis of the sample. Strain measurements were accomplished by measuring the percent displacement between optical marks made by a 50 μm tip sized marker (Copic Multiliner, Too Marker Products, Japan) on the sample and tracked by a video camera (Basler A101f, Basler Vision Technologies, Ahrensburg, Germany). Both the camera and the tensile tester were controlled by customized software (Labview 7.0, National Instruments). Each sample was tensed until fracture. Stress-strain behaviours were obtained for each sample measurement and further analysis were performed to determine characteristic material properties. Each data point tested was a mean average of three samples. All samples were kept hydrated during measurements and tensed until failure.

Scanning acoustic microscopy (SAM)

SAM measurements were performed as described elsewhere [35]. Methylmethacrylate (MMA) embedded humeri were longitudinally sectioned to medial level, showing a complete open bone marrow cavity and separated anterior and posterior cortex. Subsequently, flat sample surfaces were prepared with a grinding procedure, using silicon carbide abrasive papers (grit size 4000; Phoenix 4000, Buehler, Düsseldorf, Germany). Afterwards the surface was polished with a hard synthetic cloth, ethyleneglycol suspension and 1 μm diamond particles. Samples were measured using a custom-made scanning acoustic microscope (SAM200Ex, Q-BAM, Halle, Germany) equipped with a spherically focused transducer with a nominal center frequency of 200 MHz (FHI 200/60°: Frauenhofer Institut für Biomedizinische Technik, St. Ingbert, Germany), providing a spatial resolution of approximately 8 μm in the focal plane. All measurements were performed in distilled and degassed water at 26±0.3°C. The sample surfaces were aligned in the focal plane of the transducer. A scan increment of 4 μm in x and y direction was chosen. For each (x,y) position the entire pulse echo signal $V_{x,y}(t)$ was stored. After the x,y scan, another x-scan with variable transducer-sample distance (z-scan) was performed for each sample within a bone area to perform a defocus correction. The confocal reflection amplitude was converted to values of the reflection coefficient R and acoustic impedance Z (in Mrayl; 1 rayl = 1 $kgm^{-2}s^{-1}$), as described elsewhere [35]. The latter is equivalent to the square root of the product of mass density and apparent stiffness coefficient c [36]. For bone tissue, Z has been shown to be strongly correlated with the apparent stiffness ($R^2 = 0.996$) [37,38] and can therefore be used as a surrogate to assess variations of tissue stiffness.

Small-angle X-ray scattering (SAXS) and energy dispersive X-ray spectroscopy (EDX)

SAXS measurements were performed as described elsewhere [39]. Longitudinal sections of MMA embedded humerus with a thickness in the order of the beam size (around 200 μm) were mounted on an automatic sample holder for polishing such that the longitudinal cross section is exposed at the surface. An X-ray beam with a wavelength of $\lambda = 0.154$ nm was generated using an X-ray generator (Bruker, AXS, Karlsruhe, Germany) with a rotating copper anode (40 kV/100 mA). The SAXS signal was measured with a 2D area detector (Bruker). Measurements were performed within cortical bone, following the bone cortex from proximal to distal in ~400 μm step size. Two-dimensional SAXS patterns were evaluated for mean mineral particle thickness (T-parameter) and degree of particle alignment (Rho-parameter). The T-parameter measures the average thickness of mineral particles and higher values suggest increased volume of mineral platelets. The Rho-parameter indicates the relative orientation of mineral particles, where value "0" specifies no predominant orientation while "1" suggests parallel alignment.

EDX measurements were performed with a desktop scanning electron microscope (SEM) device (Hitachi TM-3000, Hitachi High-Technologies Europe GmbH, Krefeld Germany) on MMA embedded humeri that were prepared in a similar fashion to SAXS samples. Samples were mounted onto double sided carbon tape and subsequently, placed in the SEM sample holder and moved approximately until 1 mm away from the source of the primary beam. An accelerating voltage of 15 kV was used to examine the greyscale levels of the mineral content in the respective Nf1Prx1 and Nf1Col1 samples. An EDX unit (Bruker SAXS GmbH, Berlin Germany) was used to collect elemental spectra, specifically at energies corresponding to 2.0 and 3.7 keV, representing spectral signals for phosphorus and calcium, respectively. Whole EDX maps were created to map mineralization degree and element gradients in whole humeri tissues from respective Nf1Prx1 samples. Analysis of EDX images was performed with ImageJ (Rasband WS. ImageJ, U.S. National Institutes of Health, Bethesda, Maryland, USA, imagej.nih.gov/ij/ , 1997–2012).

Results

Blood vessel associated mineralization defects destabilize Nf1Prx1 bone diaphysis

Long bones of Nf1Prx1 mice show significant shortening, bowing and reduced trabecular bone mass [11]. To get insights into the cortical bone quality, we analyzed diaphyseal bone morphology at three months of age with high resolution micro-computed tomography (microCT). Since hind limb movement in Nf1Prx1 mice is compromised due to a hip joint fusion, we focused our analysis on the humerus. Control humeri had a straight shape with a pronounced *tuberositas deltoideus* (A1), a distinct *arteria nutriens* traversing channel (A2) and solid bone cortex (A3) (Fig. 1A). By histology, the left and right bone cortex (A4, A5) appeared fully mineralized and rarely populated by blood vessels (Fig. 1A). In Nf1Prx1 mice microCT scans revealed enlarged and porous *tuberositas deltoideus* (B1) compared to controls (Fig. 1B). The main artery *arteria nutriens* (B2), which supplies blood to the bone marrow cavity, was strikingly enlarged in Nf1Prx1 mutants (Fig. 2B). Additionally, massive cortical bone defects (B3) were present in the distal humerus (Fig. 2B) of Nf1Prx1 mice that were absent in controls. Histological analysis (von Kossa/Masson&Goldner) demonstrates that these bone lesions were in fact regions of non-mineralized bone matrix (osteoid) adjacent to ectopic blood vessels (B4, B5) (Fig. 2B). In Nf1Col1 mice, characterized by *Nf1* inactivation in osteoblasts, the *tuberositas deltoideus* was enlarged and irregularly shaped (C1); however, the *arteria nutriens* had normal size (C2) (Fig. 2C). Fewer and smaller non-mineralized areas were observed in Nf1Col1 mice in the region where large demineralization spots were present in Nf1Prx1 humeri (C3, C4, C5) (Fig. 2C). Next, we quantified macro-porosities using histological and microCT methods. The relative osteoid area (O.Ar/B.Ar) and relative blood vessel area (BlVes.Ar/B.Ar) per bone area were increased in Nf1Prx1 mice by 25- and 12-fold, respectively (O.Ar/B.Ar: ctrl $= 0.0035 \pm 0.0026\%$; Nf1Prx1 $= 0.0908 \pm 0.1254\%$; BlVes.Ar/B.Ar: ctrl $= 0.0003 \pm 0.0003\%$; Nf1Prx1 $= 0.0037 \pm 0.0028\%$), in the ROI E2 (Fig. 1D). Quantitative microCT analysis corroborated these results. Both the relative summed lacunae volume (Lc.V/Ct.BV) and the relative lacunae number (Lc.N/Ct.BV) per cortical bone volume were increased (Lc.V/Ct.BV: ctrl $= 0.0022 \pm 0.0006$; Nf1Prx1 $= 0.0079 \pm 0.0011$, Lc.N/Ct.BV: ctrl $= 23.0 \pm 8.0 * 10^{-9}$ n/μm^3; Nf1Prx1 $= 62.0 \pm 21.0 * 10^{-9}$ n/μm^3) (Fig. 1E; Table S1). In contrast, no significant increase in blood vessel related bone porosity was observed in Nf1Col1 mice (Lc.V/Ct.BV: ctrl $= 0.0039 \pm 0.0003$; Nf1Col1 $= 0.0041 \pm 0.0017$; Lc.N/Ct.BV: ctrl $= 28.2 \pm 7.3 * 10^{-9}$ n/μm^3; Nf1Col1 $= 36.2 \pm 13.4 * 10^{-9}$ n/μm^3) (Table S1).

We confirmed the vascular endothelial identity of the cells within macro-porotic bone defects in Nf1Prx1 mice using immune-staining against pan-endothelial antigen (Fig. 1F). Additionally, vessel associated bone lesions were detected in humerus sections from all analyzed stages (P14, P35 and P49), suggesting a developmental origin of the phenotype (Fig. 1G). In addition, significant presence of these lesions in Nf1Prx1 mice (limb knock-out) but less voluminous in Nf1Col1 mice (osteoblast knock-out) suggests an endothelial lineage involvement in the pathogenesis of these changes.

Reduced thickness and packaging of collagen in the proximity of diaphyseal blood vessels

Organic matrix appearance in blood vessel proximity was analyzed with picrosirus red and AgNOR histology. Similar to other matrix demineralization areas in *Nf1* deficient bones, the matrix near blood vessels stained pale-green with picrosirus red in polarized light indicating presence of collagen with reduced thickness as well as packaging (Fig. 2A). The AgNOR method gave intensive staining at the mineralization front, surrounding blood vessels, but the mineral-free zone in direct contact with the vessel was not stained (Fig. 2B). A possible cartilaginous nature of this organic matrix was excluded by Toluidin and Safranin O histology (Fig. 2C). Moreover, Toluidin and Safranin O staining demonstrated viability of osteocytes within mineralized and non-mineralized bone tissue. In summary, vessel-associated diaphyseal bone lesions contain collagen with reduced thickness and packaging that may, due to their large volumes, weaken cortical bone stability.

Micro-dissected slices of NfPrx1 bone tissue are mechanically fragile

Since large matrix mineralization defects in the Nf1Prx1 diaphysis were local, we asked if micro-scale properties of the mineralized bone tissue were also altered. In order to measure mechanical strength of the bone material, we performed tensile analysis on bone tissue slices obtained by laser micro-dissection (Fig. 3A). Typical tensile test traces are composed of three phases, the elastic modulus, yield point, and ultimate strength. The linear slope gives the elastic modulus (Young's or E-modulus), the yield point is where the stress-strain curve levels off and inelastic sample deformation begins to occur and the ultimate strength is obtained from the stress point where the bone material ruptures (Fig. 3B). Bone tissue slices from adult Nf1Prx1 humeri showed a 50% reduction of E-modulus (ctrl $= 27.5 \pm 9.9$ GPa; Nf1Prx1 $= 15.0 \pm 6.7$ GPa) and 35% decrease of ultimate strength compared to controls (ctrl $= 103.9 \pm 35.8$ MPa; Nf1Prx1 $= 67.8 \pm 27.5$ MPa) (Fig. 3C–D). A similar reduction of the bone material mechanical strength was observed in samples from other developmental stages (P4, P18, P60, P120) (Table S2). Although cortical bone slices with large defects were excluded from the analysis, mutant bone slices often contained microscopically visible large porosities that were not observed in controls (data not shown). The increased macro-porosity could explain mechanical instability. However, other factors including micro-porosity, degree of bone tissue mineralization and organic matrix quality are also likely to be involved [16,17,23,24,25,26].

Increased micro-porosity in Nf1Prx1 and Nf1Col1 bone tissue due to osteocyte lacunae enlargement

To understand the cause of decreased bone material mechanical resistance, we analyzed osteocyte (Ot.) lacunae size and number in Nf1Prx1 and Nf1Col1 humeri using high resolution microCT. We analyzed cortical bone within the diaphyseal ROI E2 (Fig. 1A). The summed Ot. lacunae volume per bone volume (Lc.V/BV) was almost doubled in Nf1Prx1 and significantly increased in Nf1Col1 mice compared to respective controls (level E2: ctrl $= 0.020 \pm 0.007\%$, Nf1Prx1 $= 0.034 \pm 0.011\%$; ctrl $= 0.036 \pm 0.003\%$, Nf1Col1 $= 0.041 \pm 0.002\%$) (Fig. 3E, Table S1). Lacunae volume distribution (the summed lacunae volume within a 100 μm^3 size

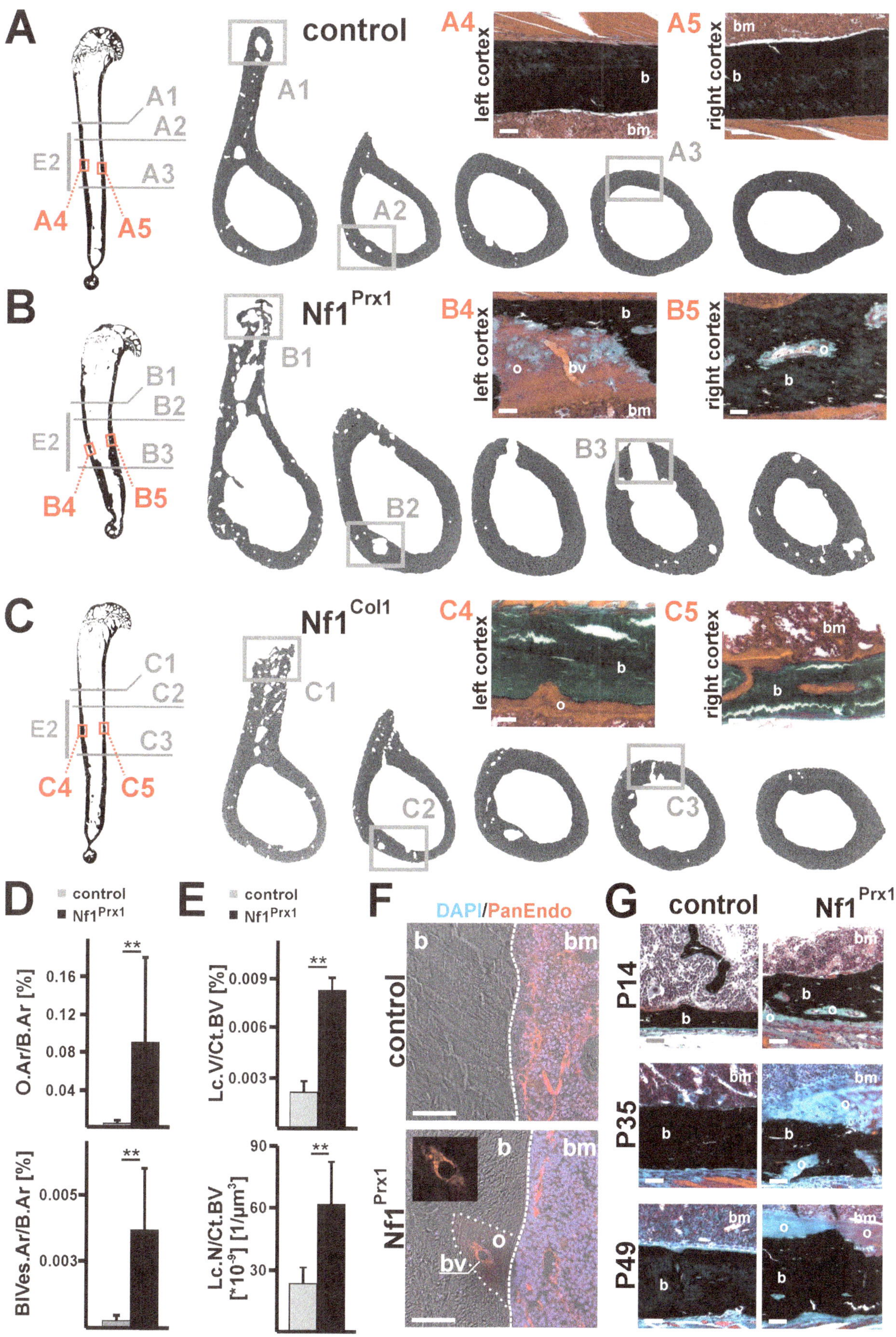
A
control
A1
A2
A3
A4
A5
E2
left cortex
right cortex
b
bm
B
Nf1 Prx1
B1
B2
B3
B4
B5
o
bv
C
Nf1 Col1
C1
C2
C3
C4
C5
D
control
Nf1 Prx1
O.Ar/B.Ar [%]
BlVes.Ar/B.Ar [%]
**
E
Lc.V/Ct.BV [%]
Lc.N/Ct.BV [*10^-9] [1/µm^3]
F
DAPI/PanEndo
G
P14
P35
P49

Figure 1. Nf1Prx1 mice show increased macro-porosity and ectopic blood vessels associated mineralization defects. (**A–C**) High-resolution micro-CT (skyscan) and von Kossa/Masson-Goldner histology of adult humeri. Consecutive cross-sections of the mid-shaft region (E2) in Nf1Prx1, Nf1Col1 and control mice representing following morphological sites: deltoid tuberosity (1), nutrient artery (2), bone cortex between deltoid tuberosity and epicondylus medialis (3), left cortex (4), and right cortex (5). (**A**) (A1) Deltoid tuberosity of controls showed solid appearance and smooth mineralization front. (A2) The site of nutrient artery bone cortex traverse. Note a fully mineralized, solid cortical bone in proximity of blood vessel. (A3, A4, A5) Diaphyseal cortical bone in control mice was free of macro-pores. (**B**) Morphology of Nf1Prx1 humeri. (B1) Note a broadened and inhomogeneously mineralized tuberosity with rough mineralization boundaries and increased porosity. (B2) A massively enlarged nutrient artery traversing site and (B3) a large ectopic lesions were observed in the cortical bone of Nf1Prx1 mice. (B4, B5) von Kossa/Masson Goldner histology of the diaphyseal bone cortex in blood vessel proximity. Note, unmineralized bone matrix (osteoid) surrounding the centrally localized blood vessel. (**C**) Nf1Col1 mouse humeri. (C1) Mutant deltoid tuberosity is widened with inhomogeneous mineral distribution and uneven bone boundaries. (C2-3) The size of the nutrient artery traversing site within diaphyseal bone cortex was normal in Nf1Col1 mice. (C4-5) In Nf1Col1 cortical bone small mineralization defects show a narrow osteoid rim surrounding blood vessels. These changes were of much smaller size compared to the Nf1Prx1 model. (**D**) Histomorphometric analysis of humerus cortical bone in the region E2 of Nf1Prx1 mice. Increased relative unmineralized bone tissue area (O.Ar/B.Ar) and blood vessel area (BlVes.Ar/B.Ar) (control n = 3, Nf1Prx1 n = 5). (**E**) Volume and number of mineralization defects (lacunae range 0.05–$1*10^6$ μm^3) in Nf1Prx1 cortical bone (region E2). High-resolution scans were evaluated with CTan (skyscan) software. Increased relative cortical bone porosity (summed lacunae volumes per cortical bone volume, Lc.V/Ct.BV) as well as lacunae number (Lc.N/Ct.BV) (control and Nf1Prx1 n = 5) in Nf1Prx1 humeri. Statistical significance - t-test, ** $p \leq 0.001$. (**F**) Immunostaining with pan-endothelial antibody confirms presence of blood vessels within mineralization defects in Nf1Prx1 cortical bone. (**G**) Nf1Prx1 cortical bone in the region E2, von Kossa/Masson-Goldner histology showing mineralization defects through developmental stages P14, P35 and P49. Scale bars - 50 μm. Abbreviations: blood vessels (bv), bone (b), bone marrow (bm), osteoid (o).

interval) was shifted toward larger size intervals within Nf1Prx1 and Nf1Col1 mutant diaphysis (Fig. 3F). Nf1Prx1 mutants showed a peak maximum at 600 μm^3 whereas control samples had a peak maximum at 300 μm^3. Statistical significance of these changes was illustrated for the selected size intervals 100–300 μm^3 and 700–900 μm^3 (Fig. 3F, insets c and d). Similar changes of lacunae volume distribution were observed in Nf1Col1 bones (Fig. 3F, insets a and b). In contrast, relative Ot. number (Ot.N) per bone tissue volume was not altered in the Nf1Prx1 humerus (Fig. 3G). We further assessed lacunae morphology by measuring the x, y and z dimensions. In both mouse models, Nf1Prx1 and Nf1Col1, osteocyte lacunae morphology was enlarged in all measured dimensions (Fig. 3H). Collectively these data indicate that Ot. viability is not impaired by *Nf1* inactivation in bone, but causes increased osteocyte volume and abnormal morphology.

Global defect of bone matrix formation and bone mineral content in *Nf1* deficient cortical bone

To further characterize bone matrix quality in the *Nf1* deficient humerus cortex, we performed acoustic impedance measurements

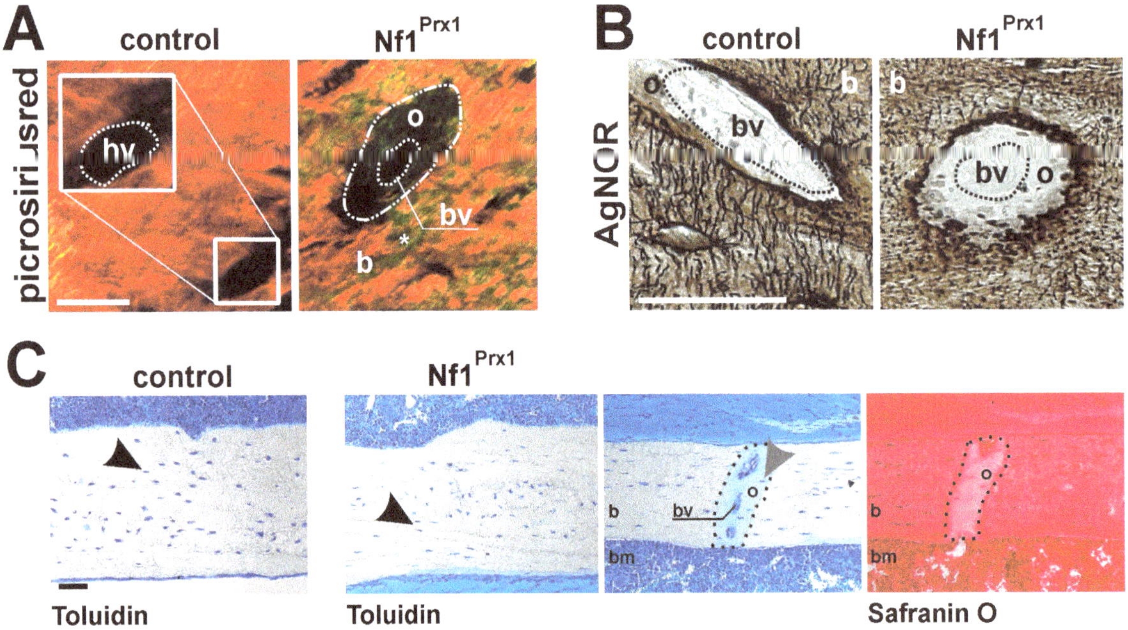

Figure 2. Diminished organic matrix properties in Nf1Prx1 mice. (**A**) Picrosirius red stained bone sections imaged with polarized light. Homogenous red staining in controls indicates highly packed and thick collagen. Heterogeneous red-yellow-green staining of Nf1Prx1 bone sections is indicative of diminished packaging and thickness of bone collagen. Note, there is no picrosirius red staining within non-mineralized bone tissue (osteoid) surrounding blood vessels. Scale bar shows 20 μm. (**B**) Silver staining (AgNOR) detects the osteocytic network and other accumulations of acidic matrix proteins. Note the large unstained area around blood vessels in Nf1Prx1 humerus. Scale bar shows 50 μm. (**C**) Sections of humerus cortex stained with Toluidin and Safranin O. Toluidin stained osteocyte (Ot.) appear blue with dark blue nuclei (black arrowhead). Presence of nuclei suggests vitality of cells in the bone cortex. Osteoid (dotted line) near to the blood vessel was stained light blue (Toluidin) or light red (Safranin O). Light blue or red staining indicates that bone lesions are not composed of cartilaginous matrix, which with these methods stains purple (Toluidin) or dark red (Safranin O) (not shown). Ot. in non-mineralized areas are viable (nuclei marked with grey arrow head). Scale bar represents 50 μm. Abbreviations: blood vessels (bv), bone (b), bone marrow (bm), osteoid (o).

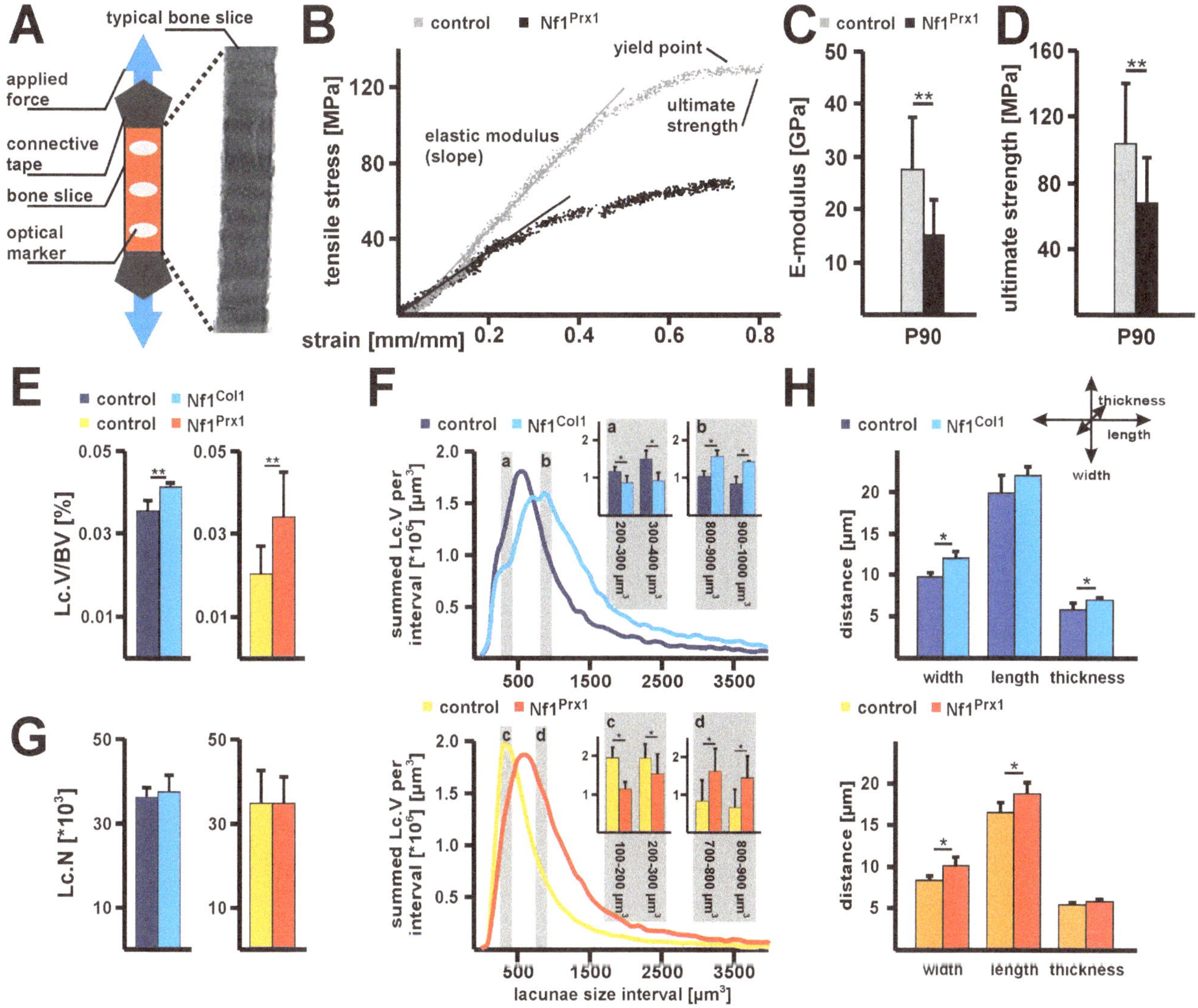

Figure 3. Nf1Prx1 bone tissue shows diminished mechanical strength and increased micro-porosity due to increased osteocyte lacuna size. (A) Diagram of the analytical setup used for tensile experiment. Measurements were done on laser dissected cortical bone slices from P90 mice. (B) A typical tensile stress-strain pattern in controls showed a linear elastic modulus (E-modulus) phase that is followed by the yield point plateau and the ultimate stress point. Note, increased elasticity and diminished ultimate strength in bone slices of Nf1Prx1 humerus compared to controls. (C) Diminished E-modulus (slope of tensile curve) and (D) ultimate stress point (point of maximal load before tissue failure) in bone tissue slices from 3 months old Nf1Prx1 (n = 14) and control (n = 15) mice. (E) Quantitative microCT analysis of the total (summed) lacunae porosity (Lc.V/BV) within the lacunae range from 100-4000 μm^3. Note the significant increase of Lc.V/BV in Nf1Col1 and Nf1Prx1 mice. (F) The summed volume of Ot. lacunae (Lc.V) within the size range 100–4000 μm^3 with an increment of 100 μm^3 (histogram). Note the shift of summed Lc.V fractions towards higher volume range in Nf1Col1 and Nf1Prx1 mutants. Insert (a) - Nf1Col1 mice demonstrated reduced summed Lc. volume in the intervals 200–300 and 300–400 μm^3 and (b) - summed Lc.V in fractions 800–900 and 900–1000 μm^3. Insert (c) - Nf1Prx1 mice showed reduced summed Lc. volume in the intervals 100–200 and 200–300 μm^3 and (d) - summed Lc.V in fractions 700–800 and 800–900 μm^3. (G) The total number of Ot. lacunae (Lc.N) was unaffected in both mouse models. (H) Ot. lacunae morphology (range from 100–4000 μm^3) assessed by measuring the x, y and z axis length in a selected volume of ROI E2. Note, lacunae size is increased in all dimensions in Nf1Col1 and Nf1Prx1 mice. The number of analyzed bone samples: Nf1Prx1 n = 5, controls n = 5; Nf1Col1 n = 3, controls n = 3. Statistical analysis was performed with unpaired Student t-test, * $p \leq 0.05$ ** $p \leq 0.01$.

by scanning acoustic microscopy (SAM). High (red) acoustic impedance values (Z) indicate high stiffness and low Z-values (greenish/blue) soft material properties (Fig. 4A). Selected regions represent the heterogeneity of matrix stiffness throughout the entire humerus bone cortex. Quantitative analysis was performed within six ROIs in anterior and posterior bone cortex (E1–E3). Z-values were heterogeneous throughout humerus cortex length (Fig. 4B). Nf1Prx1 mutant bones had reduced Z-values in ROIs E2 and E3 indicating softening of the mineralized organic matrix in the mid shaft humerus (average Z of all ROI: ctrl = 6.83±0.59 MRayl; Nf1Prx1 = 5.96±0.70 MRayl) (Fig. 4B). However, in Nf1Col1 mice the acoustic impedance was unaffected (average Z of all ROI: ctrl = 5.92±0.69 MRayl; Nf1Col1 = 5.90±0.73 MRayl) (Fig. 4B, Table S3). These results indicate that loss of neurofibromin induces impairment of the bone matrix stiffness that is most pronounced in the bowed part of Nf1Prx1 bones but not in Nf1Col1 bones.

Phantom calibrated microCT was used to assess bone mineral density (BMD) throughout cortical bone in Nf1Prx1 and Nf1Col1 humerus (Fig.S1A). Significant reduction of BMD was detected in Nf1Prx1 (ctrl = 1.299±0.020 g/cm^3, Nf1Prx1 = 1.102±0.027 g/cm^3)

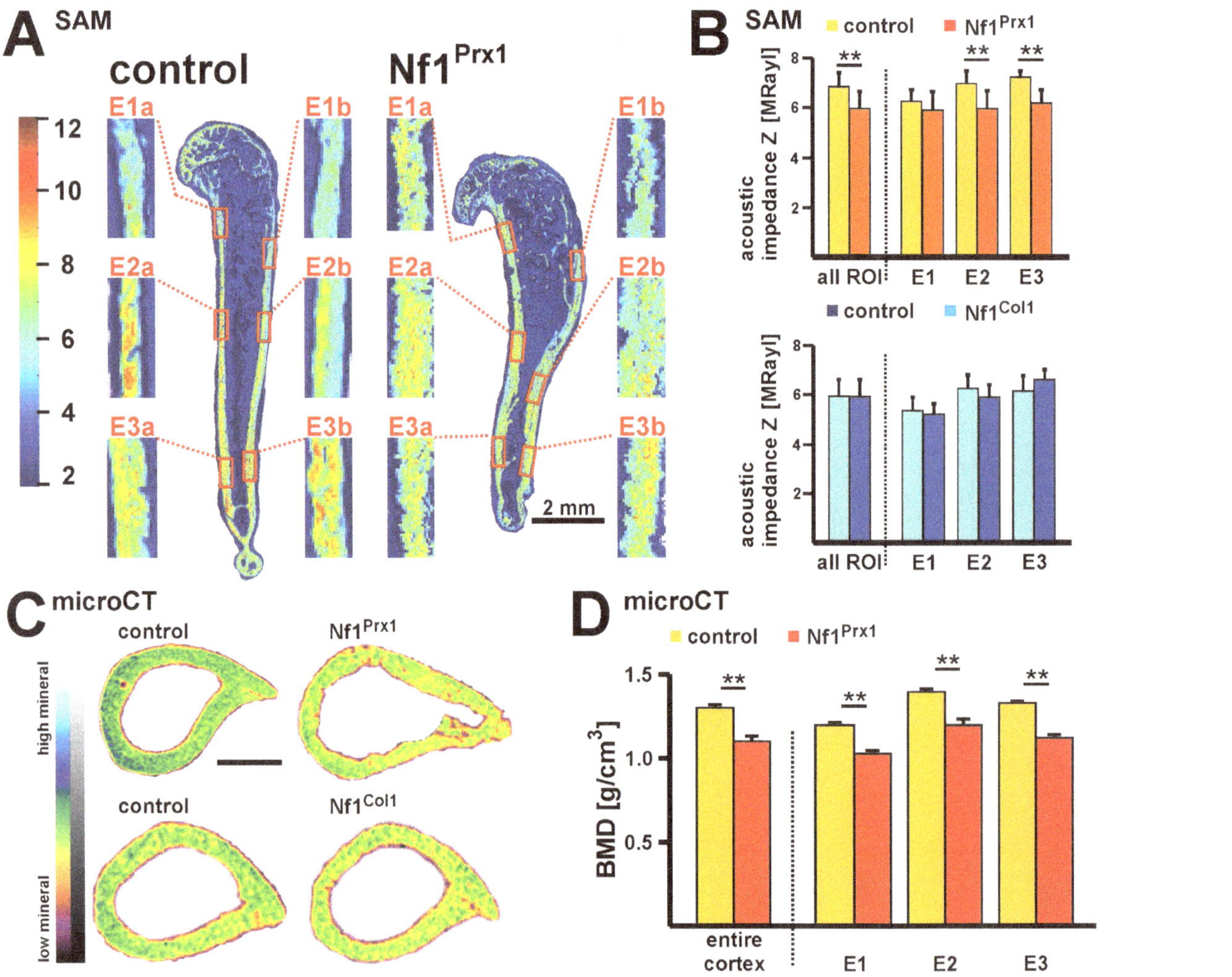

Figure 4. Diminished bone stiffness, bone mineralization and organic matrix formation in Nf1Prx1 mice. (**A**) Scanning acoustic microscopy (SAM) was applied to show elastic properties of the bone matrix. SAM measurements were performed within six ROIs E1a–E3b on anterior (a) and posterior (b) bone cortex. Images illustrate impedance values (Z in MRayl) according to the color scale (left). Nf1Prx1 mutants show diminished impedance values within all analyzed ROIs. (**B**) Quantitative evaluation of SAM measurements reveals decreased Z values in Nf1Prx1 humerus in all analyzed ROIs (control n = 4, Nf1Prx1 n = 4). Nf1Col1 humeri did not demonstrate diminished Z values (control n = 5, Nf1Col1 n = 4). (**C**) The cross sections of humerus at the level E2 with color coded BMD values measured by phantom calibrated microCT. The yellow and green coloring indicates low and high BMD values, respectively. Scale bar - 600 μm. (**D**) Cortical bone mineral density (BMD) was assessed by microCT within region E1–E3 in humeri of Nf1Prx1 (control n = 5, Nf1Prx1 n = 5) mice. BMD was reduced in the Nf1Prx1 model in all ROIs (for definition see Fig.S1). Statistical significance - t-test, * $p \leq 0.05$ and ** $p \leq 0.01$.

and Nf1Col1 mice (ctrl = 1.369±0.007 g/cm^3, Nf1Col1 = 1.271±0.024 g/cm^3) (Fig. 4C–D, Fig.S1A). Similarly to changes in Ot. lacuna size, the degree of BMD reduction was higher in the Nf1Prx1 mice than in the Nf1Col1 model. Low bone mineral content in Nf1Prx1 humerus was confirmed by energy dispersive X-ray spectroscopy (EDX) on three ROIs (E1–E3) (Fig.S1B). The calcium to phosphorus ratio was unaffected in Nf1Prx1 humerus compared to controls (ctrl = 1.9680±0.0772, Nf1Prx1 = 1.9670±0.0636). To obtain information about mineral particle size and orientation, small-angle X-ray scattering (SAXS) imaging was applied. The mean mineral particle thickness and the degree of particle alignment were similar in mutant and control samples (Fig.S1C–D). Thus, *Nf1* deficiency causes low bone mineral density without affecting mineral particle size and orientation.

Bone tissue from individuals with NF1 and tibial dysplasia shows inhomogeneous mineralization, increased micro-porosity and diminished collagen fiber thickness

We analyzed human cortical bone samples that were surgically removed from three individuals with NF1 tibial dysplasia. The samples included a fracture/pseudarthrosis lesion and a cortical bone sample removed pre-fracture. Age matched cortical bone samples were used as controls. Low-resolution microCT analysis of a pre-fracture NF1 tibial dysplasia sample showed thickening of the tibia bone cortex and increased macro-porosity (Fig. 5A). In the control bone sample, bone mineral density (BMD) distribution was homogeneous as revealed by even yellow/red coloring (Hounsfield unit [HU] calibration) and similar BMD values were measured at two distant sites within the bone shaft (ROI1 5028

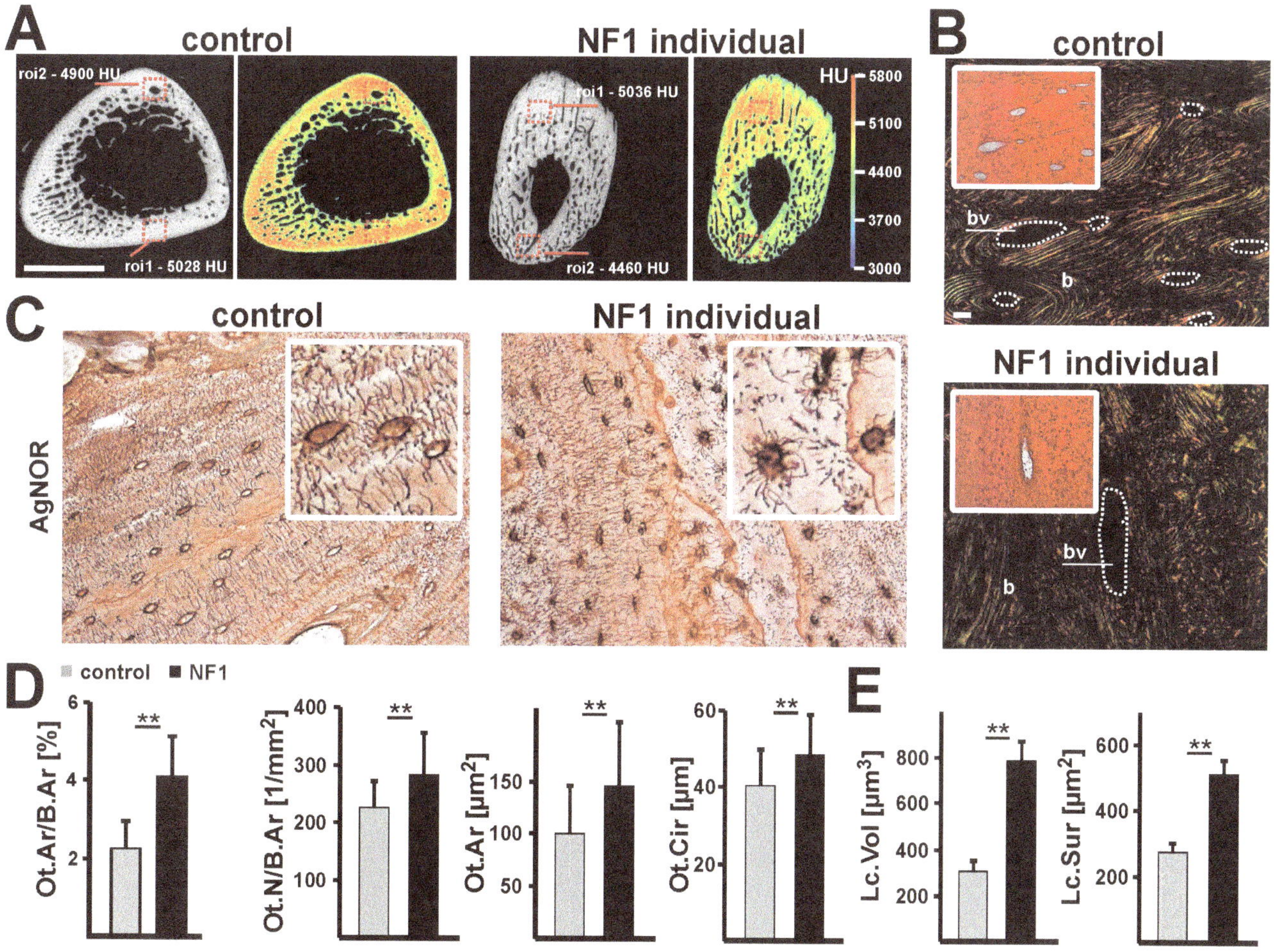

Figure 5. Cortical bone in NF1 tibial dysplasia is characterized by heterogeneous mineralization, diminished collagen thickness and increased micro-porosity. (A) MicroCT analysis of human cortical bone samples (tibia). Bone mineral density was calibrated according to Houndsfield units (HU) and color coded (see HU scale). HU values measured in ROI1 (cortical bone without blood vessels) and ROI2 (cortical bone near blood vessel) were in control specimen similar. However, in the NF1 bone sample HU values were in proximity of large vessels decreased (ROI2). The analyzed bone sample was obtained pre-fracture from an individual affected by NF1 with tibial bowing. (B) Two further mineralized bone samples were obtained from cortical bone of NF1 individuals with pseudarthrosis. Samples were analyzed by picrosirius red histology and imaged in polarized light (large image) and bright light (inset). Collagen fibers follow osteonal organization in control specimens. Note that in the NF1 cortical bone sample collagen fiber organization appears less orderly with abundant thin (green) collagen fibers. (C) Ot. morphology was visualised with AgNOR staining. Ot. are spindle shaped (inset) and regularly distributed in control cortical bone. In contrast, Ot. are round and irregularly distributed in NF1 cortical bone. (D) Histomorphometry of AgNOR stained bone sections showing: relative Ot. area (Ot.Ar/B.Ar), Ot. number per bone area (Ot.N/B.Ar), individual Ot. area (Ot.Ar) and individual Ot. circumference (Ot.Cir). Presented data are mean values with standard deviations (control n = 3, NF1 n = 2). (E) Volumetric microCT analysis showing increased specific lacunae (Ot.) volume (Lc.Vol) and surface (Lc.Sur) in NF1 tibial dysplasia cortical bone as compared to controls. Statistical analysis was performed with unpaired t-test, ** $p \leq 0.01$. Abbreviations: blood vessels (bv) and bone (b). All scale bars represent 50 µm.

and ROI2 4900 HU). In contrast, the NF1 cortical bone sample showed unbalanced mineral distribution with a BMD decrease of approx. 20% between ROI1 (5036 HU) and ROI2 (4460 HU). Picrosirius red stained control bone sections appeared red and yellow under polarized light, which is indicative of highly ordered and thick collagen fibers that followed circular osteonal organization (Fig. 5B). Two further surgically removed bone samples from individuals with NF1 tibial dysplasia, originating from cortical bone adjacent to a pseudarthrotic bone lesion, were analyzed histologically and with microCT. Picrosirius red stained NF1 bone biopsies stained in shades of orange, yellow and green, suggesting presence of less thick and packed collagen fibers. The overall Ot. morphology in NF1 bone samples analyzed by the AgNOR method appeared more heterogeneous and their lacunae size was increased (Fig. 5C). Histomorphometry revealed increased relative Ot. occupied area (Ot.Ar/B.Ar) in NF1 biopsies compared to controls (ctrl 2.25±0.72%; NF1 4.12±1.00%) (control n = 3, NF1 n = 2; analyzed cell number >1500 each group) (Fig. 5D). We also detected a statistically significant increase of Ot. number (Ot.N), individual Ot. area (Ot.Ar) and individual Ot. circumference (Ot.Cir) in NF1 bone samples. Accordingly, volumetric microCT analysis revealed increased Ot. lacunae volume (Lc.Vol) and Ot. surface (Lc.Sur) in NF1 bone samples (Fig. 5E). Thus, NF1 tibial dysplasia cortical bone samples show heterogeneous mineral distribution, poor collagen fiber thickness and increased micro-porosity, which is similar to changes in Nf1Prx1 and Nf1Col1 mice (Fig. 6A–B).

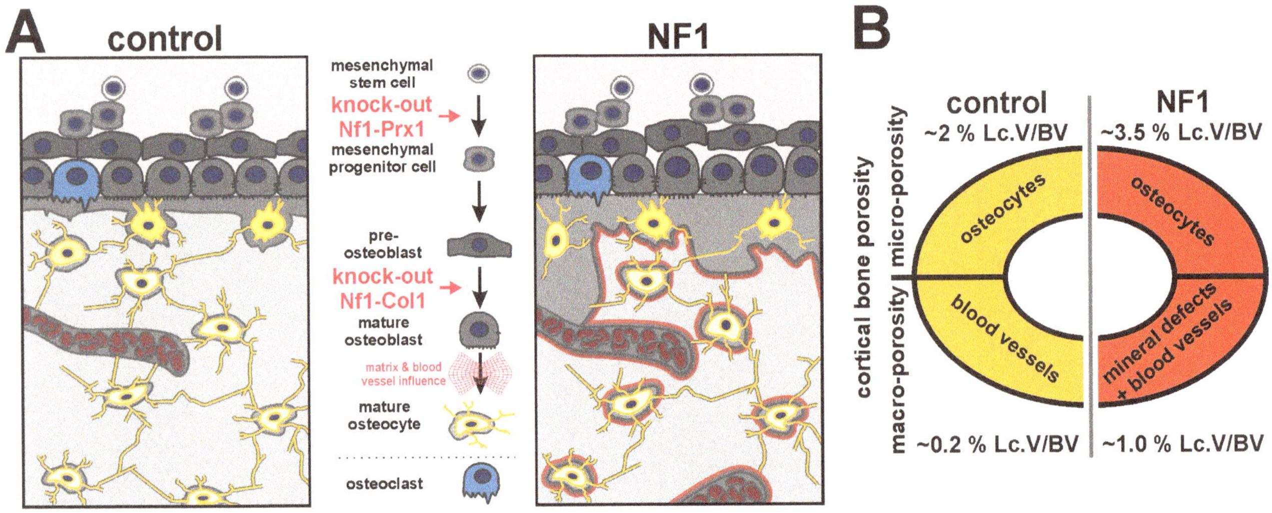

Figure 6. Neurofibromin is a critical regulator of cortical bone integrity and function. (**A**) Ablation of *Nf1* in pre-osteoblasts (Nf1Col1) results in low bone mass phenotype with hyperosteoidosis. Loss of *Nf1* in mesenchymal progenitor cells (Nf1Prx1) produces a complex phenotype characterized by low bone mass, hyperosteoidosis, increased micro-porosity (Ot.), macro-porotic mineralization lesions, and persistence of blood vessels. Moreover, loss of neurofibromin causes defective inorganic and organic bone matrix formation especially in proximity of blood vessels. (**B**) Micro- and macro-porosity contributes differentially to overall structural destabilisation in NF1 bone. In controls micro- (Ot.) and macro-porosity (blood vessels) encompasses approx. 2% and 0.2% of cortical bone volume, respectively. In Nf1Prx1 mutant bone micro-porosity is elevated to approx. 3.5%. Importantly macro-porosity is amplified to 1.0% due to blood vessel persistence and bone mineral lesions.

Discussion

Our analysis indicates that multiple changes contribute to the reduction of bone mechanical strength upon loss of neurofibromin. Previous studies documented dysregulated osteoblast and osteoclast activity in *Nf1* deficient bone, yielding a high-turnover phenotype, reduced bone mass and low bone mineral content [11,13,14,15]. We now show that *Nf1* inactivation affects osteoblasts and osteocytes to various extents, depending on the localization in the cortical bone, with the most dramatic effects seen in the proximity of blood vessels. In blood vessel regions, osteoblast and osteocyte function is compromised, triggering formation of local osteomalatic lesions (Fig. 6A–B).

Based on the localization of these changes within the long bone diaphysis and general long bone bowing, we postulate that one of the factors exacerbating matrix mineralization defects in NF1 is mechanical strain. Mechanical stimuli are required for normal osteoblast and bone development [40]. Upon *Nf1* ablation, diaphyseal accumulation of defective organic bone matrix is most likely triggered by mechanical loads on an already poor bone cortex structure. Mechanical stimulation has been recently shown to induce ERK activation and osteoblast proliferation through integrins [41]. It has also been shown that FGFs control expression of matrix mineralization genes essential for osteocyte differentiation through ERK signaling [41]. Consequently, various aspects of the bone phenotype in Nf1Prx1 mice are linked to hyperactivation of the MAPK pathway throughout bone ontogeny [11,13,28,42]. The net outcome of MAPK signaling in bone appears to be dependent on signal intensity as well as the stage of osteoblast differentiation, with an inhibitory effect in early osteoblasts [43,44], and pro-osteogenic effect in mature osteoblasts [45]. In support of this notion, *Nf1* ablation in early osteoblasts causes decreased matrix mineralization, while inactivation in late osteoblasts has opposite effects [46]. Thus, adequate intensity and timing of MAPK activation are prerequisite for normal bone formation [47].

Loss of *Nf1* has a pro-osteogenic effect in mature osteoblasts in the absence of excessive mechanical stimulation or blood vessel influences. This is strikingly different in areas of high mechanical load (diaphysis) as well as in proximity of blood vessels. In diaphyseal cortical bone, the loss of *Nf1* results in catastrophic deterioration of organic matrix quality and mineralization, resulting in local osteolysis/osteomalacia. Perhaps the most important observation of this study is the discovery of collagen with reduced thickness and packaging in proximity of ectopic blood vessels. Blood vessel-associated diaphyseal defects (macro-porosities) by proportion, contribute the most to the overall reduction of Nf1Prx1 bone structural stability (Fig. 6B). The size of these lesions and localization within the mid-shaft of bone, where the torsion and longitudinal forces coalesce, seems to pre-determine potential fracture sites. We have previously shown that *Nf1* excision rates in endothelial cells isolated from Nf1Prx1 tissue were high [11]. Thus, we hypothesize that the consequent deregulation of signaling in endothelial cells contributes to the vessel-associated bone anomalies.

Another factor involved in the etiology of macro-porotic lesions in the Nf1Prx1 model is a complete absence of the acidic matrix proteins, which mediate mineral organization in the organic collagenous matrix. This is intriguing, as acidic matrix proteins are critical for mineral binding and organization. For instance, the acidic matrix protein Dmp1 binds to collagen and facilitates site-specific HA mineral deposition and controls collagen assembly *in vitro* [48,49]. An important question to answer in future studies will be the cause of acidic matrix protein exclusion from ECM in vessel proximity. It appears that changes in the properties of *Nf1*-deficient vessels contribute to the bone demineralization. This might be caused by altered blood vessel barrier and diffusion properties [50] allowing blood serum factors with matrix mineralization inhibitory properties to access the bone matrix, e.g., fetuin-A [51]. While such a hypothesis awaits future experimental verification, some of the structural defects in cortical bone in Nf1Prx1 mice and in individuals with NF1 and tibial dysplasia develop at the interface between *Nf1* deficient bone cells and endothelium.

Structural analysis revealed increased micro-porosity in Nf1Col1 and Nf1Prx1 cortical bones was associated with increased osteocyte lacunae size, but not osteocyte number. Absence of non-nucleated lacunae indicates normal osteocyte viability, which is also supported by absence of augmented cortical bone remodeling as usually observed upon osteocyte ablation [52]. However, osteocytes in Nf1Prx1 humerus and NF1 bone tissue occupy larger bone volumes, indicating defective osteoblast-to-osteocyte differentiation and altered function (Fig. 6A–B). Together with defective organic matrix formation and mineralization, increased micro-porosity contributes to the severe mechanical impairment of Nf1Prx1 bone tissue [24,26]. In light of the macro-porotic bone lesions, it is likely that increased micro-porosity is not the major determinant of bone fragility in NF1. However, interplay between osteocytes and endothelial cells leading to severe local bone lesions in sites of high mechanical force integration is possible.

On the nano-scale level, bone strength is determined by the collagen primary and secondary structure, tropocollagen assembly, formation of mineralized collagen fibrils, organization into fibril arrays, higher order patterning of collagen fibers, and lastly by mineral phase apposition [18,53]. Disturbance at any one of these stages might perturb bone function. The complete lack of collagen polarization within macro-porotic bone lesions in Nf1Prx1 mice is a key observation, suggesting a critical role of neurofibromin for collagen formation. This is supported by irregular picrosirius red polarization in mineralized bone tissue and a reduced stiffness measured by SAM. The tensile analysis showed a ~50% reduction of the E-modulus in Nf1Prx1 bone tissue, with ~10% decreased impedance values of the bone matrix by SAM. Additionally, in adult Nf1Prx1 mice a 10% reduction of mineralization was present. However, it is important to note that overall mineral orientation measured by SAXS, providing an indirect measure of collagen orientation, is unaffected. Thus, we conclude that grossly normal collagen coexists with regions of diminished collagen thickness and packaging. Together, these findings suggest that *Nf1* ablation causes a primary defect of collagen formation. However, whether this directly affects mineralization remains speculative.

Little attention has been given to the mechanisms of blood vessel invasion during early development and their subsequent exclusion from the long bone cortex in postnatal development [21,22]. Our data indicate that neurofibromin contributes to this process. Persistence of ectopic vessels together with collagenous matrix formation defects due to osteoblast dysfunction appears to drive the demineralization processes. Similar focal mineralization defects are present in cortical bone samples from individuals with NF1 and tibial dysplasia, both post-fracture and pre-fracture (one case). In these samples, we detected inhomogeneous cortical mineralization with low BMD in proximity of large vessels penetrating the bone cortex and enlarged osteocytes. Thus, increased osteocyte micro-porosity and vessel related macro-porosity are two major components of NF1 bone dysplasia pathology.

Although major observations made in Nf1Prx1 mice could be verified in human samples, our study is restricted by the limited number of analyzed NF1 patient bone samples and by the significant differences in bone organization between mouse and man. In contrast to mouse bone, human bone is supplied with blood by a canalicular system formed by Haversian and Volkmann's canals, resulting in osteonal bone organization and remodeling [17]. In human bone, collagen fibers are circularly aligned following osteonal organization. Thus, comparison of these two bone types is not straight forward. Further limitation of this study is that it does not address whether loss of neurofibromin is also associated with changes of biochemical bone tissue composition and/or alterations of collagen fiber morphology. This kind of analysis should be addressed in further studies [17,18,54], which will be instructed by the findings that loss of neurofibromin induces generalized defects of bone tissue function as well as highly localized structural alterations [11,13,15,28].

Supporting Information

Figure S1 Small-angle X-ray scattering (SAXS) analysis demonstrates normal overall mineral orientation in Nf1Prx1 humerus. (**A**) Cortical bone mineral density (BMD) was assessed by microCT within region E1–E3 in humeri of Nf1Col1 (control n = 3, Nf1Prx1 n = 3) mice. BMD was reduced in the Nf1Col1 model in all ROIs. ROIs E1, E2 and E3 were choosen as indicated. (**B**) Relative mineral content was imaged by energy dispersive X-ray spectroscopy (EDX) and mean grey value intensities were measured with AxioVision (Zeiss) (controls n = 3, mutants n = 3). All cortical regions E1–E3 of Nf1Prx1 mice showed lower degree of mineralization. (**C**) SAXS analysis revealed normal mineral particle thickness (T-parameter) within the midshaft region of control (grey) and Nf1Prx1 (black) humeri. Analyzed samples were from different postnatal stage P15, P42 and P90. (**D**) The mineral particle orientation (Rho-parameter) appeared also unaffected between controls and Nf1Prx1 humerus. Position of measured points according to the distance from the growth plate is indicated at the abscissa and the vertical lines indicate centre of humerus cortex. For each developmental stage, one humerus was analyzed. Horizontal lines and adjacent numbers represent the mean value of appropriated individual measurements. Measurements at different developmental time points showed no differences between control and Nf1Prx1 humeri for the T- or Rho-parameter suggesting normal mineral particle thickness and alignment.

Table S1 Cortical volume parameter in P90 humeri level E2 of control, Nf1-Prx1 and Nf1-Col1 mice measured by high resolution micro-CT.

Table S2 Mechanical testing of control and Nf1-Prx1 humerus measured by tensile analysis.

Table S3 Acoustic impedance measurement of P90 humeri of control, Nf1-Prx1 and Nf1-Col1 mice measured by ultrasound microscopy.

Acknowledgments

We wish to thank the RJL Micro & Analytic GmbH for their excellent support (M. Heneka) during establishment of the microCT evaluation setup. We wish to thank Dr. Mary Gray for the critical corrections to the manuscript.

Author Contributions

Conceived and designed the experiments: JK PF UK SM MK. Performed the experiments: JK JS CL S. Schrof S. Stumpp KK DE JG NK MO MK. Analyzed the data: JK JS S. Schrof PV KR MK. Wrote the paper: JK WS DS FE UK PF SM MK. Provided clinical samples: GD ST FT TK. Read and approved the manuscript: JK JS CL S. Schroff S. Stumpp KK JG NK PV MO DE ST FT GD WS TK DAS FE UK KR PF SM MK.

References

1. Alwan S, Tredwell SJ, Friedman JM (2005) Is osseous dysplasia a primary feature of neurofibromatosis 1 (NF1)? Clin Genet 67: 378–390.
2. Stevenson DA, Carey JC, Viskochil DH, Moyer-Mileur LJ, Slater H, et al. (2009) Analysis of radiographic characteristics of anterolateral bowing of the leg before fracture in neurofibromatosis type 1. Jô Pediatr Orthop 29: 385–392.
3. Tucker T, Schnabel C, Hartmann M, Friedrich RE, Frieling I, et al. (2009) Bone health and fracture rate in individuals with neurofibromatosis 1 (NF1). Jô Med Genet 46: 259–265.
4. Wallace MR, Marchuk DA, Andersen LB, Letcher R, Odeh HM, et al. (1990) Type 1 neurofibromatosis gene: identification of a large transcript disrupted in three NF1 patients. Science 249: 181–186.
5. Cully M, Downward J (2008) SnapShot: Ras Signaling. Cell 133: 1292–1292 e1291.
6. McCubrey JA, Steelman LS, Chappell WH, Abrams SL, Montalto G, et al. (2012) Mutations and deregulation of Ras/Raf/MEK/ERK and PI3K/PTEN/Akt/mTOR cascades which alter therapy response. Oncotarget 3: 954–987.
7. Larizza L, Gervasini C, Natacci F, Riva P (2009) Developmental abnormalities and cancer predisposition in neurofibromatosis type 1. Curr Mol Med 9: 634–653.
8. Dang I, De Vries GH (2011) Aberrant cAMP metabolism in NF1 malignant peripheral nerve sheath tumor cells. Neurochem Res 36: 1697–1705.
9. Ozawa T, Araki N, Yunoue S, Tokuo H, Feng L, et al. (2005) The neurofibromatosis type 1 gene product neurofibromin enhances cell motility by regulating actin filament dynamics via the Rho-ROCK-LIMK2-cofilin pathway. Jô Biol Chem 280: 39524–39533.
10. Starinsky-Elbaz S, Faigenbloom L, Friedman E, Stein R, Kloog Y (2009) The pre-GAP-related domain of neurofibromin regulates cell migration through the LIM kinase/cofilin pathway. Mol Cell Neurosci 42: 278–287.
11. Kolanczyk M, Kossler N, Kuhnisch J, Lavitas L, Stricker S, et al. (2007) Multiple roles for neurofibromin in skeletal development and growth. Hum Mol Genet 16: 874–886.
12. Kossler N, Stricker S, Rodelsperger C, Robinson PN, Kim J, et al. (2011) Neurofibromin (Nf1) is required for skeletal muscle development. Hum Mol Genet 20: 2697–2709.
13. Elefteriou F, Benson MD, Sowa H, Starbuck M, Liu X, et al. (2006) ATF4 mediation of NF1 functions in osteoblast reveals a nutritional basis for congenital skeletal dysplasiae. Cell Metab 4: 441–451.
14. Lammert M, Kappler M, Mautner VF, Lammert K, Storkel S, et al. (2005) Decreased bone mineral density in patients with neurofibromatosis 1. Osteoporos Int 16: 1161–1166.
15. Seitz S, Schnabel C, Busse B, Schmidt HU, Beil FT, et al. (2010) High bone turnover and accumulation of osteoid in patients with neurofibromatosis 1. Osteoporos Int 21: 119–127.
16. Chappard D, Basle MF, Legrand E, Audran M (2011) New laboratory tools in the assessment of bone quality. Osteoporos Int 22: 2225–2240.
17. Weiner S, Traub W (1992) Bone structure: from angstroms to microns. Fasebô J 6: 879–885.
18. Ritchie RO (2011) The conflicts between strength and toughness. Nat Mater 10: 817–822.
19. Shapiro F (2008) Bone development and its relation to fracture repair. The role of mesenchymal osteoblasts and surface osteoblasts. Eur Cell Mater 15: 53–76.
20. Clarke B (2008) Normal bone anatomy and physiology. Clinô Jô Am Soc Nephrol 3 Suppl 3: S131–139.
21. Maes C, Kobayashi T, Selig MK, Torrekens S, Roth SI, et al. (2010) Osteoblast precursors, but not mature osteoblasts, move into developing and fractured bones along with invading blood vessels. Dev Cell 19: 329–344.
22. Maes C, Stockmans I, Moermans K, Van Looveren R, Smets N, et al. (2004) Soluble VEGF isoforms are essential for establishing epiphyseal vascularization and regulating chondrocyte development and survival. Jô Clin Invest 113: 188–199.
23. Gupta HS, Seto J, Wagermaier W, Zaslansky P, Boesecke P, et al. (2006) Cooperative deformation of mineral and collagen in bone at the nanoscale. Proc Natl Acad Sciô Uô Sô A 103: 17741–17746.
24. Currey JD (1988) The effect of porosity and mineral content on the Young's modulus of elasticity of compact bone. Jô Biomech 21: 131–139.
25. Schaffler MB, Burr DB (1988) Stiffness of compact bone: effects of porosity and density. Jô Biomech 21: 13–16.
26. Schneider P, Stauber M, Voide R, Stampanoni M, Donahue LR, et al. (2007) Ultrastructural properties in cortical bone vary greatly in two inbred strains of mice as assessed by synchrotron light based micro- and nano-CT. Jô Bone Miner Res 22: 1557–1570.
27. Turner CH (2006) Bone strength: current concepts. Annô Nô Yô Acad Sci 1068: 429–446.
28. Kolanczyk M, Kuhnisch J, Kossler N, Osswald M, Stumpp S, et al. (2008) Modelling neurofibromatosis type 1 tibial dysplasia and its treatment with lovastatin. BMC Med 6: 21.
29. Pascaretti-Grizon F, Gaudin-Audrain C, Gallois Y, Retaillaud-Gaborit N, Basle MF, et al. (2007) Osteopontin is an argentophilic protein in the bone matrix and in cells of kidney convoluted tubules. Morphologie 91: 180–185.
30. Junqueira LC, Bignolas G, Brentani RR (1979) Picrosirius staining plus polarization microscopy, a specific method for collagen detection in tissue sections. Histochemô J 11: 447–455.
31. Dayan D, Hiss Y, Hirshberg A, Bubis JJ, Wolman M (1989) Are the polarization colors of picrosirius red-stained collagen determined only by the diameter of the fibers? Histochemistry 93: 27–29.
32. Parfitt AM, Drezner MK, Glorieux FH, Kanis JA, Malluche H, et al. (1987) Bone histomorphometry: standardization of nomenclature, symbols, and units. Report of the ASBMR Histomorphometry Nomenclature Committee. Jô Bone Miner Res 2: 595–610.
33. Kawamoto T, Shimizu M (2000) A method for preparing 2- to 50-micron-thick fresh-frozen sections of large samples and undecalcified hard tissues. Histochem Cell Biol 113: 331–339.
34. Gupta HS, Wagermaier W, Zickler GA, Raz-Ben Aroush D, Funari SS, et al. (2005) Nanoscale deformation mechanisms in bone. Nano Lett 5: 2108–2111.
35. Lakshmanan S, Bodi A, Raum K (2007) Assessment of anisotropic tissue elasticity of cortical bone from high-resolution, angular acoustic measurements. IEEE Trans Ultrason Ferroelectr Freq Control 54: 1560–1570.
36. Granke M, Gourrier A, Rupin F, Raum K, Peyrin F, et al. (2013) Microfibril orientation dominates the microelastic properties of human bone tissue at the lamellar length scale. PLoS One 8: e58043.
37. Preininger B, Checa S, Molnar FL, Fratzl P, Duda GN, et al. (2011) Spatial-temporal mapping of bone structural and elastic properties in a sheep model following osteotomy. Ultrasound Med Biol 37: 474–483.
38. Raum K, Cleveland RO, Peyrin F, Laugier P (2006) Derivation of elastic stiffness from site-matched mineral density and acoustic impedance maps. Phys Med Biol 51: 747–758.
39. Lange C, Li C, Manjubala I, Wagermaier W, Kuhnisch J, et al. (2011) Fetal and postnatal mouse bone tissue contains more calcium than is present in hydroxyapatite. Jô Struct Biol 176: 159–167.
40. Tanck E, Hannink G, Ruimerman R, Buma P, Burger EH, et al. (2006) Cortical bone development under the growth plate is regulated by mechanical load transfer. Jô Anat 208: 73–79.
41. Kyono A, Avishai N, Ouyang Z, Landreth GE, Murakami S (2012) FGF and ERK signaling coordinately regulate mineralization-related genes and play essential roles in osteocyte differentiation. Jô Bone Miner Metab 30: 19–30.
42. Ono K, Karolak MR, Ndong JD, Wang W, Yang X, et al. (2013) The Ras-GTPase activity of neurofibromin restrains ERK-dependent FGFR signaling during endochondral bone formation. Hum Mol Genet.
43. Kono SJ, Oshima Y, Hoshi K, Bonewald LF, Oda H, et al. (2007) Erk pathways negatively regulate matrix mineralization. Bone 40: 68–74.
44. Xiao L, Esliger A, Hurley MM (2013) Nuclear fibroblast growth factor 2 (FGF2) isoforms inhibit bone marrow stromal cell mineralization through FGF23/FGFR/MAPK in vitro. Jô Bone Miner Res 28: 35–45.
45. Ge C, Xiao G, Jiang D, Franceschi RT (2007) Critical role of the extracellular signal-regulated kinase-MAPK pathway in osteoblast differentiation and skeletal development. Jô Cell Biol 176: 709–718.
46. El-Hoss J, Sullivan K, Cheng T, Yu NY, Bobyn JD, et al. (2011) A murine model of neurofibromatosis type 1 tibial pseudarthrosis featuring proliferative fibrous tissue and osteoclast-like cells. Jô Bone Miner Res.
47. Franceschi RT, Ge C, Xiao G, Roca H, Jiang D (2009) Transcriptional regulation of osteoblasts. Cells Tissues Organs 189: 144–152.
48. He G, George A (2004) Dentin matrix protein 1 immobilized on type I collagen fibrils facilitates apatite deposition in vitro. Jô Biol Chem 279: 11649–11656.
49. Martin A, Liu S, David V, Li H, Karydis A, et al. (2011) Bone proteins PHEX and DMP1 regulate fibroblastic growth factor Fgf23 expression in osteocytes through a common pathway involving FGF receptor (FGFR) signaling. Fasebô J 25: 2551–2562.
50. Dudley AC (2012) Tumor endothelial cells. Cold Spring Harb Perspect Med 2: a006536.
51. Kornak U (2011) Animal models with pathological mineralization phenotypes. Joint Bone Spine 78: 561–567.
52. Tatsumi S, Ishii K, Amizuka N, Li M, Kobayashi T, et al. (2007) Targeted ablation of osteocytes induces osteoporosis with defective mechanotransduction. Cell Metab 5: 464–475.
53. Seeman E, Delmas PD (2006) Bone quality—the material and structural basis of bone strength and fragility. Nô Englô Jô Med 354: 2250–2261.
54. Ascenzi MG, Liao VP, Lee BM, Billi F, Zhou H, et al. (2012) Parathyroid Hormone Treatment Improves the Cortical Bone Microstructure by Improving the Distribution of Type I Collagen in Postmenopausal Women With Osteoporosis. Journal of Bone and Mineral Research 27: 702–712.

Characterization of Mechanical and Biological Properties of 3-D Scaffolds Reinforced with Zinc Oxide for Bone Tissue Engineering

Pei Feng[1,¶], Pingpin Wei[3,¶], Cijun Shuai[1,2]*, Shuping Peng[3,4]*

1 State Key Laboratory of High Performance Complex Manufacturing, Central South University, Changsha, Hunan Province, P. R. China, **2** Department of Regenerative Medicine & Cell Biology, Medical University of South Carolina, Charleston, South Carolina, United States of America, **3** Cancer Research Institute, Central South University, Changsha, Hunan Province, P. R. China, **4** Department of Obstetrics, Gynecology and Reproductive Sciences, Yale University School of Medicine, New Haven, Connecticut, United States of America

Abstract

A scaffold for bone tissue engineering should have highly interconnected porous structure, appropriate mechanical and biological properties. In this work, we fabricated well-interconnected porous β-tricalcium phosphate (β-TCP) scaffolds via selective laser sintering (SLS). We found that the mechanical and biological properties of the scaffolds were improved by doping of zinc oxide (ZnO). Our data showed that the fracture toughness increased from 1.09 to 1.40 $MPam^{1/2}$, and the compressive strength increased from 3.01 to 17.89 MPa when the content of ZnO increased from 0 to 2.5 wt%. It is hypothesized that the increase of ZnO would lead to a reduction in grain size and an increase in density of the strut. However, the fracture toughness and compressive strength decreased with further increasing of ZnO content, which may be due to the sharp increase in grain size. The biocompatibility of the scaffolds was investigated by analyzing the adhesion and the morphology of human osteoblast-like MG-63 cells cultured on the surfaces of the scaffolds. The scaffolds exhibited better and better ability to support cell attachment and proliferation when the content of ZnO increased from 0 to 2.5 wt%. Moreover, a bone like apatite layer formed on the surfaces of the scaffolds after incubation in simulated body fluid (SBF), indicating an ability of osteoinduction and osteoconduction. In summary, interconnected porous β-TCP scaffolds doped with ZnO were successfully fabricated and revealed good mechanical and biological properties, which may be used for bone repair and replacement potentially.

Editor: Monica Soncini, Politecnico di Milano, Italy

Funding: This work was supported by the following funds: (1) the Natural Science Foundation of China (51222506, 81000972); (2) The foundation for the author of national excellent doctoral dissertation of PR China (201032); (3) Program for New Century Excellent Talents in University (NCET-12-0544); (4) The Fundamental Research Funds for the Central Universities (2011JQ005, 2012QNZT015); (5) Project supported by the Fok Ying-Tong Education Foundation, China (131050); (6) The Open-End Fund for the Valuable and Precision Instruments of Central South University. The funders had no role in study design, data collection and analysis, decision to publish, or preparation of the manuscript.

Competing Interests: The authors have declared that no competing interests exist.

* E-mail: shuai@csu.edu.cn (CS); shuping@csu.edu.cn (SP)

¶ These authors contributed equally to this work.

Introduction

Scaffold plays an important role in cells attachment, proliferation and guidance of new bone tissue formation in bone tissue engineering [1–2]. Highly interconnected porous structure and customized shape for specific bone defects are essential for ideal bone scaffold. Though porous scaffold with sufficient void volumes and surface area can be obtained by some conventional methods including freeze drying, gas foaming, solvent casting, and so on [3–5], it is difficult to realize the precise control of the pore size, pore geometry and spatial distribution or the ability to construction of internal interconnected pore network [6–8]. SLS is an additive manufacturing technique in which a high power laser was used to sinter powder material selectively, and the latter become three-dimensional (3D) objects. The sintering process is guided by the computer aided design (CAD) model and computer control [9–10]. By this technique, the bone scaffolds with well-controlled internal architectures and customized external shapes can be well realized [11].

In addition to porous structure requirements, the scaffold should also have good biocompatibility, biodegradability and adequate mechanical properties [12]. β-TCP [β-Ca_3 $(PO_4)_2$] is one of the most attractive bioceramics to produce the bone scaffold for tissue engineering because of the favorable biological compatibility, osteoconductivity and resorbability [13]. However, the low mechanical strength and toughness have restricted the application only in low- or non-load-bearing bone replacement [14]. Further, the degradation rate of pure β-TCP is too fast and uncontrolled which leads to mismatch between the degradation of scaffold and the formation of new bone [15]. Thus, it is necessary to improve mechanical and biological properties for the porous β-TCP scaffold to support bone regeneration.

It is reported that the mechanical properties and the degradation rate of β-TCP can be reinforced and modified by oxide-based dopant (such as ZnO, MgO, SiO_2) without altering its inherent

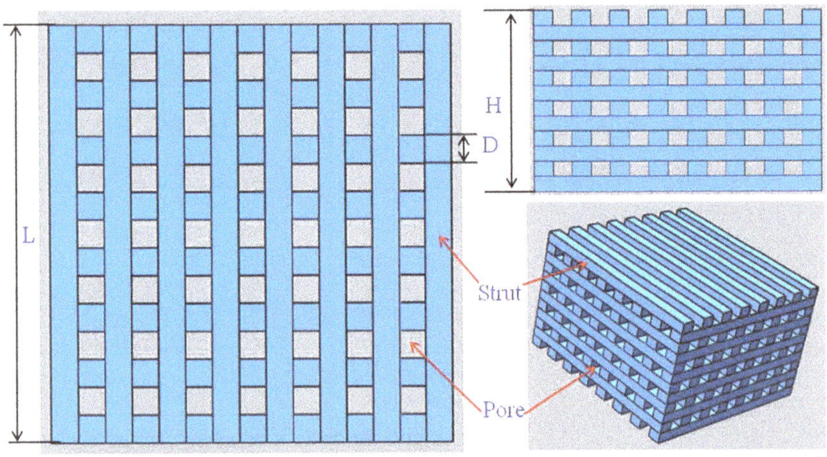

Figure 1. Scaffold model designed using SolidWorks software: D = 1.2 mm; H = 11 mm; L = 18 mm.

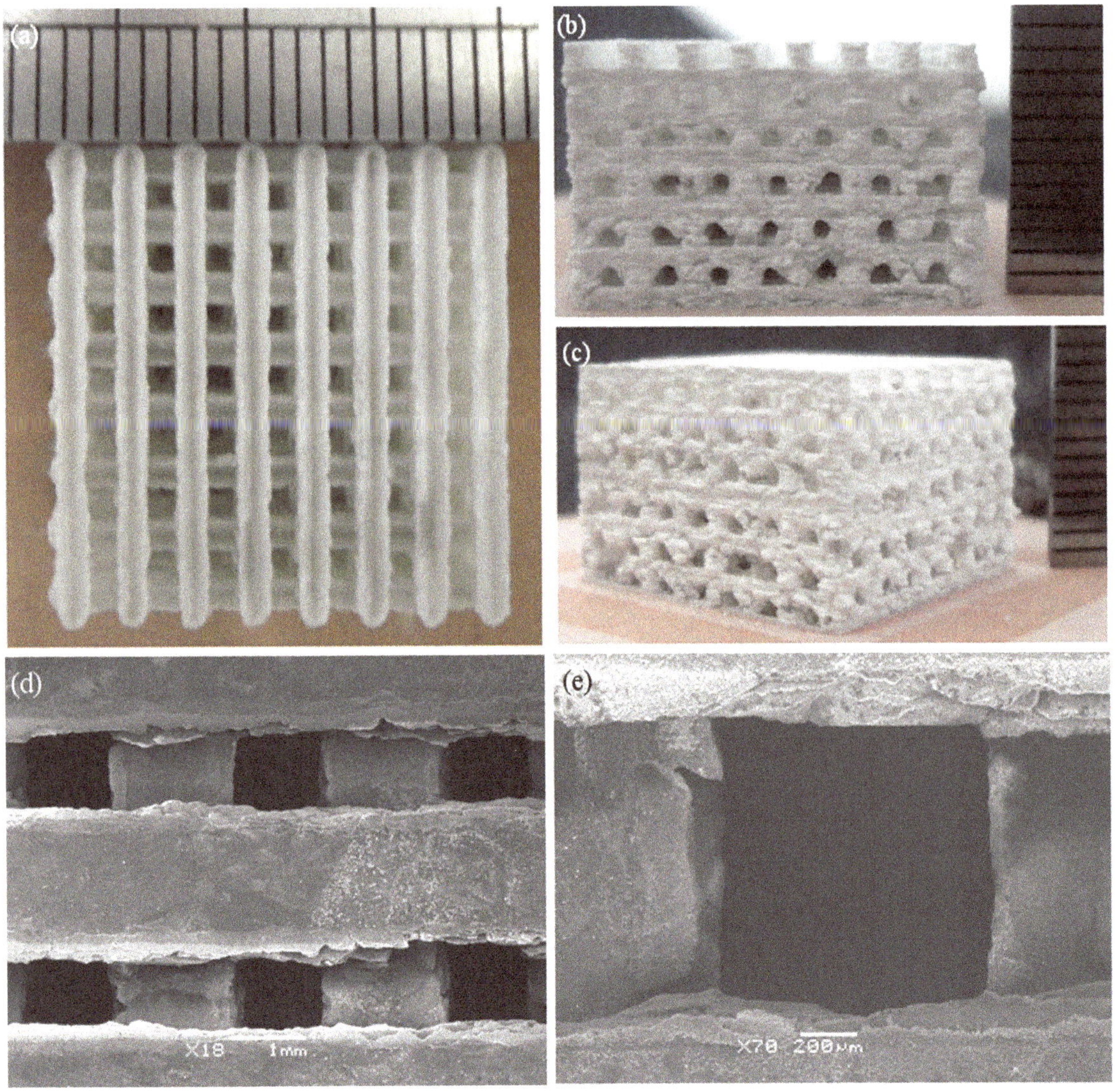

Figure 2. Optical micrographs of 3D interconnected porous scaffold prepared by SLS and SEM images of the porous structure (a) top view and (b–c) side view (d) the porous structure and (e) a single pore structure.

biocompatibility, respectively [16–17]. Zinc (Zn) was an essential trace element with a stimulatory role in bone formation and their mineralization [18]. In vitro studies showed that Zn had a direct specific proliferative role for osteoblastic cells [19] and a selective inhibitory role for osteoclastic bone resorption [20]. Jin et al. [21] produced hydroxyapatite/TCP biphasic bioceramics reinforced with ZnO-whiskers via conventional sintering and found that the addition of ZnO improved the hardness and fracture toughness. Bandyopadhyay et al. [22] fabricated TCP samples with different content of ZnO by uniaxial pressing followed by muffle furnace sintering and found that ZnO addition increased densification and hardness of ceramics. Bhatt et al. [23] conducted experiment to study the biodegradation rate of four different oxide-based β-TCP bioceramics in dynamic SBF and found that the ZnO addition could tailor the degradation rate of β-TCP. Bandyopadhyay et al. [24] had made TCP-ZnO compacts and the compacts showed an increase in densification and excellent biocompatibility with osteoblastic precursor cell line 1 cells compared with pure TCP. These investigations showed that oxide-based dopant such as ZnO could improve the mechanical properties and delay the degradation rate of β-TCP.

In this study, 3D porous bone scaffolds with controlled interconnected porous structure based on β-TCP powder with or without ZnO doping was fabricated via SLS technique. The degradation and bioactivity behavior of these porous scaffolds were studied with respect to weight loss and apatite layer formation. The in vitro biocompatibility was evaluated by the proliferation of MG-63 cells cultured on the surface of the porous scaffold. The surface morphologies were characterized using scanning electron microscope (SEM). The phase composition of the raw β-TCP powder and prepared scaffolds with different ZnO content was characterized by X-ray diffraction (XRD). The chemical composition of the scaffolds before and after SBF was analyzed using Fourier transform infrared spectrometer (FT-IR). The hardness and fracture toughness were determined by Vickers microindentor. Compressive tests were performed using an electronic universal test machine. Elemental composition of the deposits on the scaffold surface after SBF was analyzed by energy dispersive X-ray spectroscopy (EDX) spot analysis.

Materials and Methods

Materials

Raw β-TCP powder with the average particle size of 0.1~0.3 μm was acquired from Kunshan Chinese Technology New Materials Co., Ltd. High-purity ZnO powder (99.9% purity) with the average particle size of 0.1~0.2 μm was purchased from Guangdong Xilong Chemical Co., Ltd for this research. ZnO was added to β-TCP powder in proportions of 0.5, 1.5, 2.5 and 3.5 wt%, followed by mechanical mixing for 30 min. Pure β-TCP powder (i.e., 0 wt% ZnO) was also prepared and used as the control sample.

Fabrication

The scaffolds were prepared using a homemade selective laser sintering system [25]. The fabrication process began by spreading a thin layer of powder evenly onto the flat surface. The thin layer of powder could be formed by roll compaction. Then, the laser was guided to sinter the particles selectively in a powder bed layer-by-layer to fabricate the 3D scaffold based on the instructions of CAD program. A tetragonal porous scaffold model ($L \times W \times H = 18 \times 18 \times 11$ mm^3, L is the length of scaffold, W is the width of scaffold, H is the height of scaffold) with 3D orthogonal periodic porous architecture was designed using SolidWorks software (Fig. 1). The tetragonal porous scaffold model was composed of eight struts per set, with each strut of 1.2 mm in width, 0.92 mm in thickness and 2.4 mm in distance between the centerlines of the struts. The laser used in this research was a 100 W CO_2 laser (model Firestar® t-Series, Synrad Co., USA). The sintering process was performed at the power of 12 W, the scanning speed of 100 mm/min, the spot diameter of 1.2 mm and the layer thickness of 0.1–0.2 mm. After the SLS processing was completed, the scaffolds were allowed to cool to room temperature before being removed from the powder bed. Excess powder was brushed off from the exterior while the internal architecture was cleaned using compressed air.

Characterizations

The microstructures of the prepared scaffolds were examined by SEM (JEOL JSM-5600LV, JEOL Ltd., Japan). To study the effect of ZnO on grain size, the prepared samples ($18 \times 1.2 \times 0.92$ mm^3) were etched with 5% hydrofluoric acid (HF) for 5 min and then coated with a very thin layer of gold. The average grain sizes were determined from SEM images with the linear intercept method using Eq. (1) [26]:

$$Ga = (L/N) * C \tag{1}$$

Where Ga is the average grain size (μm), L is the total test line length (cm), N is the total number of intersections with grain boundaries along test line L, and C is the conversion factor (μm/cm) of the SEM picture on which the test lines were drawn as obtained from the scale bar. The phase composition was identified by XRD (D8-ADVANCE, German) with CuKα radiation (λ = 1.54056 Å) at 40 kV and 40 mA. The XRD patterns were recorded in the 2θ range of 10 to 40 degrees with a scanning rate of 8 degrees/min. Infrared spectra for the raw powder and the scaffolds were obtained using FT-IR (Thermo Scientific Nicolet™ 6700, Thermo Electron Corp., USA). For this purpose, the scaffolds were first grinded into powders, and then the powders were mixed with KBr in the proportion of 1/150 (by weight) for 15 min and pressed into a pellet using a cold press. Each infrared spectrum was obtained over the range from 500 to 4000 cm^{-1} with a resolution of 4.0 cm^{-1}.

The density of the struts ($18 \times 1.2 \times 0.92$ mm^3) was measured using the Archimedes method. The densification was calculated as the density divided by the theoretical density of the struts. The hardness and the fracture toughness were tested by Vickers Microindentor (Digital Micro Hardness Tester, HXD-1000TM/LCD, Shanghai Taiming Optical Instrument Co. Ltd) both with a load of 300 gf and a dwelling time of 15 s. The surface of strut samples ($1 \times 1.2 \times 0.92$ mm^3) was mounted in epoxy vertically, polished and subjected to indentation on the surfaces. The Vickers hardness (HV) and fracture toughness (K_{IC}) were calculated from the following Eq. (2) and (3), respectively:

$$HV = 0.1891F/d^2 \tag{2}$$

$$K_{IC} = 0.0824F/C^{3/2} \tag{3}$$

Where HV is the Vickers hardness, K_{IC} is the fracture toughness, F is the applied load, d is the diagonal of the indentation, and C the radial crack length measured from the center point of the indentation impression. Density and Vickers indentation tests were analyzed with six struts for each group. Compressive tests of the prepared scaffolds ($18 \times 18 \times 11$ mm^3) were performed at a

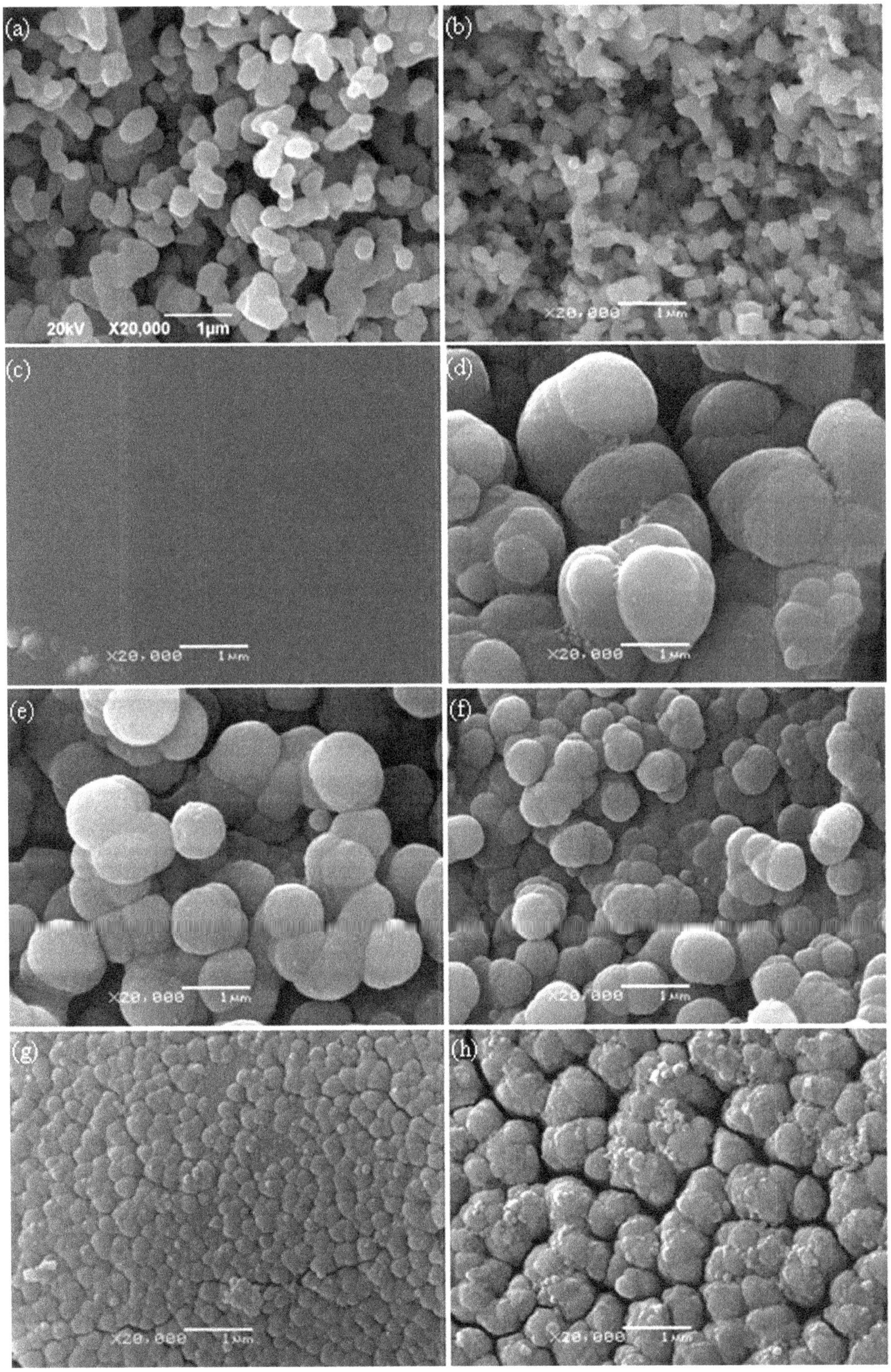

Figure 3. Micrographs of (a) raw β-TCP powder; (b) raw ZnO powder; (c) unetched surface of scaffold; etched surface of scaffold: (d) pure TCP; (e) 0.5 wt% ZnO; (f) 1.5 wt% ZnO; (g) 2.5 wt% ZnO and (h) 3.5 wt% ZnO.

crosshead speed of 0.5 mm/min using a microcomputer control electronic universal test machine (WD-D1, Shanghai zhuoji instruments Co. Ltd) to evaluate the compressive strength and stiffness. All compression tests were performed in a direction perpendicular to the circular platens. The stress versus strain responses of the scaffolds was recorded to calculate the scaffold stiffness during the compressive strength tests. Six samples for each group were used to obtain the average value along with their standard deviation.

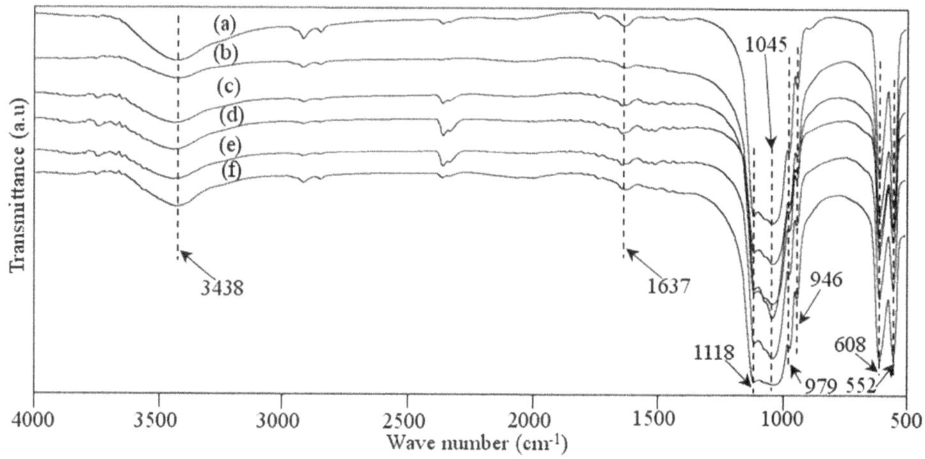

Figure 4. FT-IR spectra of the raw β-TCP powder (a) and β-TCP scaffolds with 0 wt% ZnO (b), 0.5 wt% ZnO (c), 1.5 wt% ZnO (d), 2.5 wt% ZnO (e), and 3.5 wt% ZnO (f).

Cell Culture

To evaluate the cell biocompatibility, human osteoblast-like MG-63 cells (American Type Culture Collection, Rockville, MD) were seeded on the prepared scaffolds ($18\times18\times11$ mm^3). MG-63 cells were seeded in culture flasks in Dulbecco's modified Eagle's medium (DMEM; Cell- gro by Mediatech, Inc., Manassas, VA) containing 10% fetal bovine serum (Gibco, Carlsbad, CA) and 1% penicillin/streptomycin (Gibco) at 37°C, 5% CO_2 and 100% humidity. The medium was changed every 2 days to wash off all non-adherent cells. The morphology of primary MG-63 cells was observed using a light microscope (Olympus, IX51, Japan). Prior to cell seeding, scaffolds were pre-wetted by immersing in 70% ethanol for 2 hours and exchanged by excess of phosphate buffered saline (PBS) solution. After the removal of PBS, 4×10^5 cells were seeded onto each scaffold and cultured for 5 days in DMEM. Then the scaffolds were rinsed in PBS for three times for each sample, and then fixed with a 2.5% glutaraldehyde solution for 30 min. The scaffolds were then dehydrated by a series of graded ethanol solutions before critical point dried. After dried, the scaffolds were coated with a very thin layer of gold, and the cell adhesion on the scaffolds was assessed using SEM (TESCAN, Mira 3 FEG, Tescan Co.). The MG-63 cells cultured on the scaffold and dish were digested and seeded on cover slips in six-well dishes. After incubation for 24 h under standard culture condition, the cells were washed twice with D-PBS solution. Add sufficient amount of Calcein AM/EthD-III (Invitrogen Ltd., UK) standard staining solution to cover cell monolayer. The cells were incubated for 30–45 minutes at room temperature. Calcein AM/EthD-III solution was aspirated out after incubation. Ten micro liter of the fresh Calcein AM/EthD-III solution or PBS was added to a clean microscope slide, and the cover slips seeded with the cells was reverted and mounted on the prepared slides. Fingernail polish was used to seal the cover slips and to prevent evaporation. The labeled cells were observed under the fluorescence microscope (Olympus BX51, Japan).

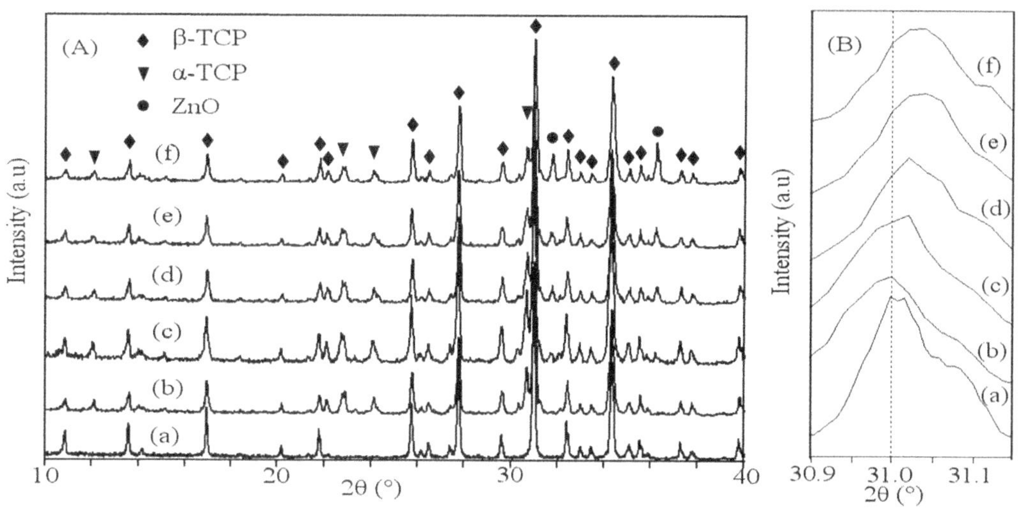

Figure 5. XRD patterns (A): 2θ from 10 to 40° and (B): 2θ from 30.9 to 31.15° of (a) the raw β-TCP powder, the scaffolds with different ratio of ZnO: (b) 0 wt%; (c) 0.5 wt%; (d) 1.5 wt%; (e) 2.5 wt% and (f) 3.5 wt%. (β-TCP, JCPDS file number 09-0169; α-TCP, JCPDS file number 09-0348; ZnO, JCPDS file number 36-1451).

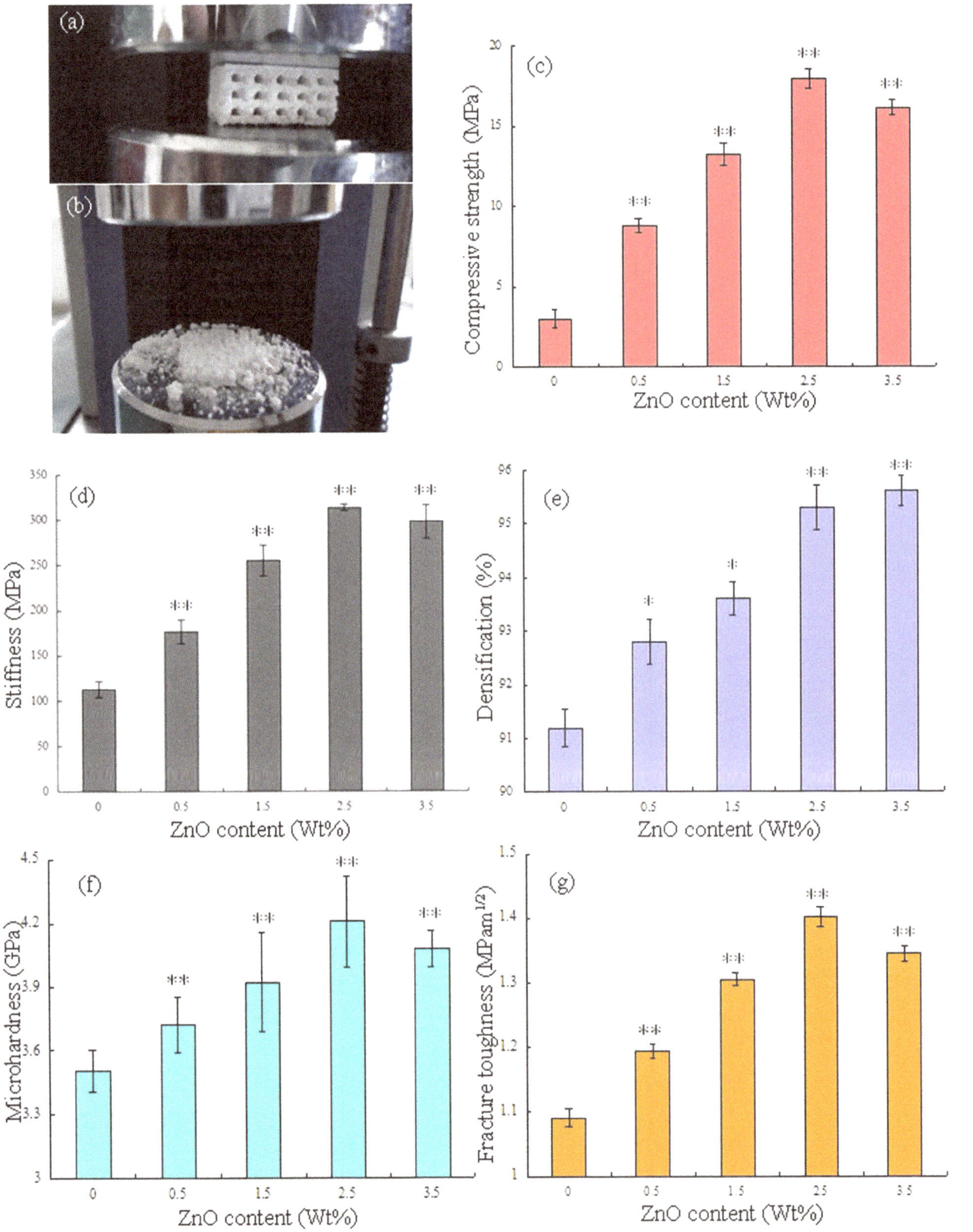

Figure 6. Representative porous TCP scaffold under compression test (a); overview of scaffold after compression test (b); Effect of ZnO contents on the compressive strength (c) and stiffness (d) of porous scaffold; Effect of ZnO contents on the densification (e), microhardness (f) and fracture toughness (g) of the strut. Data represents mean ± standard deviation for $n = 6$, $*P < 0.05$ and $**P < 0.01$ (compared with pure TCP scaffold).

Table 1. Summary of the properties of human bone.

	Density **(g/cm^3)**	**Compressive strength** **(MPa)**	**Stiffness** **(GPa)**	**Fracture toughness** **($MPam^{1/2}$)**	**Microhardness** **(GPa)**
Cortical bone	1.7–2.0	130–180	7–30	2–12	0.62–0.74
Reference	[31]	[32]	[33]	[34]	[35]
Cancellous bone	0.03–0.12	0.1–16	0.05–0.5	–	0.63±0.11
Reference	[36]	[37]	[38]	–	[39]

SBF Test

In order to evaluate the in vitro degradation behavior and bioactivity, all scaffold samples ($15\times15\times7$ mm^3) with different ZnO content were immersed in a dynamic SBF at pH 7.4. SBF was an a cellular solution with an ionic composition (in units of mM, 142.0 Na^+, 5.0 K^+, 1.5 Mg^{2+}, 2.5 Ca^{2+}, 147.8 Cl^-, 4.2 HCO_3^-, 1.0 HPO_4^{2-} and 0.5 SO_4^{2-}) almost equal to that of human plasma and buffered at a similar pH. Six scaffolds for each group were soaked in the SBF solution under dynamic condition in a thermostat at 37°C for 7, 14, 21, and 28 days, respectively. The SBF solutions were refreshed every 3 days over the course. At a predetermined time interval, the scaffolds were taken out from the SBF solution, washed with distilled water and dried at 65°C in an incubator for 2 days. Once dried, the weight of the scaffolds was carefully recorded and compared with their initial weight before immersion. The biodegradation of the scaffolds was calculated by measuring their weight loss as a function of time. The weight loss (*WL*) of sample was calculated according to Eq. (4) [27]:

$$WL(\%) = \frac{W_0 - W_d}{W_0} \times 100 \tag{4}$$

Where W_0 is the weight before immersion in SBF and W_d is the weight of the samples dried at 65°C for 2 days after removed from the SBF. Surface microstructures of these scaffolds were observed using SEM analysis to determine mineralization on the top layer. Elemental composition analysis was conducted by coupled EDX with SEM. The scaffolds surface after soaking was examined by FT-IR to confirm the formation of apatite layer.

Statistical Analysis

All experimental data were expressed as means ± standard deviation and analyzed using SPSS software. Statistical analysis was performed using Student's *t*-test and differences were considered significant for $*P<0.05$ and very significant when $**P<0.01$, respectively.

Results and Discussion

Microstructure

The prepared scaffold was approximately $18\times18\times11$ mm^3 in size (Figs. 2a–c). The porosity of the scaffolds was 56.8%. The scaffolds had well-ordered and uniform pore channel structures (Fig. 2d). There was good bonding between the adjacent layers of the scaffold. The width of the struts was 1.2 mm. The pore size of the scaffold is around 1.2 mm (Fig. 2e). The regular spatial arrangement pore channels were expected to provide osteoinductivity and guided bone tissue to grow well into the pores.

The raw powder, non-etched and etched surface of the scaffold with different ZnO content were shown in Fig. 3. It could be observed that the raw β-TCP powder (Fig. 3a) and ZnO powder (Fig. 3b) were non-uniform and micro-particle loose aggregation. The average grain size of the raw β-TCP and ZnO powder was 0.1–0.3 μm and 0.1–0.2 μm, respectively. The non-etched surface revealed a smooth and highly dense structure (Fig. 3c). The etched scaffolds surface was showed in Figs. 3d–h. Micrographs of the samples showed clear demarcation in the grain boundaries. So their grain size could be easily calculated. The average grain size of the β-TCP scaffold without ZnO doping was calculated to be 1.54 μm. For the addition of 0.5 wt% ZnO, the average grain size dropped to 1.01 μm. At 1.5 wt% and 2.5 wt%, the average grain size decreased from 0.72 μm to 0.29 μm, respectively. The average grain size decreased due to ZnO was a refractory metal oxide (melting point: 1,975°C), which had an inhibitory effect on grain grow during the sintering process. While a sudden increase in grain size was observed when ZnO content is 3.5 wt%, the average grain size was 0.83 μm. β-TCP has a hexagonal crystal structure and belongs to R3CH space group. The unit cell dimensions are: a = b = 10.4183(5) Å, c = 37.3464(23) Å, and α = β = 90°, γ = 120° [28]. The Ca^{2+} in β-TCP can be substituted by Zn^{2+} during the sintering process. The presence of Zn^{2+} in β-TCP could decrease both the *a*-axis and *c*-axis lattice when the content of ZnO increased from 0 to 2.5 wt%. The *a*-axis lattice further decreased, while the *c*-axis lattice increased when the content of ZnO was over 2.5 wt%. The sharp increase in grain size was due to the increase of the c-axis lattice. It was reported that the c-axis lattice would increase when the Zn^{2+} content in the β-TCP was higher than certain content [13].

Phase Composition

The FT-IR spectrum of raw β-TCP powder and the prepared scaffolds was presented in Fig. 4. The FT-IR pattern of raw pure β-TCP powder was shown in Fig. 4a. The characteristic absorption bands at 3438 and 1637 cm^{-1} were attributed to adsorbed water. The bands at 900–1200 cm^{-1} were the stretching vibration mode of the PO_4^{3-} group. The sharp peaks at 552 and 608 cm^{-1} represented the bend vibration mode of PO_4^{3-} in β-TCP. The FT-IR pattern of the scaffolds with 0–3.5 wt% ZnO doped was shown in Figs. 4b–f. The characteristic peaks for β-TCP at wave numbers of 1118, 1045, 609, and 552 cm^{-1} were present. It was observed that FT-IR spectrum of raw β-TCP powder and the scaffolds showed typical spectrum for TCP material. There was no presence of new functional group in the prepared scaffolds, indicating that the doping of ZnO did not change the chemical composition of TCP after sintering.

The XRD patterns of raw β-TCP powder and the prepared scaffolds with different contents of ZnO were plotted in Fig. 5. Peaks of each XRD pattern were recorded and verified using

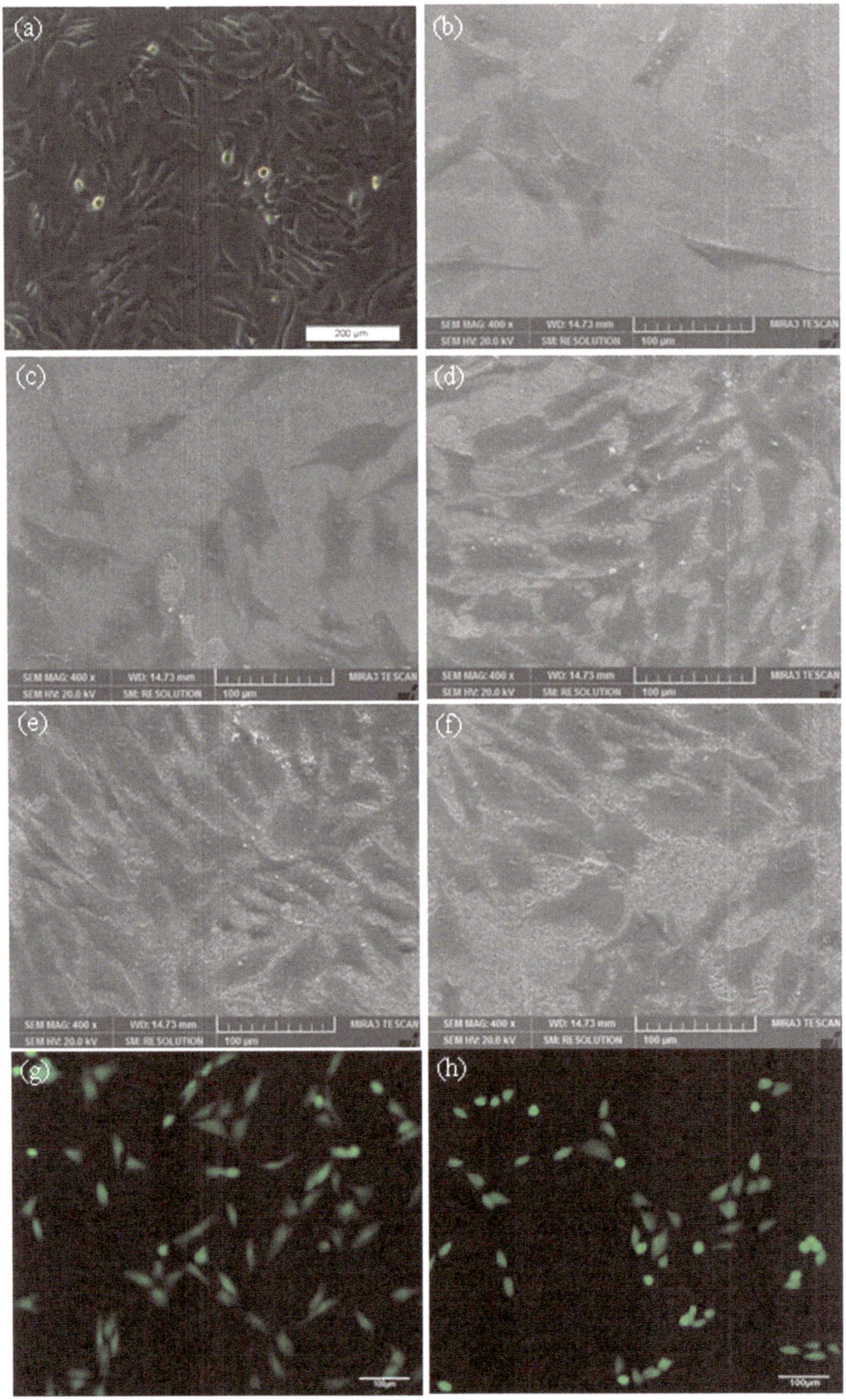
(a)
200 µm
(b)
SEM MAG: 400 x
WD: 14.73 mm
MIRA3 TESCAN
SEM HV: 20.0 kV
SM: RESOLUTION
100 µm
(c)
SEM MAG: 400 x
WD: 14.73 mm
MIRA3 TESCAN
SEM HV: 20.0 kV
SM: RESOLUTION
100 µm
(d)
SEM MAG: 400 x
WD: 14.73 mm
MIRA3 TESCAN
SEM HV: 20.0 kV
SM: RESOLUTION
100 µm
(e)
SEM MAG: 400 x
WD: 14.73 mm
MIRA3 TESCAN
SEM HV: 20.0 kV
SM: RESOLUTION
100 µm
(f)
SEM MAG: 400 x
WD: 14.73 mm
MIRA3 TESCAN
SEM HV: 20.0 kV
SM: RESOLUTION
100 µm
(g)
100µm
(h)
100µm

Figure 7. The morphology of initial MG-63 cells visualized by light microscopy (a), the morphology of MG-63 cells cultured on the scaffolds after 5 days by SEM (b) pure TCP; (c) 0.5 wt% ZnO; (d) 1.5 wt% ZnO; (e) 2.5 wt% ZnO and (f) 3.5 wt% ZnO, the fluorescence microscope images of MG-63 cells before (g) or after (h) incubation on the scaffolds with 2.5 wt% ZnO doping.

standard JCPDS files. The obtained XRD pattern of raw β-TCP powder was shown in Fig. 5A (a). The XRD pattern of raw powder was the same as the pattern of pure β-TCP, and no impurity phase was observed according to JCPDS file number 09-0169. The patterns of the scaffolds with 0–3.5 wt% ZnO doped were shown in Figs. 5A (b–f). The results revealed that the intensity of ZnO peaks became stronger with the increase of ZnO content. A few small peaks of α-TCP were observed in the XRD patterns, indicating transformation of a small amount of β-TCP to α-TCP. JCODS file number 09-0348 and 36-1451 were used to identify the peaks of α-TCP and ZnO, respectively. The characteristic peaks of ZnO were visible in all ZnO doped scaffolds. A small shift in main diffraction peak position of β-TCP was observed for ZnO doped scaffolds (Fig. 5B). It means that the Zn^{2+} ions were substituted for the Ca^{2+} ion positions of the β-TCP structure, which was in good agreement with previous studies [29–30].

Mechanical Properties

Compressive tests were carried out to evaluate the influence of ZnO content on the compressive strength and stiffness of the scaffold. The representative porous scaffold under compression test and after compression test was shown in Fig. 6 (a) and (b). The porous scaffolds were compressed between two circular platens that were sufficiently larger than the samples (Fig. 6a). The porous scaffolds were completely crushed after the compressive tests (Fig. 6b). The mechanical properties such as compressive strength, stiffness, densification, Vickers microhardness and fracture toughness were shown in Figs. 6c–g. With the content of ZnO increasing from 0 to 2.5 wt%, the compressive strength and stiffness of the scaffold increased from 3.01 to 17.89 MPa (Fig. 6c) and from 112.86 MPa to 313.48 MPa (Fig. 6d), respectively. The densification, microhardness and fracture toughness also increased from 91.2 to 95.3% (Fig. 6e), from 3.51 GPa to 4.20 GPa (Fig. 6f) and from 1.09 $MPam^{1/2}$ to 1.40 $MPam^{1/2}$ (Fig. 6g), respectively. The densification of the strut was 95.6% with ZnO content of 3.5 wt%. While the microhardness, fracture toughness, compressive strength and stiffness decreased to 4.08 GPa, 1.35 $MPam^{1/2}$, 16.12 MPa and 297.74 MPa, respectively. The compressive strength was close to the highest strength reported for human cancellous bone [37] (Table 1). The highest value of stiffness was close to the higher limit of cancellous bone (0.05–0.5 GPa) [38] but far from that of cortical bone (7–30 GPa) [33]. The maximum micro hardness was about 6 times higher than that of human bone, and the maximum fracture toughness was a little lower than that of cortical bone [34–35]. The mechanical properties (compressive strength, stiffness, Vickers microhardness and fracture toughness) of all ZnO doped scaffolds were significantly higher than that of pure TCP scaffold ($P<0.01$). Viswanath et al. [40] used the micro and nano indentation techniques to investigate the mechanical response of flux-grown β-TCP single crystals. The values of fracture toughness were measured using the longest and smallest crack lengths vary from 0.41 to 1.15 $MPam^{1/2}$, respectively. Zhang et al. [41] had applied the spark plasma sintering technique to fabricate macro porous β-TCP scaffolds from nano crystalline powders. The compressive strength of the sintered scaffolds with 66±1.0% and 55±1.0% porosity was 3.1±0.4 and 7.0±0.8 MPa, respectively. Park et al. [42] had performed the compression tests of the porous β-TCP scaffold specimens to obtain the stiffness. The stiffness of the porous scaffold with 50.9% porosity was 0.20–0.24 MPa.

These results revealed that ZnO could improve fracture toughness, compressive strength, stiffness and hardness of the scaffolds. The densification of the strut increased significantly with ZnO content increasing from 0 to 2.5 wt%, while it kept nearly the same when the ZnO content further increased to 3.5 wt%. The increase of the densification was most likely related to the presence of ZnO involved in the formation of the liquid phase that promoted high densification [21,43]. It is widely accepted that the increase of sintered density is the most effective way to improve the mechanical properties of sintered parts. The increased fracture toughness, compressive strength, stiffness and hardness may be due to the increase of sintered density of the strut. The grain size decreased with ZnO content increasing from 0 to 2.5 wt%, while the grain size increased when ZnO content increases to 3.5 wt%. Meanwhile, the mechanical properties were associated with the average grain size, the larger the grain size, the lower the mechanical properties. The fracture toughness, compressive strength, stiffness and hardness decreased due to the sudden increase in grain size when the content of ZnO was 3.5 wt%. Therefore, the scaffold with 2.5 wt% ZnO doping was optimal due to the combined effects of densification and grain size.

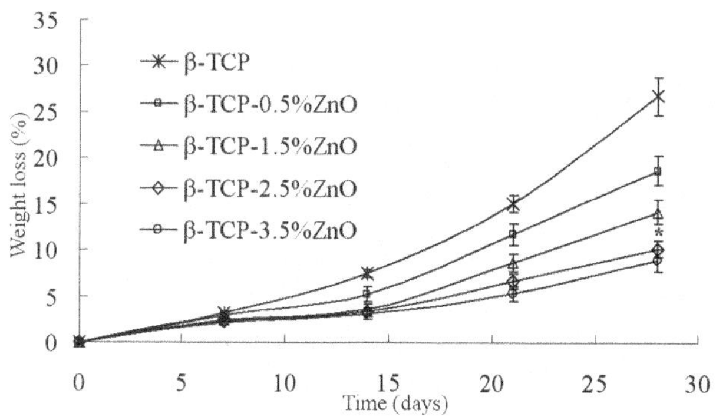

Figure 8. Weight loss assay of the scaffolds after incubation with SBF for different days. Data represents mean ± standard deviation for $n=6$, $*P<0.05$ (compared to pure TCP scaffold).

Cell Morphology on Scaffolds

The morphology of initial MG-63 cells visualized by light microscopy was shown in Fig. 7 (a). The cell morphology showed the classical fusiform shape and the size of cell was about several tens of microns. The morphologies of MG-63 cells on the surface of the scaffolds after 5 days of culture were shown in Fig. 7 (b–f). It was obviously different in the response of the cells to the different scaffold. The cells attached and proliferated well on the surface of the scaffolds when the content of ZnO was 2.5 wt% (Fig. 7e). The cells were connected together and covered most of the surfaces. While the scaffold with 3.5 wt% ZnO showed lower cell density and fewer cells adhesion (Fig. 7f). The fluorescence microscope images of MG-63 cells before and after incubation on scaffolds with 2.5 wt% ZnO doping were shown in Fig. 7 (g) and (h). It was indicated that the MG-63 cells were viable, adhered and proliferated well on the scaffold. The results showed that ZnO had a stimulating effect on osteoblastic cell proliferation. However, the scaffolds showed reduced ability to support cell attachment

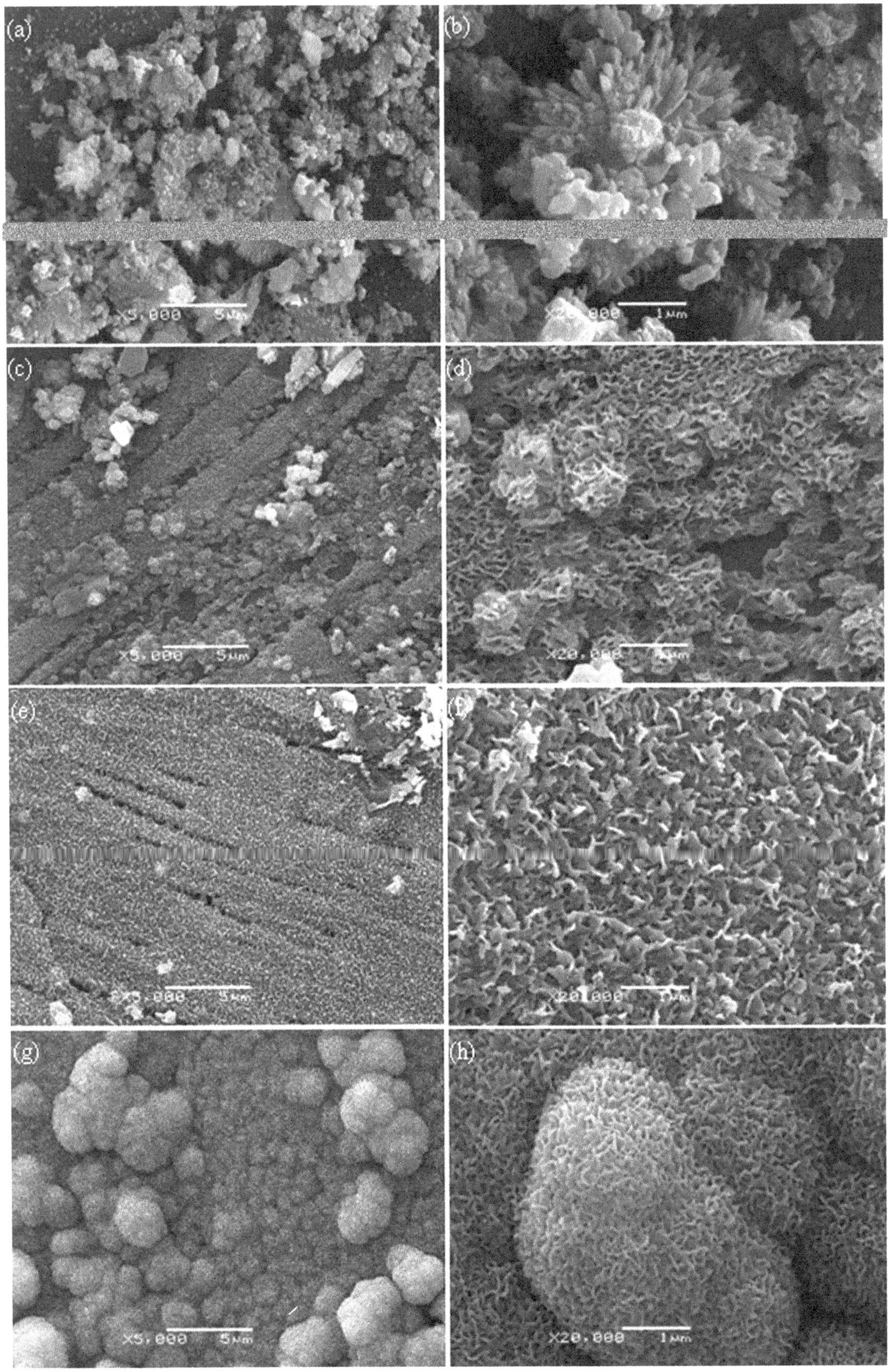

Figure 9. SEM images of bone like apatite layer formation on the surface of scaffolds with 2.5 wt% ZnO doped after SBF incubation for 7 (a, b), 14 (c, d), 21 (e, f), 28 (g, h) days.

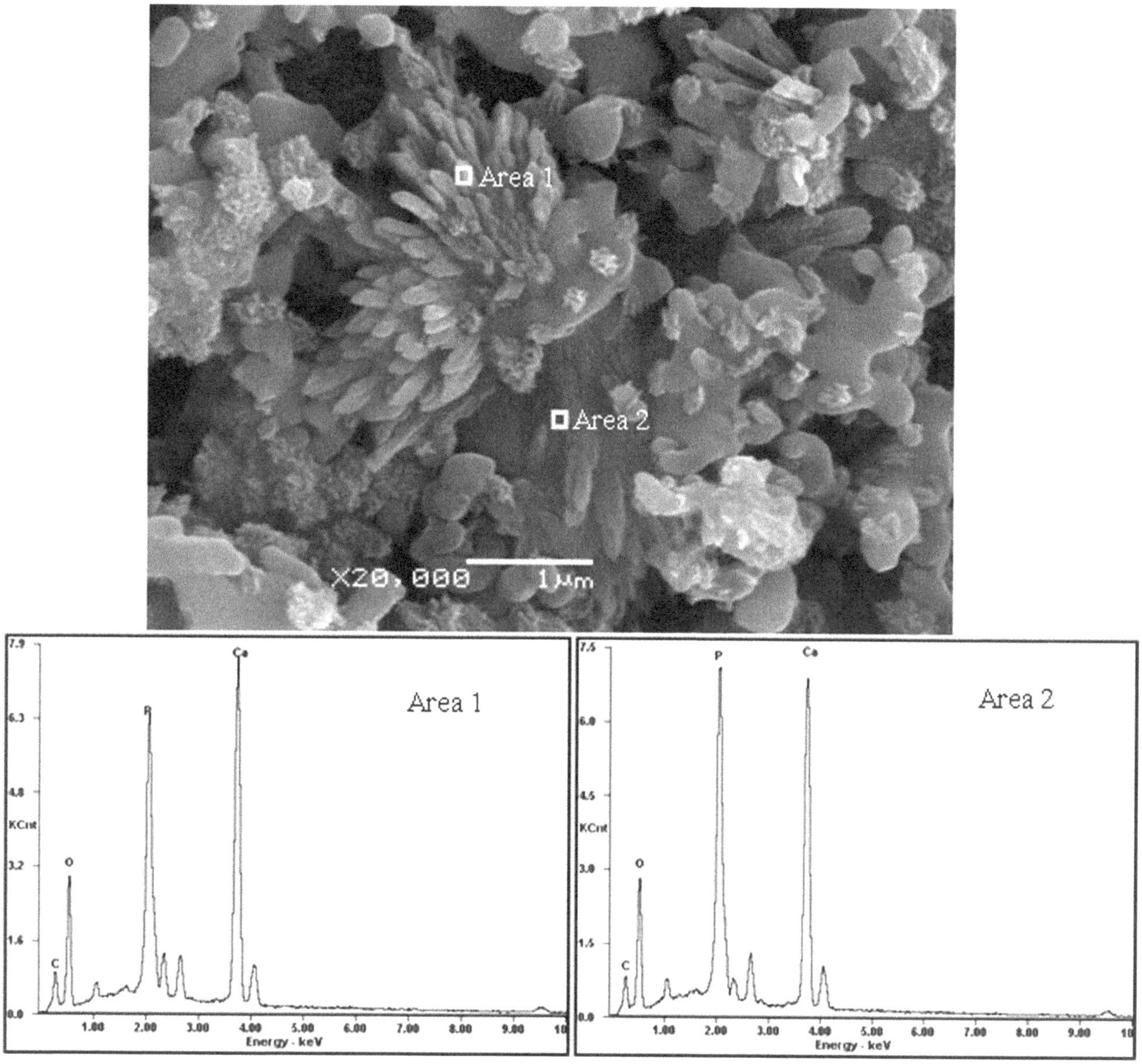

Figure 10. Images under SEM and EDX traces of the scaffold with 2.5 wt% ZnO doped after SBF incubation for 7 days.

and proliferation when ZnO content was over 2.5 wt%. It was reported that Zn promoted the activity of osteoblasts and/or inhibits the differentiation of osteoclasts, while it was harmful to cells when Zn concentration was too high [16,44]. Bandyopadhyay [22] reported that higher ZnO doping had deleterious effects on cell attachments and growth, and cell apoptosis was observed for 3.5 wt% ZnO doped TCP scaffolds.

Degradation and Bioactivity

The degradation rate of the scaffolds with different ZnO content was measured in terms of their weight loss at different time points (day 7, 14, 21, 28) after immersion in SBF (Fig. 8). It was evident that there was an increase in weight loss with time for all scaffolds. The degradation rate of the scaffolds with 2.5 wt% ZnO doping was much lower than that of pure TCP scaffolds after soaking in SBF for 28 days ($P<0.05$). ZnO could inhibit weight loss rate of the β-TCP scaffolds and delay the degradation rate in SBF solution.

As the scaffold with 2.5 wt% ZnO doping possessed good mechanical properties and excellent biocompatibility, we chose the β-TCP scaffold with 2.5 wt% ZnO doping for the bioactivity assay. The scaffolds after soaked in SBF for different time interval was observed (Fig. 9). There was an increased apatite deposition with a more crystal structure on the surface of scaffolds with the time. Numerous tiny granular apatite particles were present on the surface of scaffolds and the particles were worm-like after soaking for 7 days (Figs. 9a, b). The worm-like apatite was more obvious and the crystal layers became more compact after soaking in SBF for 14 days (Figs. 9c, d). The surface was completely covered by a rough deposit layer, and the apatite layer was composed of numerous flake-like crystals on day 21 (Figs. 9e, f). Sponge-like crystals of apatite layer formed after immersion for up to 28 days (Figs. 9g, h). The formation of a bone-like apatite layer on biomaterials was assumed to be the precondition for their

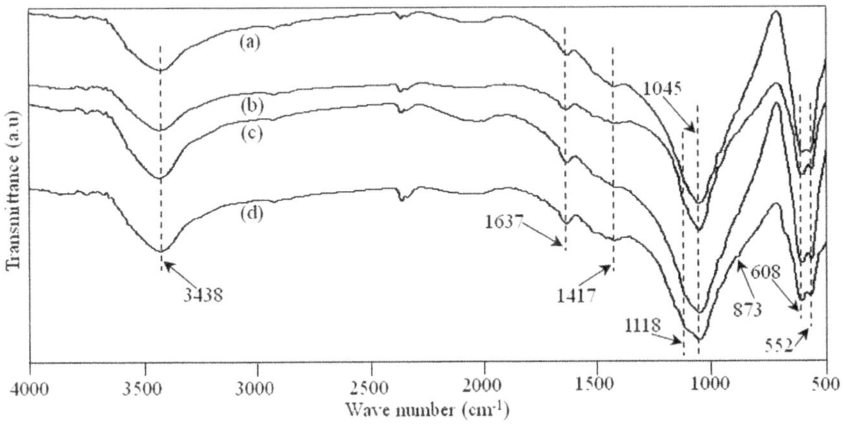

Figure 11. FT-IR spectra of the scaffold with 2.5 wt% ZnO doped after SBF incubation (a) 7 days; (b) 14 days; (c) 21 days and (d) 28 days.

osteoinduction to induce bone formation. The ability to form apatite layers in SBF had been regarded as the evidence of bioactivity for bio ceramics [45–47].

The morphology and elemental composition of the apatite deposition on the scaffold with 2.5 wt% ZnO doping after 7 days in SBF were analyzed with SEM and EDX (Fig. 10). The strong peaks of oxygen, phosphorus, and calcium plus a weaker peak of carbon were observed in the spectra. The existence of carbon in the apatite implied that the layer might be carbonate-containing apatite phase, which could be further confirmed through FT-IR analysis. The FT-IR absorption spectra of the scaffold with 2.5 wt% ZnO doping after immersion in SBF for 7, 14, 21 and 28 days were shown in Fig. 11. The characteristic peaks of phosphate for β-TCP at wave numbers of 1118, 1045, 608, and 552 cm^{-1} were all present. The peaks located at 873 and 1417 cm^{-1} were the vibration mode of carbonate [26]. It was possible that the carbonate replaced phosphate ions during the crystal growth process. The scaffolds could develop a bone like apatite layer on the surface when soaked in SBF. Such bone like apatite layer was believed to be beneficial to increase cell adhesion, proliferation and bone formation.

Conclusions

Interconnected porous β-TCP scaffolds improved by ZnO were successfully prepared with SLS technique. The scaffolds were then tested for microstructure, mechanical, and biological properties. It was found that the addition of ZnO improved the densification of the strut of β-TCP scaffolds, and the average grain size of the scaffold decreased when ZnO content increased from 0 to 2.5 wt%, while the average grain size increased with higher content of ZnO. The minimum average grain size was 0.29 μm when the content of ZnO was 2.5 wt%. The addition of ZnO could improve the mechanical properties of fracture toughness, compressive strength, stiffness and hardness. The increase in mechanical properties could be due to the combined effects of densification and grain size. In vitro cell tests showed that the scaffold with 2.5 wt% ZnO doping exhibited a good cellular viability as well as cellular proliferation. The biodegradability tests revealed that the degradation rate of the scaffolds slowed down with the increase of ZnO content. The formation of a new bone like apatite layer indicated that the scaffold demonstrated better bioactivity. So β-TCP porous scaffolds with 2.5 wt% of ZnO using SLS technique may be a good candidate for the application of bone tissue engineering.

Author Contributions

Conceived and designed the experiments: CS. Performed the experiments: PF PW. Analyzed the data: SP. Contributed reagents/materials/analysis tools: PF PW. Wrote the paper: PF SP.

References

1. Horii A, Wang X, Gelain F, Zhang S (2007) Biological designer self-assembling peptide nanofiber scaffolds significantly enhance osteoblast proliferation, differentiation and 3-D migration. Plos. One. 2(2): e190.
2. Zhang W, Ahluwalia I, Literman R, Kaplan DL, Yelick PC (2011) Human dental pulp progenitor cell behavior on aqueous and hexafluoroisopropanol (HFIP) based silk scaffolds. J. Biomed. Mater. Res. A. 97(4): 414–422.
3. Wüst S, Müller R, Hofmann S (2011) Controlled positioning of cells in biomaterials-approaches towards 3D tissue printing. J. Funct. Biomater. 2: 119–154.
4. Wang M, Zhai P, Chen X, Schreyer DJ, Sun X, et al (2011) Bioengineered scaffolds for spinal cord repair. Tissue. Eng. Part. B. Rev. 17(3): 177–194.
5. Oh S, Oh N, Appleford M, Ong JL (2006) Bioceramics for tissue engineering applications-a review. Am. J. Biochem. Biotechnol. 2(2): 49–56.
6. Soman P, Tobe BTD, Lee JW, Winquist AA, Singec I, et al (2012) Three-dimensional scaffolding to investigate neuronal derivatives of human embryonic stem cells. Biomed. Microdevices. 14(5): 829–838.
7. Bae CJ, Kim HW, Koh YH, Kim HE (2006) Hydroxyapatite (HA) bone scaffolds with controlled macrochannel pores. J. Mater. Sci:. Mater. Med. 17: 517–521.
8. Leoni L, Desai TA (2004) Micromachined biocapsules for cell-based sensing and delivery. Adv. Drug. Deliver. Rev. 56(2): 211–229.
9. Santos EC, Shiomi M, Osakada K, Laoui T (2006) Rapid manufacturing of metal components by laser forming. Int. J. Mach. Tool. Manu. 46: 1459–1468.
10. Noort RV (2012) The future of dental devices is digital. Dent. Mater. 28: 3–12.
11. Abarrategi A, Moreno-Vicente C, Martínez-Vázquez FJ, Civantos A, Ramos V, et al (2012) Biological properties of solid free form designed ceramic scaffolds with BMP-2: in vitro and in vivo evaluation. Plos. One. 7(3): e34117.
12. Cai X, Paratala BS, Hu S, Sitharaman B, Wang LV (2011) Multiscale photoacoustic microscopy of single-walled carbon nanotube-incorporated tissue engineering scaffolds. Tissue. Eng. Part. C. Meth. 18(4): 310–317.
13. Kannan S, Neunhoeffer FG, Neubauer J, Ferreira JMF (2011) Cosubstitution of Zinc and strontium in β-tricalcium phosphate: Synthesis and characterization. J. Am. Ceram. Soc. 94(1): 230–235.
14. Bose S, Darsell J, Kintner M, Hosick H, Bandyopadhyay A (2003) Pore Size and Pore Volume Effects on Calcium Phosphate Based Ceramics. Mater. Sci. Eng. C. 23: 479–486.
15. Kalita SJ, Ferguson M (2006) Fabrication of 3-D porous Mg/Zn doped tricalcium phosphate bone-scaffolds via the fused deposition modeling. Am. J. Biochem. Biotechnol. 2: 57–60.

16. Xue W, Dahlquist K, Banerjee A, Bandyopadhyay A, Bose S (2008) Synthesis and characterization of tricalcium phosphate with Zn and Mg based dopants. J. Mater. Sci:. Mater. Med. 19: 2669–2677.
17. Lin FH, Liao CJ, Chen KS, Sun JS, Lin CP (2001) Petal-like apatite formed on the surface of tricalcium phosphate ceramic after soaking in distilled water. Biomaterials 22: 2981–2992.
18. Wei X, Akinc M (2005) Si, Zn-modified tricalcium phosphates: A phase composition and crystal structure study. Key. Eng. Mater. 284–286: 83–86.
19. Hashizume M, Yamaguchi M (1993) Effect of zinc-chelating dipeptides on osteoblastic MC3T3-E1 cells: activation of aminoacyl-tRNA synthetase. Mol. Cell. Biochem. 122: 59–64.
20. Moonga BS, Dempster DW (1995) Zinc is a potent inhibitor of osteoclastic bone resorption in vitro. J. Bone. Miner. Res. 10(3): 453–457.
21. Jin HB, Oktar FN, Dorozhkin S, Agathopoulos S (2010) Sintering behavior and properties of reinforced hydroxyapatite/TCP biphasic bioceramics with ZnO-whiskers. J. Compos. Mater. 45(13): 1435–1445.
22. Bandyopadhyay A, Withey EA, Moore J, Bose S (2007) Influence of ZnO doping in calcium phosphate ceramics. Mater. Sci. Eng. C. 27: 14–17.
23. Bhatt HA, Kalita SJ (2007) Influence of oxide-based sintering additives on densification and mechanical behavior of tricalcium phosphate (TCP). J. Mater. Sci:. Mater. Med. 18: 883–893.
24. Bandyopadhyay A, Bernard S, Xue WC, Bose S (2006) Calcium phosphate-based resorbable ceramics: influence of MgO, ZnO, and SiO_2 dopants. J. Am. Ceram. Soc. 89(9): 2675–2688.
25. Shuai C, Gao C, Nie Y, Hu H, Zhou Y, Peng S (2011) Structure and properties of nano-hydroxypatite scaffolds for bone tissue engineering with a selective laser sintering system. Nanotechnol 22(28): 1–9.
26. Bose S, Tarafder S, Banerjee SS, Davies NM, Bandyopadhyay A (2011) Understanding in vivo response and mechanical property variation in MgO, SrO and SiO_2 doped β-TCP. Bone 48(6): 1282–1290.
27. Vaz CM, Fossen M, Van TRF, De GL, Reis RL, et al (2003) Casein and soybean protein-based thermoplastics and composites as alternative biodegradable polymers for biomedical applications. J. Biomed. Mater. Res. 65(1): 60–70.
28. Dorozhkin SV (2009) Calcium orthophosphates in nature, biology and medicine. Materials 2(2): 399–498.
29. Carbajal L, Caballero A, Sainz MA (2012) Design and processing of ZnO doped tricalcium phosphate based materials: Influence of β/α polymorph phase assemblage on microstructural evolution. J. Eur. Ceram. Soc. 32: 569–577.
30. Kannan S, Goetz-Neunhoeffer F, Neubauer J, Ferreira JMF (2009) Synthesis and structure refinement of zinc-doped β-tricalcium phosphate powders. J. Eur. Ceram. Soc. 92(7): 1592–1595.
31. Terrier A, Miyagaki J, Fujie H, Hayashi K, Rakotomanana L (2005) Delay of intracortical bone remodelling following a stress change: A theoretical and experimental study. Clin. Biomech. 20: 998–1006.
32. Espalin D, Arcaute K, Rodriguez D, Medina F, Posner M, et al (2010) Fused deposition modeling of patient-specific polymethylmethacrylate implants. Rapid. Prototyping. J. 16(3): 164–173.
33. Wu C, Chang J, Wang J, Ni S, Zhai W (2005) Preparation and characteristics of a calcium magnesium silicate (bredigite) bioactive ceramic. Biomaterials 26(16): 2925–2931.
34. Ramesh S, Tan CY, Sopyan I, Hamdi M, Teng WD (2007) Consolidation of nanocrystalline hydroxyapatite powder. Sci. Technol. Adv. Mater. 8: 124–130.
35. Rho JY, Roy ME, Tsui TY, Pharr GM (1999) Elastic properties of microstructural components of human bone tissue as measured by nanoindentation. J. Biomed. Mater. Res. 45(1): 48–54.
36. Campbell M, Bureau MN, Yahia L (2008) Performance of CF/PA12 composite femoral stems. J. Mater. Sci:. Mater. Med. 19: 683–693.
37. Hernandez CJ, Beaupre GS, Keller TS, Carter DR (2001) The influence of bone volume fraction and ash fraction on bone strength and modulus. Bone 29: 74–78.
38. Shi X, Wang Y, Ren L Lai C, Gong Y, Wang D (2010) A novel hydrophilic poly (lactid-co-glycolide)/lecithin hybrid microspheres sintered scaffold for bone repair. J. Biomed. Mater. Res. A. 92(3): 963–972.
39. Ni GX, Choy YS, Lu WW, Ngan AHW, Chiu KY, et al (2006) Nano-mechanics of bone and bioactive bone cement interfaces in a load-bearing model. Biomaterials 27: 1963–1970.
40. Viswanath B, Raghavan R, Gurao NP, Ramamurty U, Ravishankar N (2008) Mechanical properties of tricalcium phosphate single crystals grown by molten salt synthesis. Acta. Biomater. 4: 1448–1454.
41. Zhang F, Lin K, Chang J, Lu J, Ning C (2008) Spark plasma sintering of macroporous calcium phosphate scaffolds from nanocrystalline powders. J. Eur. Ceram. Soc. 28: 539–545.
42. Park JH, Bae JY, Shim J, Jeon I (2012) Evaluation of suitable porosity for sintered porous β-tricalcium phosphate as a bone substitute. Mater. Charact. 71: 103–111.
43. Fielding GA, Bandyopadhyay A, Bose S (2012) Effects of SiO_2 and ZnO doping on mechanical and biological properties of 3D printed TCP scaffolds. Dent. Mater. 28(2): 113–122.
44. Bettger WJ, O'dell BL (1993) Physiological roles of zinc in the plasma membrane of mammalian cells. J. Nutr. 4: 194–207.
45. Kokubo T (1991) Bioactive glass ceramics: properties and applications. Biomaterials 12: 155–163.
46. Fujibayashi S, Neo M, Kim HM, Kokubo T, Nakamura T (2003) A comparative study between in vivo bone growth and in vitro apatite formation on Na_2O-CaO-SiO_2 glasses. Biomaterials 24: 1349–1356.
47. Ragel CV, Vallet-Regi M, Rodriguez-Lorenzo LM (2002) Preparation and in vitro bioactivity of hydroxyapatite/solgel glass biphasic material. Biomaterials 23: 1865–1872.

23

Determinants of Microdamage in Elderly Human Vertebral Trabecular Bone

Hélène Follet[1,2]*, Delphine Farlay[1,2], Yohann Bala[1,2], Stéphanie Viguet-Carrin[1,2], Evelyne Gineyts[1,2], Brigitte Burt-Pichat[1,2], Julien Wegrzyn[1,2,3], Pierre Delmas[1,2], Georges Boivin[1,2], Roland Chapurlat[1,2]

1 INSERM, UMR 1033, Lyon, France, **2** Université de Lyon, UMR 1033, Lyon, France, **3** Département de Chirurgie Orthopédique, Pavillon T, Hôpital Edouard Herriot, Lyon, France

Abstract

Previous studies have shown that microdamage accumulates in bone as a result of physiological loading and occurs naturally in human trabecular bone. The purpose of this study was to determine the factors associated with pre-existing microdamage in human vertebral trabecular bone, namely age, architecture, hardness, mineral and organic matrix. Trabecular bone cores were collected from human L2 vertebrae (n = 53) from donors 54–95 years of age (22 men and 30 women, 1 unknown) and previous cited parameters were evaluated. Collagen cross-link content (PYD, DPD, PEN and % of collagen) was measured on surrounding trabecular bone. We found that determinants of microdamage were mostly the age of donors, architecture, mineral characteristics and mature enzymatic cross-links. Moreover, linear microcracks were mostly associated with the bone matrix characteristics whereas diffuse damage was associated with architecture. We conclude that linear and diffuse types of microdamage seemed to have different determinants, with age being critical for both types.

Editor: Ryan K. Roeder, University of Notre Dame, United States of America

Funding: This study was supported in part by an unrestricted educational grant from Eli Lilly to INSERM. No additional external funding received for this study. The funders had no role in study design, data collection and analysis, decision to publish, or preparation of the manuscript.

Competing Interests: This study was supported in part by an unrestricted educational grant from Eli Lilly to INSERM. This does not alter the authors' adherence to all the PLOS ONE policies on sharing data and materials, as detailed online in the guide for authors.

* E-mail: Helene.Follet@inserm.fr

Introduction

Fatigue microdamage accumulates in bone as a result of physiological loading. [1,2,3,4] Several studies have reported microdamage in human trabecular bone occurring naturally. [5,6,7,8,9,10] Increased microdamage is associated with decreased bone strength in vitro, and thus may play a role in fragility fractures. [11] Whereas microdamage appears to increase with age [6,12] and decreased with trabecular bone volume [13], few studies have examined whether bone microarchitecture and/or characteristics of the bone matrix, such as the degree of mineralization, mineral maturity, and collagen crosslink profile are associated with the accumulation of microdamage in human trabecular bone [14,15].

In cortical bone, microcracks are observed within the interstitial bone or in interstitial bone intersecting with osteonal cement lines, and are arrested by osteons. [12,16,17] In cortical bone, microdamage appears to initiate within highly mineralized regions in cortical bone, [18] which is consistent with the linear elastic fracture mechanics theory [19,20].

Nucleation of mineral occurs in the 'hole' regions of the collagen arrays and apatite crystals develop in length along the collagen long axes and in width along channels within the collagen sheets. In such a two-phase structure, a microcrack would most likely be a break or fissure not only in the mineral matrix, but also in organic matrix. [21,22]. Thus, regarding mineral matrix, the degree of mineralization, cement lines or crystal size [23] may have a specific role in the initiation of microdamage, as they are mainly located in old interstitial regions which are more mineralized. [16,17] Indeed, changes in the morphology of the mineral crystal itself may affect the bone mechanical properties and microdamage accumulation. [24,25] For example, in human femur, crystallinity explained up to 48% of the variation in monotonic mechanical properties, and up to 64% in fatigue properties. [26] In addition to the mineral phase, the type and amount of collagen cross-links by impacting strength and stability between collagen fibers may be also associated with changes in microdamage. [27,28] Recent studies showed that the extent of advanced glycation endproducts (AGEs) were negatively associated not only with mechanical parameters [29,30,31] and microarchitecture [32] but also with microdamage. [33,34] In contrast, mature enzymatic cross-links seemed to be associated with less microdamage [33].

Altogether, the relationships between *in vivo* microdamage and the intrinsic properties of human trabecular bone remain ill-defined. In particular, little is known about what factors are specifically associated with linear and/or diffuse microdamage. Thus, the primary aims of the present study were to determine whether the degree and heterogeneity of mineralization, the mineral and organic characteristics, the microhardness and the collagen cross-links are related to the amount and type of pre-existing microdamage (ie: no damage created for this study) independently of age and trabecular bone volume in human vertebral trabecular bone from older donors.

Materials and Methods

Ethics Statement

Human bone samples were obtained from French body donation to science program (Laboratory of Anatomy, Faculty of Medicine Lyon Est, University of Lyon, France).

Specimen Preparation

L2 vertebrae were taken from 53, recently deceased Caucasians donors (22 men, 30 women), mean age of 78.3±9.9 years, with a range 54–95 years of age. The sex of one subject and the age of two subjects were not known. Bone samples were wrapped in gauze soaked with saline to keep them wet, then stored at −20°C. Vertebrae were screened using medial-lateral and anterior-posterior high-definition X-rays (Faxitron X-Ray, Lincolnshire IL, USA) to exclude prevalent fracture and significant bone diseases (e.g., metastasis, Paget's disease, osteochondritis). No additional information regarding donor disease status or medication history was available. Each vertebra was sectioned in half using an Isomet Buehler 4000 microsaw (Buehler GmbH, Düsseldorf, Germany). One hemi vertebra was dedicated to mechanical tests and the bone surrounding the cores was collected for collagen cross-links quantification by HPLC [10]; the second hemi vertebra was dedicated to the detection of pre-existing microdamage and mineral analysis. The hemi vertebrae for microdamage evaluation were bulk stained for 11 days at room temperature in 0.005 M xylenol orange (Sigma-Aldrich Corp., St. Louis, MO, USA) based in 70% ethanol. In each hemi vertebrae, a cylindrical trabecular specimen (8.25 mm diameter, 25 mm length) was removed in the supero-inferior direction from the anterior quadrant using a diamond tipped coring tool. The end plate of each vertebra was removed, as previously described. [10,35] Trabecular bone volume (BV/TV, %), trabecular thickness (Tb.Th, µm), trabecular number (Tb.N, 1/mm), trabecular separation (Tb.Sp, µm), connectivity density (Conn.D, $1/mm^3$), degree of anisotropy (DA), and structure model index (SMI), which reflects the rod- versus plate-like nature of the structure, of the excised cores were assessed by microcomputed tomography, using an isotropic voxel size of 20 microns, energy (70 kVp), current (177 µA), integration time (200 ms) and a threshold corresponding to a mineral density around 0.35 $g.cm^3$ (µCT40, Scanco Medical AG, Brüttisellen, Switzerland). Structural indices of trabecular bone analysis were calculated using distance transformation (filling structure with spheres) without assuming anything about the shape of the bone (i.e. without plate model assumption). BV/TV was based on counting voxels.

Microdamage analysis

Trabecular cores for detection of microdamage were embedded in methylmethacrylate and cut parallel to the long axis to obtain at least three non-contiguous, parallel, 100±5 µm-thick sections for microdamage evaluation, as previously described. [35,36] Specimen were bulk stained with xylenol orange and general non-specific staining, morphologically different from microcracks, were easily identifiable. Three sections per specimen were measured using fluorescence (excitation/emission wavelength of 440–570/610 nm) microscopy at ×200 magnification and morphometry software (Bone Morpho; Explora Nova, La Rochelle, France). Microdamage appeared in orange under fluorescence light. [35,36] Microdamage was categorized and quantified as linear microcracks or diffuse damage (only few cross-hatching, which were counted as diffuse damage, Figure 1). Outcome assessments included the linear crack density, defined as the number of linear microcracks (Cr.N, #) per bone area (Cr.Dn, $\#/mm^2$), and the diffuse damage density, defined as the number of diffuse damage regions per bone area (Dx.Dn, $\#/mm^2$). Length was expressed as mean linear crack length (Cr.Le, µm)[1], whereas length and area density were expressed as linear length density (Cr.Le.Dn, $µm/mm^2$)[2] and diffuse damage area density defined as diffuse damage area per bone area (Dx.Ar.Dn, %).

NB: 1- Mean linear crack length is the mean of total length of linear cracks measured on three sections divided by the total number of linear cracks.

2- Crack length density is the mean crack length divided by the bone volume (BV) measured, by histomorphometry, on the same three sections: Cr.Le.Dn = Cr.Le/BV.

Mineralization Measurements

The mean degree of mineralization and heterogeneity of mineralization were assessed using quantitative microradiography on 100±1 µm thick sections, as previously described. [37,38,39] Outcomes included the mean degree of mineralization of bone (DMB, g/cm^3) and the heterogeneity index expressed as the mean of the widths at half-maximum height (HI, g/cm^3) measured on the individual DMB curves.

Hardness Analysis

Microhardness (Hv, kg/mm^2) was measured on polished remaining embedded blocks using a Vickers indenter with a 25 µg load for 10 seconds, as previously described [38].

Mineral at Crystal Level, and Organic Matrix Analysis by FTIRM

Each infrared spectra spectrum (Figure 2), performed on 2-µm-thick sections, was collected from an area of 30×100 $µm^2$ at a spectral resolution of 4 cm^{-1} and 50 scans were performed by spectrum. [40] Twenty spectra were analyzed per sample. The following variables were determined:

The mineral crystallinity index (CI) corresponds to both crystal size and perfection [40], the mineralization index (MI) is the area ratio of the bands of mineral matrix over organic matrix [41], mineral maturity (MM) was calculated as the area ratio of the apatitic phosphate over non apatitic phosphate reflecting also the age of mineral [40], carbonation was calculated as integrated area ratios ν_2CO_3 (862–894 cm^{-1}) over $\nu_1\nu_3PO_4$ (910–1184 cm^{-1}), representing the quantity of carbonates incorporated into the bone mineral, and collagen maturity (CM) was calculated as the ratio of organic matrix bands (1660/1690 cm^{-1} area ratio) [42] reflecting the evolution of the secondary structure of collagen with the mineralization [43].

Collagen Cross-links Analysis

The central part of the vertebral body around the core, containing exclusively trabecular bone, was retained for biochemical analysis. Cross-links measurements were carried out as previously described. [32,44] We assessed the content of both enzymatic nonreducible mature cross-links PYD and DPD, and the PEN induced by non-enzymatic induced, normalized to the total amount of collagen.

Statistical Analysis

Data are reported as mean values, standard deviations, ranges, median and interquartile range. As some variables were not normally distributed even after transformation, we used non-parametric tests. No significant differences between men and women were observed, consequently men and women were pooled for correlation analyses. The relationships between parameters

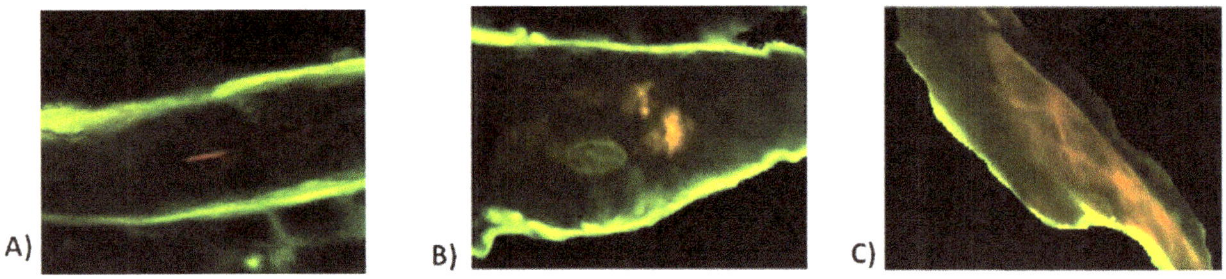

Figure 1. Pictures obtained under fluorescent light of microdamage in orange: A) Linear microcrack, B) Diffuse damage, C) Few cross-hatching microdamage were found.

were assessed by Spearman correlation coefficient (r). We used partial spearman correlation to test whether associations between parameters were significant after accounting for the contribution of BV/TV or age. All tests were two-tailed, and significance defined as $p \leq 0.05$. All statistical analyses were performed using statistical analyses software (R & SPSS 16).

Results

Association between Age, Microdamage and its Determinants

Descriptive statistics are found in Table 1. Microdamage (crack density – Figure 3a, crack length density, and diffuse damage area density), Tb.Sp, SMI, the ratio PYD/DPD and crystallinity index increased with age, whereas carbonation, BV/TV, Tb.N and DA decreased with age (Table 2). Except the ratio PYD/DPD, collagen cross-link characteristics, mineralization parameters and microhardness were not related to age (Table 3).

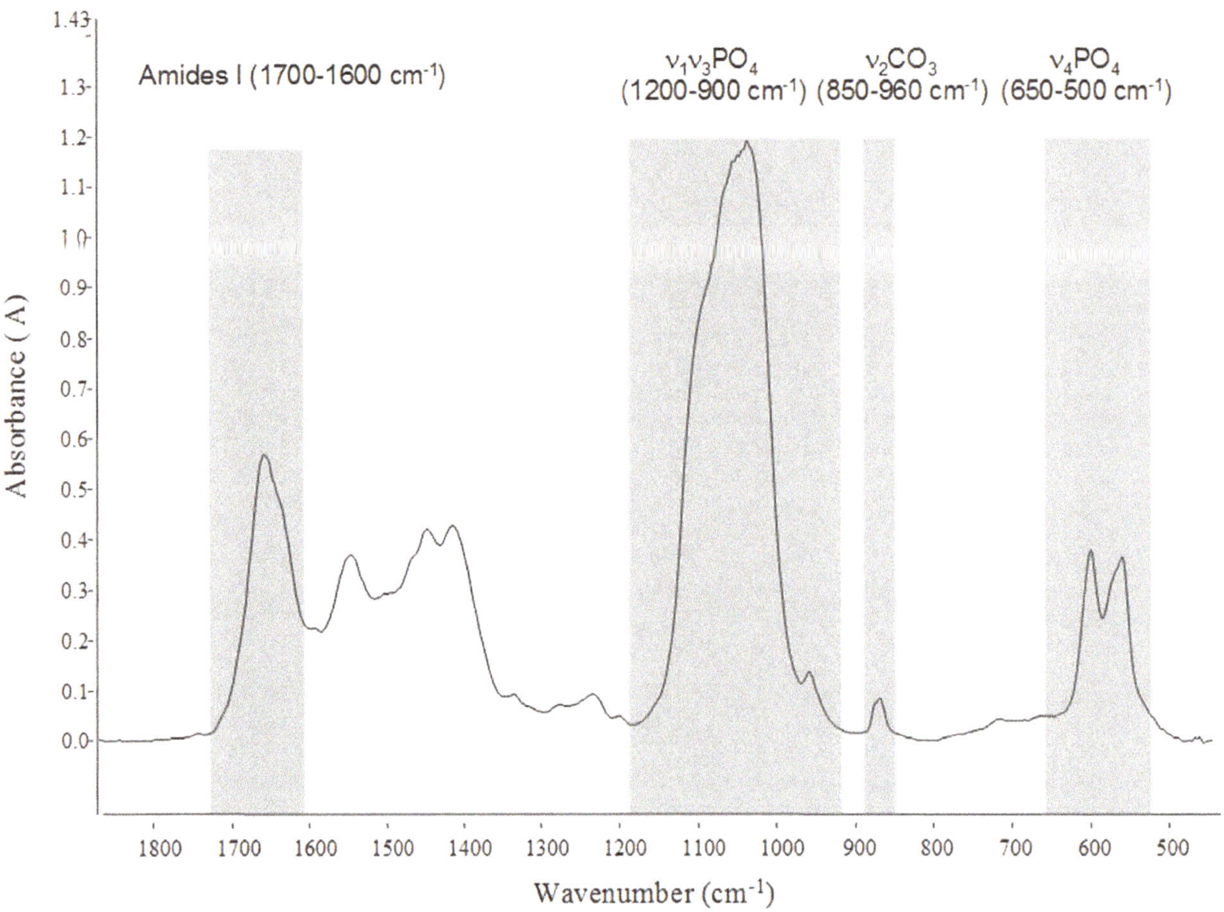

Figure 2. Infrared spectrum obtained from vertebral trabecular bone (man, 79 year-old). Spectrum is expressed as wave number (cm^{-1}) which represent the vibration modes (amide I, phosphate, carbonate).

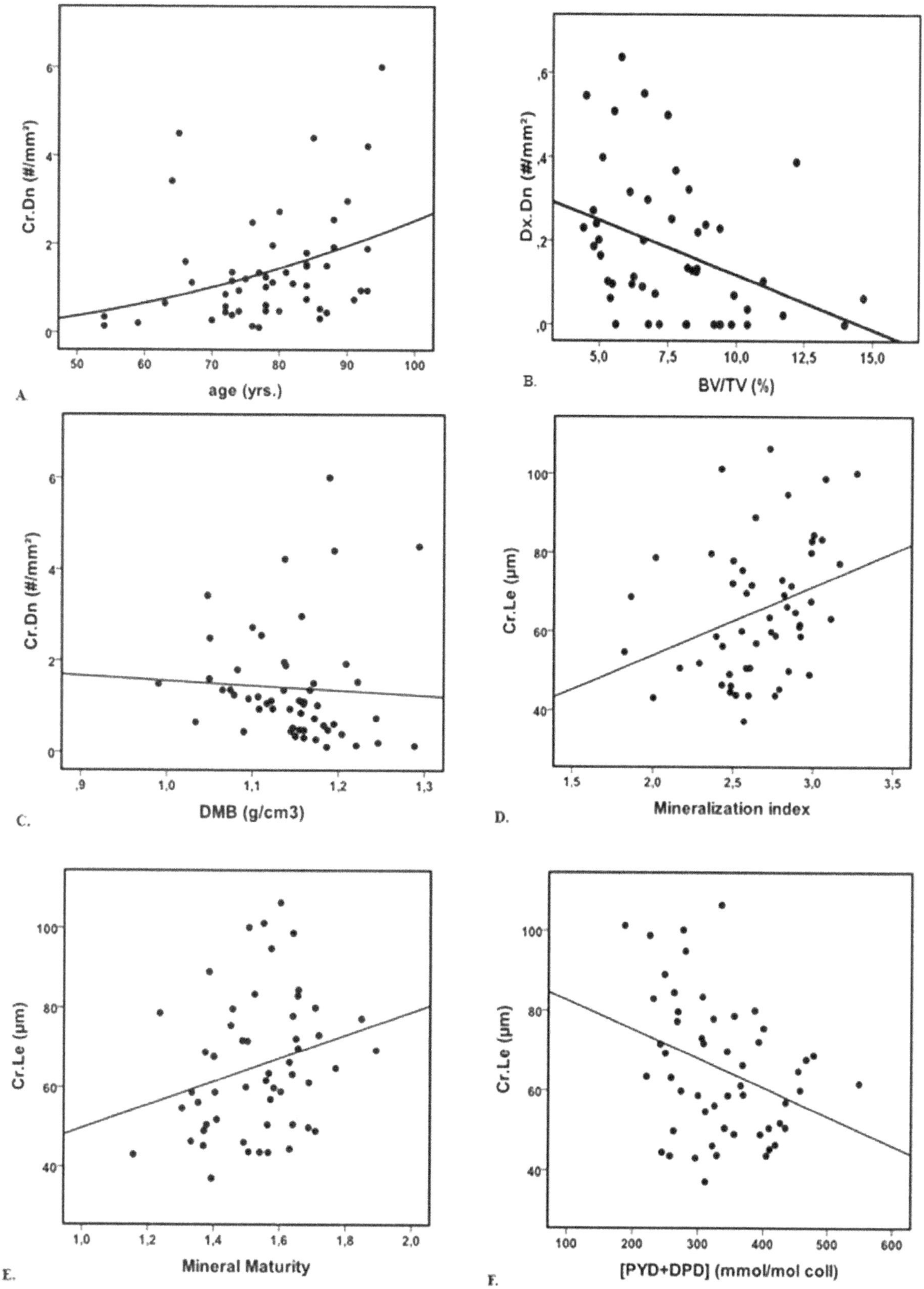

Figure 3. Bivariate Scattergrams. A) Age of donor vs Crack density – $r = 0.36$, $p = 0.010$, B) BV/TV vs Diffuse damage density, $r = -0.42$, $p = 0.003$, C) Degree of mineralization vs crack density, $r = -0.31$, $p = 0.02$, D) Mineralization index vs Crack length, $r = 0.36$, $p = 0.008$, E) Mineral maturity vs Crack length, $r = 0.30$, $p = 0.03$, F) Mature cross-links vs Crack length, $r = -0.30$, $p = 0.03$.

Table 1. Descriptive statistics, mean ± SD, range, median and interquartile range (IQR).

	n	Mean±SD	Range		Median	IQR
Age (yrs)	51	78.3±9.9	54	95	78	12.8
-FTIRM parameters	53					
Mineralization Index		2.66±0.32	1.82	3.27	2.64	0.411
Mineral Maturity		1.54±0.15	1.16	1.89	1.56	0.24
Carbonation		0.007±0.001	0.006	0.009	0.007	0.001
Collagen Maturity		4.03±0.46	2.91	5.30	3.98	0.57
Crystallinity Index		25.23±0.81	23.39	27.28	25.31	1.14
-Architecture	51					
BV/TV (%)		7.68±2.42	4.43	14.66	7.33	3.59
Tb.Th (μm)		137±18	102	187	133	28.3
Tb.Sp (μm)		1161±189	878	1932	1125	222
Tb.N (1/mm)		0.84±0.12	0.51	1.11	0.84	0.16
Connectivity density		2.03±0.80	0.74	4.32	1.87	1.14
SMI		1.77±0.49	0.33	2.52	1.80	0.74
DA		1.68±0.20	1.28	2.36	1.64	0.21
-Mineralization	53					
DMB (g/cm^3)		1.147±0.061	0.99	1.293	1.155	0.076
HI (g/cm^3)		0.287±0.087	0.122	0.525	0.274	0.111
-Hardness	53					
Hv (Kg/cm^2)		45.97±1.65	42.37	48.91	45.74	2.83
-Microdamage	53					
Cr.N (#)		22±24	1	109	15	20.3
Dx.N (#)		2.54±2.7	0	11	2.0	2.5
Cr.Dn (#/mm^2)		1.408±1.24	0.114	6.012	1.109	1.132
Dx.Dn (#/mm^2)		0.172±0.168	0	0.637	0.128	0.216
Cr.Le (μm)		65.37±17.15	37.1	106.37	63.24	26.79
Cr.Le.Dn (μm/mm^2)		93.1±92.8	7.68	430.3	69.33	66.0
Dx.Ar.Dn (%)		0.034±0.065	0	0.344	0.013	0.024
-Collagen X-Links	53					
PYD (mmol/mol coll)		232.1±61	126	406	225	91
DPD (mmol/mol coll)		103.6±25.9	61	192	103	32
PYD/DPD		2.30±0.65	1.398	5.65	2.184	0.635
PYD+DPD(mmol/mol coll)		335.7±78	187	548	128	91
PEN (mmol/mol coll)		20.85±9.41	6.19	54.5	18.4	11.71
Collagen (%)		22.77±2.49	15.30	28.74	23.27	3.197

After adjustment for BV/TV, crack length density, PYD/DPD, carbonation, mineral maturity and crystallinity index remained significantly correlated with age (Table 4).

Association between Bone Volume Fraction, Microarchitecture and Microdamage

Linear crack density was not associated with BV/TV. Linear crack length was positively associated with trabecular thickness (Tb.Th) and the degree of anisotropy (DA) (Table 2), even after adjusting for age (Table 3). After adjusting for BV/TV, Cr.Le remained strongly associated with Tb.Th (Table 4). In comparison, diffuse damage density was negatively correlated with BV/TV (Figure 3b), connectivity density and Tb.N, and positively correlated with Tb.Sp. After adjusting for age, diffuse damage density remained associated with BV/TV, Tb.Sp, Tb.N and connectivity, and association appeared with DA. After adjusting for BV/TV, all these associations disappeared, except for DA, which was positively correlated with damage density (Table 4). Diffuse damage area density was negatively correlated with BV/TV and Tb.N, and positively with Tb.Sp. (Table 2). After adjusting for BV/TV or age, all these associations disappeared (Table 3, Table 4).

Association between Mineral Traits and Microdamage

Crack length was positively correlated with mineralization index, mineral maturity and DMB, whereas crack density was negatively correlated with DMB (Table 2, Figure 3c). After adjusting for age, these correlations remained significant (Table 3). After adjusting for BV/TV, only mineralization index and mineral maturity remained significantly associated with crack length (Table 4, Figure 3d,e) even if it was borderline for DMB ($p = 0.056$). Carbonation and crystallinity index were not correlated to microdamage, neither before nor after adjusting for age or BV/TV. Neither heterogeneity index (HI) nor the microhardness (Hv) was associated with microdamage in vertebral trabecular bone.

Association between Collagen Cross-links, Organic Matrix Properties, and Microdamage

Crack density was positively correlated with PYD, (PYD/DPD), and tended to decrease with the percentage of collagen. Crack length was also negatively associated with PYD, DPD and (PYD+DPD), (Table 2, Figure 3f). After adjusting for age, only the relations between PYD, DPD, (PYD+DPD) and crack length remained significant (Table 3), whereas after adjusting for BV/TV, only the PYD/DPD ratio remained significantly associated to crack density and crack length density (Table 4). Crack length density was only correlated with the PYD/DPD ratio. Collagen maturity was not correlated with microdamage, even after adjusting for age or BV/TV. The non-enzymatic glycation product, PEN, was not associated with any parameters of microdamage.

Discussion

In this study, we found that microdamage in human vertebral trabecular bone was associated with age, microarchitecture, mineral characteristics and mature enzymatic cross-links, with different factors associated with linear versus diffuse damage.

Determinants of Linear Microcracks

Our finding that microdamage increases with age is in agreement with prior data reporting that linear microcracks (Cr.Dn, Cr.Le and Cr.Le.Dn) in trabecular bone from the femoral head, [11,13] the neck, [6] and vertebrae [9,35] increase exponentially with the age of the donors. [6,7,9,11,12,13,35,45] In contrast with our previous study in only 23 vertebrae, [35] but similarly to work of Fazzalari et al [6], in the current study, microarchitecture was not associated with linear crack density. Compared to Arlot et al [35], statistical difference is found in the crack density (same age, BV/TV, crack length), the measurement of damage area (in the current study, when no damage was found, a value of "zero" was indicated contrary to previous study where a "none" value was indicated) and the number of samples (23 compared to 53 presently). But the main difference is found in the architectural measurement of trabecular bone. In the previous study [35], structural parameters (BV/TV, Tb.Th, Tb.Sp, Tb.N)

Table 2. Bivariate spearman coefficient correlation (r_{sp}) between microdamage, age, architecture, mineralization degree, microhardness, mineral at crystal level, organic matrix and collagen cross-links.

	Age	Cr.Dn	Dx.Dn	Cr.Le	Cr.Le.Dn	Dx.Ar.Dn
	r_{sp}	r_{sp}	r_{sp}	r_{sp}	r_{sp}	r_{sp}
Age		**0.357***	0.232	0.02	**0.353***	**0.345***
-FTIRM parameters						
Mineralization	0.223	−0.106	−0.043	**0.358****	0.021	−0.007
Mineral Maturity	0.144	0.018	−0.11	**0.298***	0.109	−0.091
Carbonation	**−0.353***	0.053	0.082	−0.079	−0.002	−0.009
Collagen Maturity	0.045	0.025	0.034	−0.039	0.006	−0.045
Crystallinity Index	**0.336***	0.074	−0.093	0.22	0.152	−0.049
-Architecture						
BV/TV	**−0.574****	−0.20	**−0.417****	0.160	−0.151	**−0.379****
Tb.Th	0.10	0.025	0.032	**0.456****	0.157	0.034
Tb.Sp	**0.36***	−0.20	**0.424****	−0.052	0.005	**0.321***
Tb.N	**−0.34***	0.005	**−0.431****	−0.070	−0.018	**−0.317***
Conn density	−0.199	−0.187	**−0.356***	−0.102	−0.195	−0.194
SMI	**0.513****	0.085	0.213	−0.057	0.086	0.237
DA	**−0.348***	−0.043	0.216	**0.277***	0.008	0.064
-Mineralization						
DMB	0.030	**−0.314***	−0.172	**0.319***	−0.237	−0.108
HI	−0.033	−0.058	−0.075	−0.071	−0.097	−0.033
-Hardness						
Hv	0.136	−0.035	−0.087	0.233	0.024	−0.100
-Collagen X-Links						
PYD	0.272	**0.326***	0.164	**−0.30***	0.229	0.101
DPD	0.119	0.057	0.197	**−0.275***	−0.032	0.213
PYD/DPD	**0.307***	**0.326***	−0.011	−0.12	**0.279***	−0.005
PYD+DPD	0.222	0.269	0.21	**−0.296***	0.170	0.134
PEN	0.071	0.001	−0.063	0.074	0.036	−0.065
Collagen	−0.131	−0.261	−0.040	0.122	−0.180	0.008

*$p<0.05$,
**$p<0.01$.

were based on triangularization[1] of surface (ie: one more interpolation step in comparison to VOX, based on counting voxels). In present study, we used the called "Direct" measurement (DT)[2], based on distance transformation, which is more accurate. In prior study, Cr.Dn was linked with respectively TRI-BV/TV ($r=-0.51$, $p=0.017$), TRI-Tb.N ($r=-0.54$, $p=0.012$) and TRI-Tb.Sp ($r=0.53$, $p=0.013$). Using the direct measurement (DT), as in the current study, (for the same subset of samples), those previous associations does not remain, except for BV/TV: Cr.Dn and, respectively, Vox-BV/TV ($r=-0.51$, $p=0.018$), indeed, DT-Tb.N ($r=-0.31$, $p=0.17$) and DT-Tb.Sp ($r=0.32$, $p=0.15$). Furthermore, if the direct measurement was used for the previous study, crack length was also associated to the direct trabecular thickness.

NB: 1- Triangularization or TRI corresponds to traditional 2D histomorphometry, but this plate-model assumption leads to a bias in most cases. Scanco® recommends to use DT-Tb.N, DT-Tb,Sp for truly 3D results.

2- Direct measurement or DT indices are calculated using distance transformation (filling structure with spheres) without assuming anything about the shape of the bone (i.e. without plate model assumption).

The way of analysis the data is also essential. Indeed, depending of the analytical model used, Yeni et al., [46] who also studied human vertebral trabecular bone, found two different trends. A power law relationship between Cr. Dn and BV/TV was significant ($r^2=0.14$, $p=0.025$). However, a three-parameter exponential fit was not significant for the relationship between Cr. Dn and BV/TV ($p>0.07$). [46] There are too few papers on damaged aged human vertebrae to accurately compare with literature.

Average length of linear microcracks was associated with mineralization index, degree of mineralization and mineral maturity. The more mature the mineral, the longer the cracks. However, the crystallinity index was not associated with crack length. Linear microcrack density was not associated with any of the variables measured by FTIRM, suggesting that mineral maturity and/or mineralization does not influence microdamage accumulation in trabecular bone. [47] However, the degree of mineralization was inversely associated with Cr.Dn, and positively

Table 3. Spearman partial coefficient after adjustment for age; dependent variables shown along the top and independent variables along the side of the table.

	Cr.Dn	Dx.Dn	Cr.Le	Cr.Le.Dn	Dx.Ar.Dn
	r	r	r	r	r
-FTIRM parameters					
Mineralization Index	−0.197	−0.092	0.352**	−0.071	−0.087
Mineral Maturity	−0.043	−0.179	0.292*	0.054	−0.165
Carbonation	0.195	0.141	−0.04	0.153	0.120
Collagen Maturity	−0.005	−0.024	−0.067	−0.009	−0.087
Crystallinity Index	−0.054	−0.191	0.212	0.034	−0.195
-Architecture					
BV/TV	−0.011	−0.389**	0.246	0.064	−0.254
Tb.Th	−0.005	0.04	0.451**	0.114	0.031
Tb.Sp	−0.165	0.393**	0.025	−0.159	0.232
Tb.N	0.139	−0.398**	−0.043	0.131	−0.230
Conn density	−0.123	−0.316*	−0.09	−0.119	−0.127
SMI	−0.093	0.173	−0.07	−0.108	0.109
DA	0.074	0.297*	0.328*	0.147	0.199
-Mineralization					
DMB	−0.355**	−0.194	0.327*	−0.270	−0.124
HI	−0.056	−0.077	−0.090	−0.095	−0.019
-Hardness					
Hv	−0.096	−0.128	0.243	−0.032	−0.165
-Collagen X-Links					
PYD	0.242	0.061	−0.315*	0.151	−0.017
DPD	0.0012	0.130	−0.281*	−0.082	0.160
PYD/DPD	0.24	−0.12	−0.10	0.21	−0.14
PYD+DPD	0.197	0.120	−0.309*	0.104	0.038
PEN	−0.04	−0.094	0.09	0.005	−0.111
Collagen	−0.224	0.034	0.090	−0.166	0.079

*p<0.05,
**p<0.01.

associated with Cr.Le, meaning the more mineralized the bone was, the fewer but longer the cracks were, consistently with the positive association between elastic modulus and crack length. [10] The ensuing discrepancy between the mineralization index and DMB might be explained. Indeed, while quantitative microradiography provides results reflecting the entire bone surface of the sample, FTIRM reflects a smallest proportion of analyzed area. Therefore, the number of measurements in trabecular bone did not cover the entire bone surface, explaining the discrepancy obtained between DMB and mineralization index. It has been suggested that the more bone was mineralized, the lower the plastic deformation was and more cracks were initiated. [48] The level of mineralization might be an important factor influencing the cracks morphology. [48] Degree of mineralization and mineral maturity do not influence number or length the cracks in the same way. This finding leads to the conclusion that mineral quantity rather than mineral characteristics (maturity or crystallinity) should be used to explain cracks number.

Recent *in vitro* [49] and *ex vivo* studies [33,34] show that AGEs altered the extent of accumulated microdamage in bone tissue. Nevertheless, no association was found between PEN content and microdamage parameters, but an unexpected relationship between mature enzymatic cross-links and crack density was noted. Indeed, we found the same association between mature enzymatic cross-links and cracks density already than Saito et al [34] in cortical rib from dogs treated for 3 years with bisphosphonate. These discrepancies may be explained by the fact that microdamage may be site specific. Also, the collagen characteristic is bulk assessment (<10 mg of bone) compared to microdamage, a very localized process (thin sections). However an interesting association between mature enzymatic cross-link content and crack length was found suggesting that these cross-links, by providing strength and stability between collagen fibers, may avoid crack propagation in bone tissue. This result confirms that enzymatic cross-linking in bone is a favorable process. Lastly, collagen maturity, measured by FTIRM, was not related to microdamage whereas the collagen content, measured by HPLC, showed a negative trend with linear cracks density. This suggested that lower collagen content may be associated with numerous microcracks. Nevertheless, the orientation of the collagen fiber [50], the sacrificial bonds [51] may also participate to the propagation of microdamage and alter bone quality.

Determinants of Diffuse Damage

We found that diffuse damage in human vertebral trabecular bone was associated with age, and microarchitecture. The surface density of diffuse damage was positively associated with age, conversely to Vashishth et al. [8] who found that age did not influence the accumulation of diffuse damage in men or women. [8] However, this is partly explained by the mean age of their female population (56 years-olds) near the onset of menopause, and associated with high turnover rates. In our study, diffuse damage was only associated with microarchitecture, but not a with either characteristics of the mineral matrix nor the variables measured by FTIRM [47].

Relationship between Microcracks and Local Mechanical Properties Linked to Mineral Phase

Wang et al. showed that nanoindentation hardness was a very good predictor of bone tissue elastic modulus for both normal and osteoporotic bone tissues. [52] In another study, the same authors discussed the fact that postfailure properties of hard tissue had strong effects on bone microdamage morphology and the rate of change in apparent mechanical properties. [53] In our study, no relationship was found between hardness and microdamage, or between DMB and collagen maturity. Those hardness measurements were done at the tissue level (global level), and not at the local level of the microdamage itself. Thus, more precise measurements of hardness should be done around the microcracks to better understand the association between contact hardness and microdamage [54].

Our study has some limitations. An important limitation to the discussion of our results is that we have no information regarding medical history of persons, and therefore we cannot rule out the presence of diseases or medications that may have influenced our outcome variables. However, the anatomical specimens were radiographed to exclude bone diseases or tumors, and bone histology allowed to exclude specimens with osteomalacia. We acknowledge that many of our study subjects were old so our results are only representative of an elderly population. This

Table 4. Spearman partial coefficient after adjustment for BV/TV; dependent variables shown along the top and independent variables along the side of the table.

	Age	Cr.Dn	Dx.Dn	Cr.Le	Cr.Le.Dn	Dx.Ar.Dn
	r	r	r	r	r	r
Age		0.268	−0.056	0.194	**0.311***	0.132
-FTIRM parameters						
Mineralization	0.240	−0.151	−0.089	**0.418****	−0.008	−0.028
Mineral Maturity	**0.333***	0.021	−0.084	**0.334***	0.110	−0.062
Carbonation	**−0.326***	−0.018	0.195	−0.149	0.060	0.080
Collagen Maturity	0.106	−0.0176	0.047	0.001	−0.043	−0.072
Crystallinity Index	**0.350***	0.0286	−0.160	0.256	0.117	−0.122
-Architecture						
Tb.Th	0.240	0.045	0.129	**0.452*****	0.167	0.111
Tb.Sp	0.046	−0.169	0.242	0.216	−0.103	0.165
Tb.N	−0.037	0.140	−0.262	−0.222	0.079	−0.168
Conn density	0.084	−0.146	−0.213	−0.214	−0.168	−0.060
SMI	0.217	−0.067	−0.165	0.115	−0.010	−0.024
DA	−0.161	0.042	**0.431***	0.232	0.078	0.249
-Mineralization						
DMB	0.205	−0.269 BL	−0.049	0.258	−0.204	−0.011
HI	−0.121	−0.083	−0.157	−0.035	−0.118	−0.094
-Hardness						
Hv	0.093	−0.046	−0.154	0.246	0.028	−0.133
-Collagen X-Links						
PYD	0.1648	0.266 BL	0.045	−0.235	0.180	−0.026
DPD	0.003	−0.011	0.116	−0.223	−0.095	0.135
PYD/DPD	**0.301***	**0.327***	−0.064	−0.103	**0.285***	−0.60
PYD+DPD	0.109	0.207	0.109	−0.233	0.116	0.020
PEN	0.129	0.026	−0.002	0.030	0.050	−0.060
Collagen	−0.011	−0.229	0.025	0.110	−0.137	0.122

*p<0.05,
**p<0.01.
***p<0.001.

group, however, is most susceptible to fragility fractures. We are conscious that some donors may have received an osteoporosis therapy (i.e. estrogen or bisphosphonate) which may alter the relationships with microdamage. For example, bisphosphonate has an effect on the crystal characteristics as shown in BSUs of similar DMB and mineral maturity, the crystallinity was decreased in patients long-term treated with alendronate. [55] This was also shown for zoledronate, when crystallinity was measured between tetracycline labels (same chronology in both groups), it was lower in patients treated for 3 years once yearly. Moreover, another bisphosphonate (risedronate) has been associated with changes in collagen maturity assessed by FTIRM. [56] Furthermore, we did not quantify the reducible cross-links which may contribute to skeletal fragility and we only analyzed pentosidine, which explained 40% of the variance in bulk fluorescent AGE and comprise only a portion of total fluorescent AGEs that accumulate with tissue age in bone [33].

Our study also has a number of strengths. First, we have analyzed a relatively large number of sample, and only one sample per donor (compared to other studies using cadaveric tissues) comprising old donors whose age distribution reflected the population in which the majority of fragility fractures occur. Furthermore, this is among the few studies to assess mineral characteristics, collagen cross-links, and microdamage analyses on the same vertebral body.

In conclusion, trabecular microdamage increases with age, but this association is driven, at least in part, by declining BV/TV. We also found that linear and diffuse damage have different determinants. Linear microcracks are mostly influenced by the bone matrix quality whereas diffuse damage seems to be influenced by bone microarchitecture. The second finding is that, within the linear microcracks, there are also different factors that influence the density and the length of cracks.

Acknowledgments

The authors thank C. Bertholon, INSERM U1033, for her technical help for collagen crosslink analysis and J-P. Roux, INSERM U1033, for his help during the dissection of the vertebral blocs.

The authors also thank Dr. M. Arlot, INSERM U1033, for her contribution to microdamage analysis, and Dr M.L. Bouxsein, Orthopedic Biomechanics Laboratory, Beth Israel Deaconess Medical Center and

Harvard Medical School, Boston, MA, USA for her contribution in this study.

Author Contributions

Conceived and designed the experiments: HF PD. Performed the experiments: HF DF YB SVC EG BBP. Analyzed the data: HF DF YB SVC EG. Contributed reagents/materials/analysis tools: HF JW PD. Wrote the paper: HF DF YB SVC GB RC.

References

1. Donahue SW, Galley SA (2006) Microdamage in bone: implications for fracture, repair, remodeling, and adaptation. Crit Rev Biomed Eng 34: 215–271.
2. Burr DB, Turner CH, Naick P, Forwood MR, Ambrosius W, et al. (1998) Does microdamage accumulation affect the mechanical properties of bone? J Biomech 31: 337–345.
3. Luo Q, Leng H, Acuna R, Neil Dong X, Rong Q, et al. (2010) Constitutive relationship of tissue behavior with damage accumulation of human cortical bone. J Biomech 43: 2356–2361.
4. Taylor D, Hazenberg JG, Lee TC (2007) Living with cracks: damage and repair in human bone. Nat Mater 6: 263–268.
5. Fazzalari NL, Forwood MR, Manthey BA, Smith K, Kolesik P (1998) Three-dimensional confocal images of microdamage in cancellous bone. Bone 23: 373–378.
6. Fazzalari NL, Forwood MR, Smith K, Manthey BA, Herreen P (1998) Assessment of cancellous bone quality in severe osteoarthrosis: bone mineral density, mechanics, and microdamage. Bone 22: 381–388.
7. Fazzalari NL, Kuliwaba JS, Forwood MR (2002) Cancellous bone microdamage in the proximal femur: influence of age and osteoarthritis on damage morphology and regional distribution. Bone 31: 697–702.
8. Vashishth D, Koontz J, Qiu SJ, Lundin-Cannon D, Yeni YN, et al. (2000) In vivo diffuse damage in human vertebral trabecular bone. Bone 26: 147–152.
9. Wenzel TE, Schaffler MB, Fyhrie DP (1996) In vivo trabecular microcracks in human vertebral bone. Bone 19: 89–95.
10. Follet H, Viguet-Carrin S, Burt-Pichat B, Depalle B, Bala Y, et al. (2010) Effects of preexisting microdamage, collagen cross-links, degree of mineralization, age, and architecture on compressive mechanical properties of elderly human vertebral trabecular bone. J Orthop Res: Doi:10.1002/jor.21275.
11. Burr DB, Forwood MR, Fyhrie DP, Martin RB, Schaffler MB, et al. (1997) Bone microdamage and skeletal fragility in osteoporotic and stress fractures. J Bone Miner Res 12: 6–15.
12. Schaffler MB, Choi K, Milgrom C (1995) Aging and matrix microdamage accumulation in human compact bone. Bone 17: 521–525.
13. Mori S, Harruff R, Ambrosius W, Burr DB (1997) Trabecular bone volume and microdamage accumulation in the femoral heads of women with and without femoral neck fractures. Bone 21: 521–526.
14. Shi X, Liu XS, Wang X, Guo XE, Niebur GL (2010) Effects of trabecular type and orientation on microdamage susceptibility in trabecular bone. Bone 46: 1260–1266.
15. Hernandez CJ, Tang SY, Baumbach BM, Hwu PB, Sakkee AN, et al. (2005) Trabecular microfracture and the influence of pyridinium and non-enzymatic glycation-mediated collagen cross-links. Bone 37: 825–832.
16. Norman TL, Wang Z (1997) Microdamage of human cortical bone: incidence and morphology in long bones. Bone 20: 375–379.
17. Martin RB, Burr DB (1982) A hypothetical mechanism for the stimulation of osteonal remodelling by fatigue damage. J Biomech 15: 137–139.
18. Wasserman N, Yerramshetty J, Akkus O (2005) Microcracks colocalize within highly mineralized regions of cortical bone tissue. Eur J Morphol 42: 43–51.
19. Najafi AR, Arshi AR, Eslami MR, Fariborz S, Moeinzadeh MH (2007) Micromechanics fracture in osteonal cortical bone: a study of the interactions between microcrack propagation, microstructure and the material properties. J Biomech 40: 2788–2795.
20. Vashishth D, Behiri JC, Bonfield W (1997) Crack growth resistance in cortical bone: concept of microcrack toughening. J Biomech 30: 763–769.
21. Landis WJ (1995) The strength of a calcified tissue depends in part on the molecular structure and organization of its constituent mineral crystals in their organic matrix. Bone 16: 533–544.
22. Lee TC, Mohsin S, Taylor D, Parkesh R, Gunnlaugsson T, et al. (2003) Detecting microdamage in bone. J Anat 203: 161–172.
23. Augat P, Schorlemmer S (2006) The role of cortical bone and its microstructure in bone strength. Age Ageing 35 Suppl 2: ii27–ii31.
24. Burr DB (2002) Bone material properties and mineral matrix contributions to fracture risk or age in women and men. J Musculoskelet Neuronal Interact 2: 201–204.
25. Mongiorgi R, Romagnoli R, Olmi R, Moroni A (1983) Mineral alterations in senile osteoporosis. Biomaterials 4: 192–196.
26. Yerramshetty JS, Akkus O (2008) The associations between mineral crystallinity and the mechanical properties of human cortical bone. Bone 42: 476–482.
27. Fantner GE, Birkedal H, Kindt JH, Hassenkam T, Weaver JC, et al. (2004) Influence of the degradation of the organic matrix on the microscopic fracture behavior of trabecular bone. Bone 35: 1013–1022.
28. Fantner GE, Rabinovych O, Schitter G, Thurner P, Kindt JH, et al. (2006) Hierarchical interconnections in the nano-composite material bone: Fibrillar cross-links resist fracture on several length scales. Composites Science and Technology 66: 1205–1211.
29. Viguet-Carrin S, Roux JP, Arlot ME, Merabet Z, Leeming DJ, et al. (2006) Contribution of the advanced glycation end product pentosidine and of maturation of type I collagen to compressive biomechanical properties of human lumbar vertebrae. Bone 39: 1073–1079.
30. Tang SY, Zeenath U, Vashishth D (2007) Effects of non-enzymatic glycation on cancellous bone fragility. Bone 40: 1144–1151.
31. Wang X, Shen X, Li X, Agrawal CM (2002) Age-related changes in the collagen network and toughness of bone. Bone 31: 1–7.
32. Viguet-Carrin S, Follet H, Gineyts E, Roux JP, Munoz F, et al. (2010) Association between collagen cross-links and trabecular microarchitecture properties of human vertebral bone. Bone 46: 342–347.
33. Karim L, Vashishth D (2012) Heterogeneous glycation of cancellous bone and its association with bone quality and fragility. PLoS One 7: e35047.
34. Saito M, Mori S, Mashiba T, Komatsubara S, Marumo K (2008) Collagen maturity, glycation induced-pentosidine, and mineralization are increased following 3-year treatment with incadronate in dogs. Osteoporos Int 19: 1343–1354.
35. Arlot ME, Burt-Pichat B, Roux JP, Vashishth D, Bouxsein ML, et al. (2008) Microarchitecture influences microdamage accumulation in human vertebral trabecular bone. J Bone Miner Res 23: 1613–1618.
36. Burt-Pichat B, Follet H, Toulemonde G, Arlot M, Delmas P, et al. (2011) Methodological approach for the detection of both microdamage and fluorochrome labels in ewe bone and human trabecular bone. J Bone Miner Metab 29: 756–764.
37. Bala Y, Farlay D, Delmas PD, Meunier PJ, Boivin G (2010) Time sequence of secondary mineralization and microhardness in cortical and cancellous bone from ewes. Bone 46: 1204–1212.
38. Boivin G, Bala Y, Doublier A, Farlay D, Ste-Marie LG, et al. (2008) The role of mineralization and organic matrix in the microhardness of bone tissue from controls and osteoporotic patients. Bone 43: 532–538.
39. Boivin G, Meunier PJ (2002) The degree of mineralization of bone tissue measured by computerized quantitative contact microradiography. Calcif Tissue Int 70: 503–511.
40. Farlay D, Panczer G, Rey C, Delmas PD, Boivin G (2010) Mineral maturity and crystallinity index are distinct characteristics of bone mineral. J Bone Miner Metab 28: 433–445.
41. Paschalis EP, DiCarlo E, Betts F, Sherman P, Mendelsohn R, et al. (1996) FTIR microspectroscopic analysis of human osteonal bone. Calcified Tissue International 59: 480–487.
42. Paschalis EP, Verdelis K, Doty S, Boskey A, Mendelsohn R, et al. (2001) Spectroscopic characterization of collagen cross-links in bone. J Bone Miner Res 16: 1821–1828.
43. Farlay D, Duclos M-E, Gineyts E, Bertholon C, Viguet-Carrin S, et al. (2011) The ratio 1660/1690 cm-1 measured by Infrared Microspectroscopy is not specific of enzymatic collagen cross-links in bone tissue. PLoS ONE 6: e28736.
44. Viguet-Carrin S, Gineyts E, Bertholon C, Delmas PD (2009) Simple and sensitive method for quantification of fluorescent enzymatic mature and senescent crosslinks of collagen in bone hydrolysate using single-column high performance liquid chromatography. J Chromatogr B Analyt Technol Biomed Life Sci Jan 1: 1–7.
45. Kuliwaba JS, Tsangari H, Davies R, Fazzalari NL (2009) Bone microdamage accumulates in the central region of the human lumbar vertebra. Bone 44: S151–S151.
46. Yeni YN, Hou FJ, Ciarelli T, Vashishth D, Fyhrie DP (2003) Trabecular shear stresses predict in vivo linear microcrack density but not diffuse damage in human vertebral cancellous bone. Ann Biomed Eng 31: 726–732.
47. Soicher MA, Wang X, Zauel RR, Fyhrie DP (2011) Damage initiation sites in osteoporotic and normal human cancellous bone. Bone 48: 663–666.
48. Allen MR, Burr D (2007) Mineralization, Microdamage, and Matrix: How Bisphosphonates Influence Material Properties of Bone. BoneKEy-Osteovision 2007 February; 4(2): 49–60.
49. Tang SY, Vashishth D (2010) Non-enzymatic glycation alters microdamage formation in human cancellous bone. Bone 46: 148–154.
50. Peterlik H, Roschger P, Klaushofer K, Fratzl P (2006) From brittle to ductile fracture of bone. Nat Mater 5: 52–55.
51. Yeni YN, Kim DG, Dong XN, Turner AS, Les CM, et al. (2006) Do sacrificial bonds affect the viscoelastic and fracture properties of bone? Clin Orthop Relat Res 443: 101–108.
52. Wang X, Sudhaker Rao D, Ajdelsztajn L, Ciarelli TE, Lavernia EJ, et al. (2008) Human iliac crest cancellous bone elastic modulus and hardness differ with bone formation rate per bone surface but not by existence of prevalent vertebral fracture. J Biomed Mater Res B Appl Biomater 85: 68–77.

53. Wang X, Zauel RR, Fyhrie DP (2008) Postfailure modulus strongly affects microcracking and mechanical property change in human iliac cancellous bone: a study using a 2D nonlinear finite element method. J Biomech 41: 2654–2658.
54. Bala Y, Depalle B, Douillard T, Meille S, Clément P, et al. (2011) Respective roles of organic and mineral components of human cortical bone matrix in micromechanical behavior: an instrumented indentation study. J Mech Behav Biomed Mater 4: 1473–1482.
55. Bala Y, Depalle B, Farlay D, Douillard T, Meille S, et al. (2012) Bone micromechanical properties are compromised during long-term alendronate therapy independently of mineralization. J Bone Miner Res 27: 825–834.
56. Durchschlag E, Paschalis EP, Zoehrer R, Roschger P, Fratzl P, et al. (2006) Bone material properties in trabecular bone from human iliac crest biopsies after 3- and 5-year treatment with risedronate. J Bone Miner Res 21: 1581–1590.

Permissions

All chapters in this book were first published in PLOS ONE, by The Public Library of Science; hereby published with permission under the Creative Commons Attribution License or equivalent. Every chapter published in this book has been scrutinized by our experts. Their significance has been extensively debated. The topics covered herein carry significant findings which will fuel the growth of the discipline. They may even be implemented as practical applications or may be referred to as a beginning point for another development.

The contributors of this book come from diverse backgrounds, making this book a truly international effort. This book will bring forth new frontiers with its revolutionizing research information and detailed analysis of the nascent developments around the world.

We would like to thank all the contributing authors for lending their expertise to make the book truly unique. They have played a crucial role in the development of this book. Without their invaluable contributions this book wouldn't have been possible. They have made vital efforts to compile up to date information on the varied aspects of this subject to make this book a valuable addition to the collection of many professionals and students.

This book was conceptualized with the vision of imparting up-to-date information and advanced data in this field. To ensure the same, a matchless editorial board was set up. Every individual on the board went through rigorous rounds of assessment to prove their worth. After which they invested a large part of their time researching and compiling the most relevant data for our readers.

The editorial board has been involved in producing this book since its inception. They have spent rigorous hours researching and exploring the diverse topics which have resulted in the successful publishing of this book. They have passed on their knowledge of decades through this book. To expedite this challenging task, the publisher supported the team at every step. A small team of assistant editors was also appointed to further simplify the editing procedure and attain best results for the readers.

Apart from the editorial board, the designing team has also invested a significant amount of their time in understanding the subject and creating the most relevant covers. They scrutinized every image to scout for the most suitable representation of the subject and create an appropriate cover for the book.

The publishing team has been an ardent support to the editorial, designing and production team. Their endless efforts to recruit the best for this project, has resulted in the accomplishment of this book. They are a veteran in the field of academics and their pool of knowledge is as vast as their experience in printing. Their expertise and guidance has proved useful at every step. Their uncompromising quality standards have made this book an exceptional effort. Their encouragement from time to time has been an inspiration for everyone.

The publisher and the editorial board hope that this book will prove to be a valuable piece of knowledge for researchers, students, practitioners and scholars across the globe.

List of Contributors

Erfan Aref-Eshghi, Yuhua Zhang, Andrew Furey, Glynn Martin, Guang Sun and Proton Rahman
Faculty of Medicine, Memorial University of Newfoundland, St. John's, Newfoundland, Canada

Guangju Zhai
Faculty of Medicine, Memorial University of Newfoundland, St. John's, Newfoundland, Canada
Department of Twin Research & Genetic Epidemiology, King's College London, London, United Kingdom

Deborah Hart, Ana M. Valdes and Tim D. Spector
Department of Twin Research & Genetic Epidemiology, King's College London, London, United Kingdom

Nigel Arden
Musculoskeletal Epidemiology and Biobank, University of Oxford, Oxford, United Kingdom

Ian J. Wallace and Carrie Mongle
Department of Anthropology, Stony Brook University, Stony Brook, New York, United States of America

Brigitte Demes
Department of Anatomical Sciences, Stony Brook University, Stony Brook, New York, United States of America

Osbjorn M. Pearson
Department of Anthropology, University of New Mexico, Albuquerque, New Mexico, United States of America

John D. Polk
Department of Anthropology, University of Illinois at Urbana-Champaign, Urbana, Illinois, United States of America

Daniel E. Lieberman
Department of Human Evolutionary Biology, Harvard University, Cambridge, Massachusetts, United States of America

Sara Temiyasathit
Bone and Joint Rehabilitation R&D Center, Department of Veterans Affairs, Palo Alto, California, United States of America
Department of Bioengineering, Stanford University, Stanford, California, United States of America

W. Joyce Tang
Bone and Joint Rehabilitation R&D Center, Department of Veterans Affairs, Palo Alto, California, United States of Americ

Christopher R. Jacobs
Bone and Joint Rehabilitation R&D Center, Department of Veterans Affairs, Palo Alto, California, United States of America
Department of Bioengineering, Stanford University, Stanford, California, United States of America
Department of Biomedical Engineering, Columbia University, New York, New York, United States of America

Tim Stearns
Department of Biological Sciences, Stanford University, Stanford, California, United States of America
Department of Genetics, Stanford University, Stanford, California, United States of America

Alesha B. Castillo
Bone and Joint Rehabilitation R&D Center, Department of Veterans Affairs, Palo Alto, California, United States of America
Department of Mechanical Engineering, Stanford University, Stanford, California, United States of America

Philipp Leucht
Department of Orthopaedic Surgery, Stanford University, Stanford, California, United States of America

Stefanie D. Monica and Jill A. Helms
Department of Surgery-Plastic and Reconstructive Surgery, Stanford University, Stanford, California, United States of America

Charles T. Anderson
Energy Biosciences Institute, University of California, Berkeley, California, United States of America

Hossam M. Abdallah and Ali M. El-halawany
Department of Natural Products, Faculty of Pharmacy, King Abdulaziz University, Jeddah, Saudi Arabia
Department of Pharmacognosy, Faculty of Pharmacy, Cairo University, Cairo, Egypt

Ahmed M. Al-Abd
Pharmacology Department, Medical Division, National Research Center, Giza, Egypt
Department of Pharmacology and Toxicology, Faculty of Pharmacy, King Abdulaziz University, Jeddah, Saudi Arabia

Gihan F. Asaad
Pharmacology Department, Medical Division, National Research Center, Giza, Egypt
Pharmacology Department, Faculty of Pharmacy, Jazan University, Jazan, Saudia Arabia

Ashraf B. Abdel-Naim
Department of Pharmacology and Toxicology, Faculty of Pharmacy, King Abdulaziz University, Jeddah, Saudi Arabia

Narita L. Leong, Jonathan M. Hurng, Sabra I. Djomehri and Sunita P. Ho
Division of Biomaterials & Bioengineering, University of California San Francisco, San Francisco, California, United States of America

Stuart A. Gansky
Division of Oral Epidemiology & Dental Public Health, Department of Preventive and Restorative Dental Sciences, University of California San Francisco, San Francisco, California, United States of America

Mark I. Ryder
Division of Periodontology, Department of Orofacial Sciences, University of California San Francisco, San Francisco, California, United States of America

Jeremy F. Magland, Ning Zhang, Chamith S. Rajapakse and Felix W. Wehrli
Laboratory for Structural NMR Imaging, Department of Radiology, University of Pennsylvania Medical Center, Philadelphia, Pennsylvania, United States of America

Lamya Karim and Deepak Vashishth
Center for Biotechnology and Interdisciplinary Studies, Department of Biomedical Engineering, Rensselaer Polytechnic Institute, Troy, New York, United States of America

Michael D. Brodt, Michelle A. Lynch and Daniel J. Wood
Department of Orthopaedic Surgery, Washington University, St. Louis, Missouri, United States of America

Matthew J. Silva and Abby L. Stephens
Department of Orthopaedic Surgery, Washington University, St. Louis, Missouri, United States of America
Department of Biomedical Engineering, Washington University, St. Louis, Missouri, United States of America

Roberto Civitelli
Department of Internal Medicine, Washington University, St. Louis, Missouri, United States of America

Tomasz D. Szwedowski, William R. Taylor, Markus O. Heller, Carsten Perka, Michael Müller and Georg N. Duda
Julius Wolff Institute (JWI), Center for Musculoskeletal Surgery (CMSC), Center for Sports Science and Sports Medicine Berlin (CSSB), Charité – Universitätsmedizin Berlin, Berlin, Germany

Behzad Javaheri
Department of Oral Biology, UMKC School of Dentistry, Kansas City, Missouri, United States of America

Andrew Sunters, Gul Zaman, Rosemary F. L. Suswillo, Leanne K. Saxon and Lance E. Lanyon
Department of Veterinary Basic Sciences, The Royal Veterinary College, Royal College Street, London, United Kingdom

Joanna S. Price
Bristol Veterinary School, Langford House, Langford, Bristol, United Kingdom

Christopher L. Newman and Matthew R. Allen
Department of Anatomy and Cell Biology, Indiana University School of Medicine, Indianapolis, Indiana, United States of America

Neal X. Chen
Division of Nephrology, Department of Medicine, Indiana University School of Medicine, Indianapolis, Indiana, United States of America

Sharon M. Moe
Division of Nephrology, Department of Medicine, Indiana University School of Medicine, Indianapolis, Indiana, United States of America
Roudebush VA Medical Center, Indianapolis, Indiana, United States of America

Max A. Hammond
Weldon School of Biomedical Engineering, Purdue University, West Lafayette, Indiana, United States of America

Joseph M. Wallace
Weldon School of Biomedical Engineering, Purdue University, West Lafayette, Indiana, United States of America
Department of Biomedical Engineering, Indiana University—Purdue University, Indianapolis, Indiana, United States of America

Jeffry S. Nyman
Department of Orthopaedic Surgery and Rehabilitation and Vanderbilt Center for Bone Biology, Vanderbilt University Medical Center, Nashville, Tennessee, United States of America
Department of Veterans Affairs, Tennessee Valley Healthcare System, Nashville, Tennessee, United States of America

Richard F. Loeser
Department of Internal Medicine, Section of Molecular Medicine, Wake Forest University School of Medicine, Winston-Salem, North Carolina, United States of America

Amy L. Olex
Department of Computer Science, Wake Forest University, Winston-Salem, North Carolina, United States of America

Margaret A. McNulty and Cathy S. Carlson
Department of Veterinary Population Medicine, College of Veterinary Medicine, University of Minnesota, St. Paul, Minneapolis, United States of America

Michael Callahan and Cristin Ferguson
Department of Orthopedic Surgery, Wake Forest University School of Medicine, Winston-Salem, North Carolina, United States of America

Jacquelyn S. Fetrow
Department of Computer Science, Wake Forest University, Winston-Salem, North Carolina, United States of America
Department of Physics, Wake Forest University, Winston-Salem, North Carolina, United States of America

Scott C. Sibole and Ahmet Erdemir
Computational Biomodeling (CoBi) Core and Department of Biomedical Engineering Lerner Research Institute, Cleveland Clinic, Cleveland, Ohio, United States of America

Dawn E. Clendenning and Douglas P. Mortlock
Department of Molecular Physiology and Biophysics, Center for Human Genetics Research, Vanderbilt University School of Medicine, Nashville, Tennessee, United States of America

Jacqueline Nguyen
Graduate Program in Oral and Craniofacial Sciences, University of California San Francisco, San Francisco, California, United States of America

Simon Y. Tang and Daniel Nguyen
Department of Orthopaedic Surgery, University of California San Francisco, San Francisco, California, United States of America

Tamara Alliston
Graduate Program in Oral and Craniofacial Sciences, University of California San Francisco, San Francisco, California, United States of America
Department of Orthopaedic Surgery, University of California San Francisco, San Francisco, California, United States of America
Department of Bioengineering and Therapeutic Sciences, University of California San Francisco, San Francisco, California, United States of America
Department of Otolaryngology Head and Neck Surgery, University of California San Francisco, San Francisco, California, United States of America
Eli and Edythe Broad Center of Regeneration Medicine and Stem Cell Research, University of California
San Francisco, San Francisco, California, United States of America

Julia M. Hum, Richard N. Day and Fredrick M. Pavalko
Department of Cellular and Integrative Physiology, Indiana University School of Medicine, Indianapolis, Indiana, United States of America

Joseph P. Bidwell
Department of Anatomy and Cell Biology, Indiana University School of Medicine, Indianapolis, Indiana, United States of America

Yingxiao Wang
School of Engineering, University of California San Diego, San Diego, California, United States of America

Ahmed E. Elbanna
Department of Physics, University of California Santa Barbara, Santa Barbara, California, United States of America
Department of Civil and Environmental Engineering, University of Illinois at Urbana- Champaign, Urbana, Illinois, United States of America

Jean M. Carlson
Department of Physics, University of California Santa Barbara, Santa Barbara, California, United States of America

Sundar Srinivasan, Dewayne Threet, Leah E. Worton, Brandon J. Ausk, Steven D. Bain, Edith M. Gardiner, Ronald Y. Kwon and Ted S. Gross
Department of Orthopaedics and Sports Medicine, University of Washington, Seattle, Washington, United States of America

Toshiyuki Tsurumoto, Kazunobu Saiki, Keishi Okamoto and Tetsuaki Wakebe
Department of Macroscopic Anatomy, Graduate School of Biomedical Science, Nagasaki University, Nagasaki, Japan

Takeshi Imamura and Junichiro Maeda
Department of Orthopaedic surgery, Graduate School of Biomedical Science, Nagasaki University, Nagasaki, Japan

Yoshitaka Manabe
Department of Oral Anatomy and Dental Anthropology, Graduate School of Biomedical Science, Nagasaki University, Nagasaki, Japan

Pere Ibáñez-Gimeno and Assumpció Malgosa
Unitat d'Antropologia Biológica, Departament de Biologia Animal, Biologia Vegetal i Ecologia, Universitat Autónoma de Barcelona, Bellaterra, Barcelona, Catalonia, Spain

Ignasi Galté
Centre de Patologia Forense de Collserola, Institut de Medicina Legal de Catalunya, Montcada I Reixach, Barcelona, Catalonia, Spain
Unitat de Medicina Legal I Forense, Departament de Psiquiatria i de Medicina Legal, Universitat Autónoma de Barcelona, Bellaterra, Barcelona, Catalonia, Spain

Xavier Jordana
Departament de Paleobiologia, Institut Català de Paleontologia Miquel Crusafont (ICP), Universitat Autónoma de Barcelona, Bellaterra, Barcelona, Catalonia, Spain

Joan Manyosa
Unitat de Biofísica, Departament de Bioquímica i de Biologia Molecular, and Centre d'Estudis en Biofísica, Universitat Autónoma de Barcelona, Bellaterra, Barcelona, Catalonia, Spain

Sabine Stumpp
Institute for Medical Genetics and Human Genetics, Charité - Universitätsmedizin Berlin, Berlin, Germany

Jirko Kühnisch, Denise Emmerich, Uwe Kornak and Mateusz Kolanczyk
Institute for Medical Genetics and Human Genetics, Charité - Universitätsmedizin Berlin, Berlin, Germany
FG Development & Disease, Max Planck Institute for Molecular Genetics, Berlin, Germany

Karolina Kobus, Julia Grohmann, Nadine Kossler and Monika Osswald
FG Development & Disease, Max Planck Institute for Molecular Genetics, Berlin, Germany

Jong Seto
Department of Biomaterials, Max Planck Institute for Colloids and Interfaces, Potsdam, Germany
Department of Chemistry, Universität Konstanz, Konstanz, Germany

Claudia Lange
Department of Biomaterials, Max Planck Institute for Colloids and Interfaces, Potsdam, Germany
Institut für Physiologische Chemie, MTZ, Medizinische Fakultät Carl Gustav Carus, Technische Universität Dresden, Dresden, Germany

Susanne Schrof, Peter Varga and Kay Raum
Julius Wolff Institute & Brandenburg School of Regenerative Therapies, Charité - Universitätsmedizin Berlin, Berlin, Germany

Sigrid Tinschert
Division für Humangenetik, Medizinische Universität Innsbruck, Innsbruck, Austria
Institut für Klinische Genetik, Medizinische Fakultät Carl Gustav Carus, Technische Universität Dresden, Dresden, Germany

Falk Thielemann
Klinik für Orthopädie, Medizinische Fakultät Carl Gustav Carus, Technische Universität Dresden, Dresden, Germany

Georg Duda
Julius Wolff Institute & Brandenburg School of Regenerative Therapies, Charité - Universitätsmedizin Berlin, Berlin, Germany
Berlin-Brandenburg Center for Regenerative Therapies, Berlin, Germany

Wenke Seifert
Institute for Vegetative Anatomy, Charité - Universitätsmedizin Berlin, Berlin, Germany

Thaqif el Khassawna
Laboratory of Experimental Trauma Surgery Giessen, Justus-Liebig University Giessen, Giessen, Germany

David A. Stevenson
University of Utah, Department of Pediatrics, Division of Medical Genetics, Salt Lake City, Utah,United States of America

Florent Elefteriou
Department of Medicine, Pharmacology and Cancer Biology, Center for Bone Biology, Vanderbilt University - Medical Center, Nashville, Tennessee, United States of America

Peter Fratzl
Department of Biomaterials, Max Planck Institute for Colloids and Interfaces, Potsdam, Germany
Berlin-Brandenburg Center for Regenerative Therapies, Berlin, Germany

Stefan Mundlos
Institute for Medical Genetics and Human Genetics, Charité - Universitätsmedizin Berlin, Berlin, Germany
FG Development & Disease, Max Planck Institute for Molecular Genetics, Berlin, Germany
Berlin-Brandenburg Center for Regenerative Therapies, Berlin, Germany

Pei Feng
State Key Laboratory of High Performance Complex Manufacturing, Central South University, Changsha, Hunan Province, P. R. China

Cijun Shuai
State Key Laboratory of High Performance Complex Manufacturing, Central South University, Changsha, Hunan Province, P. R. China
Department of Regenerative Medicine & Cell Biology, Medical University of South Carolina, Charleston, South Carolina, United States of America

Pingpin Wei
Cancer Research Institute, Central South University, Changsha, Hunan Province, P. R. China

Shuping Peng
Cancer Research Institute, Central South University, Changsha, Hunan Province, P. R. China
Department of Obstetrics, Gynecology and Reproductive Sciences, Yale University School of Medicine, New Haven, Connecticut, United States of America

Héléne Follet, Delphine Farlay, Yohann Bala, Stéphanie Viguet-Carrin, Evelyne Gineyts, Brigitte Burt-Pichat, Pierre Delmas, Georges Boivin and Roland Chapurlat
INSERM, UMR 1033, Lyon, France
Université de Lyon, UMR 1033, Lyon, France

Julien Wegrzyn
INSERM, UMR 1033, Lyon, France
Université de Lyon, UMR 1033, Lyon, France
Département de Chirurgie Orthopédique, Pavillon T, Hôpital Edouard Herriot, Lyon, France

Index